Biobehavioral Assessment of the Infant

Biobehavioral Assessment of the Infant

LYNN TWAROG SINGER
PHILIP SANFORD ZESKIND

Editors

THE GUILFORD PRESS
New York   London

© 2001 The Guilford Press
A Division of Guilford Publications, Inc.
72 Spring Street, New York, NY 10012
www.guilford.com

Printed in the United States of America

This book is printed on acid-free paper.

Last digit is print: 9   8   7   6   5   4   3   2   1

Library of Congress Cataloging-in-Publication Data

Biobehavioral assessment of the infant / edited by Lynn Twarog
   Singer, Philip Sanford Zeskind.
         p. cm.
   Includes bibliographical references and index.
   ISBN 1-57230-669-6 (hardcover)
   1. Infants—Psychological testing. 2. Psychological tests for
children. 3. Behavioral assessment of infants. I. Singer, Lynn T.
II. Zeskind, Philip Sanford.

BF719.6 .B56 2001
618.92'0075—dc21

                                             2001023247

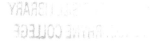

*For Tony and Betty, Mark, Maureen, and Michael,
who have propelled and sustained me.*
—L. T. S.

For my loving parents, Stanley and Shirley.
—P. S. Z.

About the Editors

Lynn Twarog Singer, PhD, is Professor of Pediatrics and Psychiatry at Case Western Reserve University School of Medicine, Cleveland, Ohio. She is the Director of Project GLAD (Growth, Learning, and Development), a 10-year longitudinal study of infants with bronchopulmonary dysplasia and very low birthweight, and Project Newborn—Next Steps, a longitudinal study of cocaine-exposed infants and their mothers, now in its seventh year. These studies reflect her interests in the effects of high-risk conditions of infancy on child development.

Philip Sanford Zeskind, PhD, is Research Professor of Pediatrics at the University of North Carolina–Chapel Hill, Professor of Psychology at the University of North Carolina–Charlotte, and Director of Neurodevelopmental Research at Carolinas Medical Center in Charlotte, North Carolina. For over 25 years, Dr. Zeskind has studied the effects of various prenatal and early postnatal experiences on the biobehavioral development of the fetus and young infant at risk, and how these variations in biobehavioral organization affect the future social experiences and subsequent course of infant development. Dr. Zeskind also directs the Carolinas Preterm Nursery Intervention Program (CPNIP), a family-centered program designed to improve the biobehavioral development of preterm infants while they continue to reside in the high-risk nurseries.

Contributors

Robert E. Arendt, PhD, Department of Pediatrics, Case Western Reserve University School of Medicine, Cleveland, Ohio

Margaret Bendersky, PhD, Institute for the Study of Child Development, University of Medicine and Dentistry of New Jersey, Robert Wood Johnson Medical School, New Brunswick, New Jersey

Rosemarie Bigsby, ScD, OTR/L, Infant Development Unit, Department of Pediatrics, Women and Infants' Hospital, Providence, Rhode Island

Jane Case-Smith, EdD, OTR/L, Division of Occupational Therapy, School of Allied Medical Professions, The Ohio State University, Columbus, Ohio

Kean H. Chew, PhD, Demand Planning and Forecasting, Perseco, Downers Grove, Illinois

Alan B. Cobo-Lewis, PhD, Interdisciplinary Studies Program and Department of Psychology, University of Maine, Orono, Maine

Janet C. Constantinou, MA, Division of Neonatal and Developmental Medicine, Pediatrics, Stanford University School of Medicine, Stanford, California

Janet A. DiPietro, PhD, Department of Population and Family Health Sciences, Johns Hopkins University, Baltimore, Maryland

Rebecca E. Eilers, PhD, Department of Psychology, University of Maine, Orono, Maine

Jeffrey W. Fagen, PhD, Department of Psychology, St. John's University, Jamaica, New York

Nathan A. Fox, PhD, Institute for Child Study, University of Maryland, College Park, Maryland

Robert L. Freedland, PhD, Department of Infant Development, New York State Institute for Basic Research in Developmental Disabilities, Staten Island, New York

Judith M. Gardner, PhD, Department of Infant Development, New York State Institute for Basic Research in Developmental Disabilities, Staten Island, New York

Maria Amy Gartstein, PhD, Pacific Graduate School of Psychology, Palo Alto, California

Susan Goldberg, PhD, Psychiatry Research Unit, Hospital for Sick Children, and University of Toronto, Toronto, Ontario, Canada

Megan R. Gunnar, PhD, Institute of Child Development, University of Minnesota, Minneapolis, Minnesota

Bernard Z. Karmel, PhD, Department of Infant Development, New York State Institute for Basic Research in Developmental Disabilities, Staten Island, New York

Anneliese F. Korner, PhD, Department of Psychiatry and Behavioral Sciences, Division of Child Psychiatry and Child Development, Stanford University School of Medicine, Stanford, California

Katharine R. Lawson, PhD, Department of Pediatrics, Rose F. Kennedy Center for Research in Mental Retardation and Human Development, Albert Einstein College of Medicine/Children's Hospital at Montefiore, Bronx, New York

Barry M. Lester, PhD, Department of Psychiatry and Department of Pediatrics, Brown Medical School; Infant Development Center, Women and Infants' Hospital; and E. P. Bradley Hospital, Providence, Rhode Island

Michael Lewis, PhD, Institute for the Study of Child Development, University of Medicine and Dentistry of New Jersey, Robert Wood Johnson Medical School, New Brunswick, New Jersey

Dalit Himmelfarb Marshall, PhD candidate, Institute for Child Study, University of Maryland, College Park, Maryland

D. Luisa Mayer, PhD, Department of Ophthalmology, Children's Hospital; Harvard University School of Medicine, Boston, Massachusetts

Dennis L. Molfese, PhD, Department of Psychological and Brain Sciences, University of Louisville, Louisville, Kentucky

Victoria J. Molfese, PhD, Center for Research in Early Childhood, School of Education, University of Louisville, Louisville, Kentucky

Julia S. Noland, PhD, Department of Pediatrics, Case Western Reserve University, Cleveland, Ohio

Phyllis S. Ohr, PhD, Department of Psychology, Hofstra University, Hempstead, New York

Esther K. Orlian, PhD, Department of Psychology, Bar-Ilan University, Ramat-Gan, Israel

Fran Lang Porter, PhD, Department of Psychology, Washington University, St. Louis, Missouri

Susan A. Rose, PhD, Department of Pediatrics, Rose F. Kennedy Center for Research in Mental Retardation and Human Development, Albert Einstein College of Medicine/Children's Hospital at Montefiore, Bronx, New York

Mary K. Rothbart, PhD, Department of Psychology, University of Oregon, Eugene, Oregon

Holly A. Ruff, PhD, Department of Pediatrics, Rose F. Kennedy Center for Research in Mental Retardation and Human Development, Albert Einstein College of Medicine/Children's Hospital at Montefiore, Bronx, New York

Ronald Seifer, PhD, Department of Psychiatry and Human Behavior, Brown University School of Medicine, E. P. Bradley Hospital, East Providence, Rhode Island

Lynn Twarog Singer, PhD, Departments of Pediatrics and Psychiatry, Case Western Reserve University School of Medicine, Cleveland, Ohio

Evelyn B. Thoman, PhD, Biobehavioral Sciences Graduate Degree Program, University of Connecticut, Storrs, Connecticut

Edward Z. Tronick, PhD, Child Development Unit, Children's Hospital, and Department of Pediatrics, Harvard University Medical School, Boston, Massachusetts

Barbara Prudhomme White, PhD, School of Health and Human Services, University of New Hampshire, Durham, New Hampshire

Philip Sanford Zeskind, PhD, Department of Pediatrics, Carolinas Medical Center, Charlotte, North Carolina, and Department of Pediatrics, University of North Carolina–Chapel Hill, Chapel Hill, North Carolina

Preface

Beginning in the late 1960s, conceptualizations of development began to emphasize the role of infants as partial producers of their own developmental pathways. By the mid-1970s, much research focused on infants who were at high risk for poor developmental trajectories based on biological insults suffered during pregnancy and childbirth. This research greatly enhanced the prevailing conceptual models. Rather than focusing on the structural defect alone, development of these infants was seen as strongly influenced by the quality of the caregiving environment, an environment also impacted by the infant via the functional consequences of the biological insult and behavior. These changes in conceptualizations of development and their application to the infant at risk contributed to a considerable rise in the number of assessment tools developed to measure the biobehavioral integrity of the newborn and young infant. The growing number of biobehavioral assessments has been matched only by the hunger of scientists and practitioners to employ these measures for their respective needs. Some assessments were created by those interested in basic questions of development as a way to conduct increasingly sophisticated measurements of changes in behavior. Increasingly sensitive assessments of newborn and young infants have also been developed and employed by those who study the wide range of adverse medical conditions and potential teratogens that affect early development and place the infant at risk for subsequent handicap. Further, practitioners use a wide variety of assessments to diagnose the severity of biobehavioral insult, prognose the infant's developmental course, and/or evaluate the effectiveness of interventions designed to aid recovery.

The purpose of this volume is to provide a source that describes the historical, diagnostic, methodological, and conceptual utility of tools used to assess the biobehavioral integrity of the newborn and young infant—and their implications for understanding the development of the infant at risk.

The term "biobehavioral" is used to emphasize the biological basis of behavior within a given environmental context. Perhaps it should be emphasized that "biology" at one level of analysis is "behavior" at another, as seen, for example, when we talk about the behavior of a cell and its environment or how the infant's autonomic nervous system "behaves." These measures can be compared to those emphasizing the developmental context, per se, such as prenatal risk factors or parenting or social class. Chapters in this volume explore assessments that vary in age appropriateness (from prenatal period to 1 year of postnatal development), level of analysis (from cortical electrophysiology to infant attachment), and technological advancement (from well-established tests of sensorimotor skills to more recent measures of neurobehavioral function). The selection of chapters and assessment tools is somewhat arbitrary—there are certainly other valuable biobehavioral assessment tools being used. The assessment tools in this volume, however, reflect an important range in utility and sometimes may represent alternatives to one another. The organization of chapters into their respective sections could also be seen as rather arbitrary but is based on the level of analysis and function for which the assessment tools were designed.

To help readers compare and contrast various assessment tools to meet their needs, each chapter has been organized around the presentation of eight common sections:

1. A brief history of the development of the assessment, including what events and conceptual and/or technical changes occurred in a field to bring about the development of the assessment tool.
2. A general description of the assessment that provides sufficient detail for readers to understand whether they have the facilities, expertise, and/or support to conduct clinical and/or research activity with the assessment procedures.
3. The biobehavioral basis of the assessment, or what it is about the biological integrity of the infant that the assessment tool is supposed to be measuring. Depending on the method of assessment, and its level of analysis, this section may describe the neural, endocrine, and/or organizational basis of the assessment tool.
4. A consideration of the reliability and validity of the assessment tool. Although some tools come from a tradition of needing to have established psychometric properties, other tools have not addressed this issue empirically.
5. An explicit discussion of the developmental model underlying the utility of the biobehavioral assessment. Implicit in the concept of being "at risk" is the fact that, although the infant has an increased probability of showing subsequent developmental problems, not all infants with some biological insult have poor outcomes. We are interested in how the assessment tool addresses this issue. Does the as-

sessment reflect only the current status of the infant as it has been affected by previous developmental conditions? Is the measure conceptualized as being predictive of subsequent development? Most important, if so—why? How does the tool reflect a researcher's implicit model of development?

6. A discussion of the theoretical constraints and limitations of the tool, as well as the uses and misuses of the tool and when it should and should not be used.
7. A discussion of the training requirements necessary to use the biobehavioral assessment tool.
8. A discussion of the implications of this assessment tool for the future, specifically for the understanding of the development of the infant at risk.

As such, we are interested in what these measures tell us about development and why. These chapters comprise a volume that uniquely covers a range of assessments that not only are at the forefront of research and clinical practice today but also hold promise for the future.

This volume is organized around functional infant developmental domains and the psychophysiological and behavioral assessments thought to measure those functional domains.

First, general issues in infant assessment and development are addressed in a chapter by Lynn Twarog Singer, including the historical antecedents of current infant assessment efforts, the neuroimaging and neurophysiological technologies that have documented our current understanding of fetal and postnatal neurobiological development, psychometric issues to be considered in the use of infant assessments, and the potential for the development of specific measures of infant functioning to influence public health efforts. Also in this introductory section, Ronald Seifer identifies crucial methodological issues in the behavioral assessment of infants at risk. His chapter covers broad-based developmental models, issues specific to understanding risk in a developmental context, and the conceptualization of growth, stability, and continuity. The role of developmentalists in understanding the interface of biology and behavior and factors important to interpretation of data in this research domain are considered.

Part II focuses on prenatal growth and sensory development. Janet A. DiPietro illustrates how exploitation of the Doppler effect is used to assess a variety of domains of fetal functioning including the heart rate, activity level, state concordance, and responsivity. She argues that a single assessment instrument for measuring fetal behavior is not yet warranted and that more empirical data are needed to establish normative behavior and to select the best ways to quantify functioning within domains of behavior.

Visual acuity assessment is now possible in infants, and methods for obtaining measures of visual acuity are described in Chapter 4 by D. Luisa Mayer and Robert E. Arendt. Given the important role vision plays in the development of infants, these authors express surprise that measures of visual acuity are so infrequently included in studies of processes that require visual ability. The Teller Acuity Cards are described as a useful method of obtaining such data. Similarly, in a corollary chapter on auditory assessments, Alan B. Cobo-Lewis and Rebecca E. Eilers identify relatively inexpensive screening methods for infants at risk for hearing impairment. Current assessment tools for infant hearing employ acoustic, electrophysiological, and behavioral phenomena to assess progressively more central aspects of the auditory system.

Assessments of arousal and regulation, covered in Part III, have received growing consideration by developmentalists as these functions have been conceptualized to underlie skills important for cognitive and emotional development. Fran Lang Porter describes the use of vagal tone, a cardiorespiratory measure, to assess biobehavioral integrity of the newborn and young infant. Vagal tone has been explored as a means to investigate attention, emotion, visual memory, stress, pain, temperament, developmental regulation disorders, and the impact of early clinical compromise. As an assessment tool, vagal tone has revealed much about the heart, its rhythmycity, and its link to the neurophysiological integrity of the developing organism. It holds promise to provide information about the behavioral and cognitive potential of the individual before those domains can be directly assessed. Porter suggests that further investigations can illustrate the factors that seem to contribute to the presence or absence of stable measures of vagal tone early in life. Chapter 7, by Evelyn B. Thoman, addresses the way sleep–wake states in infancy can serve as basic indices of neurobehavioral regulatory controls. In Chapter 8, Philip Sanford Zeskind and Barry M. Lester describe their extensive research on the diagnostic utility of infant crying. The physical properties of the cry, comprised of temporal and acoustic attributes, can be captured through a computerized, digital spectrogram. Continued development of cry analysis as a research tool suggests that it may provide a sensitive measure of alterations in biobehavioral organization, important information about the perceptual set the caregiver may bring to the child's environment, and insights in processes underlying other assessment tools.

Cortisol, a psychobiological measure, has been used as a measure of observed and perceived stress linked to the hypothalamic–pituitary–adrenal (HPA) axis system. Chapter 9, by Megan R. Gunnar and Barbara Prudhomme White, presents lines of evidence that support the conceptual relationships of changes in cortisol levels as reflecting the attachment relationship. They express a need for further research to investigate early stress experiences and subsequent neurobiological development in the child that may affect regulation of the HPA axis system.

In Chapter 10, Mary K. Rothbart, Kean H. Chew, and Maria Amy Gartstein define temperament as the constitutionally based individual differences in reactivity and self-regulation influenced over time by heredity, maturation, and experience. They demonstrate that behavioral observational measures of infant temperament are related to physiological measures of the same construct, such as vagal tone, cortisol levels, and hemispheric asymmetries. They feel that much additional work is needed to improve current laboratory caregiver reports and home observational assessments of infant temperament, and urge cooperation among researchers to develop the best scales and laboratory assays to benefit the field. In Chapter 11, Susan Goldberg discusses the evolutionary biological perspectives of attachment theory and the social and developmental contexts of attachment from which the Strange Situation assessment has stemmed. She evaluates the limitations and the controversies surrounding the use of the Strange Situation as a measure of child attachment but notes its immense value as a heuristic research tool. Its approach of examining the organization of behavior rather than specific behaviors or outcomes coincided with the general historical shift in the study of behavioral development. Goldberg notes that as the psychometric properties of this measure are refined, the debates and disagreement have pressed researchers to "sharpen and refine their constructs and to conduct increasingly sophisticated studies."

Part IV emphasizes areas considered to be reflective of more general cognitive and attentional processes. In Chapter 12, Jeffrey W. Fagen and Phyllis S. Ohr provide detailed looks at three measures of learning and information processing in infancy, namely, habituation, learned expectancies, and instrumental conditioning. The three paradigms reviewed are demonstrated to reliably tap areas of cognitive development. Fagen and Ohr attempt to show how early measures of infant learning and memory can provide important diagnostic information about the infant's current and future cognitive functioning. The efficient engagement of attentional processes is considered pivotal in permitting both the selection and storage of attributes corresponding to important events and associations in the infant's world.

Susan A. Rose and Esther K. Orlian, in Chapter 13, address how the paired-comparison paradigm is used to assess an infant's attentional encoding and memory processes through the use of novelty preferences, and cite evidence linking infant recognition memory as measured with the paired-comparison task to the same brain substrate that underlies explicit memory in adults. Cross-modal transfer of shape from touch to vision can be accomplished by infants by 6 months of age, and this capability has also been exploited to assess individual differences. Katharine R. Lawson and Holly A. Ruff have been interested in focused attention, addressed in Chapter 14, during active hands-on exploration in their laboratory, a function that traditionally has been regarded as basic to early cognitive development. They have developed global ratings of focused attention during object-related free play and have found that higher risk to the infant is associated with delayed onset and less efficient and disordered focused attention toward objects. Their future studies will assess whether ratings obtained in clinical settings are predictive of aspects of the later functioning of high-risk infants. Piaget's observations that infants' ability to search for hidden objects advances with age from 6 to 12 months led to standardized assessment of these emerging abilities. In Chapter 15, Julia S. Noland describes the competing conceptual interpretations of the A-not-B task, in which infants are challenged to find a hidden object after a time delay. This task is relatively new as an assessment tool but has been empirically investigated as a measure of working memory supported by prefrontal lobe functioning.

Aspects of cortical electrophysiological functioning and developmental processes are explored in Chapter 16 by Dennis L. Molfese and Victoria J. Molfese and in Chapter 17 by Dalit Himmelfarb Marshall and Nathan A. Fox. Event-related potentials (ERPs) and synchronized portions of an ongoing electroencephalographic (EEG) pattern allow researchers to evaluate the relationship between a neuroelectrical response and a time-locked stimulus event. Although not clear-cut, these investigators have found strong relationships to exist between ERPs and discrimination of speech-related stimuli and later language skills. Their findings raise exciting possibilities about the early identification of children with potential language problems as these measures are furthered developed. Marshall and Fox describe the use of quantified EEG assessments (qEEG), particularly the role of frontal EEG asymmetry and its relationship to expression of emotions. Lateralized changes in EEGs are associated with emotions, with differing patterns of EEG asymmetry found dependent on the type of affect in facial and vocal expressions. They cite the noninvasiveness, accuracy, and relatively low cost of the EEG as advantages that lend this technique to the study of psychophysiological processes.

Part V reviews several standard developmental assessments that measure a variety of behaviors and processes. In Chapter 18, Barry M. Lester and Edward Z. Tronick describe the historical developments of several neurobehavioral assessments including the Neonatal Behavioral Assessment Scale, the most widely used assessment of neonatal behavior; the Assessment of the Preterm Infant's Behavior; and the recently developed NICU Network Neurobehavioral Scale, which was designed for use in the large, multisite "Maternal Lifestyles" longitudinal study to assess effects of drug exposure and prematurity on infant development. In Chapter 19, Anneliese F. Korner and Janet C. Constantinou describe the extensive psychometric and conceptual underpinnings of the development of the Neurobehavioral Assessment of the Preterm Infant (NAPI). This is one of the few scales developed from a psychometric perspective, including the compilation of normative data and longitudinal testing for developmental validity. In addition, the authors developed a neonatal medical index to quantify the adverse perinatal and/or postnatal medical complications the infant experienced in the neonatal intensive care unit. The authors recommend the NAPI for assessment of the effects of interventions, monitoring developmental progress of individual infants, and studying basic questions about the development of preterm infants.

In Chapter 20, Judith M. Gardner, Bernard Z. Karmel, and Robert L. Freedland describe the relatively newly developed Neonatal Neurobehavioral Assessment Scale. In contrast to other measures, this procedure was developed to evaluate behaviors likely to differentiate at-risk infants and to achieve an accurate assessment of the different typologies and severity of central nervous system injury. The authors sought to develop a clinically useful tool to enable decisions about neurobehavioral abnormalities associated with the known structural and functional injuries to the central nervous system experienced by sick infants. The procedure was developed to have a minimum number of tasks so as to provide less stress to the sick infant. Attentional and sensory capacities, asymmetries of tone, state control, jitteriness, and feeding behaviors are evaluated through this assessment.

In Chapter 21, Jane Case-Smith and Rosemarie Bigsby highlight several scales used to describe aspects of motor development. Newly developed infancy motor assessments use Thelen's dynamic systems theory, which acknowledges the important role of the environment in motor development. In Chapter 22, Margaret Bendersky and Michael Lewis take on the task of synthesizing assessment issues related to the gold standard of infancy tests, the Bayley Scales of Infant Development.

Since the inception of work for this volume, the coeditors have relied on the support and talents of many people. As we progressed in this work, it became apparent that many areas of assessment could only be touched on; thus, this is by no means a comprehensive volume. Our editors at The Guilford Press, Seymour Weingarten and Carolyn Graham, have been extraordinarily patient and helpful. We thank the chapter authors for their dedication to writing, rewriting, and updating their work. One person in particular deserves special acknowledgment for her organization, detective work, secretarial assistance, and sense of humor in getting this work completed: Terri Lotz-Ganley has done an amazing job of editorial assistance, fact finding, and shepherding of this volume over the course of many years.

Contents

IV. LEARNING AND ATTENTION

V. STANDARD ASSESSMENTS

I

Introductory Issues

General Issues in Infant Assessment and Development

LYNN TWAROG SINGER

The ability to compile so large a volume devoted solely to the biobehavioral assessment of newborn and young infants is testimony to the continuing and undiminished growth of interest, research, and knowledge in this area of developmental psychology. By necessity, infant psychometrics and the study of individual differences and normative processes in infancy have developed in a mutually dependent fashion, each furthering and fueling greater advances in the other. As noted by Thompson (1990), in a seminal volume edited by Colombo and Fagen, a primary factor inhibiting developmental psychologists from studying individual differences in infancy has been, in addition to the highly canalized nature of some aspects of infant development, the fact that "behavioral differences among infants are difficult to measure reliably and accurately" (p. 45). The impetus for the compilation of this handbook is simple: to describe and critique some of the various infant assessment instruments that have proliferated in the past two decades, and, with a critical lens, to promote further research and refinement of these assessments.

Attempts to assess neonatal neurological and behavioral status have an extensive history (St. Clair, 1978) derived from a combination of medical and psychological/behavioral orientations. The evaluation of reflexes in a neonatal neurological evaluation had several purposes, including diagnosis of an immediate neurological problem, the evaluation of day-to-day changes concomitant with a pathological process, and the determination of long-term prognosis (Parmelee & Michaelis, 1971). Gesell (1925) expanded on this interest in reflex maturation and developmental progression. His developmental schedules were used to study normal infant mental and motor capacities longitudinally. Description of the orderly developmental sequences of reflexes and their relationships to brain injury underlay the introduction of numerous evaluations of the neonate and young infant which followed, such as those of Prechtl and Andre-Thomas (St. Clair, 1978).

By the 1950s and 1960s, behaviorally oriented examinations became prominent, reflecting the belief that maturational status and neuromotor status were interrelated, and reflecting the burgeoning psychological interest in individual differences in behavior. This period saw the development of neonatal behavioral assessments, such as the Graham–Rosenblith Scale (Rosenblith, 1966) and the Cambridge Newborn Behavioral and Neurological Scales (Brazelton & Freedman, 1971). The latter has since become the most popular and well studied neonatal assessment exam in both medical and psychological research under its more well-known name, the Brazelton Neonatal Behavioral Assessment Scale (see Lester & Tronick, Chapter 18, this volume).

In this same period, the methodological advances achieved by Robert Fantz in reliably assessing neonatal capacity to look at and prefer varying stimuli allowed inferences to be drawn about infant visual perception, discrimination, memory, and cognition. Fantz's methodological achievement initiated generations of innovative studies, many of which have culminated in the assessments described in this volume, including the Teller Acuity Cards (see Mayer & Arendt, Chapter 4, this volume); visual recognition memory tests (see Rose & Orlian, Chapter 13, this volume), and visual habituation measures (see Fagen & Ohr, Chapter 12, this volume).

The assessment of change and continuity in neurobehavioral development, one of the central and most challenging tasks of developmental psychology, continues to be rapidly influenced by data derived from the procedures described earlier and elsewhere in this volume, as well as from a growing understanding of basic neurological development. Sameroff and Chandler (1975) introduced the concept of the transactional model of development which stressed the dynamic nature of the mutual influences of child and environment. Two of the bedrocks of an assessment instrument, stability and predictive validity, have often proved to be elusive psychometric properties in neonatal and infant assessments, and they underlie the lengthy ongoing debate among developmentalists about whether there is continuity in cognitive development (Fagan & Singer, 1983; McCall & Carriger, 1993).

Our understanding of infant development and its assessment has been informed by major advances in neurobiology which have delineated the structure and processes of the long trajectory of brain development initiated prenatally. Brain development occurs in a highly complex, orderly sequence, beginning in the earliest days after conception and continuing postnatally, with continued rapid development until 2–3 years of age and extending well into adolescence (Huttenlocher, 1994). Four major stages of development have been identified (see Nelson, 1999, and Volpe, 2000, for reviews): (1) neural tube induction, which results in the formation of the brain and spinal cord and occurs in a peak period of the third and fourth weeks of gestation; (2) neuronal proliferation, occurring between 2 and 4 months gestation, in which all neurons and glia, the two major classes of brain cells, are derived; (3) neuronal migration, occurring primarily from 3 to 5 months gestation, in which millions of cells leave their places of origin to be permanently settled; and (4) cell differentiation, which includes cell death (apoptosis), synaptogenesis, and myelination, in which a sheathing substance forms to protect nerve cells and to allow faster transmission of information.

Much cortical development is postnatal due to the growth of neurons and their connections. An overabundance of synaptic connections is produced as functionally unspecific to allow for the development of complex neural circuits. Synapse elimination subsequently occurs from the pruning of these same circuits and is thought to be dependent on experience. This process of pruning is thought to underlie the greater plasticity of the brain in infancy and at "sensitive" or "critical" periods (Huttenlocher, 1994; Nelson, 2000).

The predominant causes of neurological or behavioral deficits are known to occur prenatally (Thoresen, 1999), and disruptions in the processes occurring at any of the stages noted previously can have profound developmental consequences. As an example, delayed myelination refers to an immature pattern of myelination commonly caused by prematurity, and characteristic of children with hydrocephalus (Porter & Tennekoon, 2000). Some studies have demonstrated that the quantity of myelin is associated with the child's level of cognitive functioning (Fletcher et al., 1992), but currently these functional correlates can be reliably ascertained only at older ages. Apparently, with treatment by shunting, age-appropriate myelination patterns can be attained in some children with hydrocephalus (Porter & Tennekoon, 2000). The eventual ability to link such treatment changes to functional behaviors in infancy is dependent on the continued psychometric refinement of the biobehavioral assessments described in this volume and others.

PARALLEL NEUROLOGICAL ASSESSMENTS

Our current understanding of developmental neurobiology has also been markedly advanced by technological tools which allow the study of brain development *in vivo*. Among the most salient are X-ray computed tomography (CT), magnetic resonance imaging (MRI), functional magnetic resonance imaging (fMRI), and positron emission tomography (PET). MRI techniques are noninvasive methodologies which provide information about the structure, metabolism, and function of the developing brain. The earliest

MRI has now been done with preterm infants as young as 24 weeks gestation (Battin et al., 1998), whereas, prior to the development of these techniques, only autopsy studies were possible (Inder & Huppi, 2000). Fetal MRI imaging has also been undertaken, although the safety of conducting MRI on both the pregnant mother and her fetus constitutes a major concern (Rivkin, 2000).

MRI provides spatial resolution of brain structure and avoids many limitations posed by CT scan, especially for the study of infants. These limitations include radiation exposure, which limits CT scan to clinically indicated use, and poorer anatomic resolution (Filipek, Kennedy, & Caviness, 1992). Similarly, PET, which measures regional cerebral blood flow directly, requires injecting subjects with radiopharmaceuticals, also limiting its use to adults and seriously ill children. PET studies have demonstrated that the ascending phase of the synaptogenesis curve is paralleled by a concurrent increase in metabolic activity in cortical areas during the postnatal period (Chugani, Phelps, & Mazziotta, 1987). fMRI, like PET, measures brain function through assessment of metabolic changes which occur when regional brain activity increases but is an indirect measure of blood flow. Practical limitations restrict fMRI to older children, because it requires an alert, cooperative child who can overcome the fear of a strange situation and hold his or her head still (Davidson & Slayter, 2000). Studies of sedated infants have been done, however, with passive presentation of visual or auditory stimuli (Bookheimer, 2000).

Additional MRI variations include diffusion sensor magnetic imaging (DTI), which measures diffusion of water in a particular medium. DTI has been used to study the newborn brain by assessing water diffusion in cerebral white matter. MRI spectroscopy allows quantification of metabolic information by employing standard MRI scanners to measure chemical levels in brain regions.

The cerebral Doppler effect is derived from ultrasound waves emitted by a transducer which can measure cerebral blood flow, a factor in several neonatal pathological conditions and central to the fetal behavioral assessments under development (see DiPietro, Chapter 3, this volume). Single photon emission computed tomography (SPECT) is a radionuclear technique of cerebral perfusion which has also been used to measure cerebral blood flow.

Neonatal and infant brain functioning can also be evaluated through assessment of electroencephalic activity reflected in the electroencephalogram (EEG) through electrodes placed on the infant's scalp in a standard pattern. Neurological integrity as reflected in EEG sleep patterns has recently been a focus of research in neurophysiology and behaviors (Scher, 1997; Thoman, Chapter 7, this volume). EEG patterns have proved useful in a number of the assessments featured in this volume as a measure of emotional regulation, language, and communication (see Molfese & Molfese, Chapter 16, and Marshall & Fox, Chapter 17, this volume).

Evoked potentials provide information about infant sensory perceptual processes linked to neurological conditions. They are averaged electrical responses from an EEG evoked by a stimulus. Auditory brainstem responses (ABRs) measure electrical events occurring within the auditory brainstem, while visual evoked potentials are generated by visual cortex responses to visual stimuli, and somatosensory evoked potentials are generated through peripheral brain pathways (Van Baar, 1998).

Refinement of these techniques represents a growing area of research that has already resulted in greater understanding of neurobiological development. Normative brain development using volumetric MRI techniques will be soon studied through a large multisite initiative of the National Institute of Child Health and Human Development. Collaborative efforts by developmental psychologists to develop the assessments of functional behaviors which correlate with the structural and metabolic characteristics of neurobiological processes to be compiled in such efforts will eventually lead to a true understanding of brain–behavior relationships.

ASSESSMENT

Psychological research generally attempts to measure hypothetical constructs rather than concrete physical properties such as height and weight. A psychological test is "an objective and standardized measure of a sample of behavior" (Anastasi & Urbina, 1997). Traditionally, the function of psychological tests has been to measure individual differences. Depending on the number and nature of items in an assessment, the sample of behaviors assessed may or may not be representative of a construct. One way to "assess" an assessment is to determine whether it meets standards required for use in clinical trials (Cronbach, 1984; Singer, 1997), which cannot afford to be compromised by measurement error.

These requirements include that the assessment be standardized, reliable, and valid. Standardization entails the development and publishing of uniform procedures in administrating and scoring the assessment. For comparability of scores, testing conditions must be the same for all subjects. Detailed directions are a major part of test standardization, extending to the stimuli used, which should be exactly described, time limits, how and when testing of limits of performance is allowed, scoring procedures for test items, preliminary explanations, and examiner training requirements. Included under the rubric of standardization is the establishment of norms, because performance on any test is judged based on empirical data. The standardization sample, a large representative sample for whom the procedure is designed, is used to establish norms to indicate average as well as deviant performance. Norms allow individual raw scores to be interpreted with reference to the distribution of scores obtained by the standardization sample. These raw scores, when converted into a relative measure, can indicate an individual's relative standing in the normative sample, permitting an evaluation of performance in reference to others, and can provide direct comparisons of an infant's performance across different tests. Standard scores, which indicate the infant's distance from the normative mean relative to the standard deviation of the distribution, can be obtained by transformation of the original raw scores. Standard scores are characteristic of the most highly developed infant assessments, including the Bayley Mental and Motor Scales and the Neurobehavioral Assessment of the Preterm Infant.

Reliability refers to the consistency of a measurement. No assessment has perfect reliability, but the range of fluctuation of an infant's test score due to chance factors limits the extent to which an infant's performance can be considered a reflection of the behavioral characteristic measured versus error variance. Several types of reliability are usually considered, most of which rely on correlation coefficients as a measurement.

Test–retest reliability correlates the scores obtained by an infant on two separate administrations of a test. Test–retest reliability has posed special difficulties for infancy assessments. Most childhood intelligence tests, even in the preschool years, yield remarkably stable scores, achieving correlations in the .70s and .80s (Bornstein & Krasnegor, 1989). In contrast, median values of test–retest reliabilities of visual habituation measures are in the .30 to .40 ranges, and for paired comparison performance measures, in the .20s for single novelty preference tasks. Such levels of reliability do not meet the standards for adult psychometric work (Colombo, 1993). Infant assessments are often criticized for their low stability, with correlations declining at younger ages. The Brazelton scales, as well as visual recognition memory and habituation measures, for example, have all raised concerns about their validity due to the low stability of infant performance (Benasich & Bejar, 1992; Fagan & Singer, 1983).

Several factors introduce considerable variability into many infancy assessments resulting in less than acceptable intertest agreement. These factors include biological fluctuations in the infant's physiological status underlying the behavioral construct under study, as well as the attentional variability of the infant. In defense of the poor internal consistency of many infant assessments, it has been noted that some of these assessments, such as cry analysis and the Neonatal Network Neurobehavioral Scales, are designed to be sensitive to the variable physiological states of the infant. Insofar as such measures reflect the rapidly changing neurobiological status of the infant in interaction with the environment, many infant assessments would be expected to have low week-to-week or even day-to-day stability.

Additional reliability data useful to understanding an assessment include interrater agreements, and intrarater consistency, because examiner characteristics may differentially affect infant performance on some tasks compared to others. Enthusiastic, warm, or gentle examiners may elicit better performance on a neurobehavioral scale with a neonate. The Brazelton (1973) scale, for example, has been demonstrated to be quite susceptible to examiner effects (Richardson, Day, & Taylor, 1989). Even when the infant's actual behavioral output can be judged with high reliability, however, contextual factors may influence infant cooperation. When training examiners for a multisite clinical trial to use the Fagan Test of Infant Intelligence (Fagan & Singer, 1983), for example, many previously unspecified variables needed to be delineated in written form to ensure examiners' uniformity of procedure. Variables such as whether to use a pacifier during the assessment or obtaining infant attention by tapping on the apparatus, which had been incorporated into the procedure, needed specification.

Test validity entails the degree to which an assessment measures what it purports to measure. Construct validity specifies what the test measures and is undergirded by both content and predictive validation (Cronbach & Meehl, 1955).

The construct validity is the extent to which a test measures a theoretical construct or trait. Constructs explain and organize observed response consistencies. Evidence for construct validation is derived from data on the attributes of the construct, including developmental changes, relationship to other measures, and convergent or discriminant relationships with variables with which it should reasonably be related or unrelated (Anastasi & Urbina, 1997).

Predictive validity measures the extent to which an assessment "predicts" performance on an assessment of the same trait over a long period. Because intelligence is a fairly stable construct after the preschool ages and has been so well studied as a psychological construct measured by IQ tests, it may have been a natural progression for psychologists to perceive assessments of infant developmental differences as precursors of childhood IQ. However, decades of follow-up research have indicated that except at the lowest ranges of scores, standardized tests of infant development given prior to 18 months of age have poor predictive validity for later intellectual functioning (Fagan & Singer, 1983; McCall & Mash, 1997) and are close to zero.

This conclusion led to debate about the nature of intelligence, that is, whether or not a unitary construct of intelligence, or *g*, existed and whether it was continuous or discontinuous from infancy. An alternative rationale for the lack of predictive validity of infant developmental assessments was that infant developmental assessments such as the Bayley scales were measuring the wrong behaviors, namely, sensorimotor skills which bear little relationship to higher-order cognitive skills important to school-age learning. Thus, more discrete measures of attention and information processing have been examined with the hope that they would be more reflective of the attentional, discrimination, memory, and speed of information-processing skills characteristic of later intelligence. Although still evolving, tests of visual information processing in infancy, such as recognition memory, habituation, and attentional duration, have been evaluated in longitudinal studies. Predictive validity of such measures has ranged from .30 to .40 across a variety of studies and populations, suggesting that such measures may be useful in identification of infants at risk for later developmental delays (Bornstein & Sigman, 1986; Colombo, 1997; Fagan & Singer, 1983; McCall & Carriger, 1993). Indeed, in a recent study, Rose and Feldman (1997) found evidence that speed of processing and memory accounted for the relationships that they found from 7-month visual recognition memory and 1-year cross-modal transfer to 11-year IQ. It should be recognized, however, that even with specific processing measures, prediction for an individual infant (i.e., sensitivity and specificity) is still poor, and that other measures, such as parental education, bear greater relationships to child intellectual outcome than any infant assessment.

CURRENT APPLICATIONS

There is a pressing need for the further refinement and development of infant biobehavioral assessments, many of which remain in rudimentary or experimental forms. The implementation of the Education for All Handicapped Children Act Amendments (later retitled the Individuals with Disabilities Education Act), calls for early intervention services for all handicapped infants and their families (Shonkoff & Meisels, 1990; Singer, Minnes, & Arendt, 1999). Eligible for services are infants experiencing developmental delay and those with a diagnosed condition with "high risk" of developmental delay. However, identifying which infants are at risk remains a difficult problem. It is well documented that children younger than school age are highly unlikely to be identified for intervention, as there is a tenfold disparity between prevalence rates of handicapped children from infancy to school age (Meisels & Wasik, 1990). Other explanations for the differences in earlier and later age prevalence rates have been attributed to the absence of the wide range of reliable, valid assessments available for identification of delays at younger ages. Because of the poorer predictive validity of standard global assessments such as the Bayley scales, screening devices employing both psychometric and psychophysiological perspectives have been recommended. But, as yet, although there are a large number of experimental assessments in development, as described earlier, there are none with adequate standardization and predictive properties to be appropriated for large-scale screening efforts (Meisels & Wasik, 1990).

Similarly, Public Law 99-457 paved the way for the need for outcome measures to assess the effects of the early-infancy intervention programs initiated by these amendments. Global outcome measures, such as the mental or motor indices of the Bayley scales, are broad based and represent the conglomerate of a number of diverse infant skills; thus the overall score may mask benefits from intervention on a discrete area of functioning. Moreover, because such outcome measures lack predictive validity in infancy, they provide little information for the researcher about the underlying developmental processes affected by the intervention which resulted in a positive or negative outcome.

Societal concern for and public health focus on the growing numbers of high-risk infants have also contributed to an interest in developing assessments of brain–behavior relationships that can be used as early in life as possible. Currently, about 53,000 very-low-birthweight infants (< 1,500 g) are born annually in the United States, with follow-up studies indicating that as many as 50% will need some type of supportive educational services at school age, and that for some subgroups, such as those with bronchopulmonary dysplasia, 25% will have significant sensory deficits and/or mental or motor retardation (Singer, Yamashita, Lilien, Collin, & Baley, 1997). A landmark randomized clinical intervention trial for low-birthweight infants, the Infant Health and Development Project, found that higher-weight infants in this trial had significant cognitive gains from the intensive intervention at 3 years of age, but very-low-birthweight infants derived no benefit (Brooks-Gunn et al., 1994). It is likely that prematurity leads to changes in brain organizational development which affect learning and developmental outcome. Many of the assessments of sensorimotor capacities and information-processing skills described in this volume have the potential to identify the sensory deficits and behavioral characteristics specifically affected by very-low-birthweight birth and its medical and neurological correlates at earlier ages. Earlier assessment could then lead to environmental interventions specifically directed at remediation of these deficits.

The emergence of behavioral teratology as a distinct area of developmental and neuropsychological interest has also provided impetus for the development of infancy assessments (Fein, Schwartz, Jacobson, & Jacobson, 1983; Voorhees, 1986). This field has flourished concurrent with greater understanding of principles of fetal neurobiological development and the scientific demonstration that many toxic substances could cross the placental barrier to affect fetal development. Teratology was originally conceptualized as the study of gross structural malformations seen after birth and thought to be related to fetal developmental disturbances (e.g., the major limb defects attributable to maternal ingestion of thalidomide as an antinausea drug during pregnancy). This definition is expanded on in behavioral teratology to include a range of possible teratogenic effects on the developing nervous system resulting in behavioral disabilities. Neuropsychological impairments are now recognized as possible outcomes of toxic fetal exposures even in the absence of gross physical impairments. A wide range of teratogens have now been recognized as causing subtle to significant neurobehavioral disabilities. Among the most prominent are lead (Needleman & Bellinger, 1991), alcohol (Streissguth, Barr, & Sampson, 1990), nicotine and marijuana (Fried, Watkinson, & Gray, 1992), vitamin A (Adams & Lammer, 1995), antiepileptic drugs (Leavitt, Yearby, Robinson, Sells, & Erickson, 1992), and polychlorinated biphenyls (Jacobson, Fein, Jacobson, Schwartz, & Dowler, 1985).

In the early 1990s, in response to widespread public alarm and scientific concern about the epidemic use of crack cocaine by pregnant women in the United States, the National Institute on Drug Abuse initiated funding of a number of longitudinal studies of the development of cocaine-exposed infants (Smeriglio & Wilcox, 1999), many of which incorporated novel or experimental neonatal and infant behavioral assessments as outcomes. These large-scale, methodologically rigorous studies are just beginning to yield findings about the developmental correlates of fetal cocaine and polydrug exposure, but they promise also to provide much information about the psychometric properties of these measures. To date, these studies have examined numerous neonatal and infant behaviors in relation to drug exposure, including habituation (Mayes, Bornstein, Chawarska, & Granger, 1995), neonatal visual preferences (Singer, Arendt, et al., 1999), visual recognition memory (Jacobson, Jacobson, Sokol, Martier, & Chiodo, 1996), sleep EEG (Scher, Richardson, & Day, 2000), neonatal neurobehavioral assessments (Eyler, Behnke, Conlon, Woods, & Wobie, 1998; Richardson, Hamel, Goldschmidt, & Day, 1996; Singer, Arendt, Minnes, Farkas, & Salvator, 2000), and infant movement assessment (Arendt, Singer, Angelopolous, Busdieker, & Mascia, 1998). In addition to the rise in concern about cocaine, increasing numbers of pregnant and postpartum women are receiving pharmacological treatments for depression, a problem which affects about 10% of pregnant women. Data are lacking about the effects of such drugs on fetal development and infant behavioral outcomes (Wisner, Gelenberg, Leonard, Zarin, & Frank, 1999).

An interesting corollary to the concept of behavioral teratogenicity lies in the also relatively recent recognition that nutrient deficiencies prenatally or during infancy can have long-term developmental consequences. Folic acid deficiency, for example, was found to be a causal factor in the occurrence of neural tube disorders such as spina bifida (Wald, 1994). Iron deficiency anemia has been demonstrated to affect infant behavior negatively (Lozoff et al., 1987). Biochemical studies have found that certain long-chain polyunsaturated fatty acids (LCPUFAs) (which are found in human breast milk but not infant formulas) are essential components of infant nutrition. Citing studies which show breast-fed infants to have better intellectual functioning than formula-fed infants, some have proposed that adding

LCPUFAs to infant formulas would be beneficial to infant visual and cognitive functioning (see Dobbing, 1997, for comprehensive review). This proposal has led to a large number of research studies to assess the relationship of LCPUFAs to infant mental, motor, and visual development, including a number of nutritional formula industry-led randomized clinical trials to address efficacy and safety issues of adding these nutrients to infant formulas (Auestad et al., 2001). What is of interest is (1) the notion that in the absence of any known harmful effects to formula-fed infants, these additives might provide some benefit to infants' development, and (2) the use of behavioral assessments as outcomes of these studies, with extensive consultation from developmental psychologists on which functional end points should be examined and which assessments in infancy had adequate psychometric properties to be used (Dobbing, 1997).

Thus, it is clear that recent developments in our understanding of fetal and infant neurobiological development provide impetus for the tremendous research and public health interests in interventions for the developing infant. Accurate measurement of infant biobehavioral status is needed for diagnosis, evaluation of process changes, and long-term prognosis of at-risk infants, a goal which will be reached only through further refinement of specific and global assessments of infant functioning.

ACKNOWLEDGMENTS

This work was supported by Grant No. MCJ 39071 from the Maternal Child and Health Services Bureau (Title V, Social Security Act), Health Resources and Services Administration, and Grant No. RO1-07957 from the National Institute on Drug Abuse.

REFERENCES

Adams, J., & Lammer, E. J. (1995). Human isotretinoin exposure. The teratogenesis of a syndrome of cognitive deficits. *Neurotoxicology and Teratology, 17*, 386–392.

Anastasi, A., & Urbina, S. (1997). *Psychological testing* (7th ed.). Upper Saddle River, NJ: Prentice-Hall.

Arendt, R. E., Singer, L. T., Angelopoulos, J., Busdieker, O., & Mascia, J. (1998). Sensory motor development in cocaine-exposed infants. *Infant Behavior and Development, 21*, 627–640.

Auestad, N., Halter, R. A., Hall, R. T., Blatter, M., Bogle, M., Burks, W., Erikson, J. R., Fitzgerald, K. M., Dobson, V., Innis, S. M., Singer, L. T., Montalto, M. B., Jacobs, J. R., Qui, W., & Bornstein, M. H. (in press). Growth and development in term infants fed long-chain polyunsaturated fatty acids: A double-masked, randomized, parallel, prospective, longitudinal, multivariate study. *Pediatrics.*

Battin, M., Maalouf, E. F., Counsell, S., Herlihy, A., Hall, A., Azzopardi, D., & Edwards, A. D. (1998). Physiological stability of preterm infants during magnetic resonance imaging. *Early Human Development, 52*(2), 101–110.

Benasich, A., & Bejar, I. T. (1992). The Fagan Test of Infant Intelligence: A critical review. *Journal of Applied Developmental Psychology, 13,* 153–171.

Bookheimer, S. (2000). Methodological issues in pediatric neuroimaging. *Mental Retardation and Developmental Disabilities Research Review, 6,* 161–166.

Bornstein, M. H., & Krasnegor, N. A. (Eds.). (1989). *Stability and continuity in mental development: Behavioral and biological perspectives.* Hillsdale, NJ: Erlbaum.

Bornstein, M. H., & Sigman, D. (1986). Continuity in mental development from infancy. *Child Development, 57,* 251–274.

Brazelton, T. (1973). *Neonatal Behavioral Assessment Scale.* Philadelphia: Lippincott.

Brazelton, T., & Freedman, D. (1971). Manual to accompany newborn behavioral and neurological scales. In G. Stoeling & J. VanDerWerffTenBosch (Ed.), *Normal and abnormal development of brain and behaviour.* Baltimore: Williams & Wilkins.

Brooks-Gunn, J., McCarton, C., Casey, P. H., McCormick, M. C., Bauer, C. R., Bernbaum, J. C., Tyson, J., Swanson, M., Bennett, F. C., Scott, D. T., et al. (1994). Early intervention of low-birthweight-premature infants: Results through age 5 years from the Infant Health and Development Program. *Journal of the American Medical Association, 272,* 1257–1262.

Chugani, H. T., Phelps, M. E., & Mazziotta, J. C. (1987). PET study of human brain functional development. *Annals of Neurology, 22,* 487–497.

Colombo, J. (1993). *Infant cognition: Predicting later intellectual functioning.* Newbury Park, CA: Sage.

Colombo, J. (1997). Individual differences in infant cognition. In J. Dobbing (Ed.), *Developing brain and behaviour: The role of lipids in infant formula* (pp. 339–372). San Diego: Academic Press.

Cronbach, L. J. (1984). *The essentials of psychological testing.* New York: Harper & Row.

Cronbach, L. J., & Meehl, P. E. (1955). Construct validity in psychological tests. *Psychological Bulletin, 52,* 281–302.

Davidson, R. J., & Slayter, H. A. (2000). Probing emotion in the developing brain: Functional neuroimaging in the assessment of the neural substances of emotion in normal and disordered children and adolescents. *Mental Retardation and Developmental Disabilities Research Reviews, 6,* 166–170.

Dobbing, J. (Ed.). (1997). *Developing brain and behaviour: The role of lipids in infant formula.* San Diego: Academic Press.

Eyler, F. D., Behnke, M., Conlon, M., Woods, N. S., & Wobie, K. (1998). Birth outcome from a prospective, matched study of prenatal crack/cocaine use: II. Interactive and dose effects on neurobehavioral assessment. *Pediatrics, 101,* 237–241.

Fagan, J. F., & Singer, L. T. (1983). Infant recognition memory as a measure of intelligence. In L. Lipsitt (Ed.), *Advances in infancy research* (Vol. II, pp. 31–78). Norwood, NJ: Ablex.

Fein, G. G., Schwartz, P. M., Jacobson, S. W., & Jacobson, J. L. (1983). Environmental toxins and behavioral development: A new role for psychological research. *American Psychologist, 38*(11), 1188–1197.

Filipek, P. A., Kennedy, D. N., & Caviness, V. S. (1992). Neuroimaging in child neuropsychology. In I. Rapin & S. J. Segalowitz (Eds.), *Handbook of neuropsychology: Vol. 6. Child neuropsychology* (pp. 301–329). New York: Elsevier.

Fletcher, J. M., Bohan, T. P., Brandt, M. E., Brookshire, B. L., Beaver, S. R., Francis, D. J., Davidson, K. C., Thompson, N. M., & Miner, M. E. (1992). Cerebral white matter and cognition in hydrocephalic children. *Archives of Neurology 49,* 818–824.

Fried, P. A., Watkinson, B., & Gray, R. (1992). A follow-up study of attentional behavior in 6 year old children exposed prenatally to marijuana, cigarettes, and alcohol. *Neurotoxicology and Teratology, 14*, 299–311.

Gesell, A. (1925). *The mental growth of the preschool child.* New York: Macmillan.

Huttenlocher, P. R. (1994). Synaptogenesis in human cerebral cortex. In G. Davison & K. A. Fischer (Eds.), *Human behavior and the developing brain* (pp. 137–152). New York: Guilford Press.

Inder, T. E., & Huppi, P. S. (2000). *In vivo* studies of brain development by magnetic resonance techniques. *Mental Retardation and Developmental Disabilities Research Reviews, 6*, 59–67.

Jacobson, S. W., Fein, G. G., Jacobson, J. L., Schwartz, P. M., & Dowler, J. K. (1985). The effect of PCB exposure on visual recognition memory. *Child Development, 56*, 853–860.

Jacobson, S. W., Jacobson, J. K., Sokol, R. J., Martier, S. S., & Chiodo, L. M. (1996). New evidence of neurobehavioral effects of *in utero* cocaine exposure. *Journal of Pediatrics, 129*(4), 581–588.

Leavitt, A. M., Yearby, M. S., Robinson, N., Sells, C. J., & Erikson, D. M. (1992). Epilepsy in pregnancy. Developmental outcome of offspring at 12 months. *Neurology, 42*, 141–143.

Lozoff, B., Brittenham, G. M., Wolf, A. W., McClish, D. K., Kuhnert, P. M., Jimenez, E., Jimenez, R., Mora, L. A., Gomez, I., & Krauskoph, D. (1987). Iron deficiency anemia and iron therapy: Effects on infant developmental test performance. *Pediatrics, 79*, 981–985.

Mayes, L. C., Bornstein, M. H., Chawarska, K., & Granger, R. H. (1995). Information processing and developmental assessments in 3 month old infants exposed prenatally to cocaine. *Pediatrics, 95*, 539–545.

McCall, R. B., & Carriger, N. S. (1993). A meta analysis of infant habituation and recognition memory performance as predictors of later IQ. *Child Development, 64*, 57–79.

McCall, R. B., & Mash, C. W. (1997). Long-chain polyunsaturated fatty acids and the measurement and prediction of intelligence (IQ). In J. Dobbing (Ed.), *Developing brain and behaviour: The role of lipids in infant formula* (pp. 295–338). San Diego: Academic Press.

Meisels, S. I., & Wasik, B. (1990). Who should be served? Identifying children in need of early intervention. In S. J. Meisels & J. Shonkoff (Ed.), *Handbook of early intervention* (pp. 605–632). New York: Cambridge University Press.

Needleman, H. L., & Bellinger, D. (1991). The health effects of low level lead. *Annual Review of Public Health, 12*, 111–140.

Nelson, C. A. (1999). Change and continuity in neurobehavioral development: Lessons from the study of neurobiology and neural plasticity. *Infant Behavior and Development, 22*, 415–429.

Nelson, C. A. (2000). Neural plasticity and human development: The role of early experiences in sculpting memory systems. *Developmental Science, 3*, 115–136.

Parmelee, A., & Michaelis, R. (1971). Neurological examination of the newborn. In J. Hellmuth (Ed.), *Exceptional infant* (Vol. 2). New York: Brunner/Mazel.

Porter, B. E., & Tennekoon, G. (2000). Myelin and disorders that affect the formation and maintenance of this sheath. *Mental Retardation and Developmental Disabilities Research Reviews, 6*, 47–58.

Richardson, G. A., Day, N. L., & Taylor, P. M. (1989). The effect of prenatal alcohol, marijuana, and tobacco exposure on neonatal behavior. *Infant Behavior and Development, 12*, 199–209.

Richardson, G. A., Hamel, S. C., Goldschmidt, L., & Day, N. L. (1996). The effects of prenatal cocaine use on neonatal neurobehavioral status. *Neurotoxicology and Teratology, 18*, 519–528.

Rivkin, M. (2000). Developmental neuroimaging of children using magnetic resonance techniques. *Mental Retardation and Developmental Disabilities Research Reviews, 6*, 68–80.

Rose, S. A., & Feldman, J. F. (1997). Memory and speed: Their role in the relation of infant information processing to later IQ. *Child Development, 68*(4), 630–641.

Rosenblith, J. (1966). Prognostic value of neonatal assessment. *Child Development, 37*, 623–631.

Sameroff, A., & Chandler, M. (1975). Reproductive risk and the continuum of caretaking casualty. In F. Horowitz, M. Hetherington, S. Scarr-Salpatek, & G. Siegel (Eds.), *Review of child development research* (Vol. 4, pp. 187–244). Chicago: University of Chicago Press.

Scher, M. S. (1997). Neurophysiological assessment of brain function and maturation. I. A measure of brain adaptation in high risk infants. *Pediatric Neurology, 16*, 191–198.

Scher, M. S., Richardson, G., & Day, N. L. (2000). Effects of prenatal cocaine/crack and other drug exposure on electroencephalographic sleep studies at birth and one year. *Pediatrics, 105*(1), 39–48.

Shonkoff, J., & Meisels, S. J. (1990). Who should be served?: Identifying children in need of early intervention. In S. J. Meisels & J. Shonkoff (Eds.), *Handbook of early intervention* (pp. 605–632). New York: Cambridge University Press.

Singer, L. T. (1997). Methodological considerations in longitudinal studies of infant risk. In J. Dobbing (Ed.), *Developing brain and behaviour: The role of lipids in infant formula* (pp. 210–230). San Diego: Academic Press.

Singer, L. T., Arendt, R. E., Fagan, J. F., Minnes, S., Salvator, A., Bolek, T., & Becker, M. (1999). Neonatal visual information processing in cocaine-exposed and non-exposed infants. *Infant Behavior and Development, 22*(1), 1–15.

Singer, L. T., Arendt, R. E., Minnes, S., Farkas, K., & Salvator, A. (2000). Neurobehavioral outcomes of cocaine-exposed infants. *Neurotoxicology and Teratology, 22*, 653–666.

Singer, L. T., Minnes, S., & Arendt, R. E. (1999). Innovations for high risk infants. In D. E. Biegel & A. Blum (Eds.), *Innovations in practice and service delivery across the lifespan* (pp. 57–78). New York: Oxford University Press.

Singer, L. T., Yamashita, T., Lilien, L., Collin, M., & Baley, J. (1997). A longitudinal study of developmental outcome of infants with bronchopulmonary dysplasia and very low birth weight. *Pediatrics, 100*(6), 987–993.

Smeriglio, V., & Wilcox, H. C. (1999). Prenatal drug exposure and child outcome. Past, present, future. *Clinical Perinatology, 26*(1), 1–16.

St. Clair, K. (1978). Neonatal assessment procedures: A historical review. *Child Development, 49*, 280–292.

Streissguth, A., Barr, H. M., & Sampson, P. D. (1990). Moderate prenatal alcohol exposure effects on child IQ and learning problems at 7½ years. *Alcoholism: Clinical and Experimental Research, 14*, 662–669.

Thompson, L. (1990). Genetic contributions to early individual differences. In J. Colombo & J. Fagen (Eds.), *Individual differences in infancy: Reliability, stability, and prevention* (pp. 45–76). Hillsdale, NJ: Erlbaum.

Thoresen, M. (2000). Protecting the perinatal brain. *Seminars in Neonatology, 5*, 1–2.

Van Baar, A. (1998). Evaluation of the human newborn infant. In W. Slikker & L. Chang (Eds.), *Handbook of developmental neurotoxicology* (pp. 439–454). New York: Academic Press.

Volpe, J. (2000). Overview: Normal and abnormal human brain development. *Mental Retardation and Developmental Disabilities Research Reviews, 6,* 1–5.

Vorhees, C. V. (1986). Principles of behavioral teratology in E. P. Riley & C. V. Vorhees (Eds.). *Handbook of behavioral teratology* (pp. 23–48). New York: Plenum.

Wald, N. J. (1994). Folic acid and neural tube defects. In G. Bock & J. Marsh (Eds.), *Ciba Foundation Symposium 8: Neural tube defects* (pp. 70–89). London: Wiley.

Wisner, K. L., Gelenberg, A. J., Leonard, H., Zarin, D., & Frank, E. (1999). Pharmacologic treatment of depression during pregnancy. *Journal of the American Medical Association, 282,* 1264–1269.

2

Conceptual and Methodological Basis for Understanding Development and Risk in Infants

RONALD SEIFER

The task of identifying the crucial methodological issues in behavioral assessment of infants at risk is formidable. Research reviewed in this volume spans domains of physical growth, electrophysiological activity, biobehavioral regulation, cognitive processes, and interactive social behavior. Further complicating matters, some of this work is rooted in the identification of normative phenomena while other work emphasizes individual differences models. In this chapter, I do not attempt to detail every aspect of research methods unique to all of the specific domains represented in the volume. Rather, I focus on general methods issues that influence how we understand the findings from our developmental studies. My discussion covers broad-based developmental models; issues specific to understanding risk in a developmental context; conceptualization of growth, stability, and continuity; how we understand the biology–behavior interface; and factors important to interpretation of data in these research domains.

DEVELOPMENTAL MODELS

One of the first issues to consider when designing or evaluating research in human development is the model that drives the execution and interpretation of the research efforts. Unfortunately, this is an issue that is almost universally neglected in the human development literature. By developmental models, I mean the underlying assumptions about the broadly defined processes by which growth and adaptation occur across the lifespan. When stated in their purest form, these models appear to be (and indeed probably are) strawmen that are easily knocked down. However, the underlying heuristic associated with each model does correspond to a large degree with approaches to human development evident in current research literature.

APPROACHES TO CAUSE AND EFFECT

A scheme described by Sameroff (Sameroff & Chandler, 1975) is useful in articulating differences in developmental models. He identifies main-effects, interaction, and transactional models as three basic assumptions that have permeated work in human behavioral development. These models emphasize the type of causal inferences that are made from developmental data and generally are useful in describing associations of various factors potentially affecting children and their ultimate developmental outcomes.

Main-Effects Models

Main-effects models emphasize direct one-to-one associations between antecedent conditions and subsequent outcomes. The locus of the antecedent condition may vary, but the emphasis is on the relatively linear causal path from condition to outcome. For example, two variants of explaining level of behavior problems in young children might be that (1) genetic makeup predicts level of behavior problems (Cantwell, 1996) or (2) interactive experience and reinforcement predict level of behavior problems (Thomas & Chess, 1977). Both are good examples of a main-effects model to explain human variation in that a single causal explanation is involved. The fact that one explanation posits a constitutional basis for the variation while the other posits a contextual basis does not belie their underlying formal similarity.

Interaction Models

Interaction models share with main-effects models the relatively direct link between antecedent conditions and subsequent outcomes. The difference in the interactive framework is that two (or more) factors conspire to produce the outcomes. Such models may be "additive" in nature—that is, the ultimate level of behavior exhibited is determined by the sum of factors affecting the behavior. To extend the behavior problems example, a child with "high-behavior problem" genes and "average-behavior problem-promoting" social interaction might end up around the 75th percentile on activity level. Alternatively, a more "interactive" variant of the model may be considered in which not only are multiple factors involved, but these factors act synergistically to predict outcomes. In one such scenario, only the child with "high-behavior problem" genes *and* social experience will have particularly severe behavior problem outcomes; those with average precursors in either (or both) the genetic or social realms would not be notable in terms of their ultimate outcome level of behavior problems.

Transactional Models

In contrast to both main-effects and interaction models, transactional models presume that individual and social systems have the potential to undergo basic transformations such that later status is not predictable (or as predictable) from early status prior to the reorganization. Again taking the example of early behavior problems, a child with a poor constitutional predisposition (say early temperamental difficulty or colic) might in one family environment meet with interactional experience that perpetuates the expression of similar behavioral difficulty but in another family be treated in such a way that all vestiges of early dysregulated behavior are eliminated (cf. Thompson, 1994). In each case, the interim developmental outcomes proximal in time to the expression of the early difficult behavior represent a fundamentally different way that the individual child's self-regulatory capacity becomes organized. In the first case, the dysregulation is maintained within the family system and continues on a path toward higher than average risk for later expression of problem behavior. Further, the family context may be transformed by experiencing the child's behavioral difficulty so that it becomes more rigid and less capable of devising effective adaptations. In the second case, the newfound regulatory capacity makes this child indistinguishable from his or her peers who had no comparable constitutional "deficit" early in life and from this point onward the child's probability of poor developmental outcomes (in the realm of behavior problems) is quite similar to that of the "average" child.

Why is it important to make such distinctions? First and foremost, the degree to which different models identify greater or fewer numbers of relevant developmental influences will affect the focus and scope of research programs in different domains. Second, the differing emphases on periods of systemic change will drive differences in longitudinal features of research programs—when change is more basic and frequent, longitudinal assessment must match the phenomena. Finally, the hypotheses derived to guide individual studies may differ as a function of these underlying developmental models. No individual study can capture the complexity of any of the developmental processes that interest infancy researchers. Instead, each study examines one piece of the theoretical pie, and at some points in research programs, different underlying model assumptions lead the researcher in different directions.

DEVELOPMENT IN CONTEXT

Another way of characterizing developmental models is in their approach to the consideration of individual children in developmental context. On the one hand, some approaches are relatively insensitive to contextual issues, concentrating primarily on the characteristics of individual children. On the other, multiple levels of developmental context are integral to the model for understanding human growth and adaptation (Bronfenbrenner, 1986). As students of human development from a primarily psychological perspective, our emphasis is on the individual child as the key organizational unit (Sameroff, 1983). This is, however, but one of many choices of how to study human behavior—sociology and epidemiology point toward examining large social groups, anthropology focuses on organizations provided by culture, biology emphasizes organic subsystems, and ethology highlights species typical behavior over multigenerational time spans.

When viewing behavior in context we are thus examining not only "higher" levels of organization (e.g., social groups and culture) but also more basic subsystems of the organism (e.g., brain function and endocrine systems). These different levels of systemic organization have some independence and may be examined on their own terms, yet there are important boundary conditions when communication across these levels is an important focus (e.g., brain–behavior relationships). It is crucial for researchers to recognize that identifying biological correlates of behavior provide no more fundamental explanation of that behavior than does identifying a cultural correlate or another behavioral correlate (more about this in a later section).

An important feature of studying behavior in context is the appreciation of individual by context interactions. One important way this has been manifest in recent literature is in the specification of gene by environment interactions (Wachs & Gruen, 1982). What is important about this perspective is that it explicitly identifies for study the expression of similar characteristics by individuals developing within different contexts. A second type of interaction focuses on the individual construction of personal environments (Seifer & Schiller, 1995). This perspective is in some ways the converse of the gene by environment perspective. When one focuses on how constitutional features may be expressed differently in varying contexts, the other examines the individuality of incorporating contextual experience into personal organization. This constant dialectic poses formidable theoretical challenges yet also is a basis for increased understanding of human developmental phenomena.

Still another way of viewing individual development in context is in the reference for the phenomena we study. In some cases, our reference is the performance of other similar individuals in similar situations (typically called individual-differences models). The contrasting view is to examine the similarities of performance of similar individuals in similar situations (the normative view). When pursued in "isolation," individual differences and normative agendas generally proceed in an unremarkable fashion. When these approaches are mixed, however, the outcome is often less pleasing. Good examples of this dilemma are found in the information-processing field. Much of this work has historically been from a normative perspective: How do children at different developmental phases perceive and process sensory input (Haith, 1980). Such programs have been successful at identifying developmental paths (e.g., what types of processing typically occurs before others types and what kinds of errors are predictable at different stages). In contrast, when such approaches have been used in an individual-differences framework, results have been far more difficult to understand and generally less compelling. For example, in studies of habituation dropout rates are typically near 50%, which typically results from infant fatigue or crying. In the context of normative studies, such dropout rates are less vexing than if one is pursuing an individual differences agenda. What does it mean to be a dropout? Are dropouts able or more able to habituate; do they process information in a more or less sophisticated manner; do they differentially respond more poorly to structured situations; or is this simply a transient nonsystematic state related phenomenon? Further, what is the implication of having high dropout rates in studies when identification of subjects is difficult because of the frequency of inclusion criteria or when participation in longitudinal protocols makes missing data costly?

CONCEPTUALIZATIONS OF GROWTH AND CHANGE

Moving to a more narrow focus of details of developmental models, several factors associated with the assessment of change are important to consider. Often forgotten in the day-to-day implementation of human development research is that this domain of inquiry is fundamentally about change. Although our research strategies often appear to be studying change (e.g., by looking at different age groups or the same children at different ages), the real questions addressed are more often than not about static behavior at one point in time. This is understandable—we have relatively primitive technology for describing real developmental change in systematic ways. Still, in keeping with our basic agenda of understanding developmental processes, both empirical and theoretical activities must be more attentive to processes of change.

Two early works on this topic still set the standard for how different characteristics of change may be conceived (McCall, Eichorn, & Hogarty, 1977; Wolhwill, 1973). The basic distinctions they made were between changes in levels of a particular function versus changes in the basic organization of the system. This distinction is crucial for the interpretation of demonstrated associations (or lack thereof) over time, in particular when measurements are made using the same nominal measurement device. In risk research, where the follow-up of specific outcomes over time may be of interest, the identification of continuity of function is crucial to ensure that the same process is being assessed at different points in development.

Another important distinction is between group and individual models of change. It is often the case that group averages will obscure the variety of ways that individuals reach developmental end points. Most of our design and quantitative technology is applicable to groups rather than to individuals (Willett, 1988). There are, however, recent analytic methods for applying individual change analyses in longitudinal datasets that are beginning to appear more frequently in the human development literature (Burchinal & Appelbaum, 1991; Bryk & Raudenbush, 1992).

An extension of the approach to modeling individual growth patterns is to define the developmental function of a particular phenomenon. Few examples of this approach are available in the human development literature. Perhaps the best known and most widely used example is for anthropometric growth measures like height, weight, or head circumference. Growth tables have been published for these measures and the parameters of the function are well accepted (although updating of norms appears to be needed). In psychological and behavioral development, the potential exists for identifying such functions as well. The main requirement is that the behaviors in question have invariant measurement properties on the same dimension across time. Some examples in which developmental functions would be useful to describe include levels of social interaction, infant irritability, explorations of environments, reaching behavior, or looking times (among the many that might be identified). If such developmental functions were well identified, applications to risk populations might enable researchers to identify subtle differences between risk and normative individuals (e.g., see van den Boom & Hoeksma, 1994).

Rapidity of change is an important feature of developmental functions. In many individual-differences models, the key feature is whether one individual changes more rapidly than his or her peers. The classic example of this is in the intelligence testing field. Those who change more rapidly (e.g., acquire more vocabulary, hold more items in memory, and solve more complex puzzles) will attain higher scores on tests that are normed against age. On a more conceptual level, rapidity of change may be associated with periods during which discontinuity of function is highest (Emde, Gaensbauer, & Harmon, 1976). Under these circumstances, stability of individual differences with respect to a developmental function may be lowest, and in fact it may become less acceptable to conceive of the measurement as indicating the same underlying construct or function.

In such cases it is important to keep in mind the functional understanding of individual behaviors. It has become clear that there are many situations in which similar behaviors serve different functions across developmental time (e.g., maintenance of proximity to mother as adaptive attachment strategy early in life and as dependence during toddler years). Conversely, different behaviors may become indicators of the same function as children develop (e.g., proximity maintenance early in life and joint conversation later in life as attachment behaviors). Further complicating matters is that at any single point in time, multiple behaviors may serve similar functions (e.g., cry, proximity maintenance, and direction of gaze as attachment behaviors). One useful way of dealing with this dilemma was articulated by Sroufe and Waters (1977) in their definition of organizational constructs. Such constructs attempt to integrate complex behavioral systems by concentrating less on levels of individual behaviors and more on the functional meaning of multiple behaviors interpreted in context. Thus, a developmental function can be defined in terms of multiple behavioral indicators that may appear in different patterns across individuals and across time, yet these different patterns may indicate underlying similarity of function.

DEVELOPMENTAL MODELS OF RISK

Why do some children have good developmental outcomes and why do some children have poor outcomes? This is the question that motivates us to explore many of the issues raised in this volume. The previous discussion of developmental models of change provides a framework for discussing methods issues in the field of infant risk research. It goes without saying that students of human development are far from capable of predicting developmental outcomes in children with any degree of certainty. However, in the past several decades we have learned much about many factors that are associated (at least statistically) with different classes of outcomes, albeit with varying degrees of precision.

First, it is important to consider what we mean by risk, which in general usage is defined as a factor, element, or course involving uncertain danger, harm, or loss. The two most important points in the definition of risk are that of negative consequences and uncertainty. The negative consequences are typically well attended to in developmental research, but the issue of uncertainty is often obscured. Risk is in essence a statistical concept—compared with unselected members of the population, those defined at risk are more likely to have one or more negative outcomes. Statements such as "children born under 1,500 grams will have learning problems" reflect both an ignoring of the probabilistic nature of risk as well as reliance on a main-effects developmental model. While rarely stated in such terms, more reasonable sounding statements such as "children born under 1,500 grams are at high risk for learning problems" are often interpreted in the main-effects mode, particularly as one moves away from basic research to the clinical uses of risk studies.

It is also important to keep in mind that risk is not a static phenomenon.

Rather, like most developmental processes, risk is dynamic and changing. Whereas some characteristics of individuals remain with them throughout their lives (e.g., having been born preterm or minority racial status), processes associated with such features may be dramatically altered with development. Among children born preterm (with similar gestational change and health status at birth), those who have Intraventricular Hemmorage (IVH) early in life versus those who do not (perhaps as a result of differential medical treatment or by virtue of yet to be defined physical differences) will ultimately be at greater risk for more serious developmental problems. Similarly, as patterns of discrimination and prejudice evolve in our culture, being a member of one or another racial group may have differential consequences, and hence differential risk, as children develop. Still other risk factors, such as poverty or family composition, may change dramatically over the course of a child's life, perhaps affecting the risks posed by those conditions.

Most basic models of risk emanate from the field of epidemiology, where patterns of illness are the main concern. Even for physical illness, it is rare that every individual exposed to a contagious agent or every person with a particular constitutional characteristic will develop the illness associated with those agents or characteristics—classic examples of each are tuberculosis and heart disease. Thus, epidemiologists developed a language for describing risks (especially for single risks associated with single outcomes), with two indices most frequently used. *Relative risk* refers to the ratio of incidence of negative outcomes in "exposed" and "nonexposed" groups, typically identified in a prospective manner. *Odds ratio* refers to the ratio of (1) odds that someone with a negative outcome was exposed to a particular risk to (2) odds that someone without the negative outcome was exposed to the same risk—this is typically viewed in a retrospective manner. It is surprising that these highly descriptive and easy-to-calculate indices rarely appear in the human development literature.

Although such standard estimates of risk are available, it is important to recognize that their use (and the associated research designs) may mask important features of how risk factors operate. The most important oversight is the failure to identify the specificity of risk. Where it may be easy to identify circumstances when a particular risk is associated with one outcome of interest, it is equally important to identify other outcomes that may also be adversely affected by the same risk. In high-risk mental health research, parental mental illness is often demonstrated to be associated with the same illness in their children, which supports genetic transmission models. However, such studies often fail to identify other mental illness that the children have, which would belie the direct genetic transmission hypothesis. This oversight serves to inhibit full understanding of the complex developmental processes involved (Seifer, 1995).

An analogous problem is the failure to identify the multiple ways that the same outcome might be achieved. To again use the mental health example, individuals who develop a particular mental illness may have a parent with that same illness, but it is more likely that other risk factors (e.g., poverty, family dysfunction, or negative life events) are present, and these associated risks may even explain the major portions of variance in the outcome in question.

Most current treatments of risk differentiate risk versus resilience. In essence, this differentiation refers to that between an insult to the developing system as opposed to a moderator of such insults. It is important at this point to add some precision to the definitions of terms used to define risk. In particular, the distinction between factors thought of as risks and those thought to reduce risks has emerged as an important theme in the developmental literature (Masten, 1989). Four key constructs used to describe these factors are risk, protection, vulnerability, and resilience:

1. Risk: External forces that increase likelihood of poor outcome.
2. Vulnerability: Internal characteristics that increase likelihood of poor outcome.
3. Protection: External factors that buffer effects of risk and vulnerability.
4. Resilience: Internal factors that buffer effects of risk and vulnerability.

The definitions may appear precise, but the boundaries of these constructs are arbitrary and fraught with conceptual difficulty (discussed later in this chapter). However, these four constructs have provided good heuristics for integrating current knowledge in the field.

APPLICATION OF RISK MODELS TO HUMAN DEVELOPMENT

In their influential paper, Mednick and McNeil (1968) specified reasons that examination of children at risk should lead to fuller understanding of the etiology of serious mental disorder, specifically schizophrenia. Their comparative analysis of research methods was done in the context of three existing techniques for studying etiology of illness: (1) observation of already ill people, (2) observation of families of ill people, and (3) retrospective reviews of archival information of people with illness. All these approaches were fraught with serious difficulties. For example, when studying individuals who have fully developed illness, it became impossible to disentangle the effects of the illness itself from factors that might be associated with the development of the illness. In schizophrenia it is well-known that individuals with the illness often exhibit diminished social skills, even though poor social functioning is not a necessary feature of the clinical syndrome. It is thus tempting to speculate that poor social functioning may be a predisposing factor or etiological root of the disorder. However, it may also be the case that the social functioning of affected individuals is influenced by the thought disorder central to schizophrenia, the general effects of hospitalization, or the effects of chronic psychotropic medication; thus, their lower social performance may be an artifact of having the disorder.

The solution to these dilemmas proposed by Mednick and McNeil (1968) was to study prospectively the children born to a parent with schizophrenia, prior to the onset of illness. It was well-known at the time, and it has continued to be verified, that children whose parents have serious mental disorders are themselves at increased risk for development of illness (Kendler, Neale, Kessler, Heath, & Eaves, 1992). In the case of schizophrenia, about 10% of the offspring of one biological parent with the disorder will develop schizophrenia (compared with about 1% in the general population—it must also be kept in mind that only about 10% of people diagnosed with schizophrenia have a schizophrenic parent) (Watt, Anthony, Wynne, & Rolf, 1984). The advantages of the high-risk method were said to include the following: (1) subjects in studies are not yet schizophrenic and thus they will not exhibit epiphenomena associated with the illness or its treatment, (2) researchers are blind to who will eventually become schizophrenic, (3) data collected are current rather than retrospective, (4) data are obtained systematically, rather than in many different formats as is true of retrospective data, and (5) ideal control subjects are already in the target population (those who develop illness can be compared with those who do not develop illness).

Viewed more broadly in the context of infants at risk for developmental problems, some general principles are widely applicable. First, it is difficult to retrospectively disentangle causes and consequences of poor developmental outcomes. Second, bias is easily introduced into studies when subjects are identified because of poor developmental outcomes; when the outcomes are severe and obvious on mere visual inspection, there is no good way of totally blinding researchers to index and control cases. Third, when protocols are introduced prospectively, the opportunity for systematic investigation is greatly enhanced when compared with retrospective review of information often collected in widely diverse ways with little quality control. Fourth, the ability to use the most appropriate controls—those who have the risk but not the poor outcomes—is much enhanced in prospective designs. All these points conspire to push infant risk researchers more and more toward prospective longitudinal designs when etiology of poor outcomes is the central question.

CONCEPTUAL OVERLAP AMONG CONSTRUCTS USED IN RISK RESEARCH

The major constructs we have examined in prior sections (risk, vulnerability, resilience, and protection) have enabled us to make great strides forward in understanding developmental processes. However, these constructs have serious inherent problems, which may hinder efforts to continue such gains in understanding. These problems arise from the very definition of the constructs to the empirical usage of them in research settings.

Definitional Problems

Risk, vulnerability, resilience, and protection are in essence defined by a two-by-two grid, where the dimensions are internal versus external and increasing versus decreasing poor outcomes (see Figure 2.1). Each dimension of this definition poses problems. With respect to internal/external, the field of human development research has been plagued by failed attempts to reconcile this dichotomy. Distinctions such as self–other, gene–environment, or constitution–context have typically been helpful heuristics when broad ideas are the focus but have created substantial difficulty when specific mechanisms of development are the focus (Sameroff, 1983).

The fundamental problem with such dichotomies is that human development is inherently characterized by interactions among multiple systems (some "inside" and some "outside" the organism), which are organized at different levels with respect to an individual child. However, these systems (be they inner or outer) do not function in the absence of all the other systems. For example, genes do not operate in isolation; they are only expressed within particular environments of the developing individual. Conversely, environments operate on individual development only in the context of the phenotypic expression of the child's genetic makeup. To separate out the "effects" of the genes or the environments ignores the fundamental point that each organized system only has meaning within the context of the other (a point that may be generalized to adhere across all of the systemic organizations considered in human development). As we attempt to understand risk processes in more detail, distinctions between risk and vulnerability as well as resilience and protection become more difficult to support because the basic dichotomy of internal and external breaks down under close scrutiny.

Effect on Negative Developmental Outcomes

Locus of Factor	Increase	Reduce
External	Risk	Protection
Internal	Vulnerability	Resilience

FIGURE 2.1. Terms commonly used in risk research.

The distinction between increasing and reducing negative outcomes presents a similar set of difficulties. Such a dichotomy rests on the assumption that negative outcomes are discreet entities. In reality, many outcomes are better conceived as dimensional; that is, there is a range of potential outcomes across the different domains of development examined. Thus, rather than viewing risk (or vulnerability) as increasing the probability of specific events and protection (or resilience) as decreasing those events, a more accurate characterization may be that risks put pressure on individual development toward negative ends of dimensions while protection exerts pressure toward positive ends of those dimensions.

Functionally, this makes clear distinctions between risk and protection (or vulnerability and resilience) difficult because simply indicating presence or absence of a factor would arbitrarily place it under the definition of risk versus protection (or vulnerability vs. resilience). What does it mean to say that low socioeconomic status is a risk factor while high socioeconomic status is a protective factor? Ultimately, this type of distinction is of little value. It is more important for us to gain understanding of how socioeconomic status affects a particular outcome domain, and less important to characterize it as to risk versus protective status. Rather, the important point to keep in mind is how a particular factor influences development in one direction or another based on the value of that factor.

A related point is the definition of protective factors (offered by Rutter, 1987) that requires the factor to be selectively operative only under conditions of risk. This definition remains compatible with those already discussed but adds the component that there is selective activity. That is, there is no positive effect of protective factors (so defined) under ordinary circumstances. Only when adversity is present do the protective properties of the factor emerge. Some processes do appear to work in this way in some studies (e.g., Seifer, Sameroff, Baldwin, & Baldwin, 1992), but there are few instances in which such a stringently defined protective factor has been identified in more than a single empirical study or when such a limited definition was hypothesized prior to the research and later confirmed in the data.

Multiple Risk Factors

One of the striking features of the body of work examining risk and development is that studies typically examine one risk factor at a time. This research strategy persists even though it is well established in human psychological development as well as other health fields (Kannel & Schatzkin, 1983) that risk factors viewed in combination have more predictive power than those viewed in isolation (Rutter, 1979; Sameroff, Seifer, Baldwin, & Baldwin, 1993). There are several potential ways that multiple risks may combine.

- Independent specific factors (multisyndrome view)
- Partially independent specific factors (modified multisyndrome view)
- Dependent nonspecific factors (developmental process view)

The issue of specificity in risk factors works in both directions. A risk factor may be specific in that predictable effects are associated with a particular factor, but that factor may affect a nonspecific set of outcomes. For example, specific parental mental illnesses (such as schizophrenia or depression) are related to many different kinds of poor outcomes in children (e.g., the same mental illness, learning disabilities, substance abuse, or delinquency) (Beardslee, Keller, Seifer et al., 1996). Alternatively, a risk factor may be related to a specific outcome, but the way that it affects the outcome may be unpredictable. For example, constitutional insults such as HIV infection or preterm birth are known to be associated with neurological impairment. However, the effects on the nervous system may be manifest as motor dysfunction in some individuals and cognitive dysfunction in others. Finally, a risk factor may have neither a specific domain that it always affects nor a specific way in which it affects particular domains. For example, low socioeconomic status is ubiquitous in its relation to many types of negative outcomes, including poor physical health, poor mental health, delinquency, and school failure. Further, the particular manifestation in any of these domains may occur in a variety of ways. Mental health, for example, may be affected in terms of mood disorders, thought disorders, or conduct disorders.

Given all the different ways that risk factors may be operative, and our current primitive knowledge of these issues, it may be most prudent to be concerned with maximizing predictive power using multiple risk strategies while attempting to determine whether there is any evidence that individual risk factors (or particular combinations) have any degree of specificity in the outcomes they affect and the processes by which those outcomes are affected. To begin with a strategy that assumes specificity in risk may lead us to erroneous conclusions, especially in studies that examine single risk factors with respect to single outcomes. Such designs may in effect put blinders on researchers so that broader nonspecific effects of risks are obscured.

From Risk to Prevention

The most obvious practical extensions of risk research are in the areas of intervention and prevention. The fundamental distinction between these two approaches is that intervention is concerned with reversing the effects of risk once problems have emerged whereas prevention efforts are aimed at reducing the frequency with which such problems are manifest in the population (Simeonsson, 1994). Risk research provides an important focus for prevention efforts, making them more economical and feasible in our society, which has limited resources.

Research into risk and protective factors provides a wealth of information about how to target preventive efforts. Take, for example, the agenda of preventing mental illness. An unguided approach might involve implementing prevention efforts at the community at large. Clearly, the costs associated with such efforts would be large because there are no limits on who is targeted for the prevention program. By using the results of risk studies, much smaller targeted populations could be served by such programs. Groups to target would include family members of adults with serious mental illness or children who have exhibited certain premorbid signs. The cost–benefit ratio of such targeted programs is likely to be far higher than those that do not use information gained from risk studies.

A closely related issue is what the content of prevention programs should be. Again, the results of risk and protection studies are quite informative. Factors identified as resiliencies of individuals (e.g., child social and cognitive strengths) (Beardslee, Wright, Rothberg, Salt, & Versage, 1996) or contextual protectors (e.g., parenting sensitivity) (van den Boom, 1994) would be the most obvious place to start. One point worth noting here is the distinction between prevention and protection. Whereas protection or resilience is "naturally" occurring, prevention results from systematic targeted efforts to effect positive change. Still, prevention efforts are probably most efficient when they capitalize on naturally occurring protective or resilience influences (Simeonsson, 1994).

One issue that social scientists must always address is how the processes they study affect people's lives. In the case of risk factor research, this is particularly salient because the results of this work may have a direct impact on individual access to opportunities. As the results of scientific inquiry into risk become known outside the social science community (a process that happens ever faster in our culture with sophisticated communications technology), the results of those studies are put into practice. This may occur in the context of trying to ameliorate the effects of risk factors (as in the prevention agenda discussed previously) or in the context of institutions making decisions about individuals based on their risk status. It is the latter of these applications that concerns us here.

It is often the case that individuals become categorized as a result of their risk status. Perhaps the most obvious manifestation historically has been categorization according to racial status. Aside from outright prejudice based on race, there is also evidence that members of most minority racial groups in the United States have poorer outcomes and success rates than do members of the majority white culture. Thus, an overall strategy that would maximize success of individuals admitted to various institutions (be they work environments, academic centers, community organizations, etc.) would be to accept those with the fewest risk factors associated with failure (i.e., to exclude those from minority racial groups). Lost from such a probabilistic approach is an analysis of the capacities of each individual under consideration for access to one of our society's resources, which in part may explain why such forms of discrimination are now illegal.

Many of the risk factors we study are not as obvious to the casual observer as race, although many of the social risk factors that have been identified are consistent with those that have historically been the target of discrimination (e.g., low socioeconomic status). With more sophisticated screening in the work and academic environments, elements of risk are coming under increasing scrutiny when decisions of access are being made.

Examples include physical health risk factors such as HIV infection, family history of genetic illness, or individual genetic testing results. In each of these circumstances, employers or health insurers have already attempted to reduce exposure by denying employment or benefits to specific individual because of such "preexisting" conditions. Examples of psychosocial risks abound as well, such as individual or family history of substance abuse or the neighborhood in which one lives. In the former case, such history of social behavior has been treated in much the same way as physical health problems, with employers offering fewer opportunities or benefits to individuals based on these risk factors. In the latter case, insurance practices, as they have become increasingly sophisticated in their actuarial methods, routinely single out individuals in certain neighborhoods for higher rates or sometimes inability to be insured simply because of the location of their residence. These companies are, of course, employing a well-reasoned application of risk factors to their *group* interest—minimizing financial exposure in the total insurance pool—but in the process do not consider the ability of each individual to overcome the risk inherent in their social circumstance.

As noted earlier, the fundamental flaw in the application of risk factors in the decision-making process is the transformation from probabilistic to categorical attributions of an individual. Whenever decisions about individuals are made on the basis of group norms, substantial numbers of errors will be made regarding individual members of the groups in question. Further, the frequency and severity of such errors increases with the degree of uncertainty associated with any particular risk factor. The result is a highly intellectualized form of prejudice that has the same consequences as the garden-variety racism and discrimination that is illegal and undesirable in our culture.

METHODOLOGICAL IMPLICATIONS OF DEVELOPMENTAL MODELS OF RISK ASSESSMENT STRATEGIES

The vast majority of developmental assessments are done using a single time point. Standardized tests, neurobehavioral assessments, parent-report questionnaires, and social interactions (among others) are all characteristically done at one point in time. This strategy implies some assumptions: (1) the assessment technology is reliable and (2) moment-to-moment or day-to-day variability is low (which, of course, will affect reliability estimates).

Most evidence would suggest that such assumptions are probably not correct. When variability across assessment has been evaluated (which is rare) the results generally indicate modest stability in the measurements obtained (e.g., Lancioni, Horowitz, & Sullivan, 1980; Seifer, Sameroff, Barrett, & Krafchuk, 1994). This is not a phenomenon unique to infants but is found more generally for behavioral assessments across the lifespan (Epstein & O'Brien, 1985). When introducing variance associated with time of assessment, we may be obscuring the individual-differences variance that is typically the focus of developmental studies.

One simple alternative to the single-time-point assessment strategy is to measure the same phenomenon on multiple occasions. This strategy, however, introduces problems of its own. First is the reason the multiple assessments are to be done: Is it to increase reliability by using multiple measurements, to understand the individual change function over time, or to examine longitudinal patterns of stability or continuity? There are also obvious pragmatic considerations associated with multiple measurement strategies, and studies rarely have the resources to effectively manage such large undertakings. There are, however, compelling reasons to consider such strategies when research areas are mature enough to address basic questions about developmental processes. Complicating the issue of multiple measurements is whether the desired final product is an aggregate of many assessments or a profile of those assessments. Some argue that contextually sensitive profiles provide rich information not available from either single-time-point measurements or aggregated multiple measures (Mischel & Shoda, 1995).

A related concern is where measurements are done. A long-standing distinction has been between those studies conducted in laboratory settings versus those conducted in children's "natural" contexts. Whereas control and systematic presentation of stimuli are maximized in the laboratory, the home setting affords an environment that is more familiar to infants and their families and also presents stimuli that are more typical of their daily lives. As technology for field studies becomes more sophisticated and accessible (e.g., video and electronic recorders) the availability of more natural settings as the context for research is increased. We often fall into easy habits of bringing infants and families into our laboratories when in fact it may be more desirable (and not much more difficult) to examine the behavior of interest in a more familiar context.

LEVELS OF ANALYSIS AND INTERPRETATION OF FINDINGS

In prior sections I noted that there are hierarchies of systems studied by human development researchers. From a methodological perspective, the major issue is how findings from studies at different levels are conceptually integrated. The American tradition in psychology and related fields is to emphasize the importance of reductionist explanations—that is, those explanations at the lowest levels of systemic hierarchies. In human behavior research, this is manifest as the search for biological explanations of behavior.

Biology and Behavior

Developmentalists have long been interested in the interface of biology and behavior. Study of this interface takes many forms, such as psychophysiology, brain "mapping," response to psychotropic medication, neurohormonal regulation, circadian rhythms, and functional imaging, to name a few. Of importance in the present context is a discussion of how we understand the results of these empirical studies as well as their integration in larger theoretical perspective.

This connection between biology and behavior has proved to be one of the most vexing in the field of human development. On the one hand, there is no question that biological function is the substrate of all behavior. On the other, it is not clear that understanding biology provides much insight into the organization and expression of behavior, at least at current levels of understanding. For example, we have a fairly crude understanding of localization of cognitive function in the brain. In some cases, this allows for important insights, such as the potential consequences of traumatic brain injury. Extensions of such knowledge are often made, however, and confidence in the biology–behavior connection is much less clear. Examples include functional imaging studies or electroencephalograph mapping, which provides tantalizing clues (e.g., Field, Fox, Pickens, & Nawrocki, 1995) but little firm evidence about specific behavioral and psychological processes.

Perhaps of more importance is the conceptual issue of whether a biological explanation is in any way superior to a phenomenological explanation of the behavior at its own level of systemic organization. For example, it is often assumed that if one understands biological substrates, causes of the behavior have been identified. Unfortunately, this approach ignores a basic characteristic of the systems in questions, which is that reorganization at one level may affect organization at other levels (whether subordinate or superordinate). Recent evidence suggesting that experience in psychotherapy "affects" brain function in a similar manner as psychotropic medication (Schwartz, Stoessel, Baxter, Martin, & Phelps, 1996) is an excellent example of how behavioral change appears to temporally precede physiological change. Thus, researchers should carefully consider attributions regarding direction of effect when formal correspondence between biology and behavior are identified. Perhaps more important, research programs might more aggressively pursue understanding the biological changes in individuals that are associated with behavioral experience.

A related issue is the manner in which we attach the term "neuro" to our work (e.g., neuropsychology and neurobehavioral). Typically in human behavior research, when the term "neuro" is used, it does not mean that any direct examination of nervous system function has occurred. More often, specific behavioral systems are examined, with inferences made to neurological substrates underlying the behavior. For example, one might find that visual processing or motor integration is poor in a risk population, and tests of such functions are often labeled as neurobehavioral or neuropsychological. Where suggestions about underlying neurological correlates of behavioral dysfunction are useful products of such research, the inferences that neurological dysfunction or causes of the behavior have been identified are often counterproductive. Researchers need to be explicit about the boundaries between actual findings and theoretical inferences.

When studying children at risk, there is a natural tendency to look for biological explanations. Psychological and behavioral risk is often defined in terms of a constitutional insult (e.g., preterm birth, intrauterine growth retardation, birth trauma, and prenatal substance exposure). When risk is defined in more psychosocial terms (e.g., parental mental illness or poverty) there have also been attempts to identify a constitutional or genetic basis. Time and again, however, the psychosocial factors associated with the identified risks have proven to be the best predictors of child outcomes.

Direction of Effect

As noted previously, the issue of direction of effect is highlighted in the biology–behavior interface. The interpretation difficulties, however, extend to virtually all studies of human development. These issues are particularly salient in risk research, as there is usually an implicit (if not explicit) attribution about direction of effect in the identification of risk factors preceding negative outcomes. This assumption can, however, lead to misguided conclusions. Often, whether one variable is measured temporally prior to another is a simple artifact of research design. When the degree of autocorrelation over time is considered in designs in which presumed causes and effects are measured on multiple occasions, conclusions about causality will often be different, and usually obscure.

Most of our current research technology is ill suited to determining cause and effect within the complex systems we study. Rather, our results are typically more suited to defining contemporaneous associations among measures. Careful research designs, usually across many studies, and often with an experimental component, are necessary to even begin to make reasonable statements about cause and effect in developmental research.

Size of Effects in Risk Research

One vexing issue in human development work is that we typically explain only small portions of outcome variance in our studies. This often leads us to concentrate on whether an observed effect is different from the null—that is, whether or not a statistically significant result is obtained. Although important, this emphasis usually precludes examination of effect sizes in developmental research, an index that is ultimately more useful than the significance of a result in a single study.

All the standard statistical methods (which comprise 99% of the published results in human development research) are easily converted to effect sizes (Cohen, 1988, 1990; Rosnow & Rosenthal, 1996). This information provides a standard metric that is interpretable across studies and across different types of statistical procedures. Further, when many studies are combined, whether in a meta-analysis (Goldsmith & Alansky, 1987; Rosenthal, 1995) or a standard review of literature, the expectable size of the effect is more readily apparent. This will provide the researcher with better guidance about how many subjects to include in future studies, and whether results obtained are best considered replications of prior findings or as discrepant nonreplications. Finally, effect sizes help to interpret whether a particular finding is meaningful when considered in broad context. For example, a significant effect in a large-sample study that explains 1% of variance in intelligence outcomes in a high-risk population may be of academic interest but probably has little practical importance. Along these lines, one effect-size indicator used infrequently by developmental researchers is the odds ratio. Although used extensively in epidemiology, where medical risk is of interest, this approach (best used with dichotomous predictors) provides an easily understood quantitative index of how each unit of change in predictor status is associated with unit changes in the criterion variable of interest.

SUMMARY AND CONCLUSIONS

I have reviewed many issues relevant to the theoretical interpretation of studies of children at risk, focusing mainly on areas in which there is ambiguity or uncertainty. The themes that are most salient at this point in history revolve around appropriate interpretation of findings in context. These themes include clear articulation of the developmental models that have prompted the hypotheses being tested in specific studies, the appropriate application of constructs such as risk and resilience, clear understanding of when static versus dynamic processes are being examined, and use of statistical descriptors that best characterize the size of the effect to maximize comparisons across studies. Attention to these conceptual issues can only increase the integrative understanding of outcomes in infants facing various types of adversity, which are studied from a wide variety of methodological and theoretical perspectives.

REFERENCES

Beardslee, W. R., Keller, M. B., Seifer, R., Lavori, P. W., Staley, J., Podorefsky, D., & Shera, D. (1996). Prediction of adolescent affective disorder: Effects of prior parental affective disorder and child psychopathology. *Journal of the American Academy of Child and Adolescent Psychiatry, 35,* 279–288.

Beardslee, W. R., Wright, E., Rothberg, P. C., Salt, P., & Versage, E. (1996). Response of families to two preventive intervention strategies: Long-term differences in behavior and attitude change. *Journal of the American Academy of Child and Adolescent Psychiatry, 35,* 774–782.

Bronfenbrenner, U. (1986). Ecology of the family as a context for human development: Research perspectives. *Developmental Psychology, 22,* 723–742.

Bryk, A. S., & Raudenbush, S. W. (1992). *Hierarchical linear models: Applications and data analysis methods.* Newbury Park, CA: Sage.

Burchinal, M., & Appelbaum, M. I. (1991). Estimating individual developmental functions: Methods and their assumptions. *Child Development, 62,* 23–43.

Cantwell, D. (1996). Attention deficit disorder: A review of the past 10 years. *Journal of the American Academy of Child and Adolescent Psychiatry, 35,* 678–987.

Cohen, J. (1988). *Statistical power analysis for the social sciences* (2nd ed.). Hillsdale, NJ: Erlbaum.

Cohen, J. (1990). Things I have learned (so far). *American Psychologist, 45,* 1304–1312.

Emde, R. N., Gaensbauer, T. J., & Harmon, R. (1976). Emotional expression in infancy: A biobehavioral study. *Psychological Issues, 10*(Monograph No. 37).

Epstein, S., & O'Brien, E. J. (1985). The person-situation debate in historical and current perspective. *Psychological Bulletin, 98*(3), 513–537.

Field, T., Fox, N. A., Pickens, J., & Nawrocki, T. (1995). Relative right frontal EEG activation in 3– to 6–month-old infants of "depressed" mothers. *Developmental Psychology, 31,* 358–363.

Goldsmith, H. H., & Alansky, J. (1987). Maternal and infant temperamental predictors of attachment: A meta-analytic review. *Journal of Consulting and Clinical Psychology, 55,* 805–816.

Haith, M. (1980). *Rules that babies look by: The organization of newborn visual activity.* Hillsdale, NJ: Erlbaum.

Kannel, W. B., & Schatzkin, A. (1983). Risk factor analysis. *Progress in Cardiovascular Disease, 4,* 309–332.

Kendler, K. S., Neale, M. C., Kessler, R. C., Heath, A. C., Eaves, L. J. (1992). Major depression and generalized anxiety disorder: Same genes, (partly) different environments? *Archives of General Psychiatry, 49,* 716–722.

Lancioni, G. E., Horowitz, F. D., & Sullivan, J. W. (1980). The NBAS-K:I. A study of its stability and structure over the first month of life. *Infant Behavior and Development, 3,* 341–359.

Masten, A. (1989). Resilience in development: Implications of the study of successful adaptation for developmental psychopathology. In D. Cicchetti (Ed.), *The emergence of a discipline: Rochester Symposium on Developmental Psychopathology.* Hillsdale, NJ: Erlbaum.

McCall, R., Eichorn, D., & Hogarty, P. (1977). Transitions in early mental development. *Monographs of the Society for Research, 42*(Serial No. 171).

Mednick, S. A., & McNeil, T. F. (1968). Current methodology in research on the etiology of schizophrenia: Serious difficulties which suggest the use of the high-risk group method. *Psychological Bulletin, 70*, 681–693.

Mischel, W., & Shoda, Y. (1995). A cognitive-affective system theory of personality: Reconceptualizing situations, dispositions, dynamics, and invariance in personality structure. *Psychological Review, 102*, 246–268.

Rosenthal, R. (1995). Writing meta-analytic reviews. *Psychological Bulletin, 118*, 183–192.

Rosnow, R. L., & Rosenthal, R. (1996). Computing contrasts, effect sizes, and counternulls on other people's published data: General procedures for research consumers. *Psychological Methods, 1*, 331–340.

Rutter, M. (1979). Protective factors in children's responses to stress and disadvantage. In M. W. Kent & J. E. Rolf (Eds.), *Primary prevention of psychopathology: Vol. 3. Social competence in children* (pp. 49–74). Hanover, NH: University Press of New England.

Rutter, M. (1987). Psychosocial resilience and protective mechanisms. *American Journal of Orthopsychiatry, 57*, 316.

Sameroff, A. J. (1983). Developmental systems: contexts and evolution. In W. Kessen (Ed.), P. H. Mussen (Series Ed.), *Handbook of child psychology: Vol. 4. History, theories and methods* (pp. 237–294). New York: Wiley.

Sameroff, A. J., & Chandler, M. (1975). Reproductive risk and the continuum of caretaking casualty. In F. D. Horowitz (Ed.), *Review of child development research* (Vol. 4, pp. 187–244). Chicago: University of Chicago Press.

Sameroff, A. J., Seifer, R., Baldwin, A., & Baldwin, C. P. (1993). Stability of intelligence from preschool to adolescence: The influence of social and family risk factors. *Child Development, 64*, 80–97.

Schwartz, J. M., Stoessel, P. W., Baxter, L. R., Martin, K. M., & Phelps, M. E. (1996). Systematic changes in cerebral glucose metabolic rate after successful behavior modification treatment of obsessive–compulsive disorder. *Archives of General Psychiatry, 53*, 109–113.

Seifer, R. (1995). Perils and pitfalls of high risk research. *Developmental Psychology, 31*, 420–424.

Seifer, R., Sameroff, A. J., Baldwin, C. P., & Baldwin, A. (1992). Child and family factors that ameliorate risk between 4 and 13 years of age. *Journal of the American Academy of Child and Adolescent Psychiatry, 31*, 893–903.

Seifer, R., Sameroff, A. J., Barrett, L. C., & Krafchuk, E. (1994). Infant temperament measured by multiple observations and mother report. *Child Development, 65*, 1478–1490.

Seifer, R., & Schiller, M. (1995). The role of parenting sensitivity, infant temperament,and dyadic interaction in attachment theory and assessment. In E. Waters, B. E. Vaughn, G. Posada, & K. Kondo-Ikemura (Eds.), Caregiving, cultural, and cognitive perspectives on secure-base behavior and working models: New growing points of attachment theory and research. *Monographs of the Society for Research in Child Development, 60*(Serial No. 244), 146–174.

Simeonsson, R. J. (1994). *Risk, resilience, & prevention: Promoting the well-being of all children.* Baltimore: Brookes.

Sroufe, L. A., & Waters, E. (1977). Attachment as an organizational construct. *Child Development, 48*, 1184–1199.

Thomas, A., & Chess, S. (1977). *Temperament and development.* New York: Brunner/Mazel.

Thompson, R. A. (1994). Emotion regulation: A theme in search of definition. In N. Fox (Ed.), The development of emotion regulation: Biological and behavioral considerations. *Monographs of the Society for Research in Child Development, 59*(Serial No. 240), 25–52.

van den Boom, D. C. (1994). The influence of temperament and mothering on attachment and exploration: An experimental manipulation of sensitive responsiveness among lower-class mothers with irritable infants. *Child Development, 65,* 1457–1477.

van den Boom, D. C., & Hoeksma, J. B. (1994). The effect of infant irritability on mother–infant interaction: A growth-curve analysis. *Developmental Psychology, 30,* 581–590.

Wachs, T. D., & Gruen, G. (1982). *Early experience and human development.* New York: Plenum Press.

Watt, N. F., Anthony, E. J., Wynne, L. C., & Rolf, J. E. (1984). *Children at risk for schizophrenia: A longitudinal perspective.* Cambridge, UK: Cambridge University Press.

Willett, J. B. (1988). Questions and answers in the measurement of change. In E. Z. Rothkopf (Ed.), *Review of education research* (Vol. 15, pp. 345–422). Washington, DC: American Education Research Association.

Wohlwill, J. F. (1973). *The study of behavioral development.* New York: Academic Press.

II

Prenatal Growth
and Sensory Development

3

Fetal Neurobehavioral Assessment

JANET A. DIPIETRO

HISTORY OF FETAL DEVELOPMENT RESEARCH

Fetal behavior has been described by pregnant women and referenced in literary and medical sources for centuries. The first systematic study of fetal development in the United States was launched by Sontag, Wallace, and colleagues at the Fels Institute in the 1930s. Despite limitations in available technology at that time for accessing the fetus, the research methods and objectives of this project were astonishingly innovative and provide insight into the complexities of antenatal development (Sontag & Richards, 1938; Sontag & Wallace, 1934). The questions asked then still challenge current investigators. Significant academic interest in fetal behavioral development did not reemerge until the late 1970s, coincident with advances in ultrasound technology which opened a window to the uterus. At about the same time, the obstetric specialty of perinatology emerged, oriented toward the development of techniques for detecting and improving fetal well-being and optimizing pregnancy outcome. Although the developmental and obstetric literatures are not well integrated, each can serve to inform the other about the complex nature of fetal functioning. In 1996 and 1997, the National Institute of Child Health and Human Development convened conferences which included fetal researchers from the obstetric and developmental communities in the United States and abroad. These meetings offered an opportunity to consider conceptual and methodological strategies for the study of fetal development within and across clinical and academic domains (Krasnegor et al., 1998a, 1998b).

DESCRIPTION OF FETAL ASSESSMENT METHODS

Research with neonates is plagued by special challenges. Babies fall asleep, have little motor control, and behave in ways that limit their availability for testing and introduce procedural confounds. Mundane features of the environment, such as feeding schedules, further conspire to test the patience of the most dedicated researcher. Add to these challenges the additional feature of not actually being able to see the subject of the assessment and one begins to approach the realities of fetal research. Yet no other developmental period yields the same potential to reveal the complexities of human ontogeny and to understand the origins of individual differences as do the 266 days prior to birth. No other period of developmental inquiry is so heavily dependent on technology to ask even the most basic of questions.

The Doppler effect, the phenomenon that the velocity of moving objects is systematically associated with changes in emitted frequency, is the basis of both electronic fetal heart rate (FHR) monitoring and real-time ultrasound. In each, ultrasound transducers emit high-frequency signals in the shape of an inverted funnel, while paired transducers receive echoes of the interrogating beam. Higher-frequency Doppler signals (150–220 Hz) are generated by motion of the fetal heart, so FHR monitoring requires a Doppler signal sensitive enough to detect movement changes that are as small as 1–2 mm. FHR is most commonly measured using Doppler-based cardiotocographs which have been used in clinical antepartum and intrapartum assessment for decades. The current generation of FHR monitors process the returned signal through autocorrelation techniques which match small portions of sequential waveforms to detect onset of each cardiac cycle; the processed data are output in terms of beats per minute. A single external transducer is applied to the maternal abdomen to detect heart rate; an additional pressure-sensitive tocodynamometer transducer detects uterine contractility.

Real-time ultrasound provides an image of the fetus. Visualization can reveal specific behaviors (e.g., thumb sucking), qualitative aspects of movement (e.g., flexion and extension), structural features of the fetus (e.g., size), and characteristics of the uterine milieu (e.g., volume of amniotic fluid). Three-dimensional ultrasound is newly available but currently limited to static images. Because both cardiotocography and real-time ultrasound send and interpret Doppler waveforms, it can be difficult to conduct both FHR monitoring and real-time ultrasound simultaneously, particularly in smaller fetuses, without significantly degrading the FHR signal. Successful implementation of both is based on a variety of factors, which include specific properties of both transducers and maternal–fetal transmission characteristics.

Recently, several manufacturers have modified standard electronic monitors to provide Doppler-based information on fetal movements. Actocardiographs yield information about fetal movement by band-passing both the highest-frequency (i.e., fetal heart rate) and the lowest-frequency signals (i.e., maternal digestive and respiratory activity) using a single transducer. Fetal activity signals are generated by a change in the returned Doppler waveform; if there is no movement, the returned signal will retain the same frequency as the interrogating signal. If the fetus is moving, the echo will be returned at a different frequency proportional to the velocity with which the fetal body part moves toward or away from the transducer. The resultant signal provides a continuous measure of fetal movement (Maeda, Tatsumura, & Nakajima, 1991; Maeda, Tatsumura, & Utsu, 1999).

The most recent addition to the technological tools available for fetal assessment using Doppler ultrasound measures the amount of blood flow and resistance in fetal vessels, including umbilical, cerebral, and aortic arteries. The flow velocity waveform is typically characterized in terms of pulsatility or the contrast between periods of diastole and systole. Flow studies have become a component of clinical fetal care, but they have not been widely used to study fetal development. However, this technology in general, and studies of cerebral blood flow in particular, show promise for studies of fetal neurobehavioral functioning and sensory processing (Shono, Shono, & Sugimori, 2000).

Obstetric fetal assessment is oriented toward discerning markers of fetal well-being or distress to diagnose conditions that threaten perinatal outcome and are amenable to obstetric intervention (Ware & Devoe, 1994). Antepartum assessment relies heavily on evaluation of periodic changes in fetal heart rate; the cornerstone of fetal assessment is the nonstress test (NST). A negative, or "reactive," NST is achieved when the fetus has two accelerations of fetal heart rate within a specified period. Although scoring varies among clinicians, typical criteria include two accelerations of 15 bpm above baseline for 15 seconds within a 20-minute period. Antepartum fetal heart rate is also evaluated for variability and decelerations, although the standards for categorizing each are not as uniform as those for NST results (Donker, van Geijn, & Hasman, 1993). Note that although the NST is discussed as a measure of "reactivity," external stimulation is not a component of the procedure. The biophysical profile provides a second stratum of fetal assessment by adding ultrasound-derived information to the NST. Specifically, the presence or absence of fetal breathing movements, body movements, tone, and amniotic fluid volume criteria are combined with NST results. Each component is scored individually and summed, yielding an index of 0 to 10 (Manning, Platt, & Sipos, 1980; Vintzileos & Knuppel, 1994). Maternal fetal movement counting may also be used as an adjunct in evaluation of fetal well-being (Rayburn, 1990).

The orientation of clinical research, which is to establish the diagnostic boundaries of pathology, is somewhat contrary to the goals of developmental inquiry, which seeks to document normative developmental processes.

However, both are informed by study of fetal neurobehaviors, which can be grouped into four domains of function, each with its own methodological strengths and weaknesses. These include FHR, motor activity, behavioral state, and responsivity to extrauterine stimuli.

Fetal Heart Rate

Antepartum FHR is most commonly measured by Doppler detection of fetal heart motion. The accuracy of heart rate data using modern autocorrelation techniques is quite good, with resolution ranging from ±.25 to 1.9 beats per minute (bpm) (Carter, 1993; Dawes, 1993). However, because FHR monitors do not detect voltages generated by fetal R-waves, they do not provide appropriate data for computing beat to beat (as opposed to short- or longer-term) variability (Dawes, Redman, & Smith, 1985). During the intrapartum period, once the amniotic membrane has ruptured, scalp electrodes can be used to derive an electrocardiogram (ECG). Fetal ECG recording would improve the precision of antenatal heart rate data, making it comparable to methods used in infant psychophysiological research. In the past, subcutaneous abdominal electrodes have been used to extract fetal ECG (Patrick, Campbell, Carmichael, & Probert, 1986). Recently, interest in the development of more utile, noninvasive technologies to record fetal ECG at the maternal abdomen has been renewed and an increasing number of reports detail procedures which isolate and extract the fetal ECG from the maternal ECG using a grid of externally applied electrodes (Budin & Abboud, 1994; Groome, Mooney, Bentz, & Singh, 1994). These experimental methods are not available for widespread implementation but may be refined in the future to become more practical. The precision offered by R-wave detection is necessary for measures which require quantification in milliseconds (e.g., respiratory sinus arrhythmia), but the resolution of Doppler-based FHR remains sufficient for quantifying baseline and short-term, epoched measures of variability (Dawes, Moulden, Sheil, & Redman, 1992; Krasnegor et al., 1998b).

FHR monitors are designed to be used with fetuses who are within the gestational age of viability so that clinical assessment may guide obstetric management. FHR monitoring before this time is difficult. Signal artifact resulting from rapid changes in FHR or changes in fetal position is common, particularly in younger fetuses, but can be reduced by proper transducer placement and attention to maternal position. Our investigations, which are described in a later section, typically commence FHR monitoring at 20 weeks gestation. During the second half of gestation, normal FHR ranges from 120 to 160 bpm (DiPietro, Hodgson, Costigan, Hilton, & Johnson, 1996b; James, Pillai, & Smoleniec, 1995; Martin, 1978; Mathai et al., 1995; Patrick, Campbell, Carmichael, & Probert, 1982b). Rate and variability are controlled, in part, by innervation of the parasympathetic and sympathetic branches of the autonomic nervous system (Dalton, Dawes, & Patrick, 1983; Freeman, Garite, & Nageotte, 1991; Martin, 1978).

Measurement of variability in heart rate is more informative of fetal functioning than are measures of baseline or mean heart rate, as long as these are within the normal range (Dawes, Houghton, Redman, & Visser, 1982; Martin, 1978; Odendaal, 1990; Street, Dawes, Moulden, & Redman, 1991; Yeh, Forsythe, & Hon, 1973). There is no uniform way to quantify FHR variability, and measures include root mean square (Dawes et al., 1985), standard deviation (DiPietro et al., 1996b), coefficient of variation (Searle, Devoe, Phillips, & Searle, 1988), measures of entropy (Dawes et al., 1992; Fleisher, DiPietro, Johnson, & Pincus, 1997), accelerations (Swartjes, van Geijn, Mantel, & Schoemaker, 1992), and standardized definitions of periods of low and high variation (Street et al., 1991).

Quantification of respiratory sinus arrhythmia (RSA) has a distinguished history in infant research as a marker of vagal tone (Porges, 1983; Richards, 1985; see Porter, Chapter 6, this volume). The fetus exhibits diaphragmatic breathing movements as early as 10 weeks gestation which increase in frequency and then plateau later in pregnancy (deVries, Visser, & Prechtl, 1982; James et al., 1995). RSA has been documented in fetuses through interpretation of heart rate patterns (Timor-Tritsch, Zador, Hertz, & Rosen, 1977) and application of spectral analysis techniques (Groome et al., 1994). Although vagal tone is elevated during episodes of fetal breathing movements, evidence for centrally mediated RSA during periods without breathing movements has also been documented (Groome et al., 1994).

Fetal Movement

Spontaneously generated motor activity is present during the embryonic period and early fetal periods, during which time isolated movements of the extremities, diaphragm, and head and whole body movements, including startles, can be observed (deVries et al., 1982; Ianniruberto & Tajani, 1981; Sparling & Wilhelm, 1993). During gestation, more complex movement patterns emerge, including swallowing, thumb sucking, and grasping of the umbilical cord and body parts (Ianniruberto & Tajani, 1981; Roodenburg, Wladimiroff, van Es, & Prechtl, 1991). Virtually all movement patterns present at term are initiated by 15 weeks (deVries et al., 1982; Ianniruberto & Tajani, 1981), and handedness can be detected in the first trimester (Hepper, McCartney, & Shannon, 1998).

Understanding the functional significance of fetal movements to development is rudimentary (Prechtl, 1984). Some movements (e.g., sucking and breathing movements) prepare the fetus for adaptation to postnatal life. Others contribute to intrauterine conditions which foster pregnancy (e.g., fetal swallowing regulates, in part, amniotic fluid volume). The transition from breech to vertex presentation during gestation appears to be accomplished by fetal rotational maneuvers and raises speculation about hypo-tonicity in fetuses who remain breech (Suzuki & Yamamuro, 1985). The sig-nificance and implications of many other behaviors, such as a report of heart rate decelerations instigated by fetal grasping of the umbilical cord (Petri-kovsky & Kaplan, 1993), are unknown.

Although estimates vary, in the latter half of gestation fetuses move ap-proximately once per minute and are active between 10 and 30% of the time (DiPietro, Costigan, Shupe, Pressman, & Johnson, 1998; Nasello-Paterson, Natale, & Connors, 1988; Patrick, Campbell, Carmichael, Natale, & Richard-son, 1982a; Roberts, Griffin, Mooney, Cooper, & Campbell, 1980; Rooden-burg et al., 1991). Fetal activity patterns exhibit cyclic fluctuations with a periodicity of minutes (Robertson, 1985) as well as circadian rhythms, with fetal motility peaking late in the evening (Nasello-Paterson et al., 1988; Pat-rick et al., 1982a). Comparison of fetal activity results across studies is ham-pered by lack of uniform definition of what constitutes a discrete movement; that is, the duration of quiescence necessary to designate the next movement as a new movement (ten Hof et al., 1999a)

Qualitative aspects of fetal movements include the specific motor pat-terns displayed *in utero* as well as characteristics of behavior consistent with developing motor tone. Selection of the features of fetal movement to study is guided by disciplinary orientation. Characterization of movements in terms of amplitude, speed, complexity, and fluidity has been undertaken by neurologists (Sival, 1993). Physical/occupational therapists and neuroscien-tists have applied concepts of spatial use, timing, and force to fetal actions (Green & Sparling, 1993) and documented the emerging nature of spontane-ous leg movements (Almli, Mohr, Ball, & Bernhard, 1995). Animal models have provided developmental psychobiologists with a rubric to investigate the ontogeny and adaptive significance of specific behaviors prior to birth (Smotherman & Robinson, 1996). Nonspecific fetal activity level has been quantified by developmental investigators interested in the activity dimen-sion of temperament (DiPietro, Hodgson, Costigan, & Johnson, 1996c; Eaton & Saudino, 1992) and as a means of determining intrinsic properties of peri-odicity within the developing motor system (Robertson, 1985).

Women typically cannot detect fetal movement until the 16th to 18th week of pregnancy, the period of "quickening." Even in the third trimester, maternal reports of fetal movements are not reliable means of data collec-tion. Although women perceive most large-amplitude, prolonged move-ments, they are poor detectors of other spontaneous or evoked fetal move-ments (Kisilevsky, Killen, Muir, & Low, 1991) and may detect as few as 16% of movements at term (Johnson, Jordan, & Paine, 1990). In the 1930s, Sontag and colleagues used rubber sacks encased in a plaster cast molded to the maternal abdomen (Sontag & Wallace, 1935), and in the 1980s, strain-gauge tocodynamometry was modified to detect fetal movements (Robertson, 1985; Timor-Tritsch, Dierker, Zador, Hertz, & Rosen, 1978b). Such methods can detect only movements of sufficient magnitude to perturb the maternal abdominal wall.

Real-time ultrasound is necessary for qualitative analysis of fetal movement. Because only those movements that are within or impinge on the ultrasound field can be observed, the simultaneous use of two ultrasound scanners during the second half of gestation is desirable. Ultrasound-based studies of fetal movements tend to be lengthy, with observation periods of at least 60 minutes (e.g., deVries et al., 1982; Roodenburg et al., 1991). Continuous 24-hour ultrasound-based recordings have been conducted (Patrick et al., 1982a). Coding of fetal behaviors can be done in real time by trained observers, or the session may be videotaped for later review. Movement detection is typically input into one or more channels of computerized systems through event markers.

The actocardiograph has emerged as a viable and promising tool to supplement or replace real-time ultrasound in the detection of fetal movement (Arabin, Riedewald, Zacharias, & Saling, 1988; Besinger & Johnson, 1989; DiPietro et al., 1996b; James et al., 1995). Once fetal motion is detected, the manner in which the voltage generated by this event is characterized differs by manufacturer. Some monitors produce a bar on the polygraphic paper output for the duration of a detected movement. These types of data are similar to that provided by event marking of ultrasound observations. Other monitors generate a continuous output of spikes, which allows all signals generated by the transducer to be quantified and for calibration of the appropriate threshold sensitivity at which point fetal movement may be distinguished from background noise.

Behavioral State

One of the most striking discoveries concerning fetal neurobehavioral development has been the documentation of fetal behavioral states. Beginning in the late 1970s, investigators in the United States (Timor-Tritsch, Dierker, Hertz, Deagan, & Rosen, 1978a), Germany (Junge, 1979), the Netherlands (Nijhuis, Prechtl, Martin, & Bots, 1982), and Italy (Arduini et al., 1986) began to document behavioral cycles in the fetus based on models generated by infant developmental neurology and criteria for neonatal states as identified by Prechtl and colleagues (Prechtl, 1974). Four fetal behavioral states were discerned, labeled 1F, 2F, 3F, and 4F, in concert with state scoring methods developed for neonates. Although not isomorphic with newborn states, these approximate quiet sleep, rapid eye movement (REM) sleep, quiet waking, and active waking, respectively. Characteristics of electroencephalographic (EEG) activity associated with sleep states in infants have been documented in baboon fetuses (Grieve, Myers, & Stark, 1994). Analogous studies have not been conducted in human fetuses, although there is evidence that the heart rate and behavioral manifestations of 1F, 2F, and 4F in the fetus are comparable to those observed in newborns (Junge, 1979; Pillai & James, 1990a).

The conventions developed in the Netherlands in the early 1980s have remained the standard for fetal state ascertainment. State identification is based on 3-minute epochs in which fetal body movements, eye movements, and heart rate patterns are evaluated for coincidence of predefined patterns (van Vliet, Martin, Nijhuis, & Prechtl, 1985a). Table 3.1 presents these criteria. State profiles are constructed when there is stable (i.e., 3 minutes or longer) coincidence among the three parameters and when there are predictable transitions between states such that when one parameter changes, near-simultaneous changes are displayed by the other two, consistent with the established categories. As the fetus matures, state parameters gradually develop linkage (associations between two variables) and ultimate coincidence accompanied by predictable state transitions. A tenet of fetal state development is that behavioral states cannot be observed prior to 36 weeks because the neural substrate required for integration of state parameters is not sufficiently mature until this time (Arduini et al., 1986; Martin, 1981; Nijhuis & van de Pas, 1992). Prior to 36 weeks, behavioral states can be observed at times, but coincidence among all three parameters is less frequent and there are less well-defined transitions (Arduini, Rizzo, & Romanini, 1995; Nijhuis, 1986; van Vliet, Martin, Nijhuis, & Prechtl, 1985b; Visser, Poelmann-Weesjes, Cohen, & Bekedam, 1987). Periods which fulfill the criteria in Table 3.1 prior to 36 weeks are typically designated as episodes of 1F–4F "coincidence" rather than states. Approximately 10–15% of the observation time at term cannot be categorized into *a priori* state definitions (Arabin et al., 1988; Groome, Bentz, & Singh, 1995b; van Woerden et al., 1989). Other fetal behav-

TABLE 3.1. Fetal Behavioral State Parameters

	Eye movements	Body movements	Fetal heart rate[a]
1F	Absent	None, except occasional, brief startles or other gross movements	FHR pattern A: stable FHR with small oscillations around baseline. Isolated accelerations, but always associated with fetal body movement
2F	Present (rapid and slow)	Frequent and periodic	FHR pattern B: wider oscillations than above with frequent accelerations
3F	Present	None	FHR pattern C: stable, with wider ocsillations than A, and no accelerations
4F	Present	Vigorous and continuous	FHR pattern D: unstable, with large and lengthy accelerations, often fused into sustained tachycardia

Note. Based on Nijhuis, Prechtl, Martin, and Bots (1982).

[a]Examples of FHR patterns A–D are presented in Figure 3.2.

iors, such as fetal breathing movements, micturition, and mouthing occur more often in some states than others but are not state criteria because they are not continuously present (Nijhuis, 1986).

The range of the relative proportions of specific states reported both between studies and between subjects within studies is wide. At all gestational ages, state 2F is the most frequently observed, followed by 1F. Periods of high activity (4F) are relatively infrequent and emerge near term at the expense of 2F (Nijhuis et al., 1982). Reports of periods of 3F, even at term, are rare (Arabin & Riedewald, 1992; Groome et al., 1995b; Pillai & James, 1990a; van Vliet et al., 1985a; van Woerden et al., 1989), prompting some to question whether a state consistent with alertness actually exists in the fetus (Pillai & James, 1990a). However, many diurnal effects on fetal state have been noted, and the incidence of 3F has been reported to be higher in the evening than earlier in the day, when most data are typically collected (Mulder et al., 1994).

Fetal Responsivity

Fetal responsivity in FHR and movement to stimuli originating in the extrauterine environment have been documented for over 60 years. In the 1920s and 1930s, stimuli included an electronic door buzzer (Sontag & Wallace, 1935) and a warning horn (Peiper, as cited in Sontag & Wallace, 1935). More recent stimuli include the lower end of an electric toothbrush (Leader, Baillie, Martin, Molteno, & Wynchank, 1984), an artificial electronic larynx (Gagnon, Foreman, Hunse, & Patrick, 1989), and devices designed specifically for fetal stimulation (DiPietro et al., 1996b; Groome, Gotlieb, Neely, & Waters, 1993). The term "vibroacoustic" refers to stimuli activated on or at the level of the maternal abdomen. Usually the device is placed over the fetal head (determined by manual palpation or ultrasound imaging) and activated. There are no standards for stimulus properties, such as intensity, frequency, duration, or rate of repetition. Women cannot be masked for vibroacoustic stimuli applied to their abdomen. Inclusion of a control period, where the stimulus is applied but not activated, indicates that at least part of the fetal response may be mediated by maternal anticipation (DiPietro et al., 1996b; Visser, Zeelenberg, deVries, & Dawes, 1983). Fetal response decrement to repeated presentations of invariant auditory and/or vibratory stimuli has also been documented (Goldkrand & Litvack, 1991; Groome et al., 1993; Kuhlman, Burns, Depp, & Sabbagha, 1988; Leader et al., 1984; Madison, Madison, & Adubato, 1986; Sandman, Wadhwa, Hetrick, Porto, & Peeke, 1997b).

Fetal responses depend on the potency of the stimulus. Intense, broadband vibroacoustic stimuli (i.e., > 85 dB at the source) applied to the maternal abdomen produce a range of responses, including startles, elevated heart rate and accelerations, abrupt state changes, decreased fetal breathing movements, and micturition (see Visser & Mulder, 1993, and Zimmer & Divon, 1993, for reviews). Attenuated, less frequent cardiac and motor responses are produced by milder vibroacoustic and complex airborne stimuli (Kisilevsky & Muir, 1991; Lecanuet, Granier-Deferre, Cohen, Houezec, & Busnel, 1986). Both accelerations and small decelerations in heart rate have been observed as a result of intense stimuli in immature fetuses (DiPietro et al., 1996b; Kisilevsky, Muir, & Low, 1992). At term, airborne auditory stimuli can also elicit deceleratory responses, suggesting the possibility of a biphasic orienting response (Lecanuet, Granier-Deferre, Jacquet, & Busnel, 1992); such responsivity is modulated by behavioral state (Groome et al., 1999a). Biphasic and deceleratory responses have been used to investigate fetal auditory stimulus discrimination and indicate that fetuses can discern stimulus properties, including speech sounds (Fifer & Moon, 1995; Zimmer et al., 1993). Related research on fetal sensory processing capacities is beyond the scope of this chapter (see Lecanuet & Schaal, 1996, for a review).

BIOBEHAVIORAL BASIS OF ASSESSMENT

A century ago, Freud speculated that "difficult birth in itself in certain cases is merely a symptom of deeper effects that influenced the development of the fetus" (cited in Nijhuis, 1995, p. 77). During the last 15 years there has been a shift in focus on the etiology of major neurological damage, including cerebral palsy, from the intrapartum to the antenatal period following a series of empirical reports indicating that the most significant risk factors are present prior to birth (Freeman, 1985; Manning et al., 1998; Nelson & Ellenberg, 1986; Stanley, 1994).

In 1985, observation of a fetal startle response following vibroacoustic stimulation was heralded as a new "intrauterine neurological examination" in the optimistic title of an obstetric publication (Divon et al., 1985). Although the notion that a single measure of fetal behavior can index neurological function is unlikely, there is growing consensus that multidimensional information about normative fetal development will ultimately provide a means of detecting early neurological dysfunction and unfavorable pregnancy outcomes in individuals (James et al., 1995; Krasnegor et al., 1998b; Nijhuis, 1986). Identification of measurable fetal neurobehaviors which reflect neural development is one of the primary goals of fetal neurobehavioral assessment (Vindla & James, 1995).

To what extent are measures of fetal neurobehavior relevant to developmental inquiry? Study of the extrauterine development of preterm infants has contributed to the recognition that features of neurobehavioral functioning which have been measured extensively in the full-term neonate and infant, and which are integral to current theories of development, do not originate at either term or birth (Als, 1982; Brazelton, 1984; Comparetti, 1981;

Nijhuis, 1995; Prechtl, 1984), and few neurobehavioral discontinuities have been detected between the third trimester fetus and neonate. Thus, models and measures developed to study infant neurobehavioral organization and development before and after term have been extended to the fetal period. As with postnatal maturation, antenatal maturation is a function of advancing central and autonomic control. Als's (1982) model of synactive development describes functioning both within and across autonomic, motor, state, and interactive domains (see Figure 3.1). This hierachical organization is observed in the fetus as FHR first becomes integrated with fetal movements, which subsequently become integrated into organized behavioral states, ultimately resulting in periods in which the fetus is available to process environmental stimuli. It has been proposed that understanding the mechanisms underlying development prior to term may foster interventions for preterm infants that consider behavioral ramifications rather than those solely related to growth (Smotherman & Robinson, 1996). The strong model of continuity between the fetus and infant provides a foundation for hypothesis

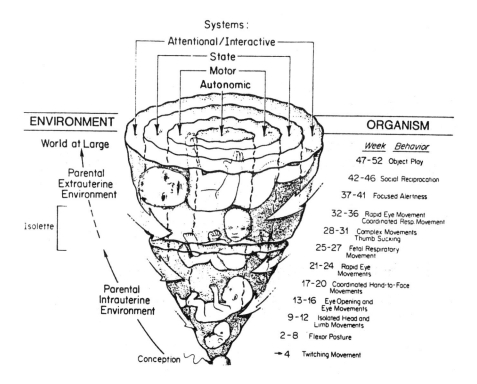

FIGURE 3.1. Als's model of synactive organization of behavioral development. From Als (1982). Copyright 1982 by Kluwer Academic/Plenum Publishers. Reprinted by permission.

generation and prediction of the existence of fetal capabilities before they are empirically documented, such as pain perception (Glover & Fisk, 1996).

Investigation of normative development during gestation has been the focus of much research to date; study of individual differences in fetal functioning and implications for predicting postnatal development have been largely relegated to clinical applications. The progression from an age-based focus to interest in individual differences among fetuses parallels that observed in infant research (Horowitz, 1990). Do individual differences begin before birth? Investigations which have attempted to predict postnatal biobehavioral development from antenatal measures are limited in number but highly provocative. These studies fall into two categories: those which attempt to document within-domain consistency between similar aspects of function and those that investigate cross-domain predictiveness. With respect to the former, FHR and variability are significantly associated with these measures through the first year of life (DiPietro, Costigan, Pressman, & Roosevelt-Doussard, 2000; Lewis, Wilson, Ban, & Baumel, 1970), and a small, but significant, relation between fetal and childhood heart rate has been found at age 10 (Thomas, Haslum, MacGillivray, & Golding, 1989). Consistencies in videotaped motor activity during sleep have been documented from the near-term fetus through the first month of life (Groome et al., 1999b). Actograph-detected fetal activity level has been associated with maternally reported infant activity level through 6 months (DiPietro et al., 1996c); this finding has been extended to include laboratory-based assessments of activity at 1 year (DiPietro, 2000). Within-subject consistency in prenatal to postnatal state expression has been reported for the duration of quiet sleep epochs (Groome, Swiber, Atterbury, Bentz, & Holland, 1997).

Cross-domain predictions have focused on the associations between fetal neurobehaviors and dimensions of subsequent infant temperament. Relations between higher FHR and lower threshold to novelty (Snidman, Kagan, Riordan, & Shannon, 1995) and lower emotional tone (DiPietro et al., 1996c) in early infancy have been documented. Maternally detected fetal movements have been demonstrated to predict infant irritability in the first few months (St. James-Roberts & Menon-Johansson, 1999). In aggregate, fetal neurobehaviors (including heart rate, motor activity, state concordance, and responsivity) account for between 22 and 60% of the variance in infant temperament scores based on maternal report (DiPietro et al., 1996c). Intrapartum and antenatal patterns of accelerations and decelerations have been associated with performance on a neonatal neurobehavioral exam (Emory & Noonan, 1984) as well as later developmental outcome (Todd, Trudinger, Cole, & Cooney, 1992). Two studies have found relations between fetal habituation performance and later development (Leader et al., 1984; Madison et al., 1986), although implementation and interpretation of fetal habituation studies present unique challenges (Hepper, 1997). The current state of knowledge regarding the genesis and measurability of stable individual differences during the prenatal period is based on modest, single-study findings which await replication and extension. However, it seems clear that fetal neurobehavioral assessment has significant potential for predicting atypical outcomes, as well as understanding the development of constitutional, biobehavioral processes which reflect nervous system function.

Developmental investigators may relish the opportunity to measure fetal behavior before postnatal environmental exposures moderate constitutional aspects of behavior. However, fetal assessment is not assessment of an individual but of a pair. The maternal psychobiological context prior to birth may exert a much more pervasive effect on development of individual differences than maternal–infant interaction after birth. The "maternal womb environment" has been estimated to account for 5–20% of variance in IQ (Devlin, Daniels, & Roeder, 1997). A growing literature indicates that psychological and environmental factors, including maternal stress and anxiety (DiPietro, Hodgson, Costigan, Hilton, & Johnson, 1996a; DiPietro et al., 1996b; Groome, Swiber, Bentz, Holland, & Atterbury, 1995c; Monk et al., 2000; Sandman, Wadhwa, Chica-DeMet, Dunkel-Schetter, & Porto, 1997a; Van den Bergh et al., 1989), influence fetal neurobehavioral development in ways that are only beginning to be understood, and their contribution to predictive models is not clear at this time.

Application to a Current Research Program

Since 1990, my colleagues and I have been developing data collection techniques and a database of normative fetal development which may ultimately make fetal neurobehavioral research more accessible to the developmental community. These procedures have been used to (1) investigate the ontogeny of fetal neurobehavioral development in normal fetuses, (2) document the stability of these measures before birth to evaluate their potential as indicators of individual differences, (3) establish prenatal to postnatal continuity and prediction, (4) investigate the relation between maternally reported stress and affect and fetal neurobehaviors, and (5) analyze the psychophysiological consequences of evoked maternal arousal on fetal functioning. The basic protocol involves 50 minutes of actocardiograph (Toitu MT320, TOFA, Malvern, Pennsylvania) monitoring, in which FHR and movement are digitized on a PC-based system. Each recording is preceded by a brief ultrasound exam to ascertain fetal position, placenta location, and amniotic fluid volume and to provide parents with photographs. Women are monitored in a semirecumbent left lateral position at the same time of day to standardize diurnal influences on both FHR and fetal movement. Artifact is minimized by constant vigilance for optimal transducer placement. Sampled FHR data undergo a series of error rejection procedures to detect values beyond acceptable ranges, which contract and expand proportionally, based on 5-point moving medians. A moving baseline is fit to the arti-

TABLE 3.2. Fetal Neurobehavioral Measures

Fetal heart rate

Epoched measures
  Mean
  Variability (*SD*)
  Range
  Tachycardia (> 165 bpm)
  Bradycardia (< 110 bpm)
  Data artifact
Periodic changes around baseline
  Accelerations (FHR ≥ 10 bpm above baseline for 15 sec)
    Number
    Duration (sec)
    Size (area)
  Decelerations (FHR < 15 bpm below baseline for 15 sec)
    Number
    Duration (sec)
    Size (area)

Fetal movement

Mean amplitude
Periodicity
Number of discrete movements
  Duration (sec)
  Amplitude
Activity level: number of movements × mean duration

FHR-FM association

Percent FHR-FM coupling
Latency (sec)
FHR-FM synchrony

Biobehavioral patterns (state)

BBP 1–4 (% observation time each)
State organization: BPP 1 + 2 + 3 + 4 (total observation time)
Noncoincidence
State changes
Longest bouts: quiescence and activity

fact-free data in order to detect episodic variation around baseline. Fetal movement data are digitized in raw voltages and calibrated into arbitrary units (AUs) which range from 0 to 100. Signals of less than 15 to 25 AUs may be produced by fetal breathing or hiccups which generate incidental fetal movement. Motor activity is thus defined as occurring whenever the actograph signal attains or exceeds 15[1] AUs. Each actograph signal that crosses this threshold and remains at or above without a 10-second break is counted as a discrete movement. Selection of criteria for distinguishing the start of one movement from the end of the previous is somewhat arbitrary; thus actograph data are also quantified continuously. A derived score, total movements multiplied by mean movement duration, yields a measure of fetal activity level. The movement data values generated using the actograph (DiPietro et al., 1998; DiPietro et al., 1996b) are consistently within the range of data reported by studies using ultrasound to observe fetal behavior (Nasello-Paterson et al., 1988; Patrick et al., 1982a; Roberts et al., 1980; Roodenburg et al., 1991). Table 3.2 provides descriptions of the measures derived by our data quantification techniques.

In addition to characterizing FHR and fetal movement (FM) separately, their interrelationship is quantified in terms of temporal contiguity, defined as whether each movement is coupled with an change in FHR. Again, because of the arbitrary nature of this definition, second-by-second FHR and movement synchrony is also analyzed using time series techniques. Consistent with other protocols, fetal state is visually coded from the polygraphic record. FHR data are coded in 3-minute windows as patterns A, B, C, or D based on the criteria developed by Nijhuis et al. (1982). We developed fetal actograph scoring to be compatible with the ultrasound movement categories that have been associated with fetal states. Four categories, also based on 3-minute epochs, are distinguished ranging from no movement to continuous, high-amplitude movement. The following FHR–FM linkage patterns are consistent with behavioral state definitions as follows: FHR A with FM 1 = 1F; FHR B with FM 1, 2, or 3 = 2F; FHR C with FM 1 = 3F; and FHR D with FM 3 or 4 = 4F. Figure 3.2 provides examples of these. Because eye movement data are not used, we refer to these as biobehavioral patterns (BBP1–BBP4; see later section for discussion). Interscorer reliability for each FHR and FM pattern is established and evaluated by kappa statistics before coding begins. Reliability maintenance is achieved in one of two ways: by either dual coding of every 10th tracing or dual coding of all tracings; disputes are resolved through consensus.

This protocol has been applied to three completed longitudinal studies of healthy fetuses of nonsmoking women with normal pregnancies. These included (1) 31 participants assessed at 20, 24, 28, 32, 36, and 38/39 weeks gestation; (2) 103 participants stratified by socioeconomic status (52 middle/upper and 51 lower socioeconomic status) assessed at 24, 30, and 36 weeks gestation; and (3) 135 participants, stratified by maternal parity and fetal sex, and assessed at the same six intervals as the first sample. The latter study has been only recently completed; its goal was to extend documentation of inter- and intrafetal neurobehavioral development but also to explicitly ascertain the relation between fetal functioning and maternal affect. In addition to the fetal data measures described in Table 3.2, this study included concurrent maternal data collection of ECG, skin conductance level and response, and respiration, digitized simultaneously with fetal functioning. Time-lag analyses are used to quantify maternal–fetal concordance among measures during undisturbed, baseline conditions. Experimental manipulations using cognitive and affective challenges (e.g., the Stroop color word test and viewing a labor and delivery documentary) are included

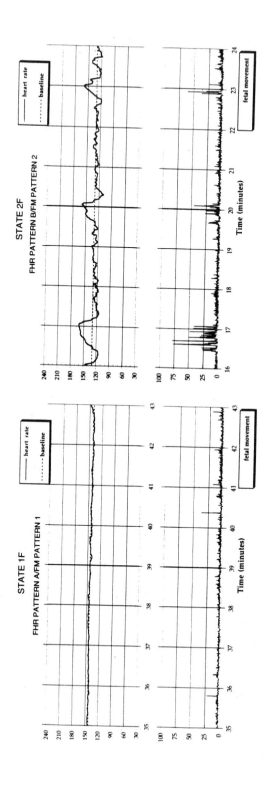

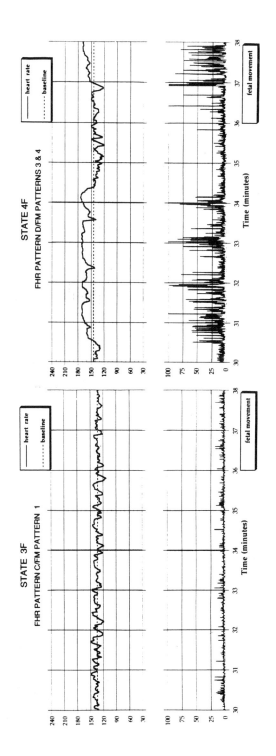

FIGURE 3.2. Fetal biobehavioral patterns based on actocardiograph-generated fetal heart rate and movement data.

to determine fetal responses to maternal arousal. Data analyses are ongoing; ultimately, these results will provide information on the influence of maternal psychophysiological functioning prior to birth on antenatal and postnatal development.

RELIABILITY AND VALIDITY

Each method of assessing fetal neurobehavioral functioning is fraught with issues pertaining to reliability and validity. Interpretation of ultrasound images requires significant training and experience, but few studies report interobserver reliability for fetal behaviors observed on ultrasound. Agreement based on visual inspection of FHR cardiograph output is known to be poor (Gagnon, Campbell, & Hunse, 1993), and reliable application of the scoring criteria for FHR patterns A through D used for distinguishing behavioral states is difficult to achieve (Arduini et al., 1993), but interscorer reliability procedures are rarely reported. Among experienced investigators, only 80% of tracings can be scored without resolution through group consensus (Nijhuis et al., 1998; van Woerden et al., 1989). However, the high degree of interindividual variation in FHR patterns associated with each state renders computerized identification ineffective (Nijhuis et al., 1998; Visser, Mulder, Stevens, & Verweij, 1993).

The most significant threat to reliability of Doppler-based heart rate data is signal artifact, generated by fetal movement, repositioning, or maternal body habitus. Artifact is not randomly generated because fetuses that move more often generate more artifact. Mean signal artifact has been reported at 6% at 20 weeks gestation but declines to between 1 to 5% by 28 weeks and beyond (Dawes et al., 1985; DiPietro et al., 1996b) and can be mitigated by proper transducer placement and vigilance during monitoring.

Interobserver reliability is not of concern when fetal movement is detected automatically by an actograph; here the monitor's ability to validly detect fetal movements is paramount. Several investigations using ultrasound-observed movements as the gold standard indicate that the Toitu actograph used in our laboratory detects from 91 to 95% of all fetal movements (Besinger & Johnson, 1989; DiPietro, Costigan, & Pressman, 1999) whether agreement is based on time intervals or individual movements and is equally reliable in detecting periods of quiescence. Most of the movements undetected by the actograph are small, isolated movements of extremities; virtually all large and sustained (i.e., greater than 1 second) movements are detected. Variability in validity among commercial brands has been observed (Melendez, Rayburn, & Smith, 1992). In all actographs, artifact can be generated by sharp maternal abdominal movements (e.g., coughing) and large excursions of the fetal diaphragm during fetal breathing and hiccuping (Maeda et al., 1991).

As with neonatal assessments, test–retest stability of measures of neuro-behavioral development is a complex issue, given the rapid rate of development, varied timing at which neurobehaviors are exhibited, and potential developmental differences in expression of the underlying neural substrate. Significant intrafetal stability in FHR and variability from 20 weeks through term has been reported (DiPietro et al., 2000; DiPietro et al., 1996c; Nijhuis et al., 1998), the magnitude of these relations is similar to that found in preterm infants (DiPietro, Caughy, Cusson, & Fox, 1994). There is wide interfetal variability in fetal movement levels, making it a relatively unstable metric for group comparisons, but moderate intrafetal stability in fetal motor activity during the first (deVries, Visser, & Prechtl, 1988) and latter (DiPietro et al., 1996c; tenHof et al., 1999b) halves of pregnancy has been documented. Stability in features of fetal behavioral state organization has been observed beginning at 36 weeks gestation (DiPietro et al., 1996c; Groome et al., 1995a).

Validation of the role of the central nervous system in mediating fetal neurobehaviors is effected through studies of jeopardized pregnancies. An accumulating body of evidence based on both case studies of individuals with anomalous structural or chromosomal conditions and group comparisons based on risk factors indicates that antenatal conditions which have postnatal developmental sequelae are accompanied by alterations in fetal neurobehavioral development. These include studies of fetuses with central nervous system abnormalities (Horimoto et al., 1993) including hydrocephalus (Arduini, Rizzo, Caforio, Romanini, & Mancuso, 1987) and anencephaly (Yoshizato et al., 1994), genetic (Pillai, Garrett, & James, 1991) and chromosomal disorders, including Down syndrome (Hepper & Shahidullah, 1992), and growth retardation (Gagnon, Hunse, Fellows, Carmichael, & Patrick, 1988; Sival, Visser, & Prechtl, 1992; van Vliet et al., 1985b). Maternal conditions which affect fetal neurobehavior include maternal diabetes (Mulder, 1993; Robertson & Dierker, 1985) and maternal substance use, such as methadone (Anyaegbunam, Tran, Jadali, Randolph, & Mikhail, 1997), cocaine (Gingras & O'Donnell, 1998), and alcohol (Mulder, Morssink, van der Schee, & Visser, 1998). Delays and/or abnormal function in one or more neurobehavioral parameters studied has been documented for each condition, lending support to the role of fetal neurobehaviors as functional manifestations of the development of the central nervous system (Hepper, 1995; Romanini & Rizzo, 1995).

DEVELOPMENTAL MODEL

All domains of fetal functioning discussed so far change over gestation. FHR increases during the first few weeks of pregnancy (van Heeswijk, Nijhuis, & Hollanders, 1990) and then declines. Variability in FHR increases during gestation; both processes reflect the increasing contribution of the parasympathetic nervous system (Freeman et al., 1991; Martin, 1978), although nonneural components have also been documented (Dalton et al., 1983). Fetal activity level peaks and then begins to decline during the mid-to-late second trimester, reflecting the mechanics of increasing uterine constraint as well as the inhibitory processes of neuromaturation (Roodenburg et al., 1991). Mature behavioral states do not coalesce until 36 weeks (Nijhuis & van de Pas, 1992). The hallmark of fetal state development is the emergence of periods of quiescence (James et al., 1995; ten Hof et al., 1999b). Fetuses become more responsive to stimuli as they mature (DiPietro et al., 1996b; Kisilevsky et al., 1992), reflecting developmental changes in both stimulus detection and response systems. Similarly, fetal response decrement to invariant stimuli becomes more rapid with advancing gestational age (Groome et al., 1993; Kuhlman et al., 1988).

Developmental Discontinuities

Just as development after birth evidences periods of discontinuities, so does maturation prior to birth. The gestational period between 28 and 32 weeks appears to be a transitional one for many aspects of fetal neurodevelopment. During this time, the fetus begins to display large-amplitude accelerations in FHR (Gagnon, Campbell, Hunse, & Patrick, 1987) and a plateau in the amount of FHR variability is attained shortly thereafter (Dawes et al., 1982). The inspiratory component of fetal breathing movements peaks between 28 and 32 weeks (Kozuma, Nemoto, Okai, & Mizuno, 1991), and fetal breathing rates plateau during this time (Pillai & James, 1990b). Beginning at about 31–32 weeks, total fetal activity stabilizes (Patrick et al., 1982a; Roberts et al., 1980), as does the frequency of specific motor patterns such as startles (Roodenburg et al., 1991). There is a significant increase in the length of periods of quiescence (James et al., 1995) during this time, and increased linkage of the parameters associated with state organization (Nijhuis et al., 1999; Visser et al., 1987). The fetus attains mature levels and patterns of responsiveness to vibroacoustic stimuli between 29 and 32 weeks (Kisilevsky et al., 1992; Kuhlman et al., 1988) and there is a concomitant increase in habituation (Groome et al., 1993).

Although there are apparent consistencies across neurobehavioral domains, most of these conclusions are based on descriptive data which were not specifically tested for developmental trends. Using a knotted spline technique which permits testing for deviations from linearity in otherwise linear regression models, evidence for a transitional period between 28 and 32 weeks was found for FHR variability, fetal activity, fetal state organization, responsivity to vibroacoustic stimuli, and the degree of coupling between fetal movements and FHR changes (DiPietro et al., 1996a, 1996b). The discontinuity can be generalized as follows: prior to 28–32 weeks, the fetus displays immature neurobehavioral patterns with a relatively steep developmental slope; after 32 weeks, the trajectory of development becomes significantly less steep. Although development in each domain continues through term, the 32-week fetus is more similar to a 40-week fetus than to a fetus prior to this period. The onset of these trends coincides with a period of rapid increase in neural development and myelination, including cortical and vagal processes (Kinney, Karthigason, Borenshteyn, Flax, & Kirschner, 1994; Sachis, Armstrong, Becker, & Bryan, 1982) as well as cortical sulcation (Lan et al., 2000). In a study designed to explicitly investigate the development of neural control of the heart, measures of FHR variability were compared between anencephalic and normal fetuses at varying gestational ages (Yoshizato et al., 1994). A critical transition period during which time higher cortical control was exerted was documented between 27 and 30 weeks gestation. The neurobehavioral maturation witnessed in the fetus by 32 weeks may underlie the successful developmental outcome of preterm infants born at this and subsequent gestational ages. Studies of fetal development in postterm fetuses (> 41 weeks gestation) have documented a linear increase in periods of wakefulness (3F and 4F)(Junge, 1979; van de Pas, Nijhuis, & Jongsma, 1994), supporting the notion first advanced by Prechtl and colleagues of a lack of discontinuity at term.

Developmentalists do not select a single age between birth and 2 years of age and consider it representative of "infancy." Similarly, the fetal period should not be considered a single stage. Measurement near term (≥ 36 weeks) ensures that the fetus has attained the most mature level of functioning. Conversely, earlier assessments yield information about the rate of maturation and disparity in the onset of neurobehaviors which may attain near universal expression at term. The rapid rate of development prior to 28–32 weeks and the discontinuities present after this time offer additional challenges in selecting periods to study. Selection of a gestational age for assessment should be guided by the nature of the research question, but it is clear that longitudinal studies offer the most complete opportunity to assess fetal neurodevelopment and provide multilevel models of development both within and across individuals. Interpretations of data generated by cross-sectional studies should be constrained to the age at which the fetus was assessed.

CONSTRAINTS AND CONTROVERSIES

A number of issues permeate the relatively new field of fetal neurobehavioral assessment and research. These include concerns about safety, spontaneous versus evoked measures, and the relevance and ascertainment of fetal behavioral states. As with the infant, fetal neurobehavioral assessment typically yields only a snapshot of performance at a given time of day.

In infant research, challenge or perturbation models have been incorporated to provide a standardized frame of reference for subsequent observations of arousal and regulation, considered to be core components of temperament and biobehavioral functioning (Derryberry & Rothbart, 1988). Fetal reactivity is usually elicited by auditory stimuli. Because sound travels better in a dense rather than weak medium, intrauterine sound pressure levels reach at least 20 dB higher than when measured in air (Gagnon, Benzaquen, & Hunse, 1992) and the sound level at the fetal ear from a common vibro-acoustic stimulus, an electronic larynx, reaches 135 decibels (Gerhardt, Abrams, Kovaz, Gomez, & Conlon, 1988). Fetal behaviors elicited by this stimulation are consistent with fetal pain (Visser, Mulder, Mulder, & Prechtl, 1989). At least two cases have been reported in the literature in which bradycardia leading to emergent delivery were the result of vibroacoustic stimulation (Sherer, Abramowicz, Hearn-Stebbins, & Woods, 1991). From a developmental perspective, application of intense stimuli elicits fetal re-sponses that can be regarded as nonphysiological (Visser et al., 1989); that is, the rise and magnitude of heart rate responses in reaction are so exaggerated as to be uninformative about normal fetal functioning. For these reasons, we have discontinued this procedure in our own research. Although there is de-bate over the safety of this procedure in clinical fetal assessment (Zimmer & Divon, 1993), stimulating the low-risk fetus in the context of academic re-search raises significant ethical and academic concerns and the use of vibroacoustic stimuli should be used only after careful deliberation.

Similarly, because habituation-oriented procedures have achieved prominence in the assessment of information processing and prediction of outcome in infancy, the value of continued investigation into fetal response decrement is apparent (Krasnegor et al., 1998a). Preliminary findings sug-gesting that individual differences in habituation *in utero* are predictive of infant outcome (Leader et al., 1984; Madison et al., 1986) and fetuses can re-tain information for at least 24 hours (van Hetteren, Boekkooi, Jongsma, & Nijhuis, 2000) heighten this interest. However, fetal habituation studies have not been as well-controlled as habituation studies in infants. Procedural cri-teria, such as stimulus characteristics, rate of stimulation, and definition of decrement, are not clearly defined. With few exceptions (Hepper & Shahidullah, 1992; Sandman et al., 1997b) dishabituation is not assessed, sig-nificantly jeopardizing the interpretation of these studies. Presentations of up to 50 stimuli have been reported in the literature (Leader et al., 1984); oth-ers have limited trials to 15 or less (Gingras & O'Donnell, 1998; Groome et al., 1993). Because the fetus cannot be observed directly, concerns about the potential harmful effects of repeated stimulations are compounded beyond those raised for single vibroacoustic applications.

Fetal research paradigms and interdisciplinary collaborations are more well established in Europe than in the United States. The single method in-stituted in Europe which has had the most pervasive influence on the nature and extent of current fetal research is the protocol for identifying fetal behavioral state. Procedures which were developed were somewhat arbitrary at their inception but have largely withstood the test of time (Pillai & James, 1990a; ten Hof et al., 1999a). The Netherlands protocol for state identification is intensive, requiring concurrent FHR recording and ultrasound visualization of both fetal body and eye movements. One transducer is used to provide a parasagittal, longitudinal section of the fetal abdomen and a lower extremity and the other oriented toward the fetal face and trained on the fetal eye. Data are generally collected for 60 to 120 minutes to allow for observation of a complete state cycle. State identification relies on post-recording visual inspection of polygraphic output resulting in construction of state profiles (Nijhuis et al., 1982). This research paradigm has generated a large body of critical findings on the nature of fetal neurobehavioral development. However, because of its procedural intensity, sample sizes are usually small, raising concerns about the replicability of reported findings, such as differences based on fetal sex or maternal parity, and limiting the number of investigators who are able or desire to initiate such an undertaking.

Under what conditions is fetal state ascertainment necessary, and what are the conditions necessary for state ascertainment? With respect to the first question, we believe that fetal behavioral state ascertainment is not requisite for every study of fetal development. FM and FHR patterns develop prior to their coalescence into organized states near term. Single-transducer ultrasound-based studies of fetal movement and studies which use only FHR monitors without ultrasound visualization also present viable research options. Knowledge about each can provide a useful contribution to advancing the field of neurobehavioral ontogeny. It is true that as term nears, FHR becomes more closely synchronized with fetal movement, and it is difficult to evaluate either in isolation. However, FHR and motor development are not necessarily dependent on state development, because the frequency of movement exhibited in each state does not remain constant over gestation (ten Hof et al., 1999b). Fetal state ascertainment seems most necessary to all procedures involving evoked responses, so that state at the time of stimulation can be controlled across subjects (Nijhuis, 1995). However, the nature of what constitutes adequate control is unclear prior to 36 weeks gestation, when fetal states are not consistently identifiable. To further confound the issue, the most common and appropriate state for eliciting responsivity in the fetus is during sleep, not wakefulness, when variability in FHR is low.

The question concerning the necessary conditions for identifying fetal state hinges on the value of knowing whether the fetal eye is moving. Fetal eye movement data are costly to collect because they require an additional ultrasound transducer dedicated to continuous visualization of the fetal eye. Doppler detection of fetal movement provides an objective, additional source of information about the fetus without the technical and logistical problems imposed by visualizing the fetus. We think that important features of fetal behavioral state organization can be discerned from FHR and reliable Doppler-based movement data alone, for several reasons. First, strong associations between periods of high FHR variability (patterns B and D) and the presence of eye movements and the lack of eye movements during low variability (pattern A) have been noted as the fetus nears term. Coincidence between FHR and body and eye movements in normal-term fetuses has been described as "so high that the different states can be recognized quite accurately by monitoring the heart rate alone" (Visser et al., 1993, p. 22). By 38 weeks, discordance between eye movements and FHR variability occurs only 12.5% of the time (Groome, Singh, Burgard, Neely, & Bartolucci, 1992); eye movements are present less than 2% of the time during FHR pattern A (Nijhuis & van de Pas, 1992).

The second means of evaluating our method is based on comparing data we have collected to those generated by ultrasound studies. State data generated by our procedures have yielded similar findings in three samples (DiPietro et al., 1998; DiPietro et al., 1996c). Comparisons of these data to others generated by ultrasound are consistent in terms of the developmental trends in periods of quiescence (1F), absolute amounts of sleep (1F + 2F observed approximately 70 to 80% of time after 36 weeks) and 4F; and the low incidence of 3F. After 36 weeks, we have found noncoincidence between parameters about 11% of the observation time, which is midrange of the values reported by others (Arabin & Riedewald, 1992; Groome et al., 1995a; Groome et al., 1995b; Martin, 1981; Nijhuis et al., 1982; Pillai & James, 1990a; van Vliet et al., 1985a; van Woerden et al., 1989). In general, we report much lower incidence of 1F; in part this is due to our absolute application of FHR pattern A across subjects rather than using relative, within-subject criteria (Visser et al., 1993). However, because the overall percentage of total sleep is consistent with other studies, this comes at the expense of 2F and not other states.

The third issue is that fetal eye visualization is the weakest procedural aspect of existing studies, particularly those which include preterm fetuses. Fetal movement and positioning interfere with eye visualization. The proportion of time in which the fetal eye cannot be visualized is rarely reported, but subject loss of 16% at term due to inadequate visualization has been noted (Groome et al., 1992). In a longitudinal study, only 48% of subjects had adequate eye visualization at each of four assessments to allow their inclusion in data analysis (Nijhuis et al., 1999); of these, fetal eye visualization loss ranged from 79% of the observation time at 24–26 weeks to 9% at term.

There are also limitations imposed by the lack of eye movement data. The two most significant pertain to fetuses younger than 36 weeks. Prior to this time a large proportion of coincidence is generated by the association of FHR and FM (Nijhuis et al., 1982), suggesting that without eye movement data prior to term, only more generalized periods of rest and activity can be discerned. By 30–32 weeks, FHR pattern A is associated with either a lack of eye and body movement or both between 53 to 72% of the time, whereas FHR B is associated with eye and/or body movements 74 to 86% of the time (Nijhuis & van de Pas, 1992; Visser et al., 1987). Although these associations are relatively high, they are not high enough to be interchangeable. Between 32 and 36 weeks, we report higher state coincidence than others (Arabin & Riedewald, 1992; Nijhuis et al., 1982; van Vliet et al., 1985a). In the only other study to extend investigation to 20 weeks, 1F and 2F coincidence is not detected until 28 and 24 weeks, respectively, and all coincidence values are consistently lower than ours until 34 weeks (Pillai, James, & Parker, 1992). Thus the first liability of the lack of eye movement data is in distinguishing which periods that have FHR and FM coincidence represent states and which do not. This is particularly true for 2F, because the FHR pattern and FM criteria are the least specific and most common; coincidence between these two are more likely to occur by chance than for any other state (van Vliet et al., 1985a). This conclusion has been confirmed by a comparison of ultrasound versus actograph-based identification of states (Arabin et al., 1988), which concludes that although the actocardiograph has high accuracy in identifying 1F, 2F, and 4F, periods in which there are no eye movements tend to be incorrectly attributed as state 2F. Second, the simultaneity of state transitioning contributes a crucial qualitative component to organization after the fetus attains 36 weeks (Arduini et al., 1995; Nijhuis et al., 1982). In one report, the combined coincidence of states 1F–4F has been reported to near 60% by 32 weeks, but no states were identifiable because the condition of transitions of all three parameters within 3 minutes was not met (Swartjes, van Geijn, Mantel, & van Woerden, 1990). Lack of eye movement data prohibits adequate ascertainment of transitioning among all three parameters.

Considering these and other issues, we have concluded that the methodological compromise provided by using a single transducer actocardiograph[2] instead of a heart rate monitor and two real-time ultrasound transducers is justified. At term we are fairly confident that our scoring system approximates true behavioral states, but the further from term the less likely this becomes. Other factors also discourage against attempts at early state attribution. In particular, FHR pattern A (low variability) is a normal indicator of immaturity in a young fetus, but as gestation advances, this same pattern, coupled with absence of movement, signifies the emergence of quiescence and indicates mature state organization. In any case, failure to evaluate coincidence and transitioning among all three variables may lead to overestimation of the developmental trajectory of state maturation. Because of this, and because our definitions do not include eye movement data, we have begun to refer to actograph-identified states as biobehavioral patterns to distinguish them from those identified by traditional, ultrasound-based scoring techniques (DiPietro et al., 1998). A similar strategy has been adopted in other studies using actograph-based state data (e.g., Gallagher, Costigan, & Johnson, 1992). As with FM data collection, methods selected for a study should be consistent with the research question.

TRAINING REQUIREMENTS

Almost all aspects of fetal research require training in areas with which developmental investigators have little experience. This includes learning the scope and variability of fetal behaviors and heart rate patterns, understanding fetal sensory capacities, and becoming familiar with the physics of the new technologies. Further, developmentalists do not usually encounter medicolegal issues in their research, but these are inherent to fetal research. Because electronic fetal monitoring and real-time ultrasound are methods of clinical fetal assessment, much of the data collected for research purposes is also clinically interpretable. Twenty to 40 minutes of FHR data without at least two accelerations within a 20-minute window represents a positive (i.e., abnormal) nonstress test. What are the implications, if any, for a researcher who fails to detect or acknowledge this situation when it is followed by a poor pregnancy outcome? The issue is further confounded by the gestational age of the fetus due to the lack of normative data for those less than 32 weeks (Gagnon et al., 1987; Ware & Devoe, 1994). The legal implications of these situations are nebulous, but ethical obligations to research participants are not. To this end, this section outlines the policy and procedures developed in my own laboratory based on our experience with more than 300 pregnant women and 1,500 sessions of fetal neurobehavioral data collection on a low-risk population.

Compliance with our longitudinal protocols has been exceptionally high. Women report that participating in the research provides them with reassurance about the fetus's well-being, despite our efforts to inform them that the research methods are not diagnostic. Because reassurance is a consequence, albeit unintended, of study participation, we feel an obligation to provide our subjects with the standard of care in routine antepartum screening. Our policy is to extend monitoring of any FHR tracing which would not pass NST criteria for fetuses at or beyond 32 weeks, using standard clinical procedures. Prior to testing, we inform women that with their consent, we will report the following circumstances to their obstetrician: (1) anomalous findings incidentally detected through ultrasound (confirmed by an external reviewer); (2) nonreassuring NST results, including FHR patterns of persistent decelerations or arrhythmias; (3) low or high levels of amniotic fluid based on standard criteria; and (4) other idiosyncratic conditions which may present. Most, although not all, physicians have been pleased to have additional information on their patients.

Based on the foregoing policy outlined, it should be clear that a highly trained research staff is essential. Ideally, fetal research should be conducted within or in close proximity to a hospital-based obstetric diagnostic facility and with collaboration by obstetric facility to provide interpretation of nonreassuring results. Research staff should include at least one person with a clinical background in obstetric and/or antenatal assessment and should have training in both ultrasound administration and interpretation of FHR tracings. The reduction in health insurance coverage for antepartum ultrasound in the absence of risk factors heightens this need. The following two anecdotes illustrate the need for this type of collaboration. In the first, ascites (i.e., fetal hydrops) was detected in a 20-week fetus during the cursory ultrasound scan conducted at the beginning of each recording. This was a potentially lethal and previously unsuspected condition. Further diagnostic testing determined this to be a result of maternal exposure to the otherwise benign parvovirus B19. The fetus subsequently received intrauterine blood transfusion for the virus-mediated anemia and recovered without subsequent physical or developmental sequelae. Had our research personnel failed to detect this condition, severe fetal compromise and death may have occurred over the ensuing days, and our ethical responsibilities to this participant would have been breached. The second incident involved identification of significant diaphragmatic hernia, also at 20 weeks. In each case, the FHR was not abnormal and without professional sonography, the subjects would have left the recording under the impression that their fetus was normal and healthy. Clearly one would never expect that all fetal conditions can be diagnosed during fetal neurobehavioral research, nor is that our goal. However, we believe that considerable effort should be directed at ensuring that data sources which have clinical relevance be examined in a manner consistent with standards of antepartum screening.

IMPLICATIONS

Thirty years of experience have provided insight into the conceptual and methodological strengths and weaknesses of neonatal neurobehavioral assessment (Brazelton, 1990). The study of fetal neurobehavioral development is subject to many of these same issues and can be informed by that history. The impetus to develop a standardized assessment for the fetus is a natural consequence of the emerging consensus that fetal neurobehavior is an integral reflection of the developing nervous system. There is universal acknowledgement among investigators of a wide range of individual differences among fetuses, which can be measured in many ways. Various approaches to developing standard assessments for the fetus have been offered. These include those that rely on undisturbed functioning, such as establishing fetal developmental milestones (James et al., 1995) and evaluating state-related processes (Nijhuis, 1986), those that are based on evoked responses to single or repeated vibroacoustic perturbations (Divon et al., 1985; Leader, 1995), and those that include a combination of both (Gingras & O'Donnell, 1998). We have not adopted the strategy of developing a single assessment instrument and do not believe such a scale is warranted at this time. A model for constructing a standardized, psychometrically sound neurobehavioral assessment for neonates includes derivation of items based on both conceptual and psychometric soundness (Korner et al., 1987); such a strategy should also be applied to a fetal assessment scale. The conceptual basis for the constituents of a fetal neurobehavioral assessment content is quite strong already, and such an instrument would include features of fetal heart rate, movement, state organization, and, perhaps, evoked responsivity. However, more empirical data are needed to establish norms across the second half of gestation, to select the best ways to quantify functioning within each domain, and to evaluate the psychometric properties, including reliability and stability of each assessment item. In the interim, the ongoing body of information that is being amassed about the psychobiological and neuromaturational features of human fetal development will directly inform such an endeavor.

ACKNOWLEDGMENTS

Preparation of this chapter was supported in part by Grant No. R01 HD27592. I thank Kathleen A. Costigan, RN, MPH, and Timothy R. B. Johnson, MD, for their insights into fetal assessment and helpful comments on this chapter.

NOTES

1. In previous research, we used the default setting of 25 AUs as the threshold setting for fetal movement. As a result of the high degree of sensitivity and specificity noted in detection of movement in a study of the validity of the Toitu MT320 actocardiograph (DiPietro et al., 1999), we have lowered this threshold to 15 AUs in current analyses.
2. All commercially available actocardiographs are not alike, and vary in reliability of movement detection. Clinically acceptable levels of reliability may be lower than those necessary in research. Investigators should carefully evaluate the performance of monitors they select.

REFERENCES

Almli, C. R., Mohr, M., Ball, R., & Bernhard, L. (1995). Human fetal and neonatal movement patterns and effects of CNS abnormality. *Neuroscience Abstracts, 21,* 1791.
Als, H. (1982). Toward a synactive theory of development: Promise for the assessment and support of infant individuality. *Infant Mental Health Journal, 3,* 229–243.

Anyaegbunam, A., Tran, T., Jadali, D., Randolph, G., & Mikhail, M. (1997). Assessment of fetal well-being in methadone-maintained pregnancies: abnormal nonstress tests. *Gynecologic and Obstetric Investigation, 43,* 25–28.

Arabin, B., & Riedewald, S. (1992). An attempt to quantify characteristics of behavioral states. *American Journal of Perinatology, 9(2),* 115–119.

Arabin, B., Riedewald, S., Zacharias, C., & Saling, E. (1988). Quantitative analysis of fetal behavioural patterns with real-time sonography and the actocardiograph. *Gynecological Obstetrical Investigation, 26,* 211–218.

Arduini, D., Rizzo, G., Caforio, L., Romanini, C., & Mancuso, S. (1987). The development of behavioral states in hydrocephalic fetuses. *Fetal Therapy, 2,* 135–143.

Arduini, D., Rizzo, G., Giorlandino, C., Dell'Acqua, S., Valensise, H., & Romanini, C. (1986). The development of fetal behavioral states: A longitudinal study. *Prenatal Diagnosis, 6,* 117–124.

Arduini, D., Rizzo, G., Piana, G., Bonalumi, R., Brambilla, P., & Romanini, C. (1993). Computerized analysis of fetal heart rate. *Journal of Maternal and Fetal Investigation, 3,* 159–164.

Arduini, D., Rizzo, G., & Romanini, C. (1995). Fetal behavioral states and behavioral transitions in normal and compromised fetuses. In J. P. Lecanuet, W. P. Fifer, N. A. Krasnegor, & W. P. Smotherman (Eds.), *Fetal development: A psychobiological perspective* (pp. 83–99). Hillsdale, NJ: Erlbaum.

Besinger, R. E., & Johnson, T. R. B. (1989). Doppler recordings of fetal movement: Clinical correlation with real-time ultrasound. *Obstetrics and Gynecology, 74,* 277–280.

Brazelton, T. B. (1984). *Neonatal Behavioral Assessment Scale* (2nd ed). Philadelphia: Lippincott.

Brazelton, T. B. (1990). Saving the bathwater. *Child Development, 61,* 1661–1671.

Budin, N., & Abboud, S. (1994). Real-time multichannel abdominal fetal ECG monitor using digital signal coprocessor. *Computers in Biology and Medicine, 24,* 451–462.

Carter, M. C. (1993). Present-day performance qualities of cardiotocographs. British *Journal of Obstetrics and Gynaecology, 100* (Suppl. 9), 10–14.

Comparetti, A. M. (1981). The neurophysiologic and clinical implications of studies on fetal motor behavior. *Seminars in Perinatology, 5(2),* 183–189.

Dalton, K., Dawes, G. S., & Patrick, J. E. (1983). The autonomic nervous system and fetal heart rate variability. *American Journal of Obstetrics and Gynecology, 146,* 456–462.

Dawes, G. S. (1993). The fetal ECG: Accuracy of measurements. *Obstetrics and Gynaecology, 100*(Suppl. 9), 15–17.

Dawes, G. S., Houghton, C. R. S., Redman, C. W. G., & Visser, G. H. A. (1982). Pattern of the normal human fetal heart rate. *British Journal of Obstetrics and Gynecology, 89,* 276–284.

Dawes, G. S., Moulden, M., Sheil, O., & Redman, C. W. G. (1992). Approximate entropy, a statistic of regularity, applied to fetal heart rate data before and during labor. *Obstetrics and Gynecology, 80*(5), 763–768.

Dawes, G. S., Redman, C. W. G., & Smith, J. H. (1985). Improvements in the registration and analysis of fetal heart rate records at the bedside. *British Journal of Obstetrics and Gynaecology, 92,* 317–325.

Derryberry, D., & Rothbart, M. K. (1988). Arousal, affect, and attention as components of temperament. *Journal of Personality and Social Psychology, 6,* 958–966.

Devlin, B., Daniels, M., & Roeder, K. (1997). The heritability of IQ. *Nature, 388,* 468–471.

deVries, J. I. P., Visser, G. H. A., & Prechtl, H. F. R. (1982). The emergence of fetal behaviour. I. Qualitative aspects. *Early Human Development, 7,* 301–322.

deVries, J. I. P., Visser, G. H. A., & Prechtl, H. F. R. (1988). The emergence of fetal behaviour. III. Individual differences and consistencies. *Early Human Development, 16,* 85–103.

DiPietro, J. A. (2000, July). Continuities in behavior and heart rate from the fetus to infant. *International Conference on Infant Studies,* Brighton, England.

DiPietro, J. A., Caughy, M. O. B., Cusson, R., & Fox, N. A. (1994). Cardiorespiratory functioning of preterm infants: Stability and risk associations for measures of heart rate variability and oxygen saturation. *Developmental Psychobiology, 27*(3), 137–152.

DiPietro, J. A., Costigan, K. A., & Pressman, E. K. (1999). Fetal movement detection: Comparison of the Toitu actograph with ultrasound from 20 weeks gestation. *Journal of Maternal-Fetal Medicine, 8,* 237–242.

DiPietro, J. A., Costigan, K. C., Pressman, E. K., & Doussard-Roosevelt, J. (2000). Antenatal origins of individual differences in heart rate. *Developmental Psychobiology, 37,* 221–228.

DiPietro, J. A., Costigan, K. A., Shupe, A. K., Pressman, E. K., & Johnson, T. R. B. (1998). Fetal neurobehavioral development: Associations with socioeconomic class and fetal sex. *Developmental Psychobiology, 33,* 79–91.

DiPietro, J. A., Hodgson, D. M., Costigan, K. A., Hilton, S. C., & Johnson, T. R. B. (1996a). Development of fetal movement—fetal heart rate coupling from 20 weeks through term. *Early Human Development, 44,* 139–151.

DiPietro, J. A., Hodgson, D. M., Costigan, K. A., Hilton, S. C., & Johnson, T. R. B. (1996b). Fetal neurobehavioral development. *Child Development, 67,* 2553–2567.

DiPietro, J. A., Hodgson, D. M., Costigan, K. A., & Johnson, T. R. B. (1996c). Fetal antecedents of infant temperament. *Child Development, 67,* 2568–2583.

Divon, M. Y., Lawrence, D., Platt, M., Cantrell, C., Smith, C., Yeh, S., & Paul, R. (1985). Evoked fetal startle response: A possible intrautrine neurological exam. *American Journal of Obstetrics and Gynecology, 153,* 454–456.

Donker, D. K., van Geijn, H. P., & Hasman, A. (1993). Interobserver variation in the assessment of fetal heart rate recordings. *European Journal of Obstetrics, Gynecology, and Reproductive Biology, 52*(1), 21–28.

Eaton, W. O., & Saudino, K. J. (1992). Prenatal activity level as a temperament dimension? Individual differences and developmental functions in fetal movement. *Infant Behavior and Development, 15,* 57–70.

Emory, E. K., & Noonan, J. R. (1984). Fetal cardiac responding: A correlate of birth weight and neonatal behavior. *Child Development, 55,* 1651–1657.

Fifer, W. P., & Moon, C. M. (1995). The effects of fetal experience with sound. In J. P. Lecanuet, W. P. Fifer, N. A. Krasnegor, & W. P. Smotherman (Eds.), *Fetal development: A psychobiological perspective* (pp. 351–366). Hillsdale, NJ: Erlbaum.

Fleisher, L. A., DiPietro, J. A., Johnson, T. R. B., & Pincus, S. (1997). Complementary and non-coincident increases in heart rate variability and irregularity during fetal development. *Clinical Science, 92,* 345–349.

Freeman, J. M. (Ed.). (1985). *Prenatal and perinatal factors associated with brain disorders* (NIH Publication No. 85–1149). National Institutes of Health.

Freeman, R. K., Garite, T. J., & Nageotte, M. P. (1991). Physiologic basis of fetal monitoring. In R. K. Freeman, T. J. Garite, & M. P. Nageotte (Eds.), *Fetal heart rate monitoring* (2nd ed., pp. 7–20). Baltimore: Williams & Wilkins.

Gagnon, R., Benzaquen, S., & Hunse, C. (1992). The fetal sound environment during vibroacoustic stimulation in labor. *Obstetrics and Gynecology, 79,* 950–955.

Gagnon, R., Campbell, K., & Hunse, C. (1993). A comparison between visual and computer analysis of antepartum fetal heart rate tracings. *American Journal of Obstetrics and Gynecology, 168,* 842–847.

Gagnon, R., Campbell, K., Hunse, C., & Patrick, J. (1987). Patterns of human fetal heart rate accelerations from 26 weeks to term. *American Journal of Obstetrics and Gynecology, 157,* 743–749.

Gagnon, R., Foreman, J., Hunse, C., & Patrick, J. (1989). Effects of low frequency vibration on human term fetuses. *American Journal of Obstetrics and Gynecology, 162,* 1479–1485.

Gagnon, R., Hunse, C., Fellows, F., Carmichael, L., & Patrick, J. (1988). Fetal heart rate and activity patterns in growth-retarded fetuses: Changes after vibratory acoustic stimulation. *American Journal of Obstetrics and Gynecology, 158,* 265–271.

Gallagher, M. W., Costigan, K., & Johnson, T. R. B. (1992). Fetal heart rate accelerations, fetal movement, and fetal behavior patterns in twin gestations. *American Journal of Obstetrics and Gynecology, 167,* 1140–1144.

Gerhardt, K. J., Abrams, R., Kovaz, B., Gomez, K., & Conlon, M. (1988). Intrauterine noise levels produced in pregnant ewes by sound applied to the abdomen. *American Journal of Obstetrics and Gynecology, 159,* 228–232.

Gingras, J. L., & O'Donnell, K. J. (1998). State control in the substance-exposed fetus: I. The fetal neurobehavioral profile: an assessment of fetal state, arousal, and regulation competency. *Annals of the New York Academy of Sciences, 846,* 262–276.

Glover, V., & Fisk, N. (1996). We don't know; better to err on the safe side from mid-gestation. *British Medical Journal, 313,* 796–797.

Goldkrand, J. W., & Litvack, B. L. (1991). Demonstration of fetal habituation and patterns of fetal heart rate response to vibroacoustic stimulation in normal and high-risk pregnancies. *Journal of Perinatology, 11,* 25–29.

Green, S., & Sparling, J. W. (1993). Q-MOVE: Development of a qualitative assessment of fetal movement. In J. W. Sparling (Ed.), *Concepts in fetal movement research* (pp. 115–137). Binghamton, NY: Haworth Press.

Grieve, P. G., Myers, M. M., & Stark, R. I. (1994). Behavioral states in the fetal baboon. *Early Human Development, 39,* 159–175.

Groome, L. J., Bentz, L. S., Holland, S. B., Swiber, M. J., Singh, K. P., & Trimm, R. F. T. (1995a). Individual consistency in behavioral state profiles in human fetuses between 38 and 40 weeks gestation. *Journal of Maternal–Fetal Medicine, 4,* 247–251.

Groome, L. J., Bentz, L. S., & Singh, K. P. (1995b). Behavioral state organization in normal human term fetuses: The relationship between periods of undefined state and other characteristics of state control. *Sleep, 18*(2), 77–81.

Groome, L. J., Gotlieb, S. J., Neely, C. L., & Waters, M. D. (1993). Developmental trends in fetal habituation to vibroacoustic stimulation. *American Journal of Perinatology, 10,* 46–49.

Groome, L. J., Mooney, D. M., Bentz, L. S., & Singh, K. P. (1994). Spectral analysis of heart rate variability during quiet sleep in normal human fetuses between 36 and 40 weeks of gestation. *Early Human Development, 38,* 1–10.

Groome, L., Mooney, D., Holland, S., Smith, L., Atterbury, J., & Dykman, R. (1999a). Behavioral state affects heart rate response to low-intensity sound in human fetuses. *Early Human Development, 54,* 39–54.

Groome, L. J., Singh, K. P., Burgard, S. L., Neely, C. L., & Bartolucci, A. A. (1992). The relationship between heart rate and eye movement in the human fetus at 38–40 weeks of gestation. *Early Human Development, 30,* 93–99.

Groome, L. J., Swiber, M. J., Atterbury, J. L., Bentz, L. S., & Holland, S. B. (1997). Similarities and differences in behavioral state organization during sleep periods in the perinatal infant before and after birth. *Child Development, 68*(1), 1–11.

Groome, L. J., Swiber, M. J., Bentz, L. S., Holland, S. B., & Atterbury, J. L. (1995c). Maternal anxiety during pregnancy: Effect on fetal behavior at 38 and 40 weeks of gestation. *Journal of Developmental and Behavioral Pediatrics, 16*(6), 391–396.

Groome, L., Swiber, M., Holland, S., Bentz, L., Atterbury, J., & Trimm, R. (1999b). Spontaneous motor activity in the perinatal infant before and after birth: Stability in individual differences. *Developmental Psychobiology, 35,* 15–24.

Hepper, P. G. (1995). Fetal behavior and neural functioning. In J. P. Lecanuet, W. P. Fifer, N. A. Krasnegor, & W. P. Smotherman (Eds.), *Fetal development: A psychobiological perspective* (pp. 105–117). Hillsdale, NJ: Erlbaum.

Hepper, P. (1997). Fetal habituation: Another Pandora's box? *Developmental Medicine and Child Neurology, 39,* 274–278.

Hepper, P. G., McCartney, G. R., & Shannon, E. A. (1998). Lateralised behavior in first trimester human foetuses. *Neuropschologia, 36,* 531–534.

Hepper, P. G., & Shahidullah, S. (1992). Habituation in normal and Down's syndrome fetuses. *Quarterly Journal of Experimental Psychology, 44,* 305–317.

Horimoto, N., Koyangi, T., Maeda, H., Satoh, S., Takashima, T., Minami, T., & Nakano, H. (1993). Can brain impairment be detected by in utero behavioural patterns? *Archives of Disease in Childhood, 69,* 3–8.

Horowitz, F. (1990). Developmental models of individual differences. In J. Colombo & J. Fagen (Eds.), *Individual differences in infancy: Reliability, stability, prediction* (pp. 3–18). Hillsdale, NJ: Erlbaum.

Ianniruberto, A., & Tajani, E. (1981). Ultrasonographic study of fetal movement. *Seminars in Perinatology, 5*(2), 175–181.

James, D., Pillai, M., & Smoleniec, J. (1995). Neurobehavioral development in the human fetus. In J. P. Lecanuet, W. P. Fifer, N. A. Krasnegor, & W. P. Smotherman (Eds.), *Fetal development: A psychobiological perspective* (pp. 101–128). Hillsdale, NJ: Erlbaum.

Johnson, T. R. B., Jordan, E. T., & Paine, L. L. (1990). Doppler recordings of fetal movement: II. Comparison with maternal perception. *Obstetrics and Gynecology, 76,* 42–43.

Junge, H. D. (1979). Behavioral states and state related heart rate and motor activity patterns in the newborn infant and the fetus antepartum: A comparative study. *Journal of Perinatal Medicine, 7,* 85–107.

Kinney, H. C., Karthigason, J., Borenshteyn, N., Flax, J., & Kirschner, D. (1994). Myelination in the developing brain: Biochemical correlates. *Neurochemical Research, 19,* 983–996.

Kisilevsky, B. S., Killen, H., Muir, D. W., & Low, J. A. (1991). Maternal and ultrasound measurements of elicited fetal movements: A methodologic consideration. *Obstetrics and Gynecology, 77,* 889–892.

Kisilevsky, B. S., & Muir, D. W. (1991). Human fetal and subsequent newborn responses to sound and vibration. *Infant Behavior and Development, 14,* 1–26.

Kisilevsky, B. S., Muir, D. W., & Low, J. A. (1992). Maturation of human fetal responses to vibroacoustic stimulation. *Child Development, 63,* 1497–1508.

Korner, A., Kraemer, H., Reade, E., Forrest, T., Dimiceli, S., & Thom, V. (1987). A methodological approach to developing an assessment procedure for testing the neuro-behavioral maturity of preterm infants. *Child Development, 58,* 1478–1487.

Kozuma, S., Nemoto, A., Okai, T., & Mizuno, M. (1991). Maturational sequence of fetal breathing movements. *Biology of the Neonate, 60,* 36–40.

Krasnegor, N. A., Fifer, W., Maulik, D., McNellis, D., Romero, R., & Smotherman, W. (1998a). Fetal behavioral development II: Measurement of habituation, state transitions and movement to assess fetal well-being and to predict outcome. *Journal of Maternal–Fetal Investigation, 8,* 51–57.

Krasnegor, N. A., Fifer, W., Maulik, D., McNellis, D., Romero, R., & Smotherman, W. (1998b). Fetal behavioral development: A transdisciplinary perspective for assessing fetal well-being and predicting outcome. *Prenatal and Neonatal Medicine, 3,* 185–190.

Kuhlman, K. A., Burns, K. A., Depp, R., & Sabbagha, R. (1988). Ultrasonic imaging of normal fetal response to external vibratory acoustic stimulation. *American Journal of Obstetrics and Gynecology, 258,* 47–51.

Lan, L. M., Yamashita, Y., Tang, Y., Sugahara, T., Takahashi, M., Ohba, T., & Okamura, H. (2000). Normal fetal brain development: MR imaging with a half-Fourier rapid acquisition with relaxation enhancement sequence. *Radiology, 215,* 205–210.

Leader, L. R. (1995). The potential value of habituation in the prenate. In J. P. Lecanuet, W. P. Fifer, N. A. Krasnegor, & W. P. Smotherman (Eds.), *Fetal development: A psychobiological perspective* (pp. 383–404). Hillsdale, NJ: Erlbaum.

Leader, L. R., Baillie, P., Martin, B., Molteno, C., & Wynchank, S. (1984). Fetal responses to vibrotactile stimulation, a possible predictor of fetal and neonatal outcome. *Australian and New Zealand Journal of Obstetrics and Gynaecology, 24,* 251–256.

Lecanuet, J. P., Granier-Deferre, C., Cohen, H., Houezec, R. L., & Busnel, M. (1986). Fetal responses to acoustic stimulation depend on heart rate variability pattern, stimulus intensity, and repetition. *Early Human Development, 13,* 269–283.

Lecanuet, J. P., Granier-Deferre, C., Jacquet, A., & Busnel, M. C. (1992). Decelerative cardiac responsiveness to acoustical stimulation in the near term fetus. *Quarterly Journal of Experimental Psychology, 44,* 279–303.

Lecanuet, J. P., & Schaal, B. (1996). Fetal sensory competencies. *European Journal of Obstetrics and Gynecology, 68,* 1–23.

Lewis, M., Wilson, C., Ban, P., & Baumel, M. (1970). An exploratory study of resting cardiac rate and variability from the last trimester of prenatal life through the first year of postnatal life. *Child Development, 41,* 799–811.

Madison, L., Madison, J., & Adubato, S. (1986). Infant behavior and development in relation to fetal movement and habituation. *Child Development, 57,* 1475–1482.

Maeda, K., Tatsumura, M., & Nakajima, K. (1991). Objective and quantitative evaluation of fetal movement with ultrasonic doppler actocardiogram. *Biology Neonate, 60*(Suppl. 1), 41–51.

Maeda, K., Tatsumura, M., & Utsu, M. (1999). Analysis of fetal movements by doppler actocardiogram and fetal B-mode imaging. *Clinics in Perinatology, 26,* 829–851.

Manning, F. A., Bondaji, N., Harman, C. R., Casiro, O., Menticoglou, S., Morrison, I., & Berck, D. (1998). Fetal assessment based on fetal biophysical profile scoring: VIII: The incidence of cerebral palsy in tested and untested perinates. *American Journal of Obstetrics and Gynecology, 178,* 696–706.

Manning, F. A., Platt, L. D., & Sipos, L. (1980). Antepartum fetal evaluation: Development of fetal biophysical profile. *American Journal of Obstetrics and Gynecology, 136,* 787–793.

Martin, C. (1978). Regulation of the fetal heart rate and genesis of FHR patterns. *Seminars in Perinatology, 2,* 131–146.

Martin, C. B. (1981). Behavioral states in the human fetus. *Journal of Reproductive Medicine, 26,* 425–432.

Mathai, M., Vijaykumar, S., Joseph, R., N. Karthikeyan, A. R., Peedicayil, A., & Jasper, P. (1995). The normal foetal heart rate pattern. *Indian Journal of Medical Research, 101,* 108–110.

Melendez, T. D., Rayburn, W. F., & Smith, C. V. (1992). Characterization of fetal body movement recorded by the Hewlett-Packard M-1350–A fetal monitor. *American Journal of Obstetrics and Gynecology, 167*(3), 700–703.

Monk, C., Fifer, W., Myers, M., Sloan, R., Trien, L., & Hurtado, A. (2000). Maternal stress responses and anxiety during pregnancy: Effects on fetal heart rate. *Developmental Psychobiology, 36,* 67–77.

Mulder, E. J. H. (1993). Diabetes in pregnancy as a model for testing behavioral teratogenicity in man. *Developmental Brain Dysfunction, 6,* 210–228.

Mulder, E. J. H., Boersma, M., Meeuse, M., van der Wal, M., van de Weerd, E., & Visser, G. H. A. (1994). Patterns of breathing movements in the near-term fetus: Relationship to behavioural states. *Early Human Development, 36,* 127–135.

Mulder, E. J., Morssink, L. P., van der Schee, T., & Visser, G. H. (1998). Acute maternal alcohol consumption disrupts behavioral state organization in the near term fetus. *Pediatric Research, 44,* 774–779.

Nasello-Paterson, C., Natale, R., & Connors, G. (1988). Ultrasonic evaluation of fetal body movements over twenty-four hours in the human fetus at twenty-four to twenty-eight weeks' gestation. *American Journal of Obstetrics and Gynecology, 158,* 312–316.

Nelson, K. B., & Ellenberg, J. H. (1986). Antecedents of cerebral palsy: multivariate analysis of risk. *New England Journal of Medicine, 315,* 61–86.

Nijhuis, I. J. M., ten Hof, J., Mulder, E. J. H., Nijhuis, J. G., Narayan, H., Taylor, D. J., & Visser, G. H. A. (1998). Fetal heart rate (FHR) parameters during FHR patterns A and B: A longitudinal study from 24 weeks gestation. *Prenatal and Neonatal Medicine, 3,* 383–393.

Nijhuis, I. J. M., ten Hof, J., Nijhuis, J. G., Mulder, E. J. H., Narayan, H., Taylor, D. J., & Visser, G. H. A. (1999). Temporal organisation of fetal behavior from 24 weeks gestation onwards in normal and complicated pregnancies. *Developmental Psychobiology, 34,* 257–268.

Nijhuis, J. G. (1986). Behavioural states: Concomitants, clinical implications, and the assessment of the condition of the nervous system. *European Journal of Obstetrics, Gynecology, and Reproductive Biology, 21,* 301–308.

Nijhuis, J. G. (1995). Physiological and clinical consequences in relation to the development of fetal behavior and fetal behavioral states. In J. P. Lecanuet, W. P. Fifer, N. A. Krasnegor, & W. P. Smotherman (Eds.), *Fetal development: A psychobiological perspective* (pp. 67–79). Hillsdale, NJ: Erlbaum.

Nijhuis, J. G., Prechtl, H. F. R., Martin, C. B., & Bots, R. S. G. (1982). Are there behavioural states in the human fetus? *Early Human Development, 6,* 47–65.

Nijhuis, J. G., & van de Pas, M. (1992). Behavioral states and their ontogeny: Human studies. *Seminars in Perinatology, 16,* 206–210.

Odendaal, H. J. (1990). More perinatal deaths associated with poor long-term variability during antenatal fetal heart rate monitoring. *South African Medical Journal, 77,* 506–508.

Patrick, J., Campbell, K., Carmichael, L., Natale, R., & Richardson, B. (1982a). Patterns of gross fetal body movements over 24–hour observation intervals during the last 10 weeks of pregnancy. *American Journal of Obstetrics and Gynecology, 142,* 363–371.

Patrick, J., Campbell, K., Carmichael, L., & Probert, C. (1982b). Influence of maternal heart rate and gross fetal body movements on the daily pattern of fetal heart rate near term. *American Journal of Obsterics and Gynecology, 144,* 533–538.

Patrick, J., Campbell, K., Carmichael, L., & Probert, C. (1986). Analysis of fetal activity and maternal and fetal heart rate using a laboratory minicomputer. *American Journal of Perinatology, 3*(2), 123–126.

Petrikovsky, B. M., & Kaplan, G. P. (1993). Fetal grasping of the umbilical cord causing variable fetal heart rate decelerations. *Journal of Clinical Ultrasound, 21*(9), 642–644.

Pillai, M., Garrett, C., & James, D. (1991). Bizarre fetal behaviour associated with lethal congenital anomalies: A case report. *European Journal of Obstetrics and Gynecology and Reproductive Biology, 39,* 215–218.

Pillai, M., & James, D. (1990a). Are the behavioural states of the newborn comparable to those of the fetus? *Early Human Development, 22,* 39–49.

Pillai, M., & James, D. (1990b). Hiccups and breathing in human fetuses. *Archives of Disease in Childhood, 65,* 1072–1075.

Pillai, M., James, D. K., & Parker, M. (1992). The development of ultradian rhythms in human fetus. *American Journal of Obstetrics and Gynecology, 167,* 172–177.

Porges, S. W. (1983). Heart rate patterns in neonates: A potential diagnostic window to the brain. In T. Field & A. Sostek (Eds.), *Infants born at risk: Physiological, perceptual, and cognitive processes* (pp. 3–22). New York: Grune & Stratton.

Prechtl, H. F. R. (1974). The behavioral states of the newborn infant. *Brain Research, 76,* 185–212.

Prechtl, H. F. R. (1984). Continuity and change in early neural development. In H. Prechtl (Ed.), *Continuity in neural functions from prenatal to postnatal life* (pp. 1–15). Philadelphia: Lippincott.

Rayburn, W. F. (1990). Fetal body movement monitoring. *Obstetrics and Gynecology Clinics of North America, 17*(1), 95–110.

Richards, J. E. (1985). Respiratory sinus arrhythmia predicts heart rate and visual responses during visual attention in 14 and 20 week old infants. *Psychophysiology, 22,* 101–108.

Roberts, A. B., Griffin, D., Mooney, R., Cooper, D. J., & Campbell, S. (1980). Fetal activity in 100 normal third trimester pregnancies. *British Journal of Obstetrics and Gynaecology, 87,* 480–484.

Robertson, S. S. (1985). Cyclic motor activity in the human fetus after midgestation. *Developmental Psychobiology, 18*(5), 411–419.

Robertson, S. S., & Dierker, L. J. (1985). The development of cyclic motility in fetuses of diabetic mothers. *Developmental Psychobiology, 19,* 223–234.

Romanini, C., & Rizzo, G. (1995). Fetal behaviour in normal and compromised fetuses: An overview. *Early Human Development, 43,* 117–131.

Roodenburg, P. J., Wladimiroff, J. W., van Es, A., & Prechtl, H. F. R. (1991). Classification and quantitative aspects of fetal movements during the second half of normal pregnancy. *Early Human Development, 25,* 19–35.

Sachis, P. N., Armstrong, D., Becker, L., & Bryan, A. (1982). Myelination of the human vagus nerve from 24 weeks postconceptional age to adolescence. *Journal of Neuropathology and Experimental Neurology, 41,* 466–472.

Sandman, C. A., Wadhwa, P. D., Chicz-DeMet, A., Dunkel-Schetter, C., & Porto, M. (1997a). Maternal stress, HPA activity, and fetal/infant outcome. *Annals of the New York Academy of Sciences, 814,* 266–275.

Sandman, C. A., Wadhwa, P., Hetrick, W., Porto, M., & Peeke, H. (1997b). Human fetal heart rate dishabituation between thirty and thirty-two weeks gestation. *Child Development, 68,* 1031–1040.

Searle, J. R., Devoe, L. D., Phillips, M. C., & Searle, N. (1988). Computerized analysis of resting fetal heart rate tracings. *Obstetrics and Gynecology, 71*(3), 407–411.

Sherer, D. M., Abramowicz, J. S., Hearn-Stebbins, B., & Woods, J. R. (1991). Sonographic verification of a nuchal cord following a vibratory acoustic stimulation-induced severe variable fetal heart rate deceleration with expedient abdominal delivery. *American Journal of Perinatology, 8,* 345–346.

Shono, M., Shono, H., & Sugimori, H. (2000). Dynamic changes in the middle cerebral artery perfusion in normal full-term human fetuses in relation to the timing of behavioral state. *Early Human Development, 58,* 57–67.

Sival, D. A. (1993). Studies on fetal motor behaviour in normal and complicated pregnancies. *Early Human Development, 34,* 13–20.

Sival, D. A., Visser, G. H., & Prechtl, H. F. (1992). The effect of intrauterine growth retardation on the quality of general movements in the human fetus. *Early Human Development, 28,* 119–132.

Smotherman, W. P., & Robinson, S. R. (1996). The development of behavior before birth. *Developmental Psychology, 32*(3), 425–434.

Snidman, N., Kagan, J., Riordan, L., & Shannon, D. (1995). Cardiac function and behavioral reactivity during infancy. *Psychophysiology, 32,* 199–207.

Sontag, L. W., & Richards, T. W. (1938). Studies in Fetal Behavior: I. Fetal heart rate as a behavioral indicator. *Monographs of the Society for Research in Child Development, 3*(Serial No. 17), 1–67.

Sontag, L. W., & Wallace, R. F. (1934). Preliminary report of the Fels Fund. *American Journal of Diseases of Children, 48,* 1050–1057.

Sontag, L. W., & Wallace, R. F. (1935). The movement response of the human fetus to sound stimuli. *Child Development, 6,* 253–258.

Sparling, J. W., & Wilhelm, I. J. (1993). Concepts in fetal movement research. In J. W. Sparling (Ed.), *Concepts in fetal movement research* (pp. 97–114). Binghamton, NY: Haworth Press.

St. James-Roberts, I., & Menon-Johansson, P. (1999). Predicting infant crying from fetal movement data: an exploratory study. *Early Human Development, 54,* 55–62.

Stanley, F. (1994). The aetiology of cerebral palsy. *Early Human Development, 36,* 81–88.

Street, P., Dawes, G. S., Moulden, M., & Redman, C. W. G. (1991). Short-term variation in abnormal antenatal fetal heart records. *American Journal of Obstetrics & Gynecology, 165*(3), 515–523.

Suzuki, S., & Yamamuro, T. (1985). Fetal movement and fetal presentation. *Early Human Development, 11,* 255–263.

Swartjes, J. M., van Geijn, H. P., Mantel, R., & Schoemaker, H. C. (1992). Quantified fetal heart rhythm at 20, 32, and 38 weeks of gestation and dependence on rest–activity patterns. *Early Human Development, 28,* 27–36.

Swartjes, J. M., van Geijn, H. P., Mantel, R., & van Woerden, E. E. (1990). Coincidence of behavioral state parameters in the human fetus at three gestational ages. *Early Human Development, 23,* 75–83.

ten Hof, J., Nijhuis, I. J., Nijhuis, J. G., Narayan, H., Taylor, D. J., Visser, G. H., & Mulder, E. J. (1999a). Quantitative analysis of fetal generalized movements: Methodological considerations. *Early Human Development, 56,* 57–73.

ten Hof, J., Nijhuis, I. J. M., Mulder, E. J. H., Nijhuis, J. G., Narayan, H., Taylor, D. J., Westers, P., & Visser, G. H. A. (1999b). *A longitudinal study of fetal body movements: Nomograms, intrafetal consistency and relationship with the rest–activity cycle.* Manuscript submitted for publication.

Thomas, P. W., Haslum, M. N., MacGillivray, I., & Golding, M. J. (1989). Does fetal heart rate predict subsequent heart rate in childhood? *Early Human Development, 19,* 147–152.

Timor-Tritsch, I. E., Dierker, L. J., Hertz, R. H., Deagan, C., & Rosen, M. G. (1978a). Studies of antepartum behavioral states in the human fetus at term. *American Journal of Obstetrics and Gynecology, 132,* 524–528.

Timor-Tritsch, I. E., Dierker, L. J., Zador, I., Hertz, R. H., & Rosen, M. G. (1978b). Fetal movements associated with fetal heart rate accelerations and decelerations. *American Journal of Obstetrics and Gynecology, 131*(3), 276–280.

Timor-Tritsch, I., Zador, I., Hertz, R., & Rosen, M. (1977). Human fetal respiratory arrhythmia. *American Journal of Obstetrics and Gynecology, 127,* 662–666.

Todd, A. L., Trudinger, B. J., Cole, M. J., & Cooney, G. H. (1992). Antenatal tests of fetal welfare and development at age 2 years. *American Journal of Obstetrics and Gynecology, 167,* 66–77.

Van den Bergh, B. R. H., Mulder, E. J. H., Visser, G. H. A., Poelmann-Weesjes, G., Bekedam, D. J., & Prechtl, H. F. R. (1989). The effect of (induced) maternal emotions on fetal behaviour: A controlled study. *Early Human Development, 19,* 9–19.

van de Pas, M., Nijhuis, J. G., & Jongsma, H. W. (1994). Fetal behaviour in uncomplicated pregnancies after 41 weeks of gestation. *Early Human Development, 40,* 29–38.

van Heeswijk, M., Nijhuis, J. G., & Hollanders, H. M. (1990). Fetal heart rate in early pregnancy. *Early Human Development, 22,* 151–156.

van Hetteren, C. F., Boekkooi, P., Jongsma, H., & Nijhuis, J. G. (2000). Fetal learning and memory. *Lancet, 356,* 1169–1170.

van Vliet, M. A., Martin, C. B., Nijhuis, J. G., & Prechtl, H. F. R. (1985a). Behavioural states in the fetuses of nulliparous women. *Early Human Development, 12,* 121–135.

van Vliet, M. A. T., Martin, C. B., Nijhuis, J. G., & Prechtl, H. F. R. (1985b). Behavioural states in growth-retarded human fetuses. *Early Human Development, 12,* 183–197.

van Woerden, E. E., vanGeijn, H. P., Caron, F. J. M., Swartjes, J. M., Mantel, R., & Arts, N. F. (1989). Automated assignment of behavioural states in the human near term fetus. *Early Human Development, 19,* 137–146.

Vindla, S., & James, D. (1995). Fetal behavior as a test of fetal well being. *British Journal of Obstetrics and Gynecology, 102,* 597–600.

Vintzileos, A. M., & Knuppel, R. A. (1994). Multiple parameter biophysical testing in the prediction of fetal acid-base status. *Clinics in Perinatology, 21*(4), 823–848.

Visser, G. H. A., & Mulder, E. J. H. (1993). The effect of vibroacoustic stimulation on fetal behavioral state organization. *American Journal of Industrial Medicine, 23,* 531–539.

Visser, G. H. A., Mulder, E. J. H., Stevens, H., & Verweij, R. (1993). Heart rate variation during fetal behavioral states 1 and 2. *Early Human Development, 34,* 21–28.

Visser, G. H. A., Mulder, H. H., Mulder, E. J. H., & Prechtl, H. F. R. (1989). Vibroacoustic stimulation of the human fetus: effect on behavioral state organization. *Early Human Development, 19,* 285–296.

Visser, G. H. A., Poelmann-Weesjes, G., Cohen, T. M., & Bekedam, D. J. (1987). Fetal behavior at 30 to 32 weeks of gestation. *Pediatric Research, 22,* 655–658.

Visser, G. H. A., Zeelenberg, H. J., deVries, J. I., & Dawes, G. S. (1983). External physical stimulation of the human fetus during episodes of low heart rate variation. *American Journal of Obstetrics and Gynecology, 145,* 579–584.

Ware, D. J., & Devoe, L. D. (1994). The nonstress test: Reassessment of the "gold standard." *Clinics in Perinatology, 21*(4), 779–796.

Yeh, S. Y., Forsythe, A., & Hon, E. H. (1973). Quantification of fetal heart beat-to-beat interval differences. *Obstetrics and Gynecology, 41*(3), 355–363.

Yoshizato, T., Koyanagi, T., Takashima, T., Satoh, S., Akazawa, K., & Nakano, H. (1994). The relationship between age-related heart rate changes and developing brain function: A model of anencephalic human fetuses in utero. *Early Human Development, 36,* 101–112.

Zimmer, E. Z., & Divon, M. Y. (1993). Fetal vibroacoustic stimulation. *Obstetrics and Gynecology, 81,* 451–457.

Zimmer, E. Z., Fifer, W. P., Kim, Y., Rey, H. R., Chao, C. R., & Myers, M. M. (1993). Response of the premature fetus to stimulation by speech sounds. *Early Human Development, 33,* 207–215.

4

Visual Acuity Assessment in Infancy

D. LUISA MAYER
ROBERT E. ARENDT

HISTORY

The study of human visual development was spurred by the fusion of research from two areas. Berlyne (1966) and Fantz (1965) independently found that using precisely controlled visual stimuli, it was possible to measure behaviorally an infant's ability to discriminate between systematically varied visual patterns. At the same time, electrophysiological and anatomical discoveries of Wiesel and Hubel (1963) showed that patterns of early visual stimulation could produce measurable differences in the developing cortex of animals.

A major challenge to any study of infant development is the infant's inability to use language to communicate. Currently a variety of test instruments and methodologies exist to evaluate visual functioning in infants and young children (Vital-Durand, Atkinson, & Braddick, 1996). At least four approaches are used to assess visual acuity in this age range: (1) tracking, (2) optokinetic response, (3) visual evoked response, and (4) preferential looking (PL) tasks. Behavioral methods with greatest practical value have their basis in the PL technique (Fantz, Fagan, & Miranda, 1975).

To measure visual acuity, Fantz (1958) presented a black-and-white grating stimulus paired with a blank stimulus. Because infants could discriminate between grating and blank stimuli on brightness differences alone, the stimulus had to be equal in space-averaged luminance to the blank stimulus. The finest grating that a group of infants of a specific age preferred significantly over the blank stimulus was taken as the average acuity for that age group.

Teller (1979) appreciated that Fantz's PL technique provided a simple and elegant means to explore infants' visual sensory abilities using their natural looking behaviors. Teller (1979), however, discerned that Fantz's PL paradigm was not objective and was susceptible to observer bias and that data from individual infants could not be obtained. She, therefore, devised a forced-choice preferential looking (FPL) paradigm using principles of adult visual psychophysics (for review, see Teller, 1979).

In FPL there is an objective stimulus referent—a grating on the right or left. The observer's task is to say whether the grating is on the right or left (thus, "forced choice") based on the infant's behavior. The observer makes this decision without prior knowledge of the grating position. Trial-by-trial feedback is given to the observer as to the correctness of right/left judgments, which is intended to improve and stabilize performance. A large number of trials of varying grating spatial frequencies[1] are presented, from well above to below threshold. Acuity is derived statistically and is defined as the grating spatial frequency corresponding to the observer's percent correct performance, typically 75% correct.

Using FPL and its variants, researchers have measured infant visual acuity in numerous studies (see review in Dobson, 1993). Other visual functions studied using FPL include color vision, night vision, and stereopsis (see review in Teller, 1982).

DESCRIPTION OF THE ACUITY CARD PROCEDURE

Following the first reports of acuity in infants, clinicians sought to apply the FPL methodology to the study of pediatric patients. FPL in its laboratory versions, however, is time-consuming, requiring several adults and relatively elaborate equipment. Attempts by researchers to modify FPL for clinical populations used short-cut psychophysical procedures to reduce testing time (see reviews in Birch & Hale, 1988; Dobson, 1993; Gwiazda, Wolfe, Brill, Mohindra, & Held, 1980; Mayer & Dobson, 1997; Teller, McDonald, Preston, Sebris, & Dobson, 1986). Although modifications of FPL were successful in clinical research studies (Birch, Stager, & Wright, 1986), they have been criticized on statistical grounds (McKee, Klein, & Teller, 1985).

To address the need for an efficient, inexpensive, and valid technique to measure visual acuity in infants, Teller et al. (1986) developed the Acuity Card Procedure (ACP). In the ACP, grating stimuli on individual rectangular cards are presented behind the window of a "stage apparatus." As in FPL, the acuity tester observes the infant's looking behaviors through a central peephole. Gratings are shown in a series ranging from suprathreshold (coarse) to progressively finer gratings, until the infant shows no detection of a grating. The number of presentations of a grating needed before the observer can make that judgment is not set. Multiple presentations of gratings around the infant's threshold are shown until the observer is confident that the finest grating that the infant detects has been reached: This is the infant's acuity.

The crucial distinction between FPL and the ACP is that the observer's role is no longer solely to judge the right/left position of the grating on each trial but to judge whether the infant detects each grating shown. The tester in the ACP controls all aspects of the test; presenting the stimuli, observing the infant's visual responses, and determining the infant's acuity. An important aspect of Teller's FPL technique is retained, however, in that the observer remains unaware of the grating position on each card until a judgment is made as to whether the infant detects that grating. Details regarding variations in ACP methods are described elsewhere (see Mayer & Dobson, 1997).

In the ACP, the observer uses differential cues as to the infant's detection of gratings (e.g., eye widening and sustained fixations for suprathreshold gratings vs. saccades and brief fixations for gratings around the infant's threshold). The flexibility of the ACP allows testing of acuity through the early years, when behavioral repertoires change markedly, from reflexive orienting to systematic scanning of the cards after 6 months to pointing and labeling responses at 2 and 3 years (see Mayer et al., 1995, Table 4).

GENERAL DESCRIPTION

The Teller Acuity Cards (TAC®) (Vistech Consultants, 1991) stimuli and ACP variation of the FPL technique provide the most sensitive, easily interpreted, noninvasive measure of infant visual acuity available. The original cards (Teller et al., 1986) were rectangular with a circular grating and a blank position on each and a central peephole, replicating the original FPL stimulus configuration. The current series of 16 commercially available cards are similar but with no discrete "blank" position. A square grating patch (12 cm × 12 cm) is situated 7.5 cm away from a central peephole on a rectangular gray card of the same space-averaged luminance as the grating. A stage apparatus is also sold in which the cards are presented behind a window in a central screen. Panels on each side of the front screen minimize infant distractions. A shield sets the test distance of the infant from the cards and also blocks the sight of the cards from the person holding the infant.

An unexpected advantage of TAC for clinical populations is that the cards can be presented out of the apparatus at any distance and in any orientation (Trueb, Evans, Hammel, Bartholomew, & Dobson, 1992). In this procedure, the cards are free-held before the infant and the tester observes the infant over the top or to one side of the cards. This feature is especially helpful for testing infants with oculomotor abnormalities (e.g., esotropia and nystagmus) or with neuromotor disabilities (e.g., cerebral palsy). Testing can usually be completed in 10 minutes or less.

BIOBEHAVIORAL BASIS OF VISUAL ACUITY ASSESSMENT IN INFANTS

Visual acuity can be theoretically and experimentally linked to the most proximal pattern-resolving elements of the visual system, cone photo-receptors and ganglion cells (Wilson, 1993). In immature primates, several models have been proposed to account for the reduced acuity of neonates versus adults (Banks & Bennett, 1988; Brown, 1994; Wilson, 1988). Models differ in assumptions regarding the immature receptoral and postreceptoral processes, and all are limited by a paucity of relevant anatomic data. However, models agree generally that prereceptoral factors (optics of the eye) and the development of cone photoreceptors (changes in morphology and distribution) can account for some but not all differences between infant and adult visual acuity. Changes in postreceptoral factors, including neural development of the lateral geniculate nucleus and striate cortex, are required to account for behavioral maturation of acuity, at least in monkeys (Jacobs & Blakemore, 1988).

RELIABILITY AND VALIDITY

Data on the reliability of acuities obtained with the ACP are expressed in terms of the interval between spatial frequencies in the acuity card set, or, more simply, in terms of the number of cards. In the full commercial TAC set, the interval between grating spatial frequencies (stripe width) is an average 0.5 octave(oct.).[2] Reliability of binocular and monocular acuities is similar.

In seven studies of normal full-term infants (Getz, Dobson, Luna, & Mash, 1996; Heersema & van Hof-van Duin, 1990; Mash & Dobson, 1995; Mayer et al., 1995; McDonald et al., 1985; McDonald, Ankrum, Preston, Sebris, & Dobson, 1986; McDonald, Sebris, Mohn, Teller, & Dobson, 1986), 86–98% of ACP acuities obtained by two testers agreed to within a *two-card* interval (1.0 oct in most studies). Within-tester agreement in the three studies reporting these data is 88–95% within a *one-card* interval (0.5 oct in most studies) (Mayer et al., 1995; Mash & Dobson, 1995; McDonald et al., 1985). This across-study comparison suggests that a second tester significantly increases (in fact, about doubles) the variability of acuity tested by a single tester. However, in studies in which both types of reliability were assessed, variability of between-tester measures was only slightly greater than within-tester variability (Mash & Dobson, 1995; Mash, Dobson, & Carpenter, 1994; Mayer et al., 1995; McDonald et al., 1985).

In clinical populations, between-tester reliability is lower than that for normal infants. Across six studies, 75–100% of between-tester comparisons were within two cards (1.0 oct) (Dobson, Carpenter, Bonvalot, & Bossler, 1990; Getz et al., 1996; Hertz & Rosenberg, 1992; Hertz, Rosenberg, Sjo, & Warburg, 1988; Mash et al., 1994; Preston, McDonald, Sebris, Dobson, & Teller, 1987). Between-tester reliability in neurologically impaired children is low and is even further reduced in more severely impaired individuals (Hertz & Rosenberg, 1992; Hertz et al., 1988).

Aside from the increased statistical "noise" expected with a second tester, the increased variability of between-tester comparisons over within-tester ones may have a systematic component. That is, some testers' acuity estimates have been reported to be systematically higher or lower than acuities estimated by other testers (Getz et al., 1996; Mash et al., 1994; Mayer et al., 1995; Quinn, Berlin, & James, 1993; Teller, Mar, & Preston, 1992). Nevertheless, in these studies significant differences among testers were not shown for all age groups nor for all tester pairs and the majority of the mean differences between testers were less than one-card interval (0.5 oct) in the TAC (Quinn et al., 1993).

Visual acuity is a function not only of an infant's pattern resolution but also of an infant's immediate attentional state. Ill or sleepy infants exhibit delayed or intermittent responses to visual stimuli, resulting in low acuity estimates. Acuities of children with neurological impairments, who may be sedated by seizure medications, show higher day-to-day variability than do normal infants (Hertz & Rosenberg, 1992; Mash et al., 1994).

Other sources of variability include test distance, lighting, and certain procedural aspects. In addition, variation of the beginning spatial frequency of the card sequence ("random start card") may cause systematic differences in acuities (Dobson et al., 1990; Mash et al., 1994).

The maturation of acuity measured with ACP and FPL techniques is similar. Variation among mean acuities at specific ages by two variants of FPL and the ACP are of a similar magnitude (see Dobson, 1994, Figure 12.7), as is the variation across studies using the ACP (Mayer & Dobson, 1997).

Grating resolution acuity and letter or symbol recognition acuity are not necessarily identical in adults and children who can be tested with both methods. The relation between these two types of acuity is complex and depends on the type of underlying visual pathology. In individuals with normal acuity or mild acuity deficits, grating and recognition acuities are in good agreement generally (Dobson, Quinn, Tung, Palmer, & Reynolds, 1995; Mayer, 1986; Mayer, Fulton, & Rodier, 1984). As acuity worsens, however, recognition acuity becomes increasingly poorer than grating acuity.

Discrepancies between grating and recognition acuities are greatest in patients with central retinal (macula, fovea) abnormalities and in those with central neural visual pathway abnormalities (amblyopia) (Dobson et al., 1995; Friendly, Jaafar & Morillo, 1990; Levi & Klein, 1982; Mayer, 1986; Mayer et al., 1984; White & Loshin, 1989). A partial explanation for this may be the different retinal areas stimulated by gratings (peripheral and central retina) versus recognition targets (central retina only). More complex explanations than stimulus size differences are required to account for discrepancies between grating and recognition acuities in amblyopia (Friendly et al., 1990; Gstalder & Green, 1971; Levi & Klein, 1982; Mayer, 1986).

Visual acuity in a small sample of children with cortical visual impairment was found to be correlated with sensorimotor skills but not with gross motor skills (Birch & Bane, 1991). In a large population of infants with severe ocular disorders, most with retinopathy of prematurity (ROP), visual acuity was correlated with scores from a parental inventory of the infant's daily life skills (Katsumi et al., 1998).

DEVELOPMENTAL MODEL

Grating acuity improves systematically with age (Dobson, 1993, 1994). Maturation can be described as a growth curve with acuity plotted on a logarithmic scale against linear age. There is an early rapid phase of improvement, from 1 cyc/deg at 1-month postnatal age to approximately 6 cyc/deg at 6 months of age. Acuity improves more slowly thereafter, to about 30 cyc/deg by 4 to 5 years of age. The rate of improvement between 6 months and 60 months is about one-tenth the rate of improvement between 1 and 6 months (Mayer & Dobson, 1997).

The average curve described previously does not, however, represent the maturation of acuity of all individual infants. Mash and Dobson (1998) identified three clusters of acuity maturation in a population of neonatal intensive care unit (NICU) survivors with mostly normal acuity. Only one of the three curves, with, notably, the largest number of individuals (33 vs. 19 in the other two groups), approximated the average maturation curve.

Grating acuity matures in healthy preterm infants at the same rate as in term infants, but the course of maturation is in better agreement with the infant's gestational (corrected) age at test rather than postnatal age (Birch & Spencer, 1991; Brown & Yamamoto, 1986; Dubowitz, Dubowitz, & Morante, 1980; Getz, Dobson, & Luna, 1992; Searle, Horne, & Bourne, 1989; van Hof-van Duin & Mohn, 1986). Slightly higher average acuity has been found in preterm than term infants when corrected ages are used (Norcia, Tyler, Piecuch, Clyman, & Grobstein, 1987; Searle et al., 1989; van Hof-van Duin & Mohn, 1986).

STRUCTURAL/THEORETICAL CONSTRAINTS

Visual acuity is the single most widely measured visual function and the most useful measure of vision for individuals with ocular disorders. It measures vision for details under photopic conditions (day vision) and is affected by damage to ocular and/or brain structures. It cannot precisely localize specific sites of abnormalities in the visual pathway, except that differences between eyes can reveal damage greater to one eye than to the other, as well as the presence of amblyopia (loss of visual acuity not attributable to structural ocular, refractive, or oculomotor causes).

Brain damage due to early (prenatal, perinatal) ischemic events can cause optic atrophy in extreme cases, as well as damage to the oculomotor control structures, misalignment of the eyes, and failure to develop normal refractive status. Thus the cause(s) of reduced visual acuity in infants with brain damage may be difficult to determine. In a study of very-low-birthweight infants with and without echolucencies (suggestive of white matter damage or periventricular leukomalacia) on cranial ultrasound, visual acuity deficits in infants with echolucencies were poorer than those without echolucencies, even after control for oculomotor and refractive anomalies (San Giovanni et al., 2000). The results of this study confirm results of other studies (Eken, de Vries, van der Graff, Meiners, & van Nieuwenhuizen, 1995; Eken, van Nieuwenhuizen, van der Graff, Schalij-Delfos, & de Vries, 1994; Gibson, Fielder, Trounce, & Levene, 1990; van Hof-van Duin, Evenhius-van Leunen, Mohn, Baerts, & Fetter, 1989), suggesting that postchiasmal factors contribute to visual acuity loss in neonatal white matter disorders independent of prechiasmal factors.

METHODS OF REDUCING VARIABILITY IN ACP/FPL

One way that variability can be minimized is to regulate procedures that directly affect visual acuity, such as illumination of the stimuli and the test distance between the infant and the stimulus. Changes in illumination can cause differences in acuity, particularly at luminances below standard room lighting. Inconsistencies in test distance can also lead to variability in acuities. For example, if the tester assumes that the acuity card is being shown at 55 cm, but the actual distance is nearer to (farther from) the infant, acuity will be overestimated (underestimated).

Use of the ACP should include testing with the screen apparatus (large version) that accompanies the TAC. The light meter provided should be used to ensure that the cards are illuminated appropriately. Additional lighting may be needed to achieve the appropriate card luminance. Monocular norms determined in the Mayer et al. (1995) study used a similar luminance level to that measured by the Vistech light meter. The Instruction Manual© (Vistech Consultants, 1991) has useful information regarding stimulus and apparatus material, controlling for distance and luminance, advice for observing infants, and training of testers.

Tester experience also contributes to variability, as do multiple testers.

Grating acuities may be higher in young infants who are turned actively toward each stimulus position, versus infants seated in a parent's lap or passively held before the stimulus (see Dobson, 1994). A holder with training in "rotating the infant" should hold the infant when infants are between birth and about 4 months of age.

Variability in acuity measures could be reduced, at least theoretically, by correction for age at test relative to gestational age at birth. However, this correction may increase variability unless estimation of gestational age is accurate. Because of the rapid maturation of acuity from birth to 6 months, correction for gestational age will have a larger effect at younger than older ages.

TRAINING REQUIREMENTS

To ensure that acuity results obtained by ACP in research studies of infants have acceptable test–retest reliability, we recommend the following:

1. Before testing, testers should read all relevant materials on ACP testing procedures, including the TAC Instruction Manual and the original papers (Courage & Adams, 1990; Dobson, 1994; Mayer et al., 1995; Salomao & Ventura, 1995).
2. Practice should begin with normal infants, followed by infants from the population and age range of study. For tests of normal infants, all acuities should be within the 99% prediction (Mayer et al., 1995) or 90% tolerance limits with 95% confidence (Salomao & Ventura, 1995) (these are identical). For monocular norms, use Mayer et al. (1995) and for binocular norms, use Courage and Adams (1990) or Salomao and Ventura (1995), and *not* the normative values in the current TAC Instruction Manual. Differences between testers' estimates in the same normal infants should differ by no more than 1 octave (two cards) in 90% of between-tester comparisons.
3. Systematic differences between testers should be monitored.
4. Tests of infants 4 months of age and younger should use a trained holder to maximize the infant's attentiveness and to keep the infant at the correct distance from the cards. Infants 5 months and older can be seated in the parent's lap. The holder or parent should be screened from seeing the acuity cards so that he or she cannot influence the infant's responses to the acuity cards.

Because young infants tend to be alert for relatively short periods and need to be fed, diapered, and so on, holders and testers should become experienced in determining whether the infant's state of arousal is appropriate before and during testing. Breaks during testing and between tests may be required to ensure a relatively constant state of alertness.

IMPLICATIONS

The important role vision plays in the development of infants is highlighted by the predominant place perceptual learning has played in the scientific investigation of human development (Spelke & Newport, 1998). It is surprising that measures of visual acuity are so infrequently included in studies that require visual ability.

Recent studies, using infant visual attention methodology, support the concept of continuity in mental development (Bornstein & Sigman, 1986; Fagan & Singer, 1983; Singer & Fagan, 1984). Stability in visual acuity might underlie both cognitive and behavioral stability in early development, thereby fostering continuity. A question arises, therefore, as to whether a visual attention task is sensitive to variations in cognitive development or is primarily assessing the ability of the infant to perceive and respond to visual stimuli. Without a measure of the latter, the former cannot be logically inferred.

Infants' performance on novelty preference/recognition memory tasks depends on their ability to discriminate between visual stimuli, for example, familiar versus novel faces or facial expressions in the Fagan Test of Infant Intelligence (Fagan & Shepard, 1983; see Rose & Orlian, Chapter 13, and Fagen & Ohr, Chapter 12, this volume). Perceptual aspects of the stimuli are deemed critical to infants' preferences. However, such visual discriminations rely on differentiating low-level stimulus information—spatial frequency, contrast, orientation—prior to encoding perceptual content. That is, an infant must be able to see the critical stimulus attributes before he or she can discriminate between them. An infant with reduced acuity may fail to perceive a novel face due solely to sensory and not perceptual visual difficulties. Thus, we recommend that visual acuity be tested in infant studies using behavioral outcomes that rely on visual discriminations.

In our prospective study of visual and neuromotor development of very-low-birthweight infants with and without abnormal neonatal cranial ultrasounds, infants with white matter damage were more likely than those without to have reduced visual acuity *and* lower Fagan test scores (Stewart, Mayer, & San Giovanni, 1999). Notable as well was a higher prevalence of oculomotor and refractive anomalies in the infants with white matter damage and reduced visual abilities (San Giovanni et al., 2000). We therefore recommend that future studies should either exclude all subjects with oculomotor, refractive, or ocular abnormalities or, more practically, control statistically for these problems. Case–control designs (with matching for potentially confounding eye problems) have significant advantages in such studies. If possible, eye examinations should be performed in all study infants near the time of outcome measurement, particularly in studies of high-risk infants (e.g., preterm infants and brain-damaged infants).

Quantitative analyses of low-level properties of visual stimulation in novelty preference/recognition memory tasks may provide insights into the aspects of these stimuli being discriminated by infants. Determining the extent to which complexity, symmetry, familiarity, and ecological salience govern infant's visual preferences will require exclusion of differences in basic visual processing. This direction of research could lead to designing visual stimuli to test specific aspects of lower- and higher-level visual processes in infant development.

Finally, even though the visual system by itself is highly complex, one of the hallmarks of early development is the integration of information from multiple sensory modalities into adaptive behavior patterns. Given that the visual system matures at a rate different from other sensory systems, how changes in visual abilities relate to other extant or emerging sensory abilities is still largely unexplored. The temporal correspondence between functional levels of different sensorimotor systems may be of particular interest in children with delays or deficits in one or more modality.

ACKNOWLEDGMENTS

We are greatly indebted to Dr. Velma Dobson, coauthor of Mayer and Dobson (1997), which provided the basis for much of this chapter. Thanks also to Terri Lotz-Ganley for her assistance in preparing the manuscript. Preparation of this chapter was supported in part by National Institute on Drug Abuse Grant No. DA-07358.

NOTES

1. Spatial frequency refers to the number of black/white bar cycles per degree of visual angle (cyc/deg). Low spatial frequencies consist of wider bars and high spatial frequencies consist of thinner bars.
2. An octave is a halving or doubling of spatial frequency, for example, from 10 to 20 cyc/deg.

REFERENCES

Banks, M. S., & Bennett, P. J. (1988). Optical and photoreceptor immaturities limit the spatial and chromatic vision of human neonates. *Journal of the Optical Society of America, 5,* 2059–2079.
Berlyne, D. E. (1966). Curiosity and exploration. *Science, 153,* 25–33.
Birch, E. E., & Bane, M. C. (1991). Forced-choice preferential looking acuity of children

with cortical visual impairment. *Developmental Medicine and Child Neurology, 33,* 722–729.

Birch, E. E., & Hale, L. A. (1988). Criteria for monocular acuity deficit in infancy and early childhood. *Investigative Ophthalmology and Visual Science, 29,* 636–643.

Birch, E. E., & Spencer, R. (1991). Monocular grating acuity of healthy preterm infants. *Clinical Vision Sciences, 6,* 331–334.

Birch, E. E., Stager, D. R., & Wright, W. W. (1986). Grating acuity development after early surgery for congenital unilateral cataract. *Archives of Ophthalmology, 104,* 1783–1787.

Bornstein, M. H., & Sigman, M. D. (1986). Continuity in mental development from infancy. *Child Development, 57,* 251–274.

Brown, A. M. (1994). Intrinsic contrast noise and infant visual contrast discrimination. *Vision Research, 34,* 1947–1964.

Brown, A. M., & Yamamoto, M. (1986). Visual acuity in newborn and preterm infants measured with grating acuity cards. *American Journal of Ophthalmology, 102,* 245–253.

Courage, M. L., & Adams, R. J. (1990). Visual acuity assessment from birth to three years using the acuity card procedure: Cross sectional and longitudinal samples. *Optometry and Vision Science, 67,* 713–718.

Dobson, V. (1993). Visual acuity testing in infants: From laboratory to clinic. In K. Simons (Ed.), *Early visual development, normal and abnormal* (pp. 318–334). New York: Oxford University Press.

Dobson, V. (1994). Visual acuity testing by preferential looking techniques. In S. J. Isenberg (Ed.), *Eye in infancy* (pp. 131–156). St Louis, MO: Mosby.

Dobson, V., Carpenter, N. A., Bonvalot, K., & Bossler, J. (1990). The acuity card procedure: Interobserver agreement in infants with perinatal complications. *Clinical Vision Sciences, 6,* 39–48.

Dobson, V., Quinn, G. E., Tung, B., Palmer, E. A., & Reynolds, J. D. (1995). Comparison of recognition and grating acuities in very-low-birth-weight children with and without retinal residua of retinopathy of prematurity. *Investigative Ophthalmology and Visual Science, 36,* 692–702.

Dubowitz, L. M. S., Dubowitz, V., & Morante, V. (1980). Visual function in the newborn: A study of preterm and full-term infants. *Brain Development, 2,* 15–29.

Eken, P., de Vries, L. S., van der Graff, Y., Meiners, L. C., & van Nieuwenhuizen, O. (1995). Haemorrhagic–ischaemic lesions of the neonatal brain: Correlation between cerebral visual impairment, neurodevelopmental outcome and MRI in infancy. *Developmental Medicine and Child Neurology, 37,* 41–55.

Eken, P., van Nieuwenhuizen, O., van der Graff, Y., Schalij-Delfos, N., & de Vries, L. S. (1994). Relation between neonatal cranial ultrasound abnormalities and cerebral visual impairment in infancy. *Developmental Medicine and Child Neurology, 36,* 3–15.

Fagan, J. F., & Shepard, P. A. (1983). *Fagan test of infant intelligence: Training manual.* Cleveland, OH: Infantest Corporation.

Fagan, J. F., & Singer, L. T. (1983). Infant recognition memory as a measure of intelligence. In L. Lipsitt & C. Rovee-Collier (Eds.), *Advances in infancy research* (Vol. 2, pp. 31–78). Norwood, NJ: Ablex.

Fantz, R. L. (1958). Pattern vision in young infants. *The Psychological Record, 8,* 43–47.

Fantz, R. L. (1965). Visual perception from birth as shown by pattern selectivity. *Annals of New York Academy of Science, 118,* 793–814.

Fantz, R. L., Fagan, J. F., & Miranda, S. B. (1975). Early visual selectivity as a function of pattern variables, previous exposure, age from birth and conception and expected cognitive deficit. In L. Cohen & P. Salapatek (Eds.), *Infant perception: From sensation to cognition* (Vol. 1, pp. 249–235). New York: Academic Press.

Friendly, D. S., Jaafar, M. S., & Morillo, D. L. (1990). A comparative study of grating and recognition visual acuity testing in children with anisometropic amblyopia without strabismus. *American Journal of Ophthalmology, 110,* 293–299.

Getz, L., Dobson, V., & Luna, B. (1992). Grating acuity development in 2-week-old to 3-year-old child born prior to term. *Clinical Vision Sciences, 7,* 252–256.

Getz, L. M., Dobson, V., Luna, B., & Mash, C. (1996). Interobserver reliability of the Teller acuity card procedure in pediatric patients. *Investigative Ophthalmology and Visual Science, 37,* 180–187.

Gibson, N. A., Fielder, A. R., Trounce, J. Q., & Levene, M. I. (1990). Ophthalmic findings in infants of very low birthweight. *Developmental Medicine and Child Neurology, 32,* 7–13.

Gstalder, R. J., & Green, D. G. (1971). Laser interferometric acuity in amblyopia. *Journal of Pediatric Ophthalmology, 8,* 251–256.

Gwiazda, J., Wolfe, J. M., Brill, S., Mohindra, I., & Held, R. (1980). Quick assessment of preferential looking acuity in infants. *American Journal of Optometry and Physiological Optics, 57,* 420–427.

Heersema, D. J., & van Hof-van Duin, J. (1990). Age norms for visual acuity in toddlers using the acuity card procedure. *Clinical Vision Sciences, 5,* 167–174.

Hertz, B. G., & Rosenberg, J. (1992). Acuity card testing of spastic children: Preliminary results. *Journal of Pediatric Ophthalmology and Strabismus, 254,* 139–144.

Hertz, B. G., Rosenberg, J., Sjo, O., & Warburg, M. (1988). Acuity card testing of patients with cerebral visual impairment. *Developmental Medicine and Child Neurology, 30,* 632–637.

Jacobs, D. S., & Blakemore, C. (1988). Factors limiting the postnatal development of visual acuity in the monkey. *Vision Research, 28,* 947–958.

Katsumi, O., Chedid, S. G., Kronheim, J. K., Henry, R. K., Jones, C. M., & Hirose, T. (1998). Visual Ability Score—A new method to analyze ability in visually impaired children. *Acta Ophthalmologica Scandinavica, 76,* 50–55.

Levi, D. M., & Klein, S. (1982). Differences in vernier discriminations for gratings between strabismic and anisometropic amblyopes. *Investigative Ophthalmology and Visual Science, 23,* 398–407.

Mash, C., & Dobson, V. (1995). The Teller Acuity Card procedure: Intraobserver agreement among a sample of infants treated in a neonatal intensive care unit (NICU). *Investigative Ophthalmology and Visual Science, 36,* S369.

Mash, C. W., & Dobson, V. (1998). Long-term reliability and predictive validity of the Teller acuity card procedure. *Vision Research, 38,* 619–626.

Mash, C., Dobson, V., & Carpenter, N. (1994). Interobserver agreement for measurement of grating acuity and interocular acuity differences with the Teller acuity card procedure. *Vision Research, 35,* 303–312.

Mayer, D. L. (1986). Acuity of amblyopic children for small field gratings and recognition stimuli. *Investigative Ophthalmology and Visual Science, 27,* 1148–1153.

Mayer, D. L., Beiser, A. S., Warner, A. F., Pratt, E. M., Raye, K. N., & Lang, J. M. (1995). Monocular acuity norms for the Teller acuity cards between ages 1 month and 4 years. *Investigative Ophthalmology and Visual Science, 76,* 671–685.

Mayer, D. L., & Dobson, V. (1997). Grating acuity cards: Validity and reliability in studies of human visual development. In J. Dobbing (Ed.), *Developing brain and behaviour: The role of lipids in infant formula* (pp. 253–292). San Diego, CA: Academic Press.

Mayer, D. L., Fulton, A. B., & Rodier, D. (1984). Grating and recognition acuities of pediatric patients. *Ophthalmology, 91,* 947–953.

McDonald, M., Ankrum, C., Preston, K., Sebris, S. L., & Dobson, V. (1986). Monocular and binocular acuity estimation in 18– to 36–month-olds: Acuity card results. *American Journal of Optometry and Physiological Optics, 63,* 181–186.

McDonald, M., Dobson, V., Sebris, S. L., Baitch, L., Varner, D., & Teller, D. Y. (1985). The acuity card procedure: A rapid test of infant acuity. *Investigative Ophthalmology and Visual Science, 26,* 1158–1162.

McDonald, M., Sebris, S. L., Mohn, G., Teller, D. Y., & Dobson, V. (1986). Monocular acuity in normal infants: The acuity card procedure. *American Journal of Optometry and Physiological Optics, 63,* 127–134.

McKee, S. P., Klein, S. A., & Teller, D. Y. (1985). Statistical properties of forced-choice psychometric functions: Implications of probit analysis. *Perception and Psychophysics, 37,* 286–298.

Norcia, A. M., Tyler, C. W., Piecuch, R., Clyman, R., & Grobstein, J. (1987). Visual acuity development in normal and abnormal preterm human infants. *Journal of Pediatric Ophthalmology and Strabismus, 24,* 70–74.

Preston, K. L., McDonald, M. A., Sebris, S. L., Dobson, V., & Teller, D. Y. (1987). Validation of the acuity card procedure for assessment of infants with ocular disorders. *Ophthalmology, 95,* 644–653.

Quinn, G. E., Berlin, J. A., & James, M. (1993). The Teller Acuity Card procedure: Three testers in a clinical setting. *Ophthalmology, 100,* 488–494.

Salomao, S. R., & Ventura D. F. (1995). Large-sample population norms for visual acuities obtained with Vistech/Teller Acuity Cards. *Investigative Ophthalmology and Visual Science, 36,* 657–670.

San Giovanni, J., Allred, E. N., Mayer, D. L., Stewart, J. E., Herrera, M. G., & Leviton, A. (2000). Reduced visual resolution acuity and cerebral white matter damage in very-low-birthweight infants. *Developmental Medicine and Child Neurology, 42,* 809–815.

Searle, C., Horne, S. M., & Bourne, K. M. (1989). Visual acuity development: A study of preterm and full-term infants. *Australian and New Zealand Journal of Ophthalmology, 17,* 23–26.

Singer, L. T., & Fagan, J. F. (1984). Cognitive development in the failure-to-thrive infant: A three year longitudinal study. *Journal of Pediatric Psychology, 9,* 363–383.

Spelke, E. S., & Newport, E. L. (1998). Nativism, empiricism, and the development of knowledge. In W. Damon (Ed.), *Handbook of child psychology: Vol. 1. Theoretical models of human development* (5th ed., pp. 275–340). New York: Wiley.

Stewart, J., Mayer, D. L., & San Giovanni, J. P. (1999). *Visual deficits in infants with echolucencies.* Unpublished raw data.

Teller, D. Y. (1979). The forced-choice preferential looking procedure: A psychophysical technique for use with human infants. *Infant Behavior and Development, 2,* 135–153.

Teller, D. Y. (1982). Scotopic vision, color vision, and stereopsis in infants. *Current Eye Research, 2,* 199–210.

Teller, D. Y., Mar, C., & Preston, K. L. (1992). Statistical properties of 500-trial infant psychometric functions. In L. A. Werner & E. W. Rubel (Eds.), *Developmental psychoacoustics* (pp. 211–227). Washington, DC: American Psychological Association.

Teller, D. Y., McDonald, M., Preston, K., Sebris, S. L., & Dobson, V. (1986). Assessment of visual acuity in infants and children: The acuity card procedure. *Developmental Medicine and Child Neurology, 28,* 779–789.

Trueb, L., Evans, J., Hammel, A., Bartholomew, P., & Dobson, V. (1992). Assessing visual acuity of visually impaired children using the Teller Acuity card procedure. *American Orthoptic Journal, 42,* 149–154.

van Hof-van Duin, J., Evenhuis-van Leunen, A., Mohn, G., Baerts, W., & Fetter, W. P. F. (1989). Effects of very low birth weight (VLBW) on visual development during the first year after term. *Early Human Development, 20,* 255–266.

van Hof-van Duin, J., & Mohn, G. (1986). The development of visual acuity in normal full-term and preterm infants. *Vision Research, 26,* 909–916.

Vistech Consultants, Inc. (1991). *Teller acuity cards: Instruction manual.* Dayton, OH: Author.

Vital-Durand, F., Atkinson, J., & Braddick, O. I. (Eds.). (1996). *Infant vision.* Oxford: Oxford University Press.

White, J. M., & Loshin, D. S. (1989). Grating acuity overestimates Snellen acuity in patients with age-related maculopathy. *Optometry and Vision Science, 66,* 751–755.

Wiesel, T. N., & Hubel, D. H. (1963). Single-cell responses in striate cortex of kittens deprived of vision in one eye. *Journal of Neurophysiology, 26,* 1003–1017.

Wilson, H. R. (1988). Development of spatiotemporal mechanisms in infant vision. *Vision Research, 28,* 611–628.

Wilson, H. R. (1993). Theories of infant visual development. In K. Simons (Ed.), *Early visual development, normal and abnormal* (pp. 560–572). New York: Oxford University Press.

5

Auditory Assessment in Infancy

ALAN B. COBO-LEWIS
REBECCA E. EILERS

HISTORY

The prevalence of childhood hearing impairment is about 1.5 per 1,000 (Parving, 1994). Currently, about 9–10% of newborns in the United States have one or more risk factors predisposing to hearing impairment, and about half the children with sensorineural hearing impairment exhibit one or more risk factors identified by the Joint Committee on Infant Hearing (1991; Mauk, White, Mortensen, & Behrens, 1991). At-risk infants are approximately 5 to 10 times more likely than infants in the population at large to exhibit hearing impairment. This statistic motivates existing programs that screen all patients in neonatal intensive care units (NICUs) for hearing impairment before discharge, because NICU infants constitute a population that greatly overlaps with those meeting the Joint Committee's risk criteria. However, focusing solely on infants at risk fails to identify fully half of hearing-impaired children. In light of the relatively inexpensive screening methods discussed in this chapter, the NIH Consensus Development Conference (1993) has recommended that *all* infants undergo hearing screening during the first 3 months of life.

GENERAL DESCRIPTION

Modern assessment tools for infant hearing exploit three classes of phenomena: acoustic, electrophysiological, and behavioral. Methods in of these three groups assess progressively more central aspects of the auditory sys-

95

tem. Assessments of otoacoustic emissions (OAEs; see Kemp, 1986) are based on an acoustic phenomenon: Normally functioning outer hair cells of the cochlea change length in response to stimulation, changing the mechanical properties of the cochlea and resulting in the emission of sound from the ear. OAEs thus offer a method for assessing the integrity of the preneural auditory system. Abnormalities located in the outer hair cells or more peripherally are usually detectable in an abnormal OAE response. Assessments of auditory brainstem responses (ABRs; Jewett, Romano, & Williston, 1970; Jewett & Williston, 1971; Lev & Sohmer, 1972) are based on an electrophysiological phenomenon: the scalp electrical potential that arises from the synchronized activity of brainstem auditory neurons. ABRs offer a method for assessing the integrity of the precortical auditory system. Abnormalities located in the brainstem or more peripherally are usually detectable in an abnormal ABR response. Behavioral tests offer a method for assessing the integrity of the entire organism's response to auditory stimulation, for central impairments as well as peripheral impairments are detectable by the appropriate behavioral test. The fact that different methods assess preneural, precortical, and total aspects of the auditory system can be useful in pinpointing the locus of a problem in auditory processing. OAEs and ABRs are applicable even for neonates, though there are important differences between infant and adult ABRs (Picton, Durieux-Smith, & Moran, 1994; see Picton, Taylor, & Durieux-Smith, 1992). The most common reliable behavioral assessment of infant hearing is applicable down to 5–6 months of age, though some laboratory-grade techniques have been applied to 1- to 2-month-olds.

Acoustic, electrophysiological, and behavioral methods provide complementary assessments of the auditory system from birth onward. Although these three groups of assessments are complementary, this volume focuses on behavioral assessments, as only behavioral testing can evaluate a subject's hearing per se. A normal ABR can only indicate that the auditory stimulus has produced a disturbance in the lower brain. A normal OAE indicates even less than that, being the product of even more peripheral components of the auditory system. Only behavioral evaluation can ensure that the subject is consciously aware of the auditory stimulation.

VISUAL REINFORCEMENT AUDIOMETRY

Most modern behavioral methods for testing infant hearing represent variations on visual reinforcement audiometry (VRA; Lidén & Kankkunen, 1969; Moore, Wilson, & Thompson, 1977; Suzuki & Ogiba, 1961), whereby a 5- to 6-month-old's orienting reflex (which manifests in a headturn toward sound) is maintained through conditioning techniques. The procedure is usually conducted with the infant sitting on a parent's lap, facing the tester.

It is important that each trial not begin until the infant's head is at midline. A loudspeaker is placed 45 degrees to the infant's right or left. In the same general position as the loudspeaker is a visual reinforcer temporarily obscured from the infant's view, usually by being placed in a dark chamber behind a sheet of smoked Plexiglas. The reinforcer is typically an animated toy (e.g., a stuffed animal playing a drum set). When a trial occurs, a stimulus is delivered through the loudspeaker. If the infant turns (orients) toward the loudspeaker in response to the stimulus, reinforcement is provided to the infant by illuminating the chamber behind the smoked Plexiglas and activating the animated toy. Before beginning trials for hearing testing per se, the tester administers several training trials in which he or she directs the infant's attention to the loudspeaker while suprathreshold stimuli are delivered, with the intention of evoking a headturn toward the loudspeaker. After the infant has been trained to criterion (e.g., three consecutive turns toward suprathreshold stimuli), testing begins. To ensure that the procedure is evaluating the infant's hearing rather than the infant's response to cues from the tester or parent, it is essential that both parent and tester be unaware of when the stimulus is being delivered. This is accomplished by having the parent and tester both wear headphones through which noise or music is delivered of an intensity sufficient to mask the auditory test stimulus. The tester indicates through an electronic switch when the infant is ready with head at midline. After a random interval, a computer (or, less commonly, another tester in a different room) initiates a signal trial or silent "catch" trial, after which the tester indicates whether the infant turned his or her head toward the stimulus. If the infant turned, the computer activates the visual reinforcer; otherwise, no reinforcement is delivered. To ensure that the infant is under stimulus control, reinforcement is never delivered unless the infant turns *in response to a stimulus.*

VRA can be used to estimate thresholds by application of adaptive staircase methods (e.g., Carhart & Jerger, 1959; Hughson & Westlake, 1944; Trehub, Bull, Schneider, & Morrongiello, 1986). However, VRA generally generates too few trials for estimating a complete audiogram (i.e., a collection of threshold measurements at several acoustic frequencies), so infant hearing testing and screening is often reduced to testing the subject's response to suprathreshold, usually wideband, signals (Widen, 1990) or testing fewer than four frequencies. However, this problem can be addressed by using computers to select stimuli judiciously, based on a dynamic trial-by-trial analysis of the responses that an infant produces. For example, we routinely use Classification of Audiograms by Sequential Testing (CAST; Özdamar, Eilers, Miskiel, & Widen, 1990), whereby a computer applies Bayesian analysis to classify the infant into one of several categories, each of which is represented by an audiogram prototypical of a specific hearing impairment. CAST exploits the fact that audibility of stimuli of similar frequency are likely to be similar, though not necessarily identical. In CAST, the computer selects not just the intensity of a VRA trial's stimulus but also its acoustic frequency. Then, after each trial, CAST uses information about baseline rates for each audiogram prototype in the population, plus information about which stimuli elicited a response from the subject, to calculate the probability that the subject's audiogram matches each prototypical audiogram, in turn. The computer discontinues testing after sufficient information has been gathered to confidently classify the subject to the appropriate audiogram prototype. Moreover, new advances in the theory of adaptive measurement (Cobo-Lewis, 1997) can be applied to CAST to allow for even more efficient selection of stimuli in the sense that the computer can select stimulus frequency and intensity in such a way that the subject's response is likely to be maximally informative about which audiogram prototype matches the subject's audiogram. This new approach, MEEE-CAST, is not yet widely used.

BEHAVIORAL OBSERVATION AUDIOMETRY

Before the development of VRA, behavioral hearing testing in infancy was usually accomplished by behavioral observation audiometry (BOA). This technique involved examining the infant for behavioral reactions to sounds. It has been empirically established that for infants old enough to make VRA an appropriate technique, VRA is more accurate than BOA (e.g., Moore et al., 1977). The problem with BOA is that it is difficult to judge reliably when an infant has responded to a sound. We therefore recommend VRA over BOA for clinical applications, whenever feasible.

OBSERVER-BASED PSYCHOACOUSTIC PROCEDURE

The primarily difficulty with BOA is that when an observer judges an infant not to have responded to a stimulus, it could be due to the infant's hearing threshold, the infant's level of interest in the sound, or the observer's failure to detect a subtle response on the part of the infant. VRA's approach to this problem is to reinforce a specific unsubtle response—headturning. Another approach, the Observer-Based Psychoacoustic Procedure (OPP; Olsho, Koch, Halpin, & Carter, 1987) typically also uses reinforcement, but does not focus attention on a headturn response, thus rendering it applicable down to even younger ages, with successful results having been obtained for 2-month-olds (Marean, Werner, & Kuhl, 1992) and even younger infants (Werner & Mancl, 1993). To deal with observer reliability, OPP explicitly acknowledges that the system being tested is the infant's response plus the observer's observation of that response. Like BOA, OPP encourages the observer to use—consciously or unconsciously—whatever cues might be effective in determining when an infant has responded to a stimulus. Like VRA, OPP reinforces correct detection of a stimulus by activating an animated toy. Although the form of an infant's response is left open, an infant is only reinforced on stimulus trials when the observer detected a response by the infant. (Half the trials are randomly selected as no-stimulus trials, and these never result in activation of the toy.) Thus, the infant is trained through operant conditioning to respond to stimuli with behaviors that the observer can reliably detect. Furthermore, because the observer is also aware of whether or not the toy was activated, the observer is also trained through operant conditioning to base his or her decisions on whatever aspects of the infant's behavior are the most reliable indicators that the infant has detected the stimulus. As in VRA, it is important that during a trial, the observer be unaware of whether or not a stimulus is being presented. This is typically accomplished by observing the infant remotely from a separate room. A modification of OPP has also been used with infants under 1 month of age, in which a three-interval forced-choice task is used without reinforcement for the infant but with feedback to the observer (Werner & Gillenwater, 1990; cf. Teller, 1979). Due to the complexity of the paradigm, OPP has not been applied in clinical settings; instead, it is being used exclusively in research settings, where the application of data analysis techniques typical of psychophysics experiments has yielded detailed information on several aspects of infant hearing, such as how their psychometric functions differ from those of adults listening to the same stimuli (Bargones, Werner, & Marean, 1995).

BIOBEHAVIORAL BASIS OF ASSESSMENT

VRA depends on the presence of an adult-like orienting response. With normally developing children, such a response is typically firmly established at 5–6 months of age. Younger infants tend to have difficulty turning their head in orientation toward a sound. OPP, on the other hand, does not focus attention on a headturn response, thus rendering it applicable down at least as far as 2 months of age (Marean et al., 1992; Werner & Mancl, 1993).

RELIABILITY AND VALIDITY

The reliability of standard VRA with normally hearing infants is well established. For infants old enough to participate in VRA, BOA is less accurate (e.g., Moore et al., 1977). With deaf infants, VRA's test–retest differences in frequency-specific thresholds can be expected to be about 10 dB (Rudmin, 1984). In clinical trials, the validity of CAST has been assessed by comparing its classifications with those based on conventional VRA and tympanometry (Eilers, Özdamar, & Steffens, 1993; Mercer & Gravel, 1997). CAST detects appropriate numbers of hearing-impaired infants based on tympanometric criteria. In a sample of children with normal hearing and mostly conductive losses, CAST was found to have overall sensitivity of 75% and specificity of 84% (Eilers et al., 1993). In a sample that included more children with sensorineural loss, CAST was found to have sensitivity of 95–100% and specificity of 43–71% (Mercer & Gravel, 1997). However, the reliability and validity of any behavioral method depend on how attentive the infant is. Moreover, the validity of methods such as CAST and MEEE-CAST depend on how well the method's assumptions about an infant's attentiveness match an infant's actual attentiveness. Because an infant's attentiveness is difficult to control even in a laboratory setting, computer simulation is useful for assessing these effects. According to such simulations of moderately attentive infants (attentive on at least 85% of trials), CAST and MEEE-CAST generally perform with sensitivity and specificity of at least 90% for 30-trial tests (Cobo-Lewis, 1997; Özdamar et al., 1990). For extremely inattentive infants, sensitivity in 30-trial tests can fall to 80%, though specificity can remain above 90% if one gives up on the ability to distinguish between normal hearing and the 15–25 dB losses commonly associated with middle-ear infections (Cobo-Lewis, 1997). This trend is consistent with the clinical trial data of Mercer and Gravel (1993), who noted that CAST's specificity increased dramatically (from 43 to 71%) when such small losses were ignored.

The reliability of OPP for assessing individual infants has not been exhaustively studied. However, it has been reported that when pairs of 30-trial OPP assessments are compared, 6-month-olds' threshold estimates rarely change by more than 5 dB. On the other hand, 3-month-olds' threshold estimates can change by as much as 10 dB (Werner & Marean, 1991).

The validity of OPP and VRA are indicated by their mutual agreement in assessing frequency-specific threshold differences between adults and 6- to 12-month-old infants. For example, for half-second tones presented through earphones, OPP indicates that typically developing 6-month-olds have thresholds 16 dB above adult levels at 1 kHz and 7 dB above adult levels at 4 kHz (Olsho et al., 1987; Olsho, Koch, Carter, Halpin, & Spetner, 1988). These thresholds are similar to respective threshold elevations of 14 and 7 dB found with VRA (Nozza & Wilson, 1984).

DEVELOPMENTAL MODEL

Between 4 and 9 months of age (most commonly at 6–7 months), normal infants begin to produce canonical syllables (Eilers, Oller, et al., 1993; Oller & Eilers, 1988). Canonical babbles, such as "mamama," "na," and "ada," represent the first manifestation of an infant's ability to form adult-like syllables (Oller, 1980; Oller & Lynch, 1992). They are easily recognized by parents (Cobo-Lewis, Oller, Lynch, & Levine, 1996; Eilers & Oller, 1994; Eilers, Oller, et al., 1993), perhaps because intuitively they sound like the baby is trying to talk (cf. Papoušek & Papoušek, 1987). Before the canonical-babbling stage, an infant's utterances sound less speech-like, with the infant producing more coos and other utterances requiring less sophisticated coordination of articulatory activity. Canonical babbling seems to be an important developmental precursor to spoken language—infants produce canonical babbles before producing their first words, and there is a relationship between characteristics of canonical babbling and later communicative development (see Stoel-Gammon, 1992; also Lynch et al., 1995). Canonical babbling is robust. It occurs on schedule in babies of all socioeconomic classes (Eilers & Oller, 1994; Oller, Eilers, Basinger, Steffens, & Urbano, 1995) and in preterm healthy infants corrected for gestational age (Eilers, Oller, et al., 1993), and it is delayed less than other important milestones in infants with Down syndrome (Cobo-Lewis et al., 1996; Lynch et al., 1995; Smith & Oller, 1981). Canonical babbling, however, is absent in severely or profoundly hearing-impaired infants before 11 months of age and is often delayed in these infants well into the third year of life (Eilers & Oller, 1994; Kent, Osberger, Netsell, & Hustedde, 1987; Oller & Eilers, 1988; Smith, 1982; Stark, 1983; Stoel-Gammon & Otomo, 1986; Vinter, 1987). Moreover, among deaf children whose hearing impairment is identified early, there is a strong relationship between the age at which hearing aids are introduced and the age of onset of canonical babbling: Such children are unlikely to babble canonically until about 8–10 months after receiving a hearing aid (Eilers & Oller, 1994).

What are the consequences of less severe hearing impairment in infancy? Although we do not yet know if canonical babbling is delayed in infants with less severe impairment, there have been some relevant studies. These address how chronic otitis media and consequent hearing loss are related to speech, language, and cognitive development (Brandes & Ehinger, 1981; Gottlieb, Zinkus, & Thompson, 1979; Jerger, Jerger, Alford, & Abrams, 1983; Sak & Ruben, 1981; Zinkus & Gottlieb, 1980). Although the presence of otitis media does not guarantee a specific depth of hearing loss (or any hearing loss at all), otitis media does tend to co-occur with hearing loss, often being associated with a fluctuating conductive loss whose depth is mild to moderately severe. Thus, in studies that document the impact of otitis media on speech and language development, otitis media serves as a proxy for hearing loss, albeit of variable depth.

Thus, the difficulty in teaching deaf children to speak, the delay in canonical babbling in deaf children, and the various consequences of otitis media in infancy all suggest that good hearing in infancy is important for subsequent vocal communicative development. Furthermore, the evidence that canonical babbling tends to emerge 8–10 months after an infant or child is fitted with a hearing aid (Eilers & Oller, 1994) suggests that early identification of hearing impairment can help assuage the negative consequences of poor hearing in infancy. In light of this evidence for the benefit of early identification and intervention, it is troubling that the average age for identification of serious hearing impairment in the U.S. pediatric population at large is over 2 years (NIH Consensus Development Conference, 1993; Stein, Clark, & Kraus, 1983). Thus, there is ample room for improvement, as the average age of identification of hearing impairment in Israeli children is 7–9 months (see Gustason, 1989).

STRUCTURAL AND/OR THEORETICAL CONSTRAINTS/CONTROVERSIES

Assessing infant hearing through behavioral paradigms might be considered inherently error-prone. Two of the biggest issues are interpreting the infant's responses and maintaining the infant's attentiveness and cooperation. VRA and OPP address these issues by operant conditioning, whereby infants (and observers as well, in the case of OPP) are trained to respond to audible stimuli. The use of conditioning procedures also addresses concerns about whether one is testing stimulus audibility or merely stimulus interest. This is especially important, for example, if one wishes to measure an infant's audiogram, when it is crucial that threshold differences be attributable to differences in audibility at the various acoustic frequencies.

Because it is important to judge audibility on the basis of the infant's response, VRA and OPP blind the observer to the presence of the stimulus by insulating the observer from the acoustic stimulus and including "catch trials" on which no acoustic stimulus is presented to the infant. Such procedures allow the assessment of false-alarm rates, which serve as a check on the assessment's validity for a specific infant–observer pair. These controls are what set VRA and OPP apart from less rigorous assessments such as BOA.

TRAINING REQUIREMENTS

In both OPP and VRA, it is important that threshold be determined by an infant's hearing rather than by the observer's skill. Because stimulus selection and presentation in these procedures are aided by modern computer control, an examiner's training can be limited to interacting with the infant and making judgments about the infant's behavior. In VRA, a single examiner must be able to (1) maintain the infant under behavioral control in a neutral affective state and (2) make accurate judgments about the direction and extent of headturns. Regarding the first task, examiners are taught to manipulate a series of visually engaging toys to keep the infant's gaze at midline between trials; however, this interaction must not be so interesting to the infant that the infant fails to respond to an audible sound presented from the loudspeaker. Regarding the second task, it is important that the examiner not record a response unless the infant turns his or her head by at least 90 degrees. Otherwise, an infant's headturns tend to get progressively subtler, and reliability and validity will suffer.

In OPP, the observer typically sits outside the testing chamber, so that one examiner need only maintain the infant under behavioral control in a neutral affective state, while the other examiner (the observer) need only judge the infant's responsiveness to the acoustic stimulus. It might seem that OPP observation would therefore require less training than VRA, but it generally requires *more,* because whereas VRA reinforces only clear headturns, OPP can reinforce subtle responses that require more practice for an examiner to detect. It might take approximately 2 months for an observer to be trained in OPP. With adequately trained examiners, OPP can be expected to yield false-alarm rates under 25%.

IMPLICATIONS

It is typically taken for granted that early hearing is important for the development of language. Results about canonical babbling provide empirical support for this hypothesis—canonical babbling represents a robust precursor to first words that is dramatically delayed by hearing impairment in infancy. Intervention can be effective in ameliorating the effects of early hearing impairment, as demonstrated by the result that hearing-impaired infants are not likely to begin canonical babbling until 8–10 months after receiving a hearing aid (Eilers & Oller, 1994). This illustrates the importance of early identification of hearing-impaired infants, as underscored by the recommendation of the NIH Consensus Development Conference (1993) that at-risk infants be screened for hearing impairment before they leave the NICU and that universal hearing screening be instituted so that all infants are screened by 3 months of age.

ACKNOWLEDGMENTS

Thanks to Rafael Delgado, Brenda Lonsbury-Martin, Michele Steffens, Lynne Werner, and Judy Gravel for helpful discussions. This chapter was supported by Grant Nos. 9896277 from the National Science Foundation (A. B. Cobo-Lewis, Principal Investigator) and DC01932 from the National Institutes of Health (D. K. Oller, Principal Investigator).

REFERENCES

Bargones, J. Y., Werner, L. A., & Marean, G. C. (1995). Infant psychometric functions for detection: Mechanisms of immature sensitivity. *Journal of the Acoustical Society of America, 98,* 99–111.

Brandes, P. J., & Ehinger, D. M. (1981). The effects of early middle ear pathology on auditory perception and academic achievement. *Journal of Speech and Hearing Disorders,* *46,* 301–307.

Carhart, R., & Jerger, J. F. (1959). Preferred method for clinical determination of pure-tone thresholds. *Journal of Speech and Hearing Disorders, 24,* 330–345.

Cobo-Lewis, A. B. (1997). An adaptive psychophysical method for subject classification. *Perception and Psychophysics, 59,* 989–1003.

Cobo-Lewis, A. B., Oller, D. K., Lynch, M. P., & Levine, S. L. (1996). Relations of motor and vocal milestones in typically developing infants and infants with Down syndrome. *American Journal on Mental Retardation, 100,* 456–467.

Eilers, R. E., & Oller, D. K. (1994). Infant vocalizations and the early diagnosis of severe hearing impairment. *Journal of Pediatrics, 124,* 199–203.

Eilers, R. E., Oller, D. K., Levine, S., Basinger, D., Lynch, M. P., & Urbano, R. (1993). The role of prematurity and socioeconomic status in the onset of canonical babbling in infants. *Infant Behavior and Development, 16,* 297–315.

Eilers, R. E., Özdamar, Ö., & Steffens, M. L. (1993). Classification of audiograms by sequential testing: Reliability and validity of an automated behavioral hearing screening algorithm. *Journal of the American Academy of Audiology, 4,* 172–181.

Gottlieb, M. I., Zinkus, P. W., & Thompson, A. (1979). Chronic middle ear disease and auditory perceptual deficits. *Clinical Pediatrics, 18,* 725–732.

Gustason, G. (1989). Early identification of hearing-impaired infants: A review of Israeli and American progress. *Volta Review, 91,* 291–295.

Hughson, W., & Westlake, H. (1944). Manual for program outline for rehabilitation of aural casualties both military and civilian. *Transactions of the American Academy of Ophthalmology and Otolaryngology Supplement, 48,* 1–15.

Jerger, S., Jerger, J., Alford, B. R., & Abrams, S. (1983). Development of speech intelligibility in children with recurrent otitis media. *Ear and Hearing, 4,* 138–145.

Jewett, D., Romano, H. N., & Williston, J. S. (1970). Human auditory evoked responses: Possible brain stem components detected on the scalp. *Science, 167,* 1517–1518.

Jewett, D., & Williston, J. (1971). Auditory evoked far fields averaged from the scalp of humans. *Brain, 94,* 681–696.

Joint Committee on Infant Hearing (1991). 1990 Position Statement. *ASHA, 33*(Suppl. 5), 3–6.

Kemp, D. T. (1986). Otoacoustic emissions, travelling waves and cochlear mechanisms. *Hearing Research, 22,* 95–104.

Kent, R. D., Osberger, M. J., Netsell, R., & Hustedde, C. G. (1987). Phonetic development in identical twins who differ in auditory function. *Journal of Speech and Hearing Disorders, 52,* 64–75.

Lev, A., & Sohmer, H. (1972). Sources of averaged neural responses recorded in animal and human subjects during cochlear audiometry. *Archiv fur klinische und experimentelle Ohren-, Nasen- und Kehlkopfheilkunde, 201,* 79–90.

Lidén, G., & Kankkunen, A. (1969). Visual reinforcement audiometry. *Acta Oto-laryngologica, 67,* 281–292.

Lynch, M. P., Oller, D. K., Steffens, M. L., Levine, S. L., Basinger, D. L., & Umbel, V. (1995). The onset of speech-like vocalizations in infants with Down syndrome. *American Journal on Mental Retardation, 100,* 68–86.

Marean, G. C., Werner, L. A., & Kuhl, P. K. (1992). Vowel categorization by very young infants. *Developmental Psychology, 28,* 396–405.

Mauk, G. W., White, K. R., Mortensen, L. B., & Behrens, T. R. (1991). The effectiveness of screening programs based on high-risk characteristics in early identification of hearing impairment. *Ear and Hearing, 12,* 312–319.

Mercer, D. M., & Gravel, J. S. (1997). Screening infants and young children for hearing loss: Examination of the CAST procedure. *Journal of the American Academy of Audiology, 8,* 233–242.

Moore, J. M., Wilson, W. R., & Thompson, G. (1977). Visual reinforcement of head-turn responses in infants under 12 months of age. *Journal of Speech and Hearing Disorders, 42,* 328–334.

NIH Consensus Development Conference. (1993, March). Early identification of hearing impairment in infants and children. *NIH Consensus Statement, 11*(1), 1–24. Available online: http://odp.od.nih.gov/consensus/cons/092/092_statement.htm

Nozza, R. J., & Wilson, W. R. (1984). Masked and unmasked pure-tone thresholds of infants and adults: Development of auditory frequency selectivity and sensitivity. *Journal of Speech and Hearing Research, 27,* 613–622.

Oller, D. K. (1980). The emergence of the sounds of speech in infancy. In G. Yeni-Komshian, J. Kavanagh, & C. Ferguson (Eds.), *Child phonology, Volume 1. Production* (pp. 93-112). New York: Academic Press.

Oller, D. K., & Eilers, R. E. (1988). The role of audition in infant babbling. *Child Development, 59,* 441–449.

Oller, D. K., Eilers, R. E.., Basinger, D., Steffens, M. L., & Urbano, R. (1995). Extreme poverty and the development of precursors to the speech capacity. *First Language, 15,* 167–187.

Oller, D. K., & Lynch, M. P. (1992). Infant vocalizations and innovations in infraphonology: Toward a broader theory of development and disorders. In C. Ferguson, L. Menn, & C. Stoel-Gammon (Eds.), *Phonological development.* Parkton, MD: York Press.

Olsho, L. W., Koch, E. G., Carter, E. A., Halpin, C. F., & Spetner, N. B. (1988). Pure-tone sensitivity of human infants. *Journal of the Acoustical Society of America, 84,* 1316–1324.

Olsho, L. W., Koch, E. G., Halpin, C. F., & Carter, E. A. (1987). An observer-based psychoacoustic procedure for use with young infants. *Developmental Psychology, 23,* 627–640.

Özdamar, Ö., Eilers, R. E., Miskiel, E., & Widen, J. (1990). Classification of audiograms by sequential testing using a dynamic Bayesian procedure. *Journal of the Acoustical Society of America, 88,* 2171–2179.

Papoušek, H., & Papoušek, M. (1987). Intuitive parenting: a dialectic counterpart to the infant's integrative competence. In J. Osofsky (Ed.), *Handbook of infant development* (2nd ed., pp. 669–720). New York: Wiley.

Parving, A. (1994). Childhood hearing disability—Epidemiology and aetiology. *Annales Nestlé, 52,* 57–61.

Picton, T. W., Durieux-Smith, A., & Moran, L. M. (1994). Recording auditory brainstem responses from infants. *International Journal of Pediatric Otorhinolaryngology, 28,* 93–110.

Picton, T. W., Taylor, M. J., & Durieux-Smith, A. (1992). Brainstem auditory evoked potentials in pediatrics. In M. J. Aminoff (Ed.), *Electrodiagnosis in clinical neurology* (3rd ed., pp. 537–569). New York: Churchill Livingstone.

Rudmin, F. W. (1984). Brief clinical report on visual reinforcement audiometry with deaf infants. *Journal of Otolaryngology, 13,* 367–369.

Sak, R., & Ruben, R. J. (1981). Recurrent middle ear effusion in childhood: Implications of temporary auditory deprivation for language and learning. *Annals of Otology, Rhinology and Laryngology, 980,* 546–551.

Smith, B. L. (1982). Some observations concerning pre-meaningful vocalizations of hearing-impaired infants. *Journal of Speech and Hearing Disorders, 47,* 439–442.

Smith, B. L., & Oller, D. K. (1981). A comparative study of premeaningful vocalizations produced by normally developing and Down's syndrome infants. *Journal of Speech and Hearing Disorders, 46,* 46–51.

Stark, R. E. (1983). Phonatory development in young normally hearing and hearing-impaired children. In I. Hochberg, H Levitt, & M. J. Osberger (Eds.), *Speech of the hearing impaired: Research, training and personnel preparation* (pp. 251–266). Baltimore: University Park Press.

Stein, L., Clark, S., & Kraus, N. (1983). The hearing-impaired infant: Patterns of identification and habilitation. *Ear and Hearing, 4,* 232–236.

Stoel-Gammon, C. (1992). Prelinguistic vocal development: Measurement and predictions. In C. A. Ferguson, L. Menn, & C. Stoel-Gammon (Eds.), *Phonological development: Models, research, implications* (pp. 439–456). Timonium, MD: York Press.

Stoel-Gammon, C., & Otomo, K. (1986). Babbling development of hearing-impaired and normally hearing subjects. *Journal of Speech and Hearing Disorders, 51,* 33–41.

Suzuki, T., & Ogiba, Y. (1961). Conditioned orientation reflex audiometry. *Archives of Otolaryngology, 74,* 192–198.

Teller, D. Y. (1979). The forced-choice preferential looking procedure: A psychophysical technique for use with human infants. *Infant Behavior and Development, 2,* 135–153.

Trehub, S. E., Bull, D., Schneider, B. A., & Morrongiello, B. A. (1986). PESTI: a procedure for estimating individual thresholds in infant listeners. *Infant Behavior and Development, 9,* 107–118.

Vinter, S. (1987). Contrôle de premières productions vocales du bébé sourd. *Bulletin d'Audiophonologie, 3*(6), 659–670.

Werner, L. A., & Gillenwater, J. M. (1990). Pure-tone sensitivity of 2- to 5-week-old infants. *Infant Behavior and Development, 13,* 355–375.

Werner, L. A., & Mancl, L. R. (1993, April). Pure-tone thresholds of 1-month-old infants. *Journal of the Acoustical Society of America, 93*(4, Pt. 2), 2367.

Werner, L. A., & Marean, G. C. (1991). Methods for estimating infant thresholds. *Journal of the Acoustical Society of America, 4,* 1867–1875.

Widen, J. E. (1990). Behavioral screening of high-risk infants using visual reinforcement audiometry. *Seminars in Hearing, 11,* 342–355.

Zinkus, P. W., & Gottlieb, M. I. (1980). Patterns of perceptual and academic deficits related to early chronic otitis media. *Pediatrics, 66,* 246–253.

III

Arousal and Regulation

6

Vagal Tone

FRAN LANG PORTER

HISTORY

One of the more novel indices to emerge in recent years to assess the biobehavioral integrity of the newborn and young infant has been vagal tone, a cardiorespiratory measure. Vagal tone has been eagerly explored as a promising means to investigate such diverse topics as attention, emotion, visual memory, stress, pain, temperament, developmental regulation disorders, and the impact of early clinical compromise.

The general psychophysiological concept that behavior is largely determined by the central nervous system has long prompted interest in identifying neurally mediated correlates of behavior. Developmental psychologists have been particularly invested in assessing the status of the nervous system to learn something abut the behavioral and even cognitive potential of the individual before those domains might be able to be directly assessed themselves. This would be particularly important for infants whose behavioral and/or cognitive potential is questionable or who might benefit from the effects of early targeted intervention.

Historically, cardiac measures have commonly been used for this purpose and have included heart rate (number of beats per minute) and its reciprocal, heart period (the time between heartbeats, measured in milliseconds). Change in either of these measures is believed to reflect the summed effects of a wide range of internally and externally derived sensory conditions, including, for example, respiration and blood pressure/vasomotor activity. However, at least in healthy mammals, neither heart rate nor heart period is fixed, but rather they undergo moment-to-moment variation, assumed to reflect the changing neural influences on the heart. Thus, it is the variability in heart rate (or heart period) which provides a more promising neurally mediated index than do either an isolated heart rate or heart period value. Although physiological survival could be considered a function of the rate at which the heart beats, the patterning of those beats reflects the varying neural influences on the heart, and thus, the functioning of the central nervous system.

Heart rate variability has been quantified as either short (beat-to-beat) or long term (the range of heart rate over time) and both measures have been used. Spectral analysis of long-term variability has emphasized the emergence of cyclicity in behavioral and motor activity (measured over periods of minutes or hours) as a function of development. In contrast, short-term variability is believed to reflect more the moment-to-moment neurally based influences. Different oscillation frequencies or patterns of beat-to-beat variability have been identified from the electrocardiographic record in adults. One relatively low-frequency oscillation (with periods of approximately 10 seconds) represents the response of the baroreceptor reflex; a second, even lower-frequency oscillation (with periods of approximately 20 seconds), may be the result of thermoregulatory fluctuations in vasomotor tone; and a third, higher-frequency oscillation—respiratory sinus arrhythmia (RSA)—reflects changes in heart rate associated with the respiratory cycle. In infants, the frequency band of the oscillation ranges from 0. 3–1. 3 Hz, the range of spontaneous breathing for infants. In adults, these frequencies would be slower. It is this higher frequency oscillation that is the basis of the vagal tone measure.

BIOBEHAVIORAL BASIS OF ASSESSMENT

Investigators have shown particular interest in developing and using measures which attempt to quantify the variability in heart rate that is primarily neurally mediated. Because the higher-frequency oscillation in the heart rate pattern is mediated via the tenth cranial nerve (commonly called the vagus nerve) by efferent innervation to the heart, RSA has been selected as a more direct representation of neural control of the heart than other measures of heart rate variability.

The original conceptualization of vagal tone was based on the proposal that respiration, either by a central mechanism or via a peripheral feedback loop to medullary areas, phasically inhibits or "gates" the source nuclei of the vagal cardioinhibitory fibers (Lopes & Palmer, 1976). Research demonstrated that the vagal cardioinhibitory neurons show a respiratory-related pattern of discharge with the primary efferent action on the heart occurring during expiration (Gilbey, Jordan, Richter, & Spyer, 1983). This manifests as a rhythmic process in which heart rate is slowed during expiration and quickened during inspiration reflecting the rhythmic gating of vagal efferents to the heart.

THE POLYVAGAL THEORY

When initially proposed, the vagal tone measure was generalized to all vagal efferent pathways. More recent examinations of both neuroanatomical data and the phylogenetic development of the neural regulation of the heart prompted Porges (1995) to propose a polyvagal theory of vagal tone. This theory emphasizes that the vagus is not one nerve with generalized effects but a family of neural pathways, originating in several different areas of the brainstem that are associated with different functions. Specifically, it suggests that the vagus nerve has two primary roles: During states of low environmental demand such as sleep, vagal activity promotes physiological homeostasis (via increased vagal activity) while during states of high environmental demand such as stress, the vagus acts to regulate metabolic output as needed (via decreased vagal activity). Thus, the vagal system responds both to the internal needs of the organism and to the external challenges in an ongoing, moment-to-moment fashion in which there is a continual trade-off between maintaining homeostasis and effectively responding to the environment. Survival can be seen as highly dependent on the success of this balancing act.

The polyvagal theory proposes that these two separate functions of the vagal network are associated with two separate and definable source nuclei in the medulla: the dorsal motor nucleus of the vagus (DMNX) and the nucleus ambiguus (NA). Most cells originating in the DMNX project to subdiaphragmatic organs (e.g., stomach and intestines) and are believed to be involved in the vegetative, homeostatic functions (e.g., digestion) while most cells in the NA project to supradiaphragmatic structures (e.g., larynx, pharynx, soft palate, esophagus, bronchi, and heart) and are believed to be associated with the more dynamic functions of attention, motion, emotion, and communication (Porges, 1995). Because the efferents originating in the NA are those which regulate the heart and bronchi, respiratory sinus arrhythmia can then be considered a measure of the general visceral efferents of the NA rather than a global measure of vagal tone or even a measure of total vagal control of the heart as previously proposed (Fouad, Tarazi, Fighaly, & Alicandri, 1984; Katona & Jih, 1975; Porges, 1992). Although the polyvagal theory acknowledges that there are other vagal and nonvagal influences on the heart which contribute to both heart rate level and to its rhythm, it emphasizes that the primary, if not sole, source of respiratory rhythms on the sinoatrial node is due to projections from the NA.

Thus, the vagal tone measure is a noninvasive estimate of the amplitude of RSA classically defined as the amplitude of the oscillation in the heart period pattern that is synchronized with respiration. Some now believe that respiratory sinus arrhythmia is reflective of a centrally mediated process that is manifest on the heart rate as RSA and on the respiratory system as a breathing frequency (Porges, 1995; Richter & Spyer, 1990). Vagal tone is usually based on normative respiratory frequency bands, not measurements of an individual's spontaneous breathing rate and, thus, is an estimate of the amplitude of RSA.

DESCRIPTION OF ASSESSMENT

To quantify vagal tone, electrocardiographic (ECG) recordings are processed, typically off-line, with software to detect each QRS complex (usually by detecting the peak of the R wave) for each heartbeat and to quantify sequential R-R intervals in milliseconds (i.e., heart periods or interbeat intervals). Vagal tone can then be computed from the interbeat intervals. The steps involved in this computation vary depending on methodology used. Using current software developed by Porges (Mxedit, Delta Biometrics, Bethesda, Maryland, 1985), the steps include (1) conversion of heart period into time-based data by sampling in 200-msec intervals; (2) detrending the periodicities in heart rate slower than RSA with a 21-point cubic polynomial moving stepwise through the data (Bohrer & Porges, 1982); (3) time-series analysis of the data to extract the variance of heart period within the frequency band of spontaneous breathing; because Porges's methods do not actually measure the synchronicity of the interbeat intervals with respiration, appropriate respiratory bandwidths need to be selected, depending on the population being studied; for neonates, respiratory frequencies range from 0. 3–1. 3 Hz or 18–78 breaths per minutes; and (4) calculation of the natural logarithm of the band-passed variance, which serves as the estimate of vagal tone. Mean vagal tone can then be computed for sequential epochs typically no shorter than 10–15 seconds in duration, which facilitates the ability to assess dynamic changes. The values of vagal tone are represented then by arbitrary units on a natural logarithmic scale. Whenever possible, normative data for different populations are presented in this chapter to provide a frame of reference. A critical step in the process of estimating the amplitude of RSA is that of ensuring that the data to be included in the analysis are physiological and not contaminated by movement or other artifact. Inclusion of such artifact would give erroneous results, principally as excessively long or short interbeat intervals. To achieve "clean" data, the duration of each interbeat interval needs to be displayed, reviewed, and, if necessary, edited. Software (Mxedit) was developed and patented by Porges for this purpose. Training to reliability criteria established by Porges's laboratory is recommended so that the vagal tone values generated from various laboratories can be considered to be comparably obtained.

Although Porges's techniques of estimating the amplitude of respiratory sinus arrhythmia are available as commercial projects and are relatively user-friendly, alternatives to his methods do exist and should be considered as options, depending on the investigator's or clinician's specific needs. For certain studies of adults, for example, when movement can be kept to a minimum, measuring the peak-to-trough height of the respiratory cycle (Grossman, 1983) could be used. This approach is less useful when the signal is of low amplitude (as it may be in neonates) (Byrne & Porges, 1993) or when measurement of the respiratory cycle is not possible (Grossman, 1983). Other researchers studying infants and children have used alternatives to Porges's methods to approximate the vagal contribution of heart rate. These include measuring the range of heart period (Garcia-Coll, Kagan, & Resnick, 1984) or the mean of the absolute value of the successive differences (Fox, 1983). Others have used alternative spectral analyses and different measures (e.g., extent of the respiratory sinus arrhythmia) to estimate vagal tone (Harper, Hoppenbrouwers, Sterman, McGinty, & Hodgman, 1976; Richards, 1987).

VALIDITY

The process of validating the amplitude of respiratory sinus arrhythmia as an index of cardiac vagal activity has been careful but complicated because there is no readily measured criterion variable for vagal tone. Direct recording from an intact vagus nerve was rejected because of the difficulties involved in recording only from the efferent fibers going to the heart and because of the complexity of decoding the resulting electrophysiological signals (Porges, McCabe, & Yongue, 1982). Instead, efforts have focused on manipulating vagal activity while trying not to affect the sympathetic nervous system. However, because the parasympathetic and sympathetic branches of the autonomic nervous system are interactive, one cannot reject the possibility that the sympathetic system responds to vagal manipulations which could indirectly change the amplitude of RSA (Porges et al., 1982).

Despite these limitations, a number of early observations indicated that the amplitude of respiratory sinus arrhythmia would be a sensitive index of vagal activity. Cardiac vagal efferents were observed to be spontaneously active only during the expiratory phase of respiration and this neural activity was accompanied by cardiac slowing (Iriuchijima & Kumada, 1964; Katona, Poitras, Barnett, & Terry, 1970; Neil & Palmer, 1975). Increases in vagal activity following a variety of different manipulations were observed only during the expiratory phase of respiration, while during normal respiratory inspiration, cardiac vagal activity was suppressed (Iriuchijima & Kumada, 1964; Jewett, 1964). Stimulation of the aortic depressor nerve in the rabbit produced a baroreceptor reflex characterized by increased vagal inhibitory action on the heart, thus increasing the amplitude of RSA. Vagal blockage with atropine removed this effect (McCabe, Yongue, Porges, & Ackles, 1984).

Similar relationships between RSA and vagal innervation were demonstrated in other anesthetized animal preparations (McCabe, Yongue, Ackles, & Porges, 1985) as well as in alert and moving preparations. In a study with alert adults, pharmacological blockade of the vagus was monotonically related to the amplitude of respiratory sinus arrhythmia. In fact, RSA was more sensitive to the vagal blockade than was heart rate (which, in response to atropine, had often been used as a criterion measure of vagal tone) (Dellinger, Taylor, & Porges, 1986; Porges, 1986). A more recent study of normal human term fetuses showed that fetal breathing was associated with an increase in vagal tone as compared to nonbreathing during quiet sleep, again supporting the relationship between respiration and vagal control of the heart (Groome, Mooney, Bentz, & Wilson, 1994).

VAGAL TONE AS A MEASURE OF BIOBEHAVIORAL STATUS

Vagal tone was initially employed to investigate the influence of development and clinical status on the biobehavioral functioning of the infant and young child. These assessments must be performed in a resting individual to ensure that they reflect the individual's homeostatic state, not the individual's response to an external stimulus. Even in a resting state, however, there can be wide differences in an individual's neurally mediated cardiorespiratory measures due to differences in behavioral state. Although this is now known, early evaluations of vagal tone and other cardiorespiratory measures rarely took behavioral state into account.

DEVELOPMENTAL MODEL

Neuroanatomic evidence indicated that the number of myelinated vagus fibers increases in a linear fashion between 24 and 40 weeks gestational age. These data were based on the morphology of the vagus nerve in premature and full-term infants who died from various causes (Sachis, Armstrong, Becker, & Bryan, 1982). To determine whether this developmental trend would be reflected in a similar maturation curve for the vagal tone measure, ECG data were collected during an undisturbed resting period from a cross-section of full-term and prematurely born infants who were free from major clinical complications. Vagal tone was estimated using Porges's methods. The correlation between vagal tone and gestational age was .82: For the youngest infants (28 weeks gestational age), vagal tone was between 1 and 2 and it increased in a linear fashion to 4 to 5 in the oldest infants (40–42 weeks gestational age) (Porges, 1986). This linear relationship is similar to the relationship observed in resting-state vagal tone ($r = .56$) in 26- to 42-week gestational age infants (Porter et al., 1989) and to the one observed between the number of weeks of pregnancy and the increase in fetal heart rate in response to atropine ($r = .74$). Although others have not observed significant developmental increases in vagal tone during the second half of the first year of life (Fracasso, Porges, Lamb, & Rosenberg, 1994), developmental regulation of vagal tone was cited by Chatow, Davidson, Reichman, and Akselrod (1995), who found that the ratio of the low- to that of the high-frequency band oscillation in the heart rate pattern decreased with increased gestational age. Thus, as the autonomic nervous system matures, vagally mediated influences on the heart appear to increase.

There is some controversy as to the effect of respiratory rate on these developmental changes. Premature infants breathe at faster rates than do full-term infants. However, Porges (1992) reported that controlling for respiratory rate differences (using an analysis of covariance) did not eliminate the significant difference in vagal tone between full-term and prematurely born infants. In contrast, Baldzer et al. (1989) observed that a difference in breathing rate does affect both heart rate variability and the low- to high-frequency band ratio. One of the obvious difficulties in understanding the relationship between respiratory rate and vagal tone for an individual is that whatever may cause the respiratory rate to change may also be influencing the vagal tone. Using experimental manipulations (e.g., pharmacological or mechanical) of respiratory rate may help resolve this problem but would likely be rather invasive. Using vagal tone in high-risk infants, particularly those who require mechanical ventilation, is an obvious concern because assumptions about the respiratory rate are built into the vagal tone calculation. As an attempt to understand how a fixed ventilatory rate might affect vagal tone, we compared vagal tone as a function of ventilatory status in premature newborn infants (Porter et al., 1989). Vagal tone was lower but not significantly different for ventilated as compared with nonventilated infants. The competing influences of a fixed respiratory rhythm and the intermittent spontaneous breaths produced by the infants themselves have not been studied with respect to their impact on the vagal tone measure.

Others, as noted previously, have emphasized the important effect behavioral state may have on measurements of vagally mediated heart rate patterns. There appears to be a predominance of sympathetic activity during active sleep and vagal activity during quiet sleep. Quiet sleep is less likely to occur in newborn infants before 35 weeks gestation and increases with increased gestational age (DeHaan, Patrick, Chess, & Jaco, 1977). Thus, the increased vagal influence and the ability to experience quiet sleep may both be reflections of autonomic maturity (Chatow et al., 1995).

RELIABILITY

Although vagal tone can be assessed in premature newborn infants and even in the fetus (Groome et al., 1994), an important question with respect to the developmental regulation of vagal tone is whether vagal tone is relatively stable over time; that is, do infants born with relatively high vagal tone maintain their vagal tone values over time? Few systematic attempts have been made to assess the stability of vagal tone across the first year of life. We observed a marked lack of systematic changes in vagal tone over the first 10 days of life in acutely ill, very-low-birthweight infants, but stability might have been masked by the clinical compromise (Porter et al., 1989). However, correlations between newborn and 5–month vagal tone values for 63 normal full-term infants were also found to be nonsignificant (Stifter & Fox, 1990). In that study, vagal tone values actually decreased over the first 5 months of life, which contrasts with previous reports. Another study which compared values of vagal tone from 3 to 13 months in 25 healthy infants reported that the early vagal tone measures (3 and 4. 5 months) were related to all subsequent (6, 9, and 13 months) measures of vagal tone (Izard et al., 1991). Others observed that vagal tone was stable between 9 months and 3 years of age (Porges, Doussard-Roosevelt, Portales, & Seuss, 1994). These data suggest that stability of vagal tone may develop sometime during the second half of the first year but perhaps not significantly before.

To examine the influence of health status on vagal tone, vagal tone was assessed during rest in a group of clinically normal newborn infants and another group of newborn infants characterized by a variety of clinical pathologies, ranging from respiratory distress syndrome, hydrocephaly, asphyxia, bronchopulmonary dysplasia, and cardiac arrest to microcephaly (Porges et al., 1982). There was a continuum of vagal tone values associated with the varying clinical pathologies; the more severe the clinical problem, the lower the vagal tone. Heart period variability calculated in the same infants differentiated between only two groups of infants, those who subsequently died (and had lower variability) and those who survived (and had higher variability). It did not distinguish among the various neural tube defects, respiratory distress syndrome, and normal neonates as did vagal tone.

In a large, prospective study, cocaine, polydrug-exposed infants were found to have lower vagal tone in the neonatal period than non-cocaine-exposed infants. Moreover, heavier drug exposure was related to lower vagal tone (Mehta et al., 2000).

The effect of therapeutic interventions on vagal tone values is an important issue, particularly among acutely ill infants. Many high-risk infants are treated with a variety of medications, some of which influence the vagal tone measure. Atropine, for example, which blocks acetylcholine at the receptor site, significantly reduces respiratory sinus arrhythmia and attenuates vagal tone in a dose-response fashion (Dellinger, Taylor, & Porges, 1987; Jansen & Dellinger, 1989; Porges, 1986). Pavulon (pancuronium bromide), which is used in some infants as a muscle relaxant to reduce the infant's struggle against mechanical ventilation, blocks vagal efferents to the heart. Vagal activity in these infants could be underestimated by the vagal tone measure. The effects of sedatives and general anesthetics on vagal tone have not been thoroughly investigated. Data suggest that vagal tone may be maintained with some but not others (Halliwill & Billman, 1992), indicating the need to document carefully the drug, its dosage, half-life, and time of administration in all infants being studied.

PREDICTION OF VAGAL TONE
FROM HOMEOSTATIC AND DYNAMIC MEASURES

Although vagal tone appeared to correlate well with concurrent assessments of the developmental and clinical status of newborn infants, all infants with the same clinical or developmental status do not respond alike or have identical outcomes. The ability to identify specific infants early in life who will subsequently exhibit developmental delays, clinical morbidities, or behavioral dysfunction would dramatically facilitate efforts to minimize these debilitating outcomes.

Prediction from Homeostatic Measures

Early work with vagal tone suggested that early individual differences in homeostatic measures of vagal tone were predictive of outcome. Fox and Porges (1985), for example, showed that infants who had higher vagal tone at birth always had positive developmental outcomes whereas infants who had lower vagal tone at birth were mixed with respect to their outcome; some had positive outcomes but some did not. Shortly thereafter it was shown that individual differences in vagal tone measured in resting 6-month-old infants were related to two measures of visual recognition memory believed to be associated with later cognitive functioning (Linnemeyer & Porges, 1986). Infants with higher vagal tone looked (i.e., paid attention) for shorter periods of time at a familiar visual stimulus during a familiarization phase and looked for longer periods at a novel stimulus during test phases. In addition, only those infants with higher vagal tone showed heart rate decelerations in response to the visual stimuli, suggesting greater neural regulation of response to stimulation. This has been further supported by studies in school-age children (Suess, Porges, & Plude, 1994); children with higher resting vagal tone performed better during sustained attention tasks.

Recently, vagal tone has again been implicated in information processing in infancy as measured by habituation. Decreases in nucleus ambiguous vagal tone consistently related to habituation efficiency in 2- and 5-month-old infants (Bornstein & Suess, 2000). Twelve-week-old infants were studied to explore the relationship between cardiac vagal tone and temperament. Infants with higher basal vagal tone were rated as having fewer negative behaviors, and infants who decreased vagal tone during a laboratory assessment were noted as having longer attention spans and being more easily soothed (Huffman et al., 1998).

Additional evidence that resting-state vagal tone may provide an early marker for outcome was provided in a study of very-low-birthweight infants at high risk for the development of chronic lung disease, diagnosed at 30 days of life (Porter et al., 1989). Vagal tone measured on the second day of life was significantly different for those who died prior to 30 days of life, for those who survived but had chronic lung disease, and for those who survived without disease. Vagal tone retained its association with outcome after controlling for other risk factors such as birthweight and ventilatory status.

All these data suggest, as proposed by the polyvagal theory, that vagal tone may be indexing individual differences in neurobehavioral functioning that facilitate or adversely affect physical and cognitive development. Individuals who are neurophysiologically flexible, responsive, and adaptive with respect to the balancing act between maintaining homeostasis and coping with external demands are more likely to develop and behave in ways that are responsive, flexible, and adaptive. These individuals would be more likely to exhibit vagal suppression or withdrawal in response to environmental demands in order to regulate their metabolic output to respond appropriately to external stressors and demands.

Prediction from Dynamic Measures

To investigate this theory, researchers expanded studies using vagal tone to include an assessment of its dynamic characteristics (i.e., how much and in what direction it changed in response to stimulation). Our laboratory, for example, was interested in identifying early individual differences in reactivity to stress and/or pain associated with commonly experienced nursery procedures. Early identification of infants at risk for adverse reactions would provide caregivers an opportunity to develop and institute more effective strategies for stress and pain management. In response to unanesthetized circumcisions, vagal tone in healthy, full-term infants was significantly reduced from its resting level, providing strong support for the theory that vagal withdrawal would accompany states of high environmental demand (Porter, Porges, & Marshall, 1988). Vagal tone also promptly returns to pre-operative levels following circumcision, suggesting that it provides a rapid and immediate index of neurophysiological functioning, more so than neuroendocrine measures could. The suppression of vagal tone was paralleled by increased cry pitch, a feature that characterizes the cries of infants born prematurely or at risk, suggesting that the vagal suppression was indeed a marker of stress reactivity. Finally, individual differences in resting state vagal tone predicted both physiological and behavioral responses to the subsequent stress of circumcision; infants with the preoperatively lowest vagal tone showed virtually no reduction in vagal tone but the highest cry pitch in response to circumcision. Thus, neonates with initially higher vagal tone had greater neurophysiological (vagal) flexibility and showed less severe behavioral distress (lower cry pitch) in response to circumcision, emphasizing that systematic changes in vagal influences provide information as to how the individual copes with environmental stress. Accounting for baseline differences in vagal tone among infants, of course, was an important component in the calculation of difference (i.e., reactivity) scores.

Further support for the idea that early individual differences in vagally mediated reactions might be markers for subsequent outcome was provided by a study of healthy premature infants during gavage feeding (DiPietro & Porges, 1991). Infants who exhibited an increase in vagal tone followed by a vagal rebound to below initial levels in response to gavage feeding had more optimal clinical courses than did those who showed either no initial reactivity or no rebound. Specifically, infants showing the systematic vagal changes were discharged an average of 20 days earlier than the other infants.

Vagally mediated heart rate reactions may predict subsequent outcome, as demonstrated by studies of the physiological basis of temperament. Temperament has been defined in terms of constitutional differences in physiological reactivity and self-regulation of reactivity (Rothbart & Derryberry, 1981, see also Rothbart, Chew, & Gartstein, Chapter 10, this volume). Extremely inhibited children exhibit high heart rate and low heart rate variability (Kagan & Snidman, 1991) and 5-month-olds with higher resting vagal tone were more emotionally reactive, both positively and negatively, than infants with lower vagal tone, but few studies have investigated the relation between vagal reactivity (as opposed to vagal tone at rest) and temperament (Stifter, Fox, & Porges, 1989). More highly reactive infants may be perceived as having more difficult temperaments. However, newborn infants who displayed greater reductions in vagal tone in reaction to a heelstick (i.e., were more reactive) were described by their mothers has having less negative temperament at 6 months (Gunnar, Porter, Wolf, Rigatuso, & Larson, 1995). Alternatively, infants who are highly reactive may be seen by their mothers as having more easily interpretable behavior and, thus, would be seen as having easier temperaments. In one study (Porges, Doussard-Roosevelt, Portales, & Greenspan, 1996) vagal regulation on an infant cognitive task predicted later behavioral problems. To investigate further, we are currently examining the relations between physiological and behavioral reactivity to routine clinical procedures during the neonatal period and temperament assessed at 6 months using both maternal assessments and a structured laboratory-based temperament assessment. The infants' facial expressions to both the clinical procedures and the temperament assessments are also being analyzed to examine the developmental course of emotional expression and its relationship to the physiological indices. In older adults we have found that individuals who are less physiologically reactive tend to be emotionally disinhibited and more facially expressive in response to stressful stimuli (Porter et al., 1996). The extent to which these different systems are coordinated in their response patterns early in development is not known.

Relationships between vagal tone and measures of temperament may be clarified by attachment status (see Chapters 10 and 11, this volume). In a study of 126 4½-year-old children, only securely attached children showed the predicted relation between low behavioral inhibition and high RSA (Stevenson-Hinde & Marshall, 1999).

FUTURE STUDIES

Throughout this chapter I have presented evidence that supports the idea that individual differences in neurobehavioral functioning as indexed by vagal tone may reflect the infant's or young child's biobehavioral status. The fact that vagal tone does seem to be related to such diverse topics as attention, stress, and pain reactions; cognitive performance; temperament; and health indicates that it is likely not a specific marker for any of these domains. Rather, it suggests that the vagal tone measure is assessing the ability of the individual organism to regulate the balance between maintaining homeostasis to support ongoing internal processes (such as digestion, growth, and metabolism) and responding appropriately to external stressors or demands. For a newborn infant, this balancing act may never be more critical than around the time of birth, a time when the newborn must perform myriad new skills such as breathing, eating, and regulating body temperature while also needing to communicate his or her needs to those nearby. For infants born prematurely or with clinical compromise, these challenges are even greater because the resources available to the infant may be even more limited, either by prematurity and/or disease or by the therapeutic interventions required to help the infant survive.

The apparent lack of stability seen in the vagal tone measure during the first half of the first year of life may simply be reflecting these dramatic developmental changes and new challenges that characterize this period of infancy. The "homeostatic" state of the infant is not the same from one day to the next; the vagal tone measure may indeed be accurately reflecting these fluctuations. Alternatively, the failure to account for differences in behavioral state could contribute to the observed lack of day-to-day stability in vagal tone. What has not been systematically explored is what we may be able to learn about the individual from his or her lack of vagal tone stability: Are there differences in the "amount of stability" that could be informative? Furthermore, because early measures of vagal tone do not exhibit stability, there may be some concern about how much value we should place on the ability of those early measures to predict later characteristics of the individual. In short, it may depend on what is being predicted. Early measures of vagal tone may not predict later measures of vagal tone, but they may still be able to provide valuable information about the consequences of individual differences in early neurobehavioral functioning.

As an assessment tool, what has vagal tone provided that is unique and valuable to our understanding of infant development? First, it has revealed much to us about the heart, its rhythmicity, and its link to the neurophysiological integrity of the developing organism. Second, it seems to provide information about the current status of the individual infant that is more comprehensive than any single demographic variable or risk factor conventionally used to characterize newborn infants. And, third, it seems to provide information about the behavioral and cognitive potential of the individual before those domains can be directly assessed themselves.

Research using vagal tone is still young. More work needs to be done to understand more precisely how variations in respiratory rhythms influence the vagal tone estimate, how changes in sympathetic components of the autonomic nervous system may be reflected in the vagal tone measure, and how a broader spectrum of pharmacological agents may influence vagal tone values. Further investigations can illustrate what factors seem to contribute to the presence or absence of stable measures of vagal tone over the first few days, weeks, or months of life and to what extent simple immaturity may be one explanation for the somewhat unreliable nature of the vagal tone measure during the neonatal period. Finally, given that an individual infant has low vagal tone or shows inappropriate vagal tone reactivity, what interventions can be identified that could directly alter that infant's vagal tone or that could alter the consequences of having low vagal tone or inappropriate vagal reactivity? Issues regarding afferent feedback are important and future research, especially associated with interventions, might be focused on the importance of visceral afferent feedback in the regulation and even in the development of vagal tone. Together, a response to these challenges will help to elucidate further how early infant development affects the future of the child and in what ways developmental psychologists, pediatricians, and parents can unite to provide better outcomes for our children.

ACKNOWLEDGMENT

Thanks are extended to Steve Porges and Cynthia Stifter for their helpful review of this chapter.

REFERENCES

Baldzer, K., Dykes, F. D., Jones, S. A., Brogan, M., Carrigan, T. A., & Giddens, D. P. (1989). Heart rate variability analysis in full-term infants: Spectral indices for study of neonatal cardiorespiratory control. *Pediatric Research, 26,* 188–195.

Bohrer, R., & Porges, S. W. (1982). The application of time-series statistics to psychological research: An introduction. In G. Kered (Ed.), *Statistical and methodological issues in psychology and social sciences research* (pp. 309–345). Hillsdale, NJ: Erlbaum.

Bornstein, M. H., & Suess, P. E. (2000). Physiological self-regulation and information processing in infancy: Cardiac vagal tone and habituation. *Child Development, 71*(2), 273–287.

Byrne, E. A., & Porges, S. W. (1993). Data-dependent filter characteristics of peak-valley respiratory sinus arrhythmia extimation: A cautionary note. *Psychophysiology, 30,* 397–404.

Chatow, U., Davidson, S., Reichman, R. L., & Akselrod, S. (1995). Development and maturation of the autonomic nervous system in premature and full-term infants using spectral analysis of heart rate fluctuations. *Pediatric Research, 37*(3), 294–302.

DeHaan, R., Patrick J., Chess, F. G., & Jaco, N. T. (1977). Definition of sleep state in the newborn infant by hr analysis. *American Journal of Obstetrics and Gynecology, 127,* 753–758.

Dellinger, J. A., Taylor, H. L., & Porges, S. W. (1986). Atropine sulfate effects on aviator performance and on respiratory-heart period interactions. *Aviation Space Environment Medicine, 943,* 1–6.

Dellinger, J. A., Taylor, H. L., & Porges, S. W. (1987). Atropine sulfate effects on aviator performance and on respiratory-heart period interactions. *Aviation, Space, and Environment Medicine, 58,* 333–338.

DiPietro, J. A., & Porges, S. W. (1991). Vagal responsiveness to gavage feeding as an index of preterm status. *Pediatric Research, 29,* 231–236.

Fouad, F. M., Tarazi, R. C., Ferrario, C. M., Fighaly, S., & Alicandri, C. (1984). Assessment of parasympathetic control of heart rate by a non-invasive method. *American Journal of Physiology, 246,* 838–842.

Fox, N. A. (1983). Maturation of autonomic control in preterm infants. *Developmental Psychobiology, 16*(6), 495–504.

Fox, N. A., & Porges, S. W. (1985). The relationship between developmental outcome and neonatal heart period patterns. *Child Development, 56,* 28–37.

Fracasso, M. P., Porges, S. W., Lamb, M. E., & Rosenberg, A. A. (1994). Cardiac activity in infancy: Reliability and stability of individual differences. *Infant Behavior and Development, 177,* 277–284.

Garcia-Coll, C., Kagan, J., & Reznick, J. S. (1984). Behavioral inhibition in young children. *Child Development, 55,* 1005–1019.

Gilbey, M. P., Jordan, D., Richter, D. W., & Spyer, K. M. (1983). The inspiratory control of vagal cardio-inhibitory neurons in the cat. *Journal of Physiology, 343,* 57–58.

Groome, L. J., Mooney, D. M., Bentz, L. S., & Wilson, J. D. (1994). Vagal tone during quiet sleep in normal human term fetuses. *Developmental Psychobiology, 27,* 453–466.

Grossman, P. (1983). Respiration, stress, and cardiovascular function. *Psychophysiology, 20,* 284–300.

Gunnar, M. R., Porter, F. L., Wolf, C. M., Rigatuso, J., & Larson, M. C. (1995). Neonatal stress reactivity: Predictions to later emotional temperament. *Child Development, 66,* 1–13.

Halliwill, J. R., & Billman, G. E. (1992). Effect of general anesthesia on cardiac vagal tone. *American Journal of Physiology, 262,* H1719–H1724.

Harper, R. M., Hoppenbrouwers, T., Sterman, M. B., McGinty, D. J., & Hodgman, J. (1976). Polygraphic studies of normal infants during the first six months of life. I. Heart rate and variability as a function of state. *Pediatric Research, 10,* 945–951.

Huffman, L. C., Bryan, Y. E., del Carmen R., Pedersen F. A., Doussard-Roosevelt, J. A., & Porges, S. T. (1998). Infant temperament and cardiac vagal tone: Assessments at twelve weeks of age. *Child Development, 69*(3), 624–635.

Iriuchijima, J., & Kumada, M. (1964). Activity of single vagal fibers efferent to the heart. *Japanese Journal of Physiology, 14,* 479–487.

Izard, C. E., Porges, S. W., Simons, R. F., Haynes, O. M., Parisi, M., & Cohen, B. (1991). Infant cardiac activity: Developmental changes and relations with attachment. *Developmental Psychology, 27,* 432–439.

Jansen, H. T., & Dellinger, J. A. (1989). Comparing the cardiac vagolytic effects of atropine and methylatropine in rhesus macaques. *Pharmacology Biochemistry and Behavior, 32,* 175–179.

Jewett, D. L. (1964). Activity of single efferent fibers in the cervical vagus nerve of the dog, with special reference to possible cardio-inhibitory fibers. *Journal of Physiology, 175,* 321–357.

Kagan, J., & Snidman, N. (1991). Temperamental factors in human development. *American Psychologist, 46*(8), 856–862.

Katona, P. G., & Jih, F. (1975). Respiratory sinus arrhythmia: non-invasive measure of parasympathetic cardiac control. *Journal of Applied Physiology, 39,* 801–805.

Katona, P. G., Poitras, J. W., Barnett, G. O., & Terry, B. S. (1970). Cardiac vagal efferent activity and heart period in the carotid sinus reflex. *American Journal of Physiology, 218,* 1030–1037.

Linnemeyer, S. A., & Porges, S. W. (1986). Recognition memory and cardiac vagal tone in 6–month-old infants. *Infant Behavior and Development, 26,* 43–56.

Lopes, O. V., & Palmer, J. F. (1976). Proposed respiratory gating mechanisms for cardiac slowing. *Nature, 264,* 454–456.

McCabe, P. M., Yongue, B. G., Ackles, P. K., & Porges, S. W. (1985). Changes in heart period, heart-period variability, and a spectral analysis estimate of respiratory sinus arrhythmia in response to pharmacological manipulation of the baroreceptor reflex in cats. *Psychophysiology, 22,* 195–203.

McCabe, P. M., Yongue, B. G., Porges, S. W., & Ackles, P. K. (1984). Changes in heart period, heart period variability, and a spectral analysis estimate of respiratory sinus arrhythmia during aortic nerve stimulation in rabbits. *Psychophysiology, 21,* 149–158.

Mehta, S. K., Super, D. M., Salvator, A., Singer, L., Connuck, D., Goetz-Fradley, L., Harcar-Sevcik, R., & Kaufman, E. S. (2000). Decreased heart rate variability in cocaine-exposed newborn infants. *Pediatric Research, 47,* 417A.

Neil, E., & Palmer, J. F. (1975). Effects of spontaneous respiration on the latency of reflex cardiac chronotropic responses to baroreceptor stimulation. *Proceedings of the Physiological Society, 247,* 16P.

Porges, S. W. (1986). Respiratory sinus arrhythmia: An index of vagal tone. In P. Grossman, K. Janssen, & D. Vaitl (Eds.), *Cardiorespiratory and cardiosomatic psychophysiology* (pp. 101–115). New York: Plenum Press.

Porges, S. W. (1992). Vagal tone: A physiologic marker of stress vulnerability. *Pediatrics, 90*(3), 498–504.

Porges, S. W. (1995). Orienting in a defensive world: Mammalian modifications of our evolutionary heritage: A polyvagal theory. *Psychophysiology, 32,* 301–318.

Porges, S. W., Doussard-Roosevelt, J. A., Portales, A. L., & Greenspan, S. I. (1996). Infant regulation of the vagal "brake" predicts child behavior problems. A psychobiological model of social behavior. *Developmental Psychobiology, 29*(8), 697–712.

Porges, S. W., Doussard-Roosevelt, J. A., Portales, A. L., & Suess, P. E. (1994). Cardiac vagal tone: Stability and relation to difficultness in infants and three-year-old children. *Developmental Psychobiology, 27,* 289–300.

Porges, S. W., McCabe, P. M., & Yongue, B. G. (1982). Respiratory-heart rate interactions: Psychophysiological implications for pathophysiology and behavior. In. J. T. Cacioppo & R. E. Petty (Eds.), *Perspectives in cardiovascular psychophysiology* (pp. 223–264). New York: Guilford Press.

Porter, F., McKee, K. M., Smith, M., Wolf, C. M., Miller, J. P., & Morris, J. (1996). Dementia and response to pain in the elderly. *Pain, 68,* 413–421.

Porter, F. L., Porges, S. W., & Marshall, R. E. (1988). Newborn pain cries and vagal tone: Parallel changes in response to circumcision. *Child Development, 59,* 495–505.

Porter, F., Ultmann, M., Miller, J. P., Arfken, C., Cohlan, B. A., & Altman, D. (1989). Vagal tone (vt) in preterm infants at risk for chronic lung disease. *Pediatric Research, 25,* 227A.

Richards, J. E. (1987). Infant visual sustained attention and respiratory sinus arrhythmia. *Child Development, 58,* 488–496.

Richter, D. W., & Spyer, K. M. (1990). Cardiorespiratory control. In A. D. Loewy & K. M. Spyer (Eds.), *Central regulation of autonomic function* (pp. 189–207). New York: Oxford University Press.

Rothbart, M. K., & Derryberry, D. (1981). Development of individual differences in temperament. In. M. E. Lamb & A. L. Brown (Eds.), *Advances in developmental psychology* (pp. 37–86). Hillsdale, NJ: Erlbaum.

Sachis, P. N., Armstrong, D. L., Becker, L. E., & Bryan, A. C. (1982). Myelination of the human vagus nerve from 24 weeks postconeptional age to adolescence. *Neurology, 41,* 466–472.

Stevenson-Hinde, J., & Marshall P. J. (1999). Behavioral inhibition, heart period, and respiratory sinus arrhythmia: An attachment perspective. *Child Development, 70*(4), 805–816.

Stifter, C. A., & Fox, N. A. (1990). Infant reactivity: Physiological correlates of newborn and 5 month temperament. *Developmental Psychology, 26,* 582–588.

Stifter, C., Fox, N., & Porges, S. (1989). Facial expressivity and vagal tone in 5– and 10–month-old infants. *Infant Behavior and Development, 12,* 127–137.

Suess, P., Porges, S., & Plude, D. (1994). Cardiac vagal tone and sustained attention in school-age children. *Psychophysiology, 31,* 17–22.

7

Sleep–Wake States as Context for Assessment, as Components of Assessment, and as Assessment

EVELYN B. THOMAN

As the result of a large and growing body of literature, it is now accepted that the sleeping and waking states of infants can be identified by distinct physiological and behavioral constellations. A number of functions of the states are also accepted, namely, that an infant's ongoing state serves to mediate perception of environmental events, states modulate the infant's behavioral output in response to those events, they are affected by those events, they constitute a major form of communication within the caregiver–infant interaction, and they reflect the effects and effectiveness of caregiving ministrations, so that parents and other caregivers may titrate their infant-directed behaviors on the basis of ongoing changes in their infant's state. Accordingly, reliable description of the sleep–wake states of infants from the earliest ages can be the basis for assessing the status of the infant's neurobehavioral regulatory controls.

"Because the nervous system of the fetus and newborn is particularly vulnerable during gestation and delivery to potentially damaging factors of biochemical and mechanical nature it is the functional integrity of the developing nervous system which must be the focus of assessment techniques" (Prechtl, 1982, p. 21). The sleep–wake states offer the potential for such assessment.

HISTORY

Parents have always attended closely to their babies' states, being eager for wide-eyed alertness in response to their coo talking, being relieved when the baby sleeps at night, watchful for cues of the baby's readiness for sleep—especially when they are themselves weary—and distressed when the baby cries inconsolably for prolonged periods. Clinicians, especially neonatal intensive care unit staff, are keenly aware of their infant patients' states. Infant states serve as an indication of times that are appropriate for intervention as well as an indication of the effects of their interventions, which may be adjusted on the basis of perceived changes in the infant's state.

The complexity of infants' states has commanded attention from researchers only since the middle of this century. At about that time, interest was aroused by two seminal papers. The first was that of Aserinsky and Kleitman (1955), who described two distinct states of sleep: periods with eye movements and periods of deep sleep with no eye movements. Then, following this lead, Wolff (1966) made intensive behavioral observations of infants and defined what he considered to be the baby's repertoire of behavioral sleeping and waking states. His categories of sleep were called active sleep (periods with eye movements) and quiet sleep (periods with no eye movements).

It is important to note that the researchers who conducted these two studies were working in very different fields. Although Aserinsky and Kleitman had noted eye movements during sleep from behavioral observations, they were primarily interested in the physiological concomitants of sleep, and their data were obtained electrophysiologically. Wolff, as a behavioral scientist, was concerned with both the sleeping and the waking states, as they express an infant's responses to the environment and play a role in interactions with the social environment. His day-long observations were made in the naturalistic circumstances of the infants' homes. Thus, the operational definitions for behavioral sleep and physiological sleep were, and continue to be, very different. However, it should be noted that behavioral observations of infants continue to accompany electroencephalograph (EEG) recordings in order to make a major state distinction, namely, that between active sleep and wakefulness.

Prechtl and Beintama (1964) were the first to provide a systematic description of infants' differential responsiveness to various stimuli as a function of the state the infant is in. Their idea came from observing that during neurological assessment, reflexes may be present, heightened, or even absent in different states. They concluded that noting or controlling for the infant's state was a prerequisite for a reliable neurological assessment. That report provided an impetus for recognition by researchers of the importance of taking an infant's state into account during testing and also during the course of infant research (e.g., Brown, 1964). In a 1972 paper, Korner took the next step and pointed to a new field of behavioral study when she argued that state should be viewed not just as a nuisance variable to be controlled in research but as a variable to be studied "in its own right."

During the intervening decades, numerous reports have described infants' sleep and wake states, although, with the exception of our own studies, more interest has been focused on the sleep states, primarily because sleep can be recorded for prolonged periods by instrumentation of the baby using polysomnography procedures. Using these procedures, Roffwarg, Muzio, and Dement (1966) published their now classic report on the developmental course of the sleep states and wakefulness from early infancy throughout the lifespan.

In 1971, Anders, Emde, and Parmelee (1971) convened and agreed on procedures for recording infants' sleep electrophysiologically: the *Manual of Standardized Terminology, Techniques, and Criteria for Scoring of States of Sleep and Wakefulness in Newborn Infants*. This important document has continued to be a guide for infant physiological sleep research. It should be noted again that the manual requires behavioral observation of the baby during these recordings, because the electrical signals during active sleep periods cannot be distinguished from those that are present during alert wakefulness. In fact, given the requisite that behavioral observations accompany EEG recordings in order to obtain valid sleep–wake information, we have argued that "behavioral sleep" be considered the "gold standard" for distinguishing the sleep states of infants rather than the EEG as is the usual presumption (Thoman & Acebo, 1995). The requisite for including behavioral observation with electrophysiological recording constitutes an important link between the operational definitions for behavioral and neurophysiological state constructs.

In the sections that follow, consideration is given to the rationale and theoretical issues that argue for sleep–wake characteristics as basic indices of neurobehavioral regulatory controls. A number of studies from our laboratory, and those of others, are summarized to illustrate these arguments.

BIOBEHAVIORAL BASIS OF ASSESSMENT FROM STATE PARAMETERS

The notion that state is an ideal behavioral characteristic for assessing infants has considerable conceptual support. Some years ago, Prechtl made a cogent argument: that from a behavioral perspective, state is the prevailing condition of an organism and it is the context within which all other behaviors occur. There are commonalities among individuals and across species in their expression of state, and these change with age. The commonalities indicate the fundamental nature of state as a consequence of evolutionary processes that have assured the survival of developing organisms. A major challenge is to explore the range of variations in state expression as they may provide clues to developmental trajectories.

From a biological perspective, the neurobehavioral underpinnings of the sleep–wake states constitute basic support for the importance of state: Physiologists have demonstrated that sleep results from a complicated series of biochemical reactions involving many parts of the brain, various kinds of cells, and the immune system. Multiple mechanisms, in widely distributed areas of the brain involving both neural and humoral processes, interact to produce sleep and wake states. Changes within and between sleep and wakefulness are accompanied by changes in systems controlling cardiovascular and respiratory function, temperature regulation, cerebral metabolism and blood flow, and renal, alimentary, and endocrine function (Orem & Barnes, 1980).

Using electrophysiological, neuropharmacological, and neuroanatomical methodologies, physiologists have also explored developmental aspects of sleep. For these studies, wakefulness has generally been scored as an undifferentiated nonsleep category. From both animal and human infant studies, Curzi-Dascalova and Challamel (2000) provide an insightful and critical review of the development of neurophysiological regulation of sleep.

At the present time, the interrelatedness of the neurophysiological controlling mechanisms for sleep states and those for wakefulness is an exciting area for sleep researchers. This is a timely endeavor in view of the growing evidence for the interactive effects of sleep quality and events occurring during waking (e.g., Acherman & Borbely, 1994; Thoman, 1990).

During the early years of electrophysiological studies, a number of associations between sleep characteristics and abnormal brain development were revealed: Autistic children show a delay in the development of sleep patterns (Tanguay, Ornitz, Forsythe, & Ritvo, 1976); newborn small-for-gestational-age infants show an immature EEG, and some also have abnormal EEG components (Schulte, Hinze, & Schremph, 1971); unstable state patterns are present in premature infants (Kopp, Sigman, Parmelee, & Jeffrey, 1975), those with Down syndrome (Prechtl, 1974), and those exposed prenatally to alcohol (Rosett et al., 1979); children with PKU or hypothyroidism show deviations in sleep patterns (Lenard & Schulte, 1974; Petre-Quadens, 1974); infants with bilirubinemia have slow breathing during sleep states (Theorell, Prechtl, & Vos, 1974); and babies with brain malformation and/or chromosomal anomalies were described as showing "poor" sleep patterns (Monod & Guidasci, 1976).

In recent years, understanding of biochemical interactions and their relationships with sleep has led to discoveries of close ties between the immune system, the endocrine network, and the brain (Krueger & Obal, 1993). As with neural activity, all the putative sleep-promoting substances thus far identified have multiple biological activities, and some of these activities pertain to functions other than sleep. The current emphasis on those multiple functions of neural and endocrine activities indicates the pervasiveness of sleep factors throughout the central nervous system, further supporting the expectation that the functional status of an infant is expressed in sleep–wake organization.

As already indicated, behavioral scientists, using direct observations, have the possibility of including the full range of waking states as well as those during sleep, but with only a few exceptions, they have not carried out developmental studies. This is the case primarily because of the time limitations on such observations. At the same time, sleep physiologists' interest in development has focused primarily on descriptive studies designed to determine the developmental course of EEG parameters or of circadian or ultradian rhythms and their central neural regulation. A few polygraphic studies have been carried out for the purpose of exploring developmental continuity in individual infants.

Clearly an integration of findings from both behavioral and physiological researchers is required for an understanding of state, the circumstances and events that effect changes, and the significance of variations, from the time of birth and even before, for the developmental course. The studies that are referred to or summarized in the following sections illustrate the potential for state to contribute to understanding infant development from each of these perspectives.

First, however, I describe the constructs that constitute a state system, and depict the repertoire of categories of infants' sleep and wakefulness.

A TAXONOMY OF THE SLEEPING AND WAKING STATES

The infant's states comprise a highly complex system, described by constructs which require rigorous operational definitions if they are to be used for reliable and valid assessment. From many years of study of the states of infants in naturalistic circumstances, we have developed such a taxonomy for the sleeping and waking states that is applicable for infants from birth, as well as the preterm period of premature infants, through the first year of life.

The states in this system of categories are defined from observer judgments of recurring behavior patterns which are distinguishable despite variations among individual infants in expression of their states. Special attention is given to the infant's eyes, face, skin coloring, motility, muscle tone, vocalization, and breathing. Judgments are based on the quality and the patterning of behaviors, not just their presence or absence, as is the case for some taxonomic categories described in the literature. For example, for coding the categories of wakefulness or sleep–wake transition, it is of little use to note whether the infant's eyes are simply open or shut—they may be opening and shutting (as during sleep–wake transition); when the eyes are open they can be fully or only partially open (as they are during drowse);

they can be very bright and scanning (i.e., during alertness) or they can have a dull vacant stare (as they are during nonalert waking). With training, observers can readily agree on these qualitative differences. Thus, it is possible to make reliable judgments of the waking states, as well as the sleep states. However, interobserver reliability for the state categories observed is rarely reported in the literature (Thoman, 1990).

Our state system consists of a set of 10 primary states, which are described in the following paragraphs. The 10-state distinctions are made for researchers who want to obtain the most detailed behavioral sleep–wake observations; then a subset of state categories are defined for observations where fewer discriminations are more appropriate to the goals of a study. Another subset of states is described for making sleep recordings using polysomnography or other physiological or recording procedures. It is important to note that in our defined categories, each of the subsets incorporates all the primary states, so that comparisons, generalizations, and meaningful assessment of reliability and validity can be made across studies.

CLASSIFICATION OF THE STATES FOR SLEEP–WAKE RECORDINGS

The following 10 waking and sleeping states (the primary categories) represent the repertoire of recurring behavioral state patterns one can observe in infants.

Awake States

• *Alert.* The infant's eyes are open, bright and shining, and attentive or scanning. Motor activity is typically low during the first 2 weeks of life, but the infant may be active.
• *Nonalert waking.* The infant's eyes are usually open but dull and unfocused. Motor activity may vary but is typically high.
• *Daze.* The infant's eyes are open but glassy and immobile. The level of motor activity is typically low. Daze typically occurs between episodes of drowse and alert.
• *Fuss.* Fuss sounds are made continuously or intermittently, at relatively low levels of intensity.
• *Cry.* Intense vocalizations occur either singly or in succession.

Transition States between Sleep and Waking

• *Drowse.* The infant's eyes are dull and unfocused and are either open but "heavy-lidded" or opening and closing slowly.

- *Sleep–wake transition.* The infant shows behaviors of both wakefulness and sleep. The level of motor activity is typically low but may vary. During periods of high-level activity, isolated fuss vocalizations may occur. This state generally occurs when the baby is awakening from sleep.

Sleep States

- *Active sleep.* The infant's eyes are closed. Respiration is uneven and primarily costal in nature. Sporadic movements may occur, but muscle tone is low between movements. Rapid eye movements (REMs) occur intermittently, ranging from a brief, light flicker of the eyelids to prolonged intense REM storms accompanied by raising of the eyelids and brief eye opening. Other behaviors that may be seen in active sleep include smiles, frowns, grimaces, mouthing, sucking, or sighing.
- *Quiet sleep.* The infant's eyes are closed. Respiration is relatively slow, regular, and abdominal in nature. A tonic level of motor tone is maintained, and motor activity is usually limited to occasional startles. Brief periods of limb or body movements may occur (these are more frequent in preterm infants). Associated behaviors include sighing or rhythmic mouthing.
- *Active–quiet transition sleep.* This state occurs between periods of active sleep and quiet sleep. Respiration is not as regular as during quiet sleep and is more regular than during active sleep. The baby shows mixed behavioral signs of active sleep and quiet sleep, with twitching or trembling movements of the extremities. The baby may emit brief, high-pitched cries as well as "straining" or grunting vocalizations during large stretching movements.

A SIMPLER CLASSIFICATION OF STATES

For many research and clinical purposes, 10 states are a large number to differentiate and record. It is reasonable to combine some of the primary states into clusters to reduce the number of categories for observation. Such combinations have been derived rationally and systematically, and the resulting construct groupings have repeatedly been demonstrated to show measurement reliability as in the case of the original 10 states. The six categories are as follows, with indications of which of the 10 primary states are included in each:

- Alert
- Nonalert waking (includes daze)
- Crying (includes fuss)
- Sleep–wake transition (includes drowse)
- Active sleep (includes active–quiet transition preceding active sleep)
- Quiet sleep (includes active–quiet transition preceding quiet sleep)

Some procedures, such as time-lapse video and actigraphy, permit recording of only the sleep states and the general category of wakefulness, as follows:

- Wake
- Sleep–wake transition or drowse
- Active sleep
- Quiet sleep

We have used this limited taxonomic description of the sleep–wake states for video recordings, and, again, all the 10 primary categories are accounted for in this set of states.

In our studies, we have consistently demonstrated measurement reliability for each of the state categories defined. Thus, the measures can be considered appropriate for characterizing individual infants.

PROCEDURES THAT HAVE USED THESE CATEGORIES FOR DESCRIBING INFANTS' SLEEP–WAKE STATES

Direct Behavioral Observations

Direct behavioral observations (as reported in Becker & Thoman, 1981, 1982, 1983; Holditch-Davis & Thoman, 1987) permit recording the full range of infants' sleeping and waking states, in the laboratory or in naturalistic circumstances—the hospital or the infants' homes. But they require the presence of an observer, which can be intrusive in the home, and they are labor intensive, which places limitations on the duration of observations.

For this procedure, the state of an infant can be code-recorded for successive 10-second epochs, and one can use an electronic timer that provides an auditory signal through an earphone. This time period is appropriate for wakefulness, when the infant's states can change within a matter of seconds. For the sleep states, which are more enduring, the 10-second epoch serves as a moving time window to attend to a change in state.

We have observed newborn babies in the hospital for as little as an hour (Thoman, Korner, & Kraemer, 1976) and found evidence for significant individual differences among infants, based on repeated observations, but such a brief period is likely to show reliability only if environmental conditions are carefully controlled. Our major studies using direct behavioral observations were of 7-hour duration, carried out in the infants' homes. Two observers made the code recordings—with each recording for 3½ hours, morning and afternoon, with a 15-minute period of both observers recording at midday (for ongoing assessment of interobserver reliability). States, as well as the occurrence of infant and mother–infant behaviors, were recorded throughout the day's activities. Infants 1 to 5 weeks old spend about half the 7-hour day in waking states and the other half in sleep.

Video Recording

Anders and Keener (1985) developed time-lapse video procedures for recording the sleep–wake states in the home during overnight periods, and they describe the developmental course of the state patterns throughout the first postnatal year. We used this technology to make time-lapse video for successive 24-hour recordings of preterm infants in the NICU (Thoman, 1990; Thoman & Acebo, 1995). The video camera was directly above the isolette, attached to a brace from an IV pole, and a miniature VCR monitor was also attached to the IV pole, so the isolette was fully mobile. Reliability of measurement was found from the repeated days' recordings.

Actigraphy

Sadeh, Acebo, Seifer, Aytur, and Carskadon (1995) have developed and explored actigraphy procedures. The major advantage of this procedure is the possibility of recording continuously over a week or longer.

Motility Monitoring

From years of experience making direct behavioral observations and scoring the accompanying respiration recordings, we developed the automated Motility Monitoring System (MMS) (Thoman & Whitney, 1989). Because most of our studies in recent years—and most of those to be referred to—were carried out with this procedure, I will describe it in some detail.

The MMS consists of a thin ($1/8$-inch) capacitance-type sensor pad that is placed in the infant's crib under the bedding. The pad is connected to a battery-driven amplifier and a 24-hour data recorder. A single channel of analog signals produced by the infant's respiration and body movements is continuously recorded. In the laboratory, the recordings are computer scored, in 30-second epochs, for sleep–wake states, using a pattern recognition program. Then the complete signal file is printed out and visually edited; thus, the scoring is considered to be "computer aided." The states scored are active sleep, active–quiet transition sleep, quiet sleep, sleep–wake transition, and wakefulness. Periods out of the crib are also scored. Because nothing is attached to the baby for the purposes of the recordings, this is a nonintrusive procedure which permits continuous 24-hour monitoring in the hospital or home without requiring changes in caregiving practices by nursing staff or parents.

For our studies, trained observers of behavior and coders of motility-monitored recordings provide reliable, valid data from infants at preterm and early postterm ages, from older infants and children, from elderly humans, from infant and adult animals, and, thus, for cross-species studies (reviewed in Thoman, 1990).

STUDIES OF STATE AS A CORRELATE, AS A PREDICTOR, AND AS A DEPENDENT VARIABLE FOR EARLY INTERVENTION

For many years, behavioral researchers have used sleep–wake states as dependent variables to assess the developmental effects of early interventions, ranging from circumcision in the newborn (Anders & Chalemian, 1974) to more general environmental manipulations (e.g., Gabriel, Grote, & Jonas, 1981; Sander, Julia, Stechler, & Burns, 1972), as well as our Breathing Bear (Thoman, 1990; Thoman & Graham, 1986; Thoman, Hammond, Afflick, & DeSilva, 1995). The Breathing (teddy) Bear serves as a "crib companion" that provides rhythmic stimulation produced by oscillation of its torso, and the rate of its breathing is made to match that of the infant's breathing in quiet sleep (Ingersoll & Thoman, 1994). Stimulation is optional for the infant, who can regulate the timing and duration of stimulation by moving to make contact with the bear, or even move away from it. We have found that experience with the Breathing Bear facilitates neurobehavioral development in preterm infants compared with infants exposed to a nonbreathing bear, and the effects include more mature sleep–wake organization (Thoman, 1999; Thoman, Ingersoll, & Acebo, 1991).

Viewing state as a predictor, from all-night video recordings in the home, Anders and collaborators (Anders & Keener, 1985; Anders, Keener, Bowe, & Shoaff, 1983) found that arousals in sleep, especially quiet sleep, were negatively related to mental development scores at 1 and 2 years of age. This finding was important because it was the first to suggest the notion of sleep fragmentation as having negative developmental implications. Studies in our laboratory and others have consistently confirmed this finding.

Based on longitudinal electrophysiological study of premature infants, Beckwith and Parmelee (1986) found that low levels of trace alternate in the EEG of term-aged prematures were predictive of lower mental development and learning problems starting at 4 months and continuing to age 8. However, the relationship did not hold in infants being reared in consistently attentive and responsive environments. These findings are of special significance because demographic indicators did not distinguish infants with later learning problems. DiPietro and Porges (1991) also report that delay in the development of EEG patterns is associated with later mental delay.

Viewing state as a correlate, we found that mode of delivery is associated with differing sleep–wake patterns of newborns (Freudigman & Thoman, 1998). Further, only vaginally delivered infants showed significant day–night differences in their patterns during the first 2 postnatal days, with the vaginally delivered infants showing more wakefulness, shorter sleep periods, and shorter longest-sleep periods during the daytime than at night on both days. The results suggest that early diurnal rhythms are disrupted by surgical delivery. I cite evidence that this irregularity in diurnal organization in surgically delivered infants may persist to later ages.

For an intensive developmental study of 95 very-low-birthweight preterm infants, we recorded sleep states and wakefulness continuously for 3 successive days, using time-lapse video, when they were 33 weeks postconceptional age A and again when they were 35 weeks postconceptional age (Ingersoll & Thoman, 1999). There were significant individual differences at each age, over age, and from day- to nighttime. The infants showed the same developmental course in state changes that continues over postterm ages. These results indicate that the premature infant is capable of a marked stability along with organized developmental changes in their states from an early preterm age.

In addition, the infants' sleep patterns showed significant relationships with the amount and distribution of caregiving activities. This was the case although, in a previous study, we did not find significant differences in preterm infants' states as a function of specific interventions prescribed by a caregiving program (Ariagno et al., 1997).

PREDICTION FROM THE EARLIEST POSTNATAL PERIOD

Few studies have aimed at prediction from the states of newborn infants. This early period has not been expected to have developmental implications because it was generally assumed that, during the first postnatal days, the infant is going through a passing phase of recovery from the birth process. Although this assumption persists, it has been contradicted in studies by Tharp (1989) and by Pezzani, Radvanyi-Bouvet, Reiler, and Monod (1986), who reported evidence that deviances in EEG seen during the early postnatal days were related to later developmental abnormalities. This notion has also been contradicted by our studies.

In one of our earliest state studies (Thoman, Miano, & Freese, 1978), the behavioral states of 2-day-old infants were observed for 1 hour during two successive midfeeding periods. Immediately after observing the baby, the observer gave a rating on a 4-point scale of how well "organized" the baby appeared to be during the observation. These ratings were found to be associated with distinct profiles of the infants' state measures. The ratings were also found to be related to mothers' general ratings of the infants' behavioral organization when they were 8 months old. This preliminary study is described here not only because it was our first clue to the importance of the earliest postnatal period for assessing neurobehavioral status and its implications for subsequent development, but because it was the first indication to us that measures which are more complex than simple amounts of the states might be required as clues to the infants' status and developmental trajectory. Other studies of state patterning as organization are described in the section that follows.

The findings from a more recent study suggest that the first postnatal day is a unique time for highly sensitive assessment of later development. From continuous sleep recordings over the first 2 postnatal days, we found that on postnatal day 1, six sleep measures were related to 6-month Bayley mental and motor scores; and by postnatal day 2, two measures showed such relationships (Freudigman & Thoman, 1993). Our inference from these findings was that given the stressfulness of the birth process, some babies may be less able neurophysiologically to cope with this challenge, and their reduced adaptive capability is expressed in deviant state regulation. Accordingly, we have proposed that the infant's sleep characteristics during the first postnatal day provide uniquely sensitive indices of developing neurobehavioral status.

Assessment Using Measures of State Organization

While measures of isolated state variables, such as the percent of time spent in a state, are of ongoing interest for comparing groups of subjects, a number of researchers have reported procedures for depicting organization of the sleep–wake states within individual infants. These procedures yield indices that can be used for group analyses.

Harper, Frostig, Taube, Hoppenbrouwers, and Hodgman (1983) assessed the periodic organization of waking, quiet sleep, and active sleep, using spectral analysis for 12-hour all-night polygraphic recordings. They used the procedure for a study of siblings of victims of sudden infant death syndromes (SIDS) and a control group of infants at 1 week and 1, 2, 3, 4, and 6 months. The results revealed "disturbed" patterns of sleep states in the siblings of sudden infant death syndrome infants (SSIDS) through the age range studied. The researchers concluded that the temporal patterning of sleep states can be used as an important neurological marker for development.

Anders (1974) and Anders and Keener (1985) have reported organizational descriptors which, though not applied, can be noted: (1) the Infant Sleep Profile for polygraphic study of sleep—dimensions of sleep are used to compare the profiles of infants for determination of deviancy; (2) a "holding time index" which represents allocation of time to active sleep and quiet sleep during each third of the night, as an indication of the degree of diurnal organization of the two sleep states; and (3) a transition probability index.

A procedure for estimating individual developmental trajectories statistically was developed by Kraemer (Kraemer, Korner, & Hurwitz, 1985), and it was illustrated with data from preterm infants. This analytic procedure makes it possible to evaluate the relative contribution of an infant's gestational age, birthweight, and conceptional and chronological ages to a developmental variable. An important aspect of the procedure is that assessing a group of infants over different age periods during the preterm stay in the hospital does not pose a problem. Transformed data are regressed on postconceptional or chronological age for each infant, producing an intercept and slope for the infant. The effects of gestational age, birthweight, and chronological age on a developmental variable can be determined by correlating these variables with the intercepts and slopes. For that study, the mathematical model was not used for the behavioral states, but it is included here because the approach is especially creative, and it would be most appropriate for assessing the three major factors as they contribute to the developmental course of the sleep–wake states, especially in preterm infants.

Holditch-Davis and collaborators describe two statistical models for examining the development of sleep–wake states in premature infants. One assesses the temporal organization of the states, and from a study of preterm infants, they found that transitional probabilities remain relatively invariant during the preterm period, while other state measures may be modified by differing environmental conditions (Holditch-Davis & Edwards, 1998). The second is "a mixed general linear model analysis" for the development of the sleep–wake states, and the researchers conclude that the developmental patterns of sleep–wake states in preterm infants are stable enough in the preterm period that infants with neurological problems may be identified (Holditch-Davis, Edwards, & Helms, 1998).

STABILITY OF STATE ORGANIZATION
AS A PREDICTOR OF DEVELOPMENT

For a major study, already referred to, for which the sleep–wake states of healthy 2- to 5-week old infants were directly observed in the home for 7-hour periods, an index of state stability was devised by Denenberg (Thoman, Denenberg, Sievel, Zeidner, & Becker, 1981). That is, in order to characterize individual subjects, a profile of the means of the sleep measures for each week was derived, and the profiles were assessed for consistency over weeks for each infant, using analysis of variance.

We found that infants with the lowest profile consistency had major developmental problems at later ages, including severe retardation and SIDS. Infants with less extreme but low consistency scores showed minor developmental delay, while none of the infants above the median on the consistency index showed evidence of any developmental dysfunction by 30 months of age. These findings indicate that developmental inconsistency in state organization during the early postnatal weeks is predictive of risk for later development. The findings of predictive validity of the State Stability Index has been replicated in more recent studies in other laboratories.

THE STATE STABILITY INDEX
PERMITS SPECIFIC PREDICTION

In another study of state organization, the MMS was used for weekly 24-hour recordings of premature infants during the first 5 postterm weeks (Whitney & Thoman, 1993). All were considered to be normally developing infants at the time of the recordings. Infants were later classified as those who, by 3 years, were still considered to be normal, those who showed mental delay, those who were diagnosed with neurological disorder, and those who were diagnosed with a major physical disorder.

The mean State Stability Index was calculated for each of the four outcome groups and these were compared. We found that each of the deviant outcome groups showed state profiles that differed significantly from the normal group, and the state profiles of each of the deviant groups differed significantly from each other. This was the first study to differentiate among groups of apparently normal infants who later show specific forms of abnormal outcomes.

A PATTERN OF STATE AND RESPIRATORY DEVIANCE
IS ASSOCIATED WITH SIDS RISK

The data for the SIDS infant in a study described earlier were examined further and included in a subsequent study (Thoman, Davis, Graham, Scholz, & Rowe, 1988). Not only did the SIDS infant have unstable state organization (low state stability score, as described earlier), he also showed deviant respiratory patterns. For the subsequent study, three siblings of SIDS infants and a group of 16 normal infants were studied prospectively using the home observation procedures. Based on the data from the early weeks for the four infants, one of the three SIDS infants was predicted to have later respiratory problems because she showed a pattern of state and respiratory deviancies similar to the SIDS infants. All three were placed on apnea monitors by their pediatricians. At 4 months, in accordance with our prediction, the one infant had prolonged apneic episodes, both at home and later in the hospital, where she required resuscitation on two occasions. The other two infants, as predicted, showed no difficulties over the year they were followed. These findings are congruent with the proposition that identifying subtle but serious central nervous system dysfunction at a very early age is possible from measures of state organization.

The study also highlighted the importance of state-related respiration patterns. More recent findings of Montgomery-Downs and Thoman (1998) provide further support. Quiet sleep respiration rates (QSRR) during the neonatal period were found to differentiate among individual infants, female infants had lower QSRR than did male infants, and QSRR at 6 months was related to mental scores of infants at 6 and 12 months.

EARLY STRESS AND ACCELERATION OF MATURATION

In our studies of the states of infants during the newborn period, we have observed a phenomenon that is of great significance for understanding infants' response to the birth process and the implications of this early response for later development. A summary of three of our studies reveals the nature of this observation (Borghese, Minard, & Thoman, 1995; Minard & Thoman, 1995; Freudigman & Thoman, 1993).

We investigated within-sleep rhythmicity in preterm infants. Our Cyclicity Index is another statistical descriptor of organization, one that is very different from the State Stability Index. For this assessment we use a modification of a statistical procedure devised by Kraemer (Kraemer, Hole, & Anders, 1984), which is designed to permit calculation of a cyclicity score for quiet sleep recurrence in individual infants. The procedure is unique in two important ways: (1) it takes into account the duration of the quiet sleep episodes, and (2) it permits determination of whether the degree of cyclicity differs significantly from chance. Other statistical procedures for assessment of within-sleep rhythmicity, as a form of ultradian rhythm, have been reported in the literature, but they were not designed to be evaluated for significance, nor have they been used to assess predictive validity.

For this study, the sleep of preterm infants was recorded on three successive days at 36 weeks postconceptional age, and then again in the home at 6 months for two successive 24-hour periods (Borghese, Minard, & Thoman, 1995). A cyclicity score was calculated for each infant at the two ages, The results indicated that preterm infants are capable of sleep rhythmicity as early as 36 weeks conceptional age: About 50% of the preterm infants showed significant cyclicity. By 6 months, most of the infants showed significant cyclicity. To our surprise, measures from the preterm period, including cycle length and the active sleep component of the cycle, were inversely related to mental development, whereas at 6 months the relationship was positive. The finding that higher cyclicity scores during the preterm period were associated with lower Bayley scores at a later age was important as an expression of the phenomenon that more mature sleep patterns in very immature infants can be an expression of stress rather than an indication of more advanced neurobehavioral development. Clearly, preterms are stressed infants whereas by the later ages maturation rather than stress is being expressed in their sleep organization.

The phenomenon of stress accelerating early development, at least temporarily, has been reported in the animal literature. We have further evidence in other studies. In another study of cyclicity, this time in full-term newborns, quiet sleep cyclicity was assessed from continuous sleep monitoring during the first 2 postnatal days (Minard & Thoman, 1995). The MMS recordings started as soon as the baby was admitted to the newborn nursery. Cyclicity measures on the first postnatal day were found to be inversely related to mental development scores obtained at 6 months. These results are consistent with the findings from the study of preterm infants just described.

Finally, in a study described earlier in this chapter, also from continuous sleep–wake recordings during the first 2 postnatal days (Freudigman & Thoman, 1993), we found that a number of sleep measures predict later cognitive competence. We did not note in the summary of that study, above, that the direction of five of the six relationships on Day 1 were contrary to what might be expected in view of the developmental course of infants' sleep state changes. Further, all significant changes in state from Day 1 to Day 2 were in the direction contrary to the developmental course. We concluded that "those newborns who show greater reactivity to the birth events are the ones who have poorer developmental outcome because the stress of the birth process may serve to accentuate and/or exacerbate an existing neural compromise" (Freudigman & Thoman, 1993, p. 377).

A DEVELOPMENTAL MODEL FOR VIEWING
THE SLEEP–WAKE STATES

Clearly, there are a variety of methods available for assessing characteristics of infants' states. As a highly complex process, there are no apparent short-cuts to describing the sleep–wake states and their development in infants.

The studies described indicate that sleep–wake assessment for very young infants can be related to later developmental status, including subsequent abnormalities, and this is the case even for infants who are considered to be "normal" at the time of their state recordings. Thus, current research supports the notion that there is continuity over development in neurobehavioral competence of infants and that the trajectory of this continuity can be predicted from the sleep–wake states.

Evidence from extensive research by neurophysiologists, neuroanatomists, and neurochemists indicating the complexity of sleep led Webb (1979) to conclude that "Sleep (we would add "Wake") is one of many complicated systems of mechanisms that protect it (the individual) against the influences of the environment and enable it to maintain itself as a living organism" (p. 30). Accordingly, we have assumed (Thoman, 1990; Thoman, Acebo, & Becker, 1983) that any theory of state development, in fact any theory of development, must be a systems theory. General systems theory is concerned with problems of organized complexity (Bertalanffy, 1933; Weiss, 1971). The characteristics of system dynamics are as follows: (1) there is ongoing feedback within the system, (2) the system functions to maintain its own equilibrium, and (3) there are simultaneous interactions of complex variables. Of major interest to systems theorists are the functions of the brain, as a hierarchically organized system, with multiple expressions, including overt behavior. The richness of state behavior derives from its complexity. Thus, the patterning of state behaviors is an emergent process from the integration of processes of the central nervous system, expressing temporal organization of the reciprocal regulatory mechanisms among different systems.

Whereas general systems theory notions have guided our own research conceptually, a number of researchers have exploited dynamic, nonlinear models to describe the state system quantitatively (Thelen, 1990). Guess and Siegel-Causey (1995) propose that it would be particularly useful to search for similar patterns of behavior state quality and significant attractor dimensions that transverse clinical syndromes and conditions. As suggested by the studies described in this chapter, such an approach holds the promise of enhancing our understanding of behavioral and physiological conditions associated with very early trauma to the central nervous system.

As emergent process, the states have a number of characteristics that must be taken into account for purposes of description, prediction, or use as a dependant variable: (1) state occurs over time and, therefore, must be observed for long enough periods to reliably depict that process, (2) the context for recording state must be taken into account in any interpretation of findings, and (3) the state process occurs in individuals, and though averages for groups may be useful for many purposes, states within individuals must be the basis of prediction for individuals. These are major issues to consider in any procedure designed to use sleep–wake states as indices of the functional integrity of an infant's developing central nervous system.

From a systems perspective, it is comprehensible that it may not be possible to identify critical state variables that will provide the clues to "normal" or "nonnormal" development. One of the characteristics of a system is that single elements within the system can vary widely without the system as a whole becoming unstable. Even more, in a biological system, brain plasticity permits reorganization as a function of stress or trauma to elements of the central nervous system. Thus, variations in single variables may not necessarily be indicative of later system central nervous system "problems." One must conclude that in addition to measuring individual state parameters, it is necessary to find ways of describing the overall organization of the states in order to detect subtle instabilities in the system at an early age.

The argument for this chapter is that a systems conception of the sleep–wake states calls for statistical procedures that provide measures that can depict the complexity of states as neurophysiological systems output. "Anything that is as complex as the central nervous system warrants comprehensive and sophisticated evaluation" (Butler, 1983, p. 305). It may seem obvious, but the point is too important not to state: System processes are not group phenomena; they occur within each individual. Thus, state systems descriptors have to depict state organization within each infant, and it is essential that the descriptors be context sensitive.

FURTHER CONSIDERATIONS OF ASSESSMENT FROM SLEEP–WAKE STATES

In 1987, Hoppenbrouwers concluded that "polygraphic monitoring of sleep and waking behavior to identify neurological deficits and predict behavioral and neurological outcome in infants does not hold great promise. There is significant diversity in results that cannot be easily reconciled, even in normal infants. . . . Conventions for analysis vary widely among investigators . . . " (p. 10). The studies described in this chapter indicate that procedures are available that do provide results contrary to this general conclusion. However, the picture is still complicated, and apparent contradictions need to be resolved.

Hoppenbruwers's quote also points to a related problem that continues to bedevil this area of study, namely, the lack of agreement among researchers on the categories and definitions of the states, whether the researchers are recording electrophysiological sleep–wakefulness or behavioral states. It was for this reason that the *Manual of Standardized Terminology, Techniques and Criteria for Scoring of States of Sleep and Wakefulness in Newborn Infants* (Anders et al., 1971) was published. However, problems persist. As a simple, but profound, example, the manual for infants (Anders et al., 1971) defined the states of active sleep and quiet sleep, rather than REM and NREM (non-REM) because young infants do not show the adult structure of sleep, which includes the four stages of NREM sleep. During early infancy, infants show states that are antecedents of the stages of NREM and REM, referred to as quiet sleep and active sleep, respectively. Researchers do not agree on the age during the first year at which the adult sleep categories appear and can be reliably identified. From 3 to 9 months, researchers may try to translate states into stages or the reverse, and the result is not consistent across studies from different laboratories.

Among the behavioral sleep researchers, a major problem derives from the fact that researchers "create" new behavioral "state scales," or they report "modifications" of those that have been recognized for many years—those of Wolff, of Prechtl, and of Thoman (Prechtl & Beintama, 1964; Thoman, 1990; Wolff, 1966). Although the states of active sleep and quiet sleep are common to all state classifications, variations in the definitions (or even exclusion) of transitional periods have effects on the resulting sleep state measures that are more than trivial.

Other issues should be mentioned. Namely, most studies in which behavioral states are measured as dependent variables have used relatively short durations of observation, and few studies include assessment of measurement reliability. Finally, most studies using physiological measures have recorded the infants in the laboratory, a circumstance which, in itself, modifies the states of the subjects. If the purpose is to assess the effects of a stress or a challenge to the infant's regulatory controls, laboratory recordings can be effective, but if the objective is to determine the infants' typical functioning, nonstressful and nonintrusive procedures are called for, and, of course, the least intrusive context is the infant's home.

Thus, despite considerable progress over recent decades, state study still seems to be a victim of many of the sins of being a new field of research. Under these circumstances, there might seem to be little encouragement for anyone to use infants' states for assessment and prediction. To the contrary, the evidence from both behavioral and biological research strongly supports the view that state should be a critical component of any comprehensive assessment of an infant. The flaws in the state picture are not fatal ones. For some of the issues raised, solutions have been found in recent research, and for others, recent research points to directions for solution. We would argue that standardized operational definitions for the sleep–wake states for both the behavioral and the physiological states are timely.

It is clear, from the current body of literature that the sleep–wake states provide a special window on central neural regulatory function. However, some might argue that the view is a bit cloudy, and there is not sufficient evidence that the window is clearing. To the extent that operational definitions are individualized to researchers, there is limited comparability of findings among research groups. Anders pointed out in 1974, when proposing a sleep polygram to depict sleep organization, that "Uniform methodologies, readily shared by others, which permit multiple avenues of exploration remain necessary requirements before the sleep polygram can attain clinical acceptability" (p. 426). More than two decades later, this issue has still not been resolved.

Definitional problems are more acute in infancy, because of the changing expression of the states, especially the sleep states, over age. At the older ages, there is little disagreement among behavioral researchers because there are so few of them. A notable exception is to be found in the studies of children and youths with profound disabilities by Guess, Siegel-Causey, and collaborators (as cited in Guess & Siegel-Causey, 1995). They spend as much as 5 hours observing the behavioral states of their subjects.

Despite differences in definitional criteria and variations in procedures for observing or recording infants' states, there is general agreement on some aspects of the developmental course. For example, all studies, behavioral and physiological, indicate that wakefulness, especially alertness, increases over age, active sleep decreases, and quiet sleep increases. The commonalities of findings attest to the robustness of the behavioral state concept. However, developmental science needs a body of state literature with comparable findings across laboratories that are relevant for testing theories and elaborating the state process—and for developing standardized assessment procedures.

CONCLUDING COMMENTS

I have described a state taxonomy that has been extensively studied and tested for reliability and validity for the range of ages, from the preterm period to 1 year, in adults—and also in infant and adult animals. The animal studies are important by way of indicating cross-species generality of the state categories defined. We have also demonstrated comparability of data using these definitions while using different procedures to obtain data simultaneously, including behavioral observation and the MMS and behavioral observations with EEG.

The findings described in this chapter point to the ultimate potential of early state assessment for identifying risk status and predicting later development. In view of the predictive potential of sleep measures and the nonintrusiveness of recordings using the new procedures described, it is now within the realm of reality (probably distant future) that the sleep–wakefulness of newborns in any hospital could be monitored throughout the infant's stay in the hospital (2 days is now federally mandated). In cases in which newborn infants show excessive sleep fragmentation, or other forms of disorganization or deviancy in their sleep–wake patterns, additional surveillance of a baby could be recommended through the early months to reduce the possibility that the baby's apparent vulnerability might lead to later problems. Such monitoring is now procedurally feasible and should soon be economically reasonable.

Continuing research will permit refinement of state predictors, with Honzik's (1976) admonition to keep in mind for these efforts: "predication of later . . . functioning is a worthy aim of infant tests but secondary to the more important objective of adding to our understanding and knowledge of the course of development of . . . abilities in infancy and early childhood" (p. 91). Such understanding should ultimately provide the context within which more reliable and valid assessment of individual infants becomes a possibility. There is work to be done.

REFERENCES

Acherman, P., & Borbely, A. A. (1994). Simulation of daytime vigilance by the additive interaction of a homeostatic and a circadian process. *Biological Cybernetics, 71*(2), 115–121.

Anders, T. F. (1974). The infant sleep profile. *Neuropaediatrie, 5,* 425–442.

Anders, T. F., & Chalemian, R. (1974). Effect of circumcision on sleep–wake states in human neonates. *Psychosomatic Medicine, 36,* 174–179.

Anders, T. F., Emde, R., & Parmelee, J. (1971). *A Manual of Standardized Terminology, Techniques, and Criteria for the Scoring of States of Sleep and Wakefulness in Newborn Infants.* Los Angeles: UCLA Brain Information Service, NINDS Neurological Information Network.

Anders, T. F., & Keener, M. (1985). Developmental course of nighttime sleep–wake patterns in full term and premature infants during the first year of life. I. *Sleep, 8*(3), 173–192.

Anders, T. F., Keener, M., Bowe, T. R., & Shoaff, B. A. (1983). A longitudinal study of nighttime sleep–wake patterns in infants from birth to one year. In J. Call, E. Galenson, & R. Tyson (Eds.), *Frontiers of infant psychiatry* (pp. 150–170). New York: Basic Books.

Ariagno, R. L., Thoman, E. B., Boeddiker, M. A., Constantinou, J. C., Baldwin, R. B., Kugener, B., Mirmiran, M. M., Fleisher, B. E. (1997). Developmental care does not alter sleep and development of premature infants. *Pediatrics, 100,* 1–7.

Aserinsky, E., & Kleitman, N. (1955). A motility cycle in sleeping infants as manifested by ocular and gross bodily activity. *Journal of Applied Physiology, 8,* 11–18.

Becker, P. T., & Thoman, E. B. (1981). Rapid eye movement storms in infants: Rates of occurrence at 6 months predicts mental development at one year. *Science, 212,* 1415–1416.

Becker, P. T., & Thoman, E. B. (1982). "Waking Activity": The neglected state of infancy. *Developmental Brain Research, 4,* 395–401.

Becker, P. T., & Thoman, E. B. (1983). Organization of sleeping and waking states in infants: Consistency across contexts. *Physiology and Behavior, 31,* 405–410.

Beckwith, L., & Parmelee, A. (1986). EEG patterns of preterm infants home environment and later IQ. *Child Development, 57,* 777–789.

Bertalanffy, L. V. (1933). *Modern theories of development: An introduction to theoretical biology.* London: Oxford University Press.

Borghese, I. F., Minard, K. L., & Thoman, E. B. (1995). Sleep rhythmicity in premature infants: Implications for developmental status. *Sleep, 18*(7), 523–530.

Butler, R. (1983). Aging, research on aging, and national policy. *American Psychologist, 38,* 300–307.

Brown, J. L. (1964). States in newborn infants. *Merrill–Palmer Quarterly, 10,* 313–327.

Curzi-Dascalova, L., & Challamel, M. (2000). Neurophysiological basis of sleep development. In G. M. Loughlin, J. L. Carroll, & C. L. Marcus (Eds.), *Sleep and breathing in children: A developmental approach* (pp. 3–37). New York: Marcel Dekker.

DiPietro, J. A., & Porges, S. W. (1991). Relations between neonatal states and 8-month developmental outcome in preterm infants. *Infant Behavior and Development, 14,* 441–450.

Freudigman, K. A., & Thoman, E. B. (1993). Infant's sleep during the first postnatal day: an opportunity for assessment of vulnerability. *Pediatrics, 92,* 373–379.

Freudigman, K. A., & Thoman, E. B. (1998). Infants' earliest sleep–wake organization differs as a function of delivery mode. *Developmental Psychobiology, 32,* 293–303.

Gabriel, M., Grote, B., & Jonas, M. (1981). Sleep–wake pattern in preterm infants under two different care schedules during four-day polygraphic recording. *Neuropediatrics, 12*(4), 366–373.

Guess, D., & Siegel-Causey, D. (1995). Attractor dimensions of behavior state changes among individuals with profound disabilities. *American Journal on Mental Retardation, 99*(6), 642–663.

Harper, R. M., Frostig, Z., Taube, D., Hoppenbrouwers, T., & Hodgman, J. E. (1983). Development of sleep–waking temporal sequencing in infants at risk for the Sudden Infant Death Syndrome. *Experimental Neurology, 79,* 821–829.

Holditch-Davis, D., & Edwards, L. J. (1998). Temporal organization of sleep–wake states in preterm infants. *Developmental Psychobiology, 33,* 257–269.

Holditch-Davis, D., Edwards, L. I., & Helms, R. W. (1998). Modeling development of sleep–wake behaviors. I. Using the mixed general linear model. *Physiology and Behavior, 63,* 311–318.

Holditch-Davis, D. H., & Thoman, E. B. (1987). Behavioral states of premature infants: Implications for neural and behavioral development. *Developmental Psychobiology, 20*(1), 25–38.

Honzik, M. P. (1976). Value and limitations of infants tests: an overview. In M. Lewis (Ed.), *Origins of intelligence: Infancy and early childhood* (pp. 59–95). New York: Plenum Press.

Hoppenbrouwers, T. (1987). Sleep in infants. In. C. Guilleminault (Ed.), *Sleep and its disorders in children* (pp. 1–15). New York: Raven Press.

Ingersoll, E. W., & Thoman, E. B. (1994). The breathing bear: Effects on respiration in premature infants. *Physiology and Behavior, 56*(5), 855–859.

Ingersoll, E. W., & Thoman, E. B. (1999). Sleep–wake states of preterm infants: Stability, developmental change, diurnal variation, and relationships with caregiving activity. *Child Development, 70,* 1–10.

Kopp, C. B., Sigman, M., Parmelee, A. H., & Jeffrey, W. E. (1975). Neurological organization and visual fixation in infants at 40 weeks conceptual age. *Developmental Psychobiology, 8,* 165–170.

Korner, A. F. (1972). State as variable, as obstacle, and as mediator of stimulation in infant research. *Merrill–Palmer Quarterly, 18,* 77–94.

Kraemer, H., Hole, W., & Anders, T. (1984). Detection of behavioral state cycles and classification of temporal structure in behavioral states. *Sleep, 7,* 3–17.

Kraemer, H., Korner, A., & Hurwitz, S. (1985). A model for assessing the development of preterm infants as a function of gestational age, conceptional age or chronological age. *Developmental Psychology, 21*(5), 806–812.

Krueger, J. M., & Obal, F. J. (1993). Growth hormone-releasing hormone and interleukin-1 in sleep regulation. *Federation of American Societies for Experimental Biology, 7*(8), 645–652.

Lenard, H., & Schulte, F. (1974). Sleep studies in hormonal and metabolic disease of infancy and childhood. In O. Petre-Quadens & J. Schalg (Eds.), *Basic sleep mechanisms*. New York: Academic Press.

Minard, K., & Thoman E. B. (1995, September 12–16). *Rhythmicity of the sleep states in newborns: Implications for later developmental status*. Paper presented at the 2nd International Congress of the World Federation of Sleep Research Societies, Nassau, The Bahamas.

Monod, N., & Guidasci, S. (1976). Sleep and brain malformation in the neonatal period. *Neuropadiatrie, 7(3),* 229–245.

Montgomery-Downs, H., & Thoman, E. B. (1998) Biological and behavioral correlates of Quiet Sleep respiration rates in infants, *Physiology and Behavior, 64,* 637–643.

Orem, J., & Barnes, C. D. (1980). *Physiology in sleep*. New York: Academic Press.

Petre-Quadens, O. (1974). Sleep in the human newborn. In O. Petre-Quadens & J. Schlag (Eds.), *Basic sleep mechanisms* (pp. 335–380). New York: Academic Press.

Pezzani, C., Radvanyi-Bouvet, M. F., Reiler, J. P., & Monod, N. (1986). Neonatal electroencephalography during the first twenty-four hours of life in full-term newborn infants. *Neuropediatrics, 17,* 11–18.

Prechtl, H. F. R. (1974). The behavioral states of the newborn infant (a review). *Brain Research, 76,* 185–212.

Prechtl, H. F. R. (1982). Assessment methods for the newborn infant, a critical evaluation. In P. Stratton (Ed.), *Psychobiology of the human newborn* (pp. 1–52). New York: Wiley.

Prechtl, H. F. R., & Beintama, D. (1964). *The neurological examination of the full-term newborn infant*. London: Spastic Society Medical Education & Information Unit and William Heinmann Medical Books.

Roffwarg, H. P., Muzio, J. N., & Dement, C. (1966). Ontogenetic development of the human sleep–dream cycle. *Science, 152,* 604–619.

Rosett, H. L., Snyder, P., Sander, L. W., Lee, A., Cook, P., Weiner, L., & Gould, J. (1979). Effects of maternal drinking on neonate state regulation. *Developmental Medicine and Child Neurology, 21,* 464–473.

Sadeh, A., Acebo, C., Seifer, R., Aytur, S., & Carskadon, M. A. (1995). Activity-based. Assessment of sleep–wake patterns during the first year of life. *Infant Behavior and Development, 18,* 329–337.

Sander, L., Julia, H., Stechler, G., & Burns, P. (1972). Continuous 24–hours interactional monitoring in infants reared in two caretaking environments. *Psychosomatic Medicine, 34,* 270–282.

Schulte, F., Hinze, G., & Schremph, G. (1971). Maternal toxemia, fetal malnutrition, and bioelectric brain activity in the newborn. *Neuropediatrics, 2,* 439–460.

Tanguay, P. E., Ornitz, E. M., Forsythe, A. B., & Ritvo, E. R. (1976). Rapid eye movement (REM) activity in normal and autistic children during REM sleep. *Journal of Autism and Child Schizophrenia, 6,* 275–288.

Tharp, B. R. (1989). Electroencephalography in the assessment of the premature and full-term infant. In. D. K. Stevenson, & P. Sunshine (Eds.), *Fetal and neonatal brain injury* (pp. 175–184). Toronto: B. C. Decker.

Thelen, E. (1990). Dynamical systems and the generation of individual differences. In J. Columbo & J. W. Fagen (Eds.), *Individual differences in infancy* (pp. 19–43). Hillsdale, NJ: Erlbaum.

Theorell, K., Prechtl, H. F. R., & Vos, J. E. (1974). A polygraphic study of normal and abnormal newborn infants. *Neuropediatrics, 5,* 279–317.

Thoman, E. B. (1990). Sleeping and waking states in infants: A functional perspective. *Neuroscience and Biobehavioral Reviews, 14,* 93–107.

Thoman, E. B. (1999). The Breathing Bear and the remarkable premature infant. In E. Goldson (Ed.), *Nurturing the premature infant: Developmental interventions in the neonatal intensive care nursery* (pp. 161–181). New York: Oxford University Press.

Thoman, E. B., & Acebo, C. (1995). Monitoring of sleep in neonates and young children. In R. Ferber & M. Kryger (Eds.), *Principles and practice of sleep medicine in the child* (pp. 55–68). Philadelphia: Saunders.

Thoman, E. B., Acebo, C., & Becker, P. T. (1983). Infant crying and stability in the mother–infant relationship: A systems analysis. *Child Development, 54,* 653–659.

Thoman, E. B., Davis, D. H., Graham, S., Scholz, J. P., & Rowe, J. C. (1988). Infants at risk for Sudden Infant Death Syndrome: Differential prediction for three siblings of SIDS infants. *Journal of Behavioral Medicine, 11,* 565–583.

Thoman, E. B., Denenberg, V. H., Sievel, J., Zeidner, L., & Becker, P. T. (1981). State organization in neonates: Developmental inconsistency indicates risk for developmental dysfunction. *Neuropediatrics, 12,* 45–54.

Thoman, E. B., & Graham, S. (1986). Self-regulation of stimulation by premature infants. *Pediatrics, 78,* 855–860.

Thoman, E. B., Hammond, K., Affleck, G., & DeSilva, H. N. (1995). The Breathing Bear with preterm infants: Effects on sleep, respiration, and affect. *Infant Mental Health Journal, 16,* 160–168.

Thoman, E. B., Ingersoll, E. W., & Acebo, C. (1991). Premature infants seek rhythmic stimulation and the experience facilitates neurobehavioral development. *Journal of Developmental and Behavioral Pediatrics, 12,* 11–18.

Thoman, E. B., Korner, A. F., & Kraemer, H. C. (1976). Individual consistency in behavioral states in neonates. *Developmental Psychobiology, 9,* 271–283.

Thoman, E. B., Miano, V. N., & Freese, M. P. (1978). The role of respiratory instability in SIDS. *Developmental Medicine and Child Neurology, 19,* 748–756.

Thoman, E. B., & Whitney, M. P. (1989). Sleep states of infants monitored in the home: Individual differences, developmental trends, and origins of diurnal cyclicity. *Infant Behavior and Development, 12,* 59–75.

Thoman, E. B., Zeidner, L. P., & Denenberg, V. H. (1981). Cross-species invariance in state related motility patterns. *American Journal of Physiology, 241,* R312–R315.

Webb, W. B. (1979). Theories of sleep functions and some clinical implications. In R. Drucker-Colin, M. Shkurovich, & M. B. Sterman (Eds.), *The functions of sleep* (pp. 19–36). New York: Academic Press.

Weiss, P. (1971). The basic concept of hierarchical systems. In P. Weiss (Ed.), *Hierarchically organized systems in theory and practice* (pp. 3–42). New York: Hafner.

Whitney, M. P., & Thoman, E. B. (1993). Early sleep patterns of premature infants are differentially related to later developmental disabilities. *Journal of Developmental and Behavioral Pediatrics, 14,* 71–80.

Wolff, P. H. (1966). The causes, controls, and organization of behavior in the neonate. *Psychological Issues, 5,* 1–106.

8

Analysis of Infant Crying

PHILIP SANFORD ZESKIND
BARRY M. LESTER

HISTORY

The cry of the newborn and young infant is unique among early behaviors for its role in the survival, health, and development of the child. In a general sense, crying is a biological siren, alerting the caregiving environment about the needs and wants of the infant and motivating the listener to respond. The physical properties of the cry, consisting of myriad temporal and acoustic attributes, conspire to create a remarkably compelling, sometimes noxious sound. This sound not only triggers autonomic reactivity that prepares the caregiver to reduce infant distress but also aids in the spatial location of the infant. A rich literature now describes how crying, in general, and specific components of the sound, in particular, affect caregivers' perceptions of, and responses to, the newborn and young infant (see Dessureau, Kurowski, & Thompson, 1998; Gustafson & Green, 1989; Lester & Boukydis, 1985; Murray, 1979; Zeskind, Klein, & Marshall, 1992). In its capacity as a salient social behavior, infant crying has been investigated for its evolutionary value, perceptual significance, and roles in social interactions, attachment, parenting, and temperament.

In a traditionally separate line of inquiry, research has focused on the diagnostic utility of infant crying. This line of investigation evolved from its clinical origins in noting the strength of crying as part of the Apgar (1953) score and considering its sound in standard neurological examinations (e.g., Prechtl & Beintema, 1964) to support the differential diagnosis of apparent and significant medical problems. Pioneering spectrum analytic studies described the acoustic characteristics of cry sounds associated with such condi-

149

tions as brain damage, genetic defects, hypoglycemia, hypothyroidism, encephalitis, asphyxia, and meningitis (see Michelsson, 1971; Wasz-Höckert, Lind, Vuorenkoski, Partanen, & Valanne, 1968). Although the goal of these studies was to determine whether specific abnormalities in the cry sound, such as a high basic pitch, were diagnostic of specific medical conditions, the same abnormalities in crying appeared in infants with different medical problems as well as in infants without medical problems. In addition, the apparent severity of the medical problem made the analysis of infant crying redundant as a diagnostic tool. The great contribution of this work, however, was establishment of the concept that wide variations in the characteristics of infant crying indicate changes in the functioning of the infant's nervous system.

A second generation of research subsequently evolved in which the concept that variations in infant crying reflect alterations in nervous system function was integrated with concepts from contemporary developmental science. In the first component, the characteristics of crying previously used to differentiate infants with obvious brain damage were applied to relatively healthy infants who were at risk due to biological insult but whose outcome was less well known or determined. Cry analysis has reliably differentiated infants suffering from drug exposure, prenatal and postnatal malnutrition, poor fetal prenatal growth and prematurity, and other conditions that put the infant at risk for nonoptimal developmental pathways (for a partial summary, see Corwin, Lester, & Golub, 1996). In some cases, the characteristics of crying have differentiated infants who show no physical or neurological abnormalities on routine examination but who are at risk for subsequent neurological problems based on poor obstetric histories (e.g., Zeskind & Lester, 1978). In other cases, the analysis of infant crying has been associated with poor autonomic regulation (Zeskind, Marshall, & Goff, 1996a) and sudden infant death syndrome (SIDS; Corwin et al., 1995), even in the absence of other identified risk factors. As such, this line of research has indicated that the analysis of crying may assess a generalized insult to the integrity of the infant's nervous system, even in the absence of other clinical signs.

A second important component of this latter generation of cry research has been its integration with developmental models that emphasize the contribution of the caregiving environment in determining the developmental pathway of the infant at risk. Two traditionally separate lines of cry research—treating crying as a social behavior that affects parenting and as a window into the integrity of the infant's nervous system—were brought together into biosocial (Lester, 1984) and other developmental models of infant crying (Zeskind, 1985). A wide range of studies has shown that parents perceive the high-pitched cries characteristic of the infant at risk in ways that could provide the basis for poor parenting that could exacerbate the biological deficit or optimal parenting that may help ameliorate the biological deficit (see Zeskind & Lester, 1978; Zeskind & Marshall, 1988). Even in response to normal patterns of infant crying, parents have a wide repertoire of responses that vary in how supportive they are for optimal early development. Thus, at this point in history, the infant's cry can be assessed both as a biological event and as a social event—two conditions that perhaps cannot be meaningful separated when attempting to understand the role of infant crying in early development.

GENERAL DESCRIPTION

Crying is a qualitative state of arousal that results from a change in homeostasis due to changes in internal and/or external sources of stimulation. At the most basic level, crying consists of a rhythmic repetition of an expiratory sound, a brief pause, an inspiratory sound, and a second pause (Wolff, 1967). Within this qualitative state, the sound of crying is dynamic over time, as acoustic characteristics change with the ebb and flow of infant arousal and alterations in biobehavioral organization. For example, the duration of expiratory components and the repetition rate of the rhythmic cycles of crying decreases and increases, respectively, as the time since feeding and presumed hunger increases (Zeskind, Parker-Price, & Barr, 1993). The amount of stimulation from internal and/or external sources that is required to produce the crying state, as well as the amount of time infants cry once they are in that state, also varies widely among infants. As such, there are broad individual differences in the quantitative and qualitative aspects of infant crying that provide the basis for infant assessment. These aspects have provided a plethora of measures of how much the infant cries and what the cry sounds like when it does, respectively. Based on descriptions provided by Corwin et al. (1996), Table 8.1 lists measures of infant crying discussed in this chapter and used in biobehavioral assessment.

Capturing the Cry

Unlike many measures of ongoing infant physiology or behavior—such as electroencephalograph (EEG), vagal tone, and behavioral state—crying must either be elicited or captured when it occurs spontaneously. Of course, the word "spontaneous" in this context simply means that the proximal cause of crying is unknown. Because variations in the intensity of the proximal cause of crying may result in different levels of infant arousal and variations in infant cry sounds, cries have typically been elicited to assess the neurobehavioral integrity of the newborn and young infant. In essence, eliciting the cry holds the cause of crying "constant," thus allowing for variations in the sound to be attributed to variations in infant nervous system function. Elicitation by presumably painful stimulation is thought to "challenge" the infant's neurobehavioral organization—much like the way a

TABLE 8.1. Some Measures of Infant Crying Used in Biobehavioral Assessment

Cry amount: amount of crying per unit time, such as by hour or day.

Cry threshold: number of applications of stimulation, such as RBS, to elicit a sustained cry.

Cry latency: time from stimulus to onset of first expiratory utterance.

Cry duration: time of total sustained crying bout before two consecutive inspirations without an expiratory cry sounds.

Cry modes: the vibratory mode of the vocal folds during an expiratory utterance. Different cry modes include:

 Phonation: cry sounds resulting from harmonic vibration, usually between 350–750 vibrations per second (Hz)

 Hyperphonation: cry sounds caused by a change in vocal register resulting from harmonic vibration, usually between 1,000 to 2,000 vibrations per second (Hz)

 Dysphonation: cry sounds caused by a change in vocal register resulting in an inharmonic (or noisy) vibration

Cry mode changes: number of times the cry modes change in an utterance.

Fundamental frequency (F_0): basic frequency, during harmonic vibration, usually heard as the pitch of the cry.

Formant frequencies ($F_1, F_2 \ldots F_n$): center frequencies of the theoretically infinite number of resonances of the vocal tract system. Only the first two or three formants are usually measured.

---

stress test is used to challenge cardiac function in adults for diagnostic purposes. This challenge appears to bring out diagnostically relevant acoustic attributes, such as an increased presence of high-pitched hyperphonation, than cries resulting from less intense eliciting conditions (Zeskind, 1983). Further, the important measures of cry threshold and latency can only be obtained from an elicited cry. Historically, for routine neurological examinations, cries were elicited by pulling the infant's hair, rubbing the infant's spine, or flicking the infant's foot with a finger. To meet the more rigorous needs of research and formal clinical assessment, the intensity of the eliciting stimulus needs to be controlled.

 Based on early methods described by Karelitz and Fisichelli (1962; Fisichelli & Karelitz, 1963), two standard procedures include the application of a controlled eliciting stimulus to the sole of the infant's foot. One procedure involves applying a rubberband snap (RBS), stretched a standard distance along a dowel, to elicit a sustained 10-second cry sound. If the duration of sustained crying does not meet that criterion, another RBS is applied, up to a maximum of five RBS. This procedure produces a measure of cry threshold that has long differentiated high-risk infants and has been related to specific measures of autonomic regulation (see Zeskind et al., 1996a). The necessary equipment is easily obtained and inexpensive and has been used in multiple research settings. The second procedure includes an automated mechanical stimulator connected electronically to a tone box and tape recorder. When the pain stimulus is delivered, a 3,300-Hz pure tone is automatically placed on the tape recorder followed by up to 30 seconds of the infant's cry. The tone is used to enable a computer to "identify" a new cry for acoustical analysis as part of an automated system described in the next section. This cry-eliciting device and system have been widely used by independent researchers and have differentiated cry threshold in high-risk infants as part of the National Institutes of Health multisite Maternal Lifestyle Study of prenatal drug exposure and child outcome (Lester, 1998). The mechanical stimulator must be individually built and purchased.

Cries are optimally elicited in both procedures with the infant in a supine position, midway between scheduled feedings and in an awake, nonfussy state. The cry is recorded with a high-quality tape recorder and microphone held at a constant distance midline to the infant's mouth. High-quality tape recordings are optimal, but limited analyses with some systems are possible with lesser-quality recordings from videotapes and other sources. In any case, there should be no background noise that will distort the cry signal. The complete elicitation and recording procedure requires approximately 5 minutes per infant, depending on recording conditions and setting.

Capturing quantitative aspects of crying outside a controlled environment, such as how many hours a day an infant has cried, has been achieved mostly by parental report and/or audiotape recordings. Parent report can be collected from an interview or having parents complete a daily diary in which a checkmark is placed in specified blocks of time in which the infant cries. Audiotape recordings have been obtained using voice-activated devices that mark the onset and offset of each cry vocalization. The association between the two methods is generally high (see St. James-Roberts, Conroy, & Wilsher, 1995). Audiotape devices have the added potential of meeting the needs of qualitative assessments, depending on the quality of the recording. Analyses of cries captured during the challenge of the NBAS have been related to other dimensions of neonatal behavior (e.g., Zeskind, 1983) and long-term developmental outcome (Lester, 1987; Lester et al., 1989a; Lester et al., 1995).

Analyzing the Cry

There have been three primary approaches to the acoustic analysis of cry sounds. The first generation of cry research was accomplished mostly using the sound spectrograph, a device that burned onto carbon paper the harmonic structure of approximately 2 seconds of infant crying. Each analysis required about 10 minutes to load the cry signal, calibrate and position the paper, and burn the sonogram. Although this unit represented a true technological and important advance, relative to methods available today, the spectrograph had poor frequency resolution and dynamic range and did not lend itself well to quantitative measures.

The second generation of research has been advanced by digital systems that either stand alone or come as software packages to be installed in a personal computer. Although these systems have primarily been designed for use with child and adult language, they have been used successfully to analyze the acoustic attributes of infant cry sounds. Cries are usually transferred to the computer via an analog-to-digital sound card. Recent systems now accept digital recordings. Depending on the program and memory limitations of the computer, up to 2 minutes or more of sound can be stored for analysis. Some programs produce a digital spectrogram that allows the user to trace a cursor across the screen to determine the frequency and amplitude at any given point in the cry with good resolution. These programs may also produce power spectra of a chosen block of time (e.g., 25 msec) with digital displays of frequency and amplitude in the power spectrum. The commercial availability and relatively low cost of these systems have allowed researchers to approach the analysis of crying from a wide variety of perspectives and measurement systems essential to a creative science.

There are several important issues to consider regarding use of these systems. First, the systems are easy to use but labor intensive. The amount of time required to analyze a cry depends on the number of 25-msec blocks the researcher chooses to analyze in order to adequately characterize the acoustic properties of a particular cry segment or bout of crying. The numerical values of selected measures, including pitch, amplitude, and any number of other characteristics, may need to be hand-recorded on paper or scored into a spreadsheet for each 25-msec block analyzed. Some programs allow the user to analyze a larger portion of sound by automatically summing across the power spectra of contiguous 25-msec blocks. However, unless phonated cry segments are differentiated from dysphonated cry segments in this summation, estimates of the fundamental frequency will be inaccurate. Further, as described in the next section, these systems are based on analytic models of the adult, rather than infant, vocal tract, thus making location of the formant frequencies inaccurate. Thus, these utilitarian systems are limited by intensive labor requirements and some of the measures that can be ascertained.

A system designed specifically by a team from CRI (Cry Research Inc., formerly Pediatric Diagnostic Service) developed the analysis of infant crying headed by Golub in collaboration with Lester. The automated mechanical cry-eliciting device described previously was designed to interface with this system. The system is fully automated and, thus, less labor intensive. The computer turns the tape recorder on and off, reads in and digitizes the cry, and provides summary calculations. Each 25-msec block in a cry expiration can be analyzed and its measures summed and averaged as chosen by the researcher. Phonated and dysphonated cry segments are clearly delineated before spectral analyses are conducted, thus improving accuracy. Unlike other systems, calculations of acoustic characteristics are based on models of the infant vocal tract and thus provide more accurate measures of formant frequencies. Some disadvantages to this system are that it is not published or commercially available and it generates a large volume of acoustic information that requires a high degree of expertise to interpret. Raw data are available if the investigator wants to determine how summary variables were computed.

BIOBEHAVIORAL BASIS OF ASSESSMENT

Crying is a complex biobehavioral phenomenon with a basis in a range of anatomical, physical, and central nervous system (CNS) components. At the peripheral level, three components determine the cry sound: the respiratory system, the larynx, and the physical construction of the vocal tract (Golub & Corwin, 1985). The actual cry sound occurs during the expiratory phase of the respiratory cycle, although inspiratory whistles may also be heard as part of the basic rhythmic temporal morphology underlying crying. The production of the phonated cry sound results when a reduction in pressure across the glottis causes the adducted vocal folds in the larynx to vibrate. As described previously, the rate of vibration is called the fundamental frequency and is what we hear as the "basic pitch" of the cry sound. Hyperphonation results when central innervation causes the vocal cords to act in a discontinuous manner and suddenly shifts vocal registers to a qualitatively higher-pitched sound (Lester, 1984). As such, the lower vocal tract, with respiratory and laryngeal sources, controls such features as the pitch, timing, and intensity of the cry and is closely tied to the autonomic nervous system and infant arousal. The sound generated at the larynx is then modified by the airways that form the upper vocal tract to produce the resonant frequencies or formants. As suggested earlier, because the size and shape of the vocal tract determine these acoustic characteristics, analysis systems based on models of the adult vocal tract may inaccurately identify these formant frequencies.

Our understanding of CNS involvement and control over these peripheral systems has developed over the years. Analysis of crying has differentiated infants with a list of conditions in which CNS insult is implicated, including asphyxia, brain damage from various causes, hypoglycemia, hydrocephalus, encephalitis, meningitis, Down syndrome and other trisomy disorders, various other genetic defects, hyperbilirubinemia, prematurity, low birthweight, nonoptimal obstetric conditions, intrauterine growth restriction and malnutrition (IUGR, SGA, low and high ponderal index), maternal drug abuse (cocaine, heroin, methadone, alcohol, marijuana, tobacco), and prenatal and perinatal lead exposure (for a partial summary, see Corwin et al., 1996). Initially, finding distinctive cry features in brain-damaged infants clearly implicated the global role of the CNS. Subsequently finding the same cry features in apparently healthy infants who show various signs of risk suggests that cry analysis provides information about the functional status of the infant rather than about a particular structural defect. The range of these insults has been associated with changes in both the quantity and quality of crying.

As suggested long ago by Parmelee (1962), measures of the quantitative aspects of crying—threshold, latency, and duration—reflect the capacity of the infant's nervous system to be activated and then to inhibit that activation. As such, problems in central and autonomic nervous system function may result in infants requiring either atypically high amounts of stimulation to elicit sustained crying or atypically low amounts of stimulation that may produce often inconsolable crying. A high cry threshold has been found in infants across the continuum of biological insult, ranging from various forms of brain damage to apparently healthy newborn infants whose mothers had poor obstetric histories that place the infant at risk (see Zeskind et al., 1996a). Whereas newborn infants typically require one RBS to elicit a sustained cry, infants at risk typically require three or more. Reflecting the capacity of the nervous system to be aroused and to inhibit that arousal, a high cry threshold has been associated with poor regulation of behavioral state and long-term heart rate variability—as well as other measures of autonomic activity (Zeskind et al., 1996a). Infants with higher cry thresholds often also have a longer cry latency, shorter cry sounds, and shorter overall bouts of crying. Less is known about conditions that produce lower cry thresholds, but infants who cry for extended periods of time to an RBS may also be "irritable" and show poor state regulation on the NBAS (e.g., Zeskind, 1981). Infant colic is also an example of lower cry threshold and inconsolability and may be related to a complex syndrome of different acoustic characteristics and behavioral temperament (see Lester, Boukydis, Garcia-Coll, Hole, & Peucker, 1992).

Variations in the qualitative aspects of crying are also based on the functional activity of the central and autonomic nervous systems. Corwin et al. (1996) have provided a summary of the association between acoustic characteristics of cries and many of the medical conditions that have been investigated. The cries of infants with conditions across the spectrum of CNS-implicated insult are most typically characterized by higher-frequency components, most notably the fundamental frequency (F_0). Whereas the F_0 of typical pain cries averages up to 600 Hz, pain cries of infants who are at risk average approximately 800 Hz but range from 1,000 to 2,000 Hz when the cry is hyperphonated. With or without differences in F_0, infants with still other conditions are characterized by higher-frequency components such as higher formant frequencies (e.g., Golub & Corwin, 1982) and dominant frequency (Zeskind & Barr, 1997). Other cry characteristics found in infants with insult to the integrity of nervous system function include higher numbers of mode changes, more variable frequency components, shorter cry utterances, lower amplitude sounds, and/or greater amounts of dysphonation. Trisomy disorders, such as Down syndrome, and hypothyroidism are cases in which the cry is characterized by a lower F_0, often averaging 300 Hz.

Lester and Boukydis (1990) described how central control of these characteristics of crying involves the brainstem, midbrain, and limbic system with later involvement by the cortex. At one level, CNS control is provided by the lower brainstem. Muscles of the larynx, pharynx, chest, and upper neck are controlled by the vagal complex of nerves (cranial nerves 9–12) and by the phrenic and thoracic nerves. Damage to these cranial nerves affects input to the muscles of the larynx that control the F_0. Brainstem input also affects the contour and airway of the vocal tract that determines the formant frequencies. Studies relating the acoustic characteristics of crying to the brain auditory-evoked response (BAER; Vohr et al., 1989) and to the vagal tone measure of heart rate variability (Porter, Porges, & Marshall, 1988) support the role of brainstem control of crying. As a measure that reflects central control of peripheral muscle activity in the vocal tract, variations in F_0 have also been directly related to the central processing of the cardiac orienting response (Lester, 1976) and motor maturity, as measured by the NBAS (Zeskind, 1983).

Although the brainstem is necessary for the production of the cry, it is not sufficient. Based on animal models (Jurgens, 1986; Jurgens & Ploog, 1981), Lester and Boukydis (1990) proposed a hierarchical model for the role of higher brain structures that describes the potential basis for individual differences in infant cry production and acoustic features. Level 1 includes the reticular formation and is responsible for the coordination of respiratory, laryngeal and articulation activity. This level serves as the motor coordination center for the cry but is not capable of initiating vocalization. Level 2 involves sections of the midbrain region and configures the cry response into a particular vocal pattern (such as a pain or hunger cry). Level 3, the limbic system/hypothalamus, is responsible for initiation of the cry (such as cry threshold) as ascending efferent traffic increases the arousal level of the infant. Level 4 consists of the motor cortex necessary for the voluntary control of vocalization that comes into play at 1–2 months when crying also becomes an instrumental response.

DEVELOPMENTAL MODELS

Biosocial (Lester, 1984) and other developmental models of infant crying in the infant at risk (Zeskind, 1985) explicitly address the dynamic and bidirectional transactions between the infant and its caregiving environment that direct developmental outcome. Crying is at once a biological signal, reflecting changes in infant homeostasis, and a social signal, affecting the caregiving environment and the care the infant receives. In contrast to conditions of "typical" development of "normal" infants, the biological and social signal values of the cry of the infant at risk are amplified and perhaps more readily apparent. As such, the analysis of infant crying may inform our understanding of the developmental process. In understanding the varied developmental outcomes of the infant at risk, the analysis of infant crying may not only help identify infants who have experienced conditions that adversely affected nervous system development, but also some of the social factors that contribute to different developmental pathways.

As a biological signal, the analysis of infant crying may provide important information regarding which infants have suffered some biological insult or been more adversely affected, either within a risk category or in the absence of some other risk classification. For example, infants of mothers who consumed alcohol during pregnancy have been reliably differentiated by a higher cry pitch, a higher cry threshold, and longer latency than comparison infants, even in the absence of any physical or neurological findings (Zeskind, Platzman, Coles, & Schuetze, 1996b). Structural-equation models have shown direct effects of cocaine to be associated with cry measures indicating greater excitation (e.g., longer duration and higher F_0) but indirect effects moderated by fetal growth retardation to be associated with CNS "depression" (longer latency, lower amplitude, fewer utterances) (Lester et al., 1991). Michelsson, Sirvio, and Wasz-Höckert (1977) showed that asphyxiated infants with the most abnormal cry sounds had the poorest neurological outcome on follow-up. In a prospective study of 21,880 asymptomatic infants, Corwin et al. (1995) found a higher F_1 and more mode changes in infants who subsequently died of SIDS.

Importantly, when considering prediction of infant development, measures of infant crying may provide information that is not redundant with, and improves on, the information provided by knowledge of the infant's risk condition. Measures of infant crying at 2 days of age were better predictors of the infant's regulation of state at 1 month of age than was the known prenatal polydrug exposure of the infant (Zeskind, Schuetze, Platzman, & Coles, 1997) and of Bayley scores at 2 years of age than was the known prenatal methadone exposure of the infant (Huntington, Hans, & Zeskind, 1990). In studies of preterm infants, measures of infant crying have been correlated with more long-term neurodevelopmental consequences (e.g., Corwin et al., 1992). Measures of infant crying have predicted 18-month Bayley and 5-year McCarthy scores (Lester, 1987) and neurological outcome, Bayley scores, memory for locations, and word comprehension at 4 years of age (Lester, McGrath, Boukydis, & Kilis, 1989c). Importantly, in both studies of preterm infants, measures of infant crying predicted outcome with medical and social factors controlled.

As a social signal, crying affects the caregiving environment and helps determine the quality of care an infant will receive, thus influencing the infant's future developmental pathway. The effects of infant crying on the caregiver can be conceived within a framework of a "synchrony of arousal" in which increases in infant arousal produce changes in infant cry sounds, such as increased pitch, that then typically act in a synchronous manner to increase the perceived arousal and motivation of the adult listener (Zeskind, Sale, Maio, Huntington, & Weiseman, 1985). As such, this model emphasizes the role of the sound of crying as one of the infant's contributions to caregiver–infant interactions. Importantly, however, the functional significance of the cry sound depends on the characteristics and perceptual set of the caregiver. For example, in contrast to typical patterns of higher perceived arousal, teenage mothers (Lester, Garcia-Coll, & Valcarel, 1989b) and young depressed women perceive higher-pitched cry sounds as less arousing (Schuetze & Zeskind, in press). In this case, the mother's emotional condition may make her actually less able to respond, as the perceived needs of the infant increase. A wide range of studies has shown how perceptual and physiological responses to cries are influenced by the caregivers' parity, gender, cultural background, age, attitudes, parenting experience, and/or emotional health. As such, caregivers bring different characteristics to the perceptual meaning of infant crying that may provide the basis for differential responsivity and variations in the infant's developmental pathway.

As reflecting a special condition of infant arousal, the high-pitched, hyperphonated cry of the infant at risk has long been shown to elicit strong perceptual and physiological reactions. A number of studies has indicated that the high-pitched cry of the infant at risk elicits at least two orthogonal perceptual dimensions: one that the infant's cry is particularly aversive, yet one that the cry may indicate that the infant sounds sick (see Zeskind & Lester, 1978; Zeskind & Marshall, 1988). Some caregivers may respond to an infant who sounds sick with ameliorative care (e.g., picking up and holding the infant) whereas others may withdraw from an infant with a particularly aversive cry, thus beginning a cycle of poor infant development and unresponsive caregiving (see Lester, 1984; Zeskind, 1985). In an extreme set of conditions, this cycle may account for anecdotal reports of high-pitched cries being a precipitating factor in cases of physical abuse and "Shaken Baby Syndrome" (see Frodi, 1985). Whereas young women typically show lower heart rates over time when listening to infant crying, young women who are at high risk for physically abusing their infants show increases in heart rate and other measures of arousal over time, even before they have children of their own (Crowe & Zeskind, 1992).

Cry perception studies provide indirect evidence of the effects of infant crying on infant development. They are based on the assumption that perception translates into comparable action on the part of the caregiver. Direct longitudinal evidence is found in a "goodness of fit" study in which infant–mother dyads were divided into groups based on the "match" between the acoustic characteristics and maternal perceptions of the infant's cries (Lester et al., 1995). Follow-up at 18 months showed higher Bayley mental scores and higher language scores in the matched groups than in the mismatched groups, suggesting that mothers who are better able to read their infant' cry signal provided parenting that facilitates cognitive and language outcome.

RELIABILITY AND VALIDITY

Group analyses have shown that infant crying differentiates the same group of high-risk infants at multiple assessments over the first postnatal month (Zeskind et al., 1996b). Overall, however, there are few reported assessments of reliability in the analysis of infant crying. With regard to engineering and mathematical formulations underlying spectral analysis, reliability is assumed to be high, although not reported in the literature, nor have results of analyses been compared across cry analysis systems. Reliability of the CRI system was found to be high when 10 cries were analyzed twice to find the same results. Similarly, little is known about interobserver reliability. Typically analysts are trained to criterion. The digital output of contemporary analysis programs has increased the amount of objective measurement. To the extent that subjective measurements are included in any analysis, investigators should be blind to group membership of the subject. Finally, test–retest reliability of the elicited cry's characteristics has also not been typically reported. To the extent that the cry is a sensitive measure of infant arousal and biobehavioral organization, changes in either of these domains would produce changes in infant cry features and thus reduce this measure of reliability. Research using cry analysis would benefit by reporting reliability estimates in the future. The external validity of the analysis of infant crying is strongly supported by the high number of biological insults associated with measures of infant crying, as well as the relations between variations in infant crying and other biobehavioral measures described previously.

THEORETICAL CONSTRAINTS

Although assessment value of the analysis of infant crying has become clearer in recent years, the study of infant crying is still in its infant stage. Our understanding at this time is that the analysis of crying is a sensitive indicator that the biobehavioral organization of the infant has been detrimentally affected. This kind of information may be particularly useful to researchers who are interested in determining whether some experience or set of conditions has had an adverse impact on early infant development, even in the absence of other signs. Because there is no known idiopathic, or one-to-one, relation between any known biobehavioral or medical condition and characteristics of infant crying, cry analysis does not provide direct evidence for differential diagnoses or information about what specific adverse condition the infant has experienced. As such, cry analysis suffers from too much sensitivity and too little specificity.

Several issues continue to cloud or limit our understanding of infant cry analysis. First, the assessment utility of crying is complicated by the fact that there are no clear criteria for what constitutes an "abnormal" cry. Although such features as hyperphonation or multiple RBS are associated with biological insult, it is unclear whether these are clear cases of "abnormality" because apparently healthy infants may also have these characteristics of crying. A related question concerns whether the significance of atypical cry characteristics increases continuously or whether there is a threshold which, when crossed, denotes that an infant has suffered a biological insult. Is an infant with a fundamental frequency of crying at 1,500 Hz necessarily in worse condition than one with a cry at 1,000 Hz, or is the severity of insult comparable once the cry exceeds 1,000 Hz, for example? Second, there has been no conceptual argument made regarding when the analysis of crying has the most assessment value. Few data are available to indicate the persistent or transient nature of distinctive cry characteristics—and, thus, their clinical significance.

Methodological constraints and inconsistencies include the lack of standardization among studies. There is no standard method of elicitation, nor is there agreement that cries should be elicited or captured, for example, during a behavioral examination. Studies also vary widely in the choice of measures of infant crying, sometimes reflecting the capabilities of the analysis system. Similarly, measures of the same aspect of crying are often created differently from laboratory to laboratory. Characterization of the F_0, for example, has been made by measuring the peak F_0 of the expiratory sound, by averaging 3 or 4 points interspersed through the expiratory sound and by averaging all phonated 25-msec points in the expiratory sound. Thus, even when the same source of biological insult is studied, differences in the way cries have been elicited or captured and analyzed have precluded direct comparisons. Despite these inconsistencies, the fact that different methods and approaches have consistently differentiated infant risk groups speaks to the strength and sensitivity of the biobehavioral phenomenon of infant crying.

Perhaps the greatest constraint that should be exercised is the interpretation of infant crying. The significance of crying needs to be interpreted in context—in the context of how the information was collected (spontaneous, elicited, parent report), in the context of the rest of the infant's medical and neurobehavioral status, and in the context of the parenting/home environment. The "goodness of fit" study reminds us that infant development is not based on the acoustic features of the infants' cry or mothers' perceptions of those cries in isolation of each other but in the context of one another.

TRAINING REQUIREMENTS

Training requirements vary depending on the methods of elicitation and analysis chosen by the researcher. Elicitation procedures are relatively straightforward and require little instruction. Both the RBS and CRI procedures have been used successfully in multiple settings after researchers have received relatively little training. The RBS procedure requires that researchers be able to judge the duration of sustained crying to determine the cry threshold. Conducting spectral analysis requires more sophisticated training if individuals choose to purchase their own systems. Training requires a basic understanding of computers and software and a few hours of direct supervision from someone trained in sound analysis and the specific software program. Some software manufacturers offer formal instruction at their training facility, but training is based on a system that was designed to analyze language—an acoustic signal that is significantly less complex and less difficult to analyze than infant cry sounds. Although a minimal level of competency is often satisfactory to meet some needs, supervision from an experienced researcher may still be required for interpretation of the more ambiguous or subjective judgments inherent in cry analysis.

Another option is for researchers to choose to have the cries analyzed for them by any of a number of laboratories. Numerous studies have been conducted in which audio recordings of the elicitation procedure and cry sound have been sent to a laboratory for analysis. To have cries analyzed, researchers may choose to collaborate or have laboratories act as paid consultants—much like having any laboratory test. It is always best to plan the cry analysis with the analyzing laboratory to ensure that the elicitation procedure is conducted correctly, that the recordings are suitable for acoustic analyses, and that data analysis can be validly interpreted. Further, the number and selection of specific measures to be extricated should be planned *a priori*.

IMPLICATIONS

As a research tool, there are several implications of the analysis of infant crying in the biobehavioral assessment of the infant at risk. First, cry analysis may be particularly useful with regard to questions concerning whether specific prenatal experiences, such as prenatal drug exposure or maternal depression, have adversely affected infant development. The analysis of infant crying provides a sensitive measure of alterations in biobehavioral organization, often in the absence of other routine clinical signs. Second, the social signal value of the cry may provide important information about the perceptual set a caregiver may bring to a wide range of settings not directly related to crying per se. Studies of the perceptions of cries varying in pitch have been used, for example, to explore cultural variations in childrearing attitudes and the perceptual set that teenage and depressed mothers may bring to interactions with their infants. Third, variations in infant crying may provide insight into processes underlying other assessment tools. Individual differences in infant crying have long been directly associated with differences in state organization (e.g., Korner, Hutchinson, Koperski, Kraemer, & Schneider, 1981), temperament (e.g., Boukydis & Burgess, 1982), heart rate variability (Porter et al., 1988; Zeskind et al., 1996a), performance on the NBAS (e.g., Lester & Zeskind, 1978; Zeskind, 1983), newborn attention (see Zeskind & Marshall, 1991), and brainstem auditory evoked potential (Vohr et al., 1989); and as evidenced throughout this volume. Fourth, as a social signal the analysis of infant crying has implications for understanding attachment, especially as it relates to infants who are at risk.

With regard to its clinical utility, the analysis of infant crying has implications for general screening. The cry may not inform us about the specific nature of a CNS insult, but it may tell us to look more closely for other significant indicators. This relationship is analogous to the way that a high temperature or white cell count would suggest the presence of an infection but not the source or specific disease. Although more empirical support is needed, clinical experience suggests that when an infant has an atypical cry sound, individual differences in such other biobehavioral domains as attention, reactivity, or sleep organization are found. In a clinical setting, it may be important to know if the infant cries too much or too little. Although the latter is not a typical complaint, informing parents that their infant may not always communicate when it is in need is solid clinical advice. For parents who find their infant's cries excessive, either in quantity or quality, clinicians may help prevent unwarranted problems in parent–infant relationships and attachment by involving parents in a discussion of the infant's behavioral repertoire, reframing its biological and social significance and helping parents cope with the concerns they raise about their infant's crying.

REFERENCES

Apgar, V. (1953). A proposal for a new method of evaluation in the newborn infant. *Current Research in Anesthesia and Analgesia, 32,* 260.

Boukydis, C. F. Z., & Burgess, R. L. (1982). Adult physiological response to infant cries: Effects of temperament of infant, parental status and gender. *Child Development, 53,* 1291–1298.

Corwin, M. J., Lester, B. M., & Golub, H. L. (1996). The infant cry: What can it tell us? *Current Problems in Pediatrics, 26*(9), 325–333.

Corwin, M. J., Lester, B. M., Sepkoski, C., McLaughlin, S., Kayne, H., & Golub, H. L. (1995). Newborn acoustical cry characteristics of infants dying of SIDS. *Pediatrics, 96,* 73–77.

Corwin, M. J., Sepkoski, C., Gross, S., Lester, B., Peucker, M., Kayne, H., & Golub, H. (1992). Early prediction of low Cognitive indices at 30 months in preterm infants. *Pediatric Research, 31,* 244A.

Crowe, H. P., & Zeskind, P. S. (1992). Psychophysiological and perceptual responses to infant cries varying in pitch: Comparison of adults with low and high scores on the Child Abuse Potential Inventory. *Child Abuse and Neglect, 16,* 19–29.

Dessureau, B. K., Kurowski, C., & Thompson, N. (1998). A reassessment of the role of pitch and duration in adults' responses to infant crying. *Infant Behavior and Development, 21,* 367–371.

Fisichelli, V., & Karelitz, S. (1963). The cry latencies of normal infants and those with brain damage. *Journal of Pediatrics, 62,* 724–734.

Frodi, A. (1985). When empathy fails: Aversive infant crying and child abuse. In B. M. Lester & C. F. Z. Boukydis (Eds.), *Infant crying: Theoretical and research perspectives* (pp. 263–277). New York: Plenum Press.

Golub, H. L., & Corwin, M. J. (1982). Infant cry: A clue to diagnosis. *Pediatrics, 69,* 197–201.

Golub, H. L., & Corwin, M. J. (1985). A physioacoustic model of the Infant Cry. In B. M. Lester & C. F. Z. Boukydis (Eds.), *Infant crying: Theoretical and research perspectives* (pp. 59–82). New York: Plenum Press.

Gustafson, G., & Green, J. (1989). On the importance of fundamental frequency and other acoustic features in cry perception and infant development. *Child Development, 60,* 772–780.

Huntington, L., Hans, S., & Zeskind, P. S. (1990). Relations among cry characteristics, demographic variables and developmental test scores in infants prenatally exposed to methadone. *Infant Behavior and Development, 13,* 533–538.

Jurgens, U. (1986). The squirrel monkey as an experimental model in the study of cerebral organization of emotional vocal utterances. *European Archive of Psychiatry and Neurological Science, 236,* 40–43.

Jurgens, U., & Ploog, D. (1981, June). On the neural control of mammalian vocalization. *Trends in Neuroscience,* 135–137.

Karelitz, S., & Fisichelli, V. (1962). The cry thresholds of normal infants and those with brain damage. *Journal of Pediatrics, 61,* 679–685.

Korner, A. F., Hutchinson, C., Koperski, J., Kraemer, H., & Schneider, P. (1981). Stability of individual differences of neonatal motor and crying patterns. *Child Development, 52,* 83–90.

Lester, B. M. (1976). Spectrum analysis of the cry sounds of well-nourished and malnourished infants. *Child Development, 47,* 237–241.

Lester, B. M. (1984). A biosocial model of infant crying In L. Lipsitt & C. Rovee-Collier (Eds.), *Advances in infant research* (pp. 167–212). Norwood, NY: Ablex.

Lester, B. M. (1987). Prediction of developmental outcome from acoustic cry analysis in term and preterm infants. *Pediatrics, 80,* 529–534.

Lester, B. M. (1998). The Maternal Lifestyles Study. *Annals of the New York Academy of Sciences, 846,* 296–306.

Lester, B. M., Anderson, L. T., Boukydis, C. F. Z., Garcia-Coll, C. T., Vohr, B. & Peucker, M. (1989a). Early detection of infants at risk for later handicap through acoustic cry analysis. *BD:OAS, 25*(6), 99–118.

Lester, B. M., & Boukydis, C. F. (Eds.). (1985). *Infant crying: Theoretical and research perspectives* New York: Plenum Press.

Lester, B. M., & Boukydis, C. F. (1990). No language but a cry. In H. Papousek, J. Jurgens, & M. Papousek (Eds.), *Nonverbal vocal communication: Comparative and developmental approaches* (pp. 41–69). New York: Cambridge University Press.

Lester, B. M., Boukydis, C. F. Z., Garcia-Coll, C. T., Hole, W., & Peucker, M. (1992). Infantile colic: Acoustic cry characteristics, maternal perception of cry, and temperament. *Infant Behavior and Development, 15*, 15–26.

Lester, B. M., Boukydis, C. F. Z., Garcia-Coll, C. T., Peucker, M., McGrath, M. M., Vohr, B. R., Brem, F., & Oh, W. (1995). Developmental outcome as a function of the goodness of fit between the infant's cry characteristics and the mother's perception of her infant's cry. *Pediatrics, 95*, 516–521.

Lester, B. M., Corwin, M. J., Sepkoski, C., Seifer, R., Peucker, M., McGlaughlin, S., & Golub, H. L. (1991). Neurobehavioral syndromes in cocaine exposed newborn infants. *Child Development, 62*, 694–705.

Lester, B. M., Garcia-Coll, C., & Valcarcel, M. (1989b). Perception of infant cries in adolescent and older mothers. *Journal of Youth and Adolescents, 18*, 231–243.

Lester, B. M., McGrath, M., Boukydis, C. F. Z., & Kilis, E. (1989c). Acoustic cry analysis at one month predicts four year cognitive outcome in preterm and term infants. *Pediatric Research, 37*, 264A.

Lester, B. M., & Zeskind, P. S. (1978). Brazelton scale and physical size correlates of neonatal cry features. *Infant Behavior and Development, 1*(4), 393–402.

Michelsson, K. (1971). Cry analysis of symptomless low birth weight neonates and of asphyxiated newborn infants. *Acta Pediatrica Scandinavia* (Suppl. 216), pp. 1–45.

Michelsson, K., Sirvio, P., & Wasz-Höckert, O. (1977). Pain cry in full term asphyxiated newborn infants correlated with later findings. *Acta Paediatrica Scandinavica, 1*–45.

Murray, A. (1979). Infant crying as an elicitor of parental behavior: an examination of two models. *Psychological Bulletin, 86*, 191–215.

Parmelee, A. (1962). Infant crying and neurological diagnosis. *Journal of Pediatrics, 61*, 801–802.

Prechtl, H. F. R., & Beintema, D. (1964). *The neurological examination of the full-term infants.* (Clinics in Developmental Medicine, No. 12.) Philadelphia: Lippincott.

Porter, F. L., Porges, S. W., & Marshall, R. E. (1988). Newborn pain cries and vagal tone: Parallel changes in response to circumcision. *Child Development, 59*, 495–505.

Schuetze, P., & Zeskind, P. S. (in press). Relations between women's depressive symptoms and perceptions of infant distress signals varying in pitch. *Infancy.*

St. James-Roberts, I., Conroy, S., & Wilsher, K. (1995). Clinical, developmental and social aspects of infant crying and colic. *Early Development and Parenting, 4*, 107.

Vohr, B. R., Lester, B., Rapisardi, G., O'Dea, C., Brown, L., Peucker, M., Cashore, W., & Oh, W. (1989). Abnormal brainstem function (brainstem auditory evoked response) correlates with acoustic cry features in term infants with hyperbilirubinemia. *Journal of Pediatrics, 115*, 296–302.

Wasz-Höckert, O., Lind, J., Vuorenkoski, V., Partanen, T., & Valanne, E. (1968). *The infant cry (Clinics in Developmental Medicine, No. 29).* Philadelphia: Lippincott.

Wolff, P. H. (1967). The role of biological rhythms in early psychological development. *Bulletin of the Menninger Clinic, 31*, 197–218.

Zeskind, P. S. (1981). Behavioral dimensions and cry sounds of infants of differential fetal growth. *Infant Behavior and Development, 4*, 321–330.

Zeskind, P. S. (1983). Production and spectral analysis of neonatal crying and its relation to other biobehavioral systems in the infant at-risk. In T. Field & A. Sostek (Eds.), *Infants born at-risk: Physiological and perceptual processes* (pp. 23–44). New York: Grune & Stratton.

Zeskind, P. S. (1985). A developmental perspective of infant crying. In B. M. Lester & C. F. Z. Boukydis (Eds.), *Infant crying: Theoretical and research perspectives* (pp. 159–185). New York: Plenum.

Zeskind, P. S., & Barr, R. (1997). Acoustic characteristics of the naturally occurring cries of infants with colic. *Child Development, 68,* 394–403.

Zeskind, P. S., Klein, L., & Marshall, T. R. (1992). Experimental modification of relative durations of pauses and expiratory sounds in infant cries alters adults' perceptions. *Developmental Psychology, 28,* 1153–1162.

Zeskind, P. S., & Lester, B. M. (1978). Acoustic features and auditory perceptions of the cries of newborns with prenatal and perinatal complications. *Child Development, 49*(3), 580–589.

Zeskind, P. S., & Marshall, T. R. (1988). The relation between mothers' perceptions and pitch of infant crying. *Child Development, 59,* 193–196.

Zeskind, P. S., & Marshall, T. R. (1991). Temporal organization in neonatal arousal: Systems, oscillations, and development. In M. Weiss & P. Zelazo (Eds.), *Newborn attention: Biological constraints and influence of experience* (pp. 22–62). Norwood, NJ: Ablex.

Zeskind, P. S., Marshall, T. R., & Goff, D. M. (1996a). Cry threshold predicts regulatory disorder in newborn infants. *Pediatric Psychology, 21,* 803–819.

Zeskind, P. S., Parker-Price, S., & Barr, R. G. (1993). Rhythmic organization of the sound of infant crying. *Developmental Psychobiology, 26,* 321–333.

Zeskind, P. S., Platzman, K., Coles, C. D., & Schuetze, P. (1996b). Cry analysis detects subclinical effects of prenatal alcohol exposure. *Infant Behavior and Development, 19,* 497–500.

Zeskind, P. S., Sale, J., Maio, M. L., Huntington, L., & Weiseman, J. (1985). Adult perceptions of pain and hunger cries: A synchrony of arousal. *Child Development, 56,* 549–554.

Zeskind, P. S., Schuetze, P. A., Platzman, K., & Coles, C. (1997). *Analysis of infant crying predicts neurobehavioral integrity in newborns with prenatal polydrug exposure.* Paper presented at the biennial meeting of the Society for Research in Child Development, Washington, DC.

9

Salivary Cortisol Measures in Infant and Child Assessment

MEGAN R. GUNNAR
BARBARA PRUDHOMME WHITE

HISTORY

Corticosteroid measures (cortisol in primates, corticosterone in rodents) have been commonly used in psychobiological studies of stress for nearly half a century (see reviews by Kirschbaum & Hellhammer, 1989, 1994; Mason, 1968; Rose, 1980). Most of the work has been conducted on either animals or human adults. Cortisol in humans is interesting to developmental researchers because varying levels and responsivity patterns have been linked with observed and perceived stress (both acute and chronic), with emotional/behavioral reactions to specific contexts, and with attributes of the caregiving environment, including the quality of attachment relationships as well as experiences of suboptimal care (Carlson & Earls, 1997; Gunnar & Barr, 1998; Gunnar, Broderson, Nachmias, Buss, & Rigatuso, 1996b; Hart, Gunnar, & Cicchetti, 1996; Ramsay & Lewis, 1994; Stansbury & Gunnar, 1994). Initially, the work in humans relied on measures of urinary metabolites (e.g., 17-OHCS) because urine could be sampled noninvasively. A few of these studies were conducted on children. Montagner et al. (1978) investigated the relations between urinary 17-OHCS concentrations over the day in preschool children and their behavioral styles. Similarly, Tennes, Downey, and Vernadakis (1977) conducted one study of urinary cortisol excretion and emotional behavior in year-old infants. Although these studies were groundbreaking, they did not have much impact on the developmental psychology community, perhaps because the problems of urine collection precluded widespread adoption of these measures.

The development of radioimmunoassay (RIA) techniques permitted the assessment of cortisol in small samples of plasma and urine. This had significant effects on corticoid–behavior research (Riad-Fahmy, Read, & Hughes, 1979). RIA procedures allowed detection of corticoids at small concentrations, requiring only a few drops of blood for analysis. Plasma sampling, unlike urine sampling, allows for punctate measures of response. Literally thousands of studies of plasma cortisol exist in the literature. Nonetheless, relatively few of these studies involved children. One reason is obvious: Blood sampling is invasive and difficult to employ in children participating in developmental research. Most of the work dealing with blood measures, therefore, has involved hospitalized children who are routinely sampled for other reasons. An example of this research is provided by a frequently cited study by Barnes, Kenny, Call, and Reinhart (1972) on plasma cortisol levels and psychological defenses in children undergoing various surgical procedures. Several early studies of newborns were also conducted, one by Anders, Sachar, Kream, Roffwarg, and Hellman (1970) and one by Tennes and Carter (1973). Both of these studies demonstrated positive correlations between plasma cortisol levels and crying in newborn babies.

Because newborns are blood-sampled for the metabolic screening exam, they offer a rare opportunity to study cortisol–behavior relations using blood measures in healthy, normal children. That is, the researcher can organize the blood sampling for the phenylketonuria test so that several extra drops of blood can be collected for cortisol analysis. Gunnar and colleagues took advantage of these procedures in the early 1980s and conducted a series of plasma cortisol studies (see Gunnar, 1989, for review). The results of this work form one basis for the use of cortisol measures in infant assessment. Despite interest in this work, few researchers incorporated plasma cortisol measures into their infant assessments. In contrast, interest in assessing cortisol has burgeoned in the last 10 years because of the refinement of RIA procedures to allow assessment of cortisol in small samples of free-flowing saliva (Kirschbaum & Hellhammer, 1989; Riad-Fahmy, Read, Joyce, & Walker, 1981). Adult studies using salivary cortisol increased from none in the mid- to late 1970s to over 140 by the late 1980s (Kirschbaum & Hellhammer, 1989). The 1990s reflected steady increases in the literature on infants, children, and adults examining the relations between physiological responses using salivary cortisol, among other measures, and behavior.

GENERAL DESCRIPTION

The attraction of salivary cortisol measures from both a practical and theoretical perspective has led to their increasingly widespread adoption in research on infants and children (Gunnar, 1989; Lewis, 1992; Spangler & Scheubeck, 1993; Stansbury & Gunnar, 1994). Saliva sampling is a simple and relatively noninvasive procedure. Furthermore, many of the initial concerns about the reliability of these measures have been abated by studies showing that (1) the time course for salivary cortisol is almost identical to that of plasma cortisol measures, (2) the flow rate of saliva does not affect cortisol concentrations, and (3) the concentrations of cortisol in saliva are a good reflection of the concentration of free cortisol in plasma (see Kirschbaum & Hellhammer, 1989, for an excellent review). This last point is important and makes salivary cortisol measures increasingly attractive to developmental researchers.

Cortisol travels in blood largely bound to protein (cortisol binding globulin, or CBG) (Tepperman & Tepperman, 1987). Once bound, cortisol is "biologically inactive," meaning that it must become unbound from CBG before it can bind to cell receptors and exert effects on the organism's physiology. Under resting conditions, approximately 5–10% of cortisol is "unbound" or "free" and available to exert effects. Only this "free fraction" can enter saliva due to the barrier provided by cells lining the salivary glands. Thus, salivary measures assess the biologically or physiologically active fraction of the hormone in circulation. This has tremendous theoretical advantages that may be particularly important in infant research. Newborns have low CBG levels initially that increase over the first 6 months of life (Hadjian, Chedin, Cochet, & Chambaz, 1975). Plasma cortisol levels (free and bound fractions) are quite low in the newborn and increase over the first half year as binding globulin levels increase. Salivary cortisol levels (the free fraction) do not show this same developmental progression and are similar, or slightly higher, in the newborn period than later in the first year (Francis et al., 1987). Thus, the use of salivary measures reduces the need to question whether changing values reflect a true change in biologically active cortisol.

There are various methods for collecting saliva. A procedure that works well with newborns and with premature infants was reported by Emory and his colleagues (Davis & Emory, 1995; Emory, Konopka, Hronsky, Tuggey, & Dave, 1988) and also used by Magnano, Gardner, and Karmel (1992). This procedure involves the use of wall or portable suction units in hospital nurseries. DeLee suction catheters are also an option and are available from most medical supply companies. Recently, a company from Germany has marketed the "salivette" (Sarstedt Inc., Rommelsdorf, Germany). This is a collection tube with a small cotton roll attached to the inside of the lid. The cotton can be used to swab the mouth and is then returned to the tube. The tube is placed in a centrifuge and the clear saliva is extracted and stored for later analysis. Centrifuging the sample has the advantage of retrieving nearly all the saliva from the cotton. Another and economical option is to use plain cotton dental rolls, also available from medical supply companies. The cotton roll is used to swab the mouth, and the moistened portion is cut and placed into a needleless plastic syringe where it can be expressed into air-tight vials for storage. Preferably, the vials should have seals that prevent leakage, especially during freezing when the expressed saliva expands.

To some individuals, particularly older infants and children, the cotton can taste or feel unpleasant, possibly provoking resistance, especially with repeated sampling. Resistance to sampling may likely interfere with the "noninvasiveness" of the procedure, possibly affecting baseline values. Previous studies used sweetened drink mix powders to reduce this possible unpleasant aspect of the cotton. However, a recent study suggested that the use of oral stimulants to collect saliva samples may compromise the validity of cortisol values (Schwartz, Granger, Susman, Gunnar, & Laird, 1998). Specifically, some currently available assay reagents appear sensitive to the pH level alterations produced by oral stimulants such as sweetened drink mixes and may likely either artificially inflate cortisol values or confound cortisol–behavior relations. The authors of this study suggested that oral stimulants should either not be used for saliva collection or be used cautiously and concurrently with carefully controlled procedures. The findings of this study support previously reported similar results (Kirschbaum & Hellhammer, 1994). An alternative method for nonintrusively introducing cotton rolls for saliva collection is to provide a number of playful, practice trials that allow for accommodation to the procedure. Infants and small children, however, must be carefully monitored each time they are introduced to cotton rolls in order to avoid any risk of the child aspirating the cotton rolls. Cotton roll lengths should remain at least 6 inches, and an adult should maintain a strong hold at all times.

Saliva samples are typically stored at –20°C until assayed. However, cortisol is a stable hormone and can remain at room temperature for several weeks without degrading (Kirschbaum & Hellhammer, 1994). The ease of sampling allows the researcher to have parents collect samples at home, keep them in the refrigerator for several days if needed, and then send them through the regular mail to the researcher for analysis.

BIOBEHAVIORAL BASIS OF ASSESSMENT

Cortisol is a glucocorticoid hormone produced in the cortices of the adrenal glands. It is generated and released spontaneously throughout the day and in response to both internal and external events (Van Cauter, 1990). Cortisol is a potent hormone, stress elevations of which begin as part of a complex neurophysiological response to actual or anticipated threats to the organism's homeostasis. Modulation of salivary cortisol production largely involves activity in limbic and hypothalamic areas of the brain (see Figure 9.1). A number of neuroregulatory peptides, or hormones, are involved in regulating the release of corticotropin releasing hormone (CRH) from cells in the

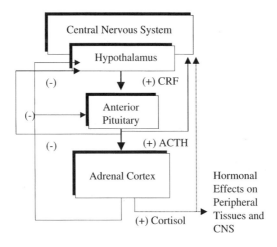

FIGURE 9.1. Hypothalamic pituitary adrenal axis and modulation of cortisol.

paraventricular area of the hypothalamus. CRH stimulates cells in the anterior pituitary to cleave the prohormone proopiomelanocortin (POMC) into the hormone adrenocorticotropin (ACTH) and other related peptides (e.g., beta-endorphin) which are then released into the bloodstream. Other neuropeptide hormones, in particular vasopressin, operate synergistically with CRH to potentiate the production and release of ACTH. Once in the bloodstream, ACTH stimulates cells of the adrenal cortex to break down cholesterol into cortisol and other related hormones (for more complete reviews, see Kandel, Schwartz, & Jessell, 1991; Tepperman & Tepperman, 1987).

Receptors for cortisol in the hypothalamus and in the hippocampus (De Kloet, 1991) regulate CRH production via negative feedback mechanisms. Cortisol levels vary throughout the day resulting in the circadian rhythm in cortisol production seen in mature organisms (Figure 9.2). Newborns do not express this rhythm, but they possess the underlying physiology for its expression. Development of an early morning peak in cortisol production occurs within the first months of life (Price, Close, & Fielding, 1983) and is influenced by patterns of sleeping, eating, physical activity, and light–dark exposure (Krieger, 1979; Moore-Ede, 1986). The neurochemicals involved in the production of cortisol are not stored by the body in large quantities and must be manufactured by cells in the pituitary (for ACTH) and the adrenal cortex (for cortisol). This means that there is considerable time between the central neural events producing a rise in CRH in the hypothalamus and peak levels of cortisol in circulation. Typical estimates are 15-plus minutes to peak plasma concentrations plus approximately 2 more minutes to peak saliva concentrations. Cortisol remains in circulation until taken up by tissues or cleared

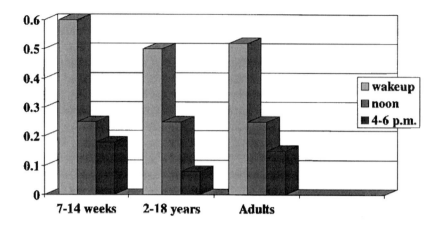

FIGURE 9.2. Circadian rhythm in salivary cortisol from infancy through adulthood. Adapted from Flinn and England (1996); Kirschbaum and Hellhammer (1989); Larson, White, Cochran, Donzella, and Gunnar (1998).

through the kidneys. The half-life of cortisol is long, being estimated at 106 to 118 minutes in saliva for adults (Kirschbaum & Hellhammer, 1989).

The time-to-peak concentrations, the duration of the response, and thus the time from peak concentrations to the reestablishment of basal concentrations vary with the intensity of the response. Thus, it is important to examine the time course typically observed in each research paradigm. Much information about psychobiological regulation is contained in individual variations from this normative time course. To date, the time-course approach has not been used in most research on salivary cortisol with infants and children. However, the ease of saliva collection makes this approach feasible.

RELIABILITY AND VALIDITY

Although cortisol concentrations in plasma and saliva are highly correlated, salivary cortisol typically reflects only 5–10% of plasma concentrations (see review by Kirschbaum & Hellhammer, 1989). The reasons for this attenuated ratio include the following: (1) salivary cortisol reflects only the free fraction of cortisol in circulation and (2) an enzyme present in large concentrations in saliva converts cortisol to cortisone. There are now a number of RIAs available for analysis of cortisol in saliva. Most were designed, however, for plasma and must be modified for saliva samples. Many companies provide protocols for adapting their assay procedures for salivary cortisol assessment (see Kirschbaum & Hellhammer,

1989). Unfortunately, because the RIA kits were designed for plasma, the quality-control samples commercially available for plasma cortisol with known cortisol concentrations are not available for salivary cortisol. This means that caution must be exercised in comparing absolute values across assays and across laboratories. Variations can be accounted for by differences among assay systems in cross-reactivity of the antiserum with different steroids that are closely related to cortisol, particularly cortisone and corticosterone. It is wise for the researcher to generate a large quantity of control samples (from the same pool of saliva) that can be used across assay batches and can be available for comparison with other assays. RIA procedures require licensing for the use of isotopes and the availability of a gamma-counter. If the researcher does not have access to a laboratory that can deal with radioactive material, there are several laboratories that accept samples for analysis. Recent advances in assay procedures and chromatography raise the prospects for saliva cortisol assays that do not require use of radioactive substances (see Kirschbaum & Hellhammer, 1994, for a brief overview). Some companies are now marketing enzyme immunoassays (EIA) for salivary cortisol that do not require the use of radioactivity (Granger, personal communication, January 1999; Salimetrics, State College, Pennsylvania).

Control over the times of day that samples are taken is an important consideration. Cortisol is produced in pulses by the adrenal cortex. Healthy individuals under resting conditions have about 15 pulses in each 24-hour period (Van Cauter, 1990). The amplitude of the pulses is highest in the early morning hours and the lowest around midnight in adults, resulting in a marked circadian rhythm in circulating basal levels of cortisol. There has been a good deal of argument over when this circadian pattern is established, and even in adults there is considerable day-to-day fluctuation in baseline levels. Initial estimates for when rhythms were established in humans was between 1 and 3 years of age (Franks, 1967). These estimates were based on hospitalized/institutionalized children. Research using saliva samples collected by mothers in the home under nonstressed conditions yielded a different picture (Price et al., 1983). At birth there appear to be two peaks in cortisol production per 24 hours that are unrelated to clock time, but by 3 months of age it is easy to detect an early-morning peak in saliva cortisol. In fact, in a recent study (Larson, White, Cochran, Donzella, & Gunnar, 1998), by 7 weeks of age, roughly 30% of infants exhibit an early-morning peak in cortisol production. By 12 weeks of age nearly all infants showed this circadian pattern. Morning concentrations in infants were similar to those reported for adults, averaging between 0.5 and 0.6 mg/dl (Kirschbaum & Hellhammer, 1989). Thus within a few weeks of birth, the time of day for sampling needs to be considered in accurately assessing the hypothalamic–pituitary–adrenal (HPA) system. Before the circadian rhythm is established, requiring the baby to be in a quiescent behavioral state for the

30 minutes prior to sampling is probably the best researchers can do to control baseline concentrations.

The need to control for time of day is often questioned because of the unfamiliar restrictions it places on child development researchers. However, the necessity to assert some control over when saliva samples are taken is clear once the rhythmicity of the system is understood. The need for circadian control is the greatest in the early-morning hours as cortisol decreases markedly within 1 to 2 hours following its circadian peak. Thus, average values between 7 and 8 A.M. may be around 0.50 to 0.60 mg/dl while by 9 to 10 A.M. the averages are typically around 0.30 mg/dl and at 3 to 4 P.M. they are around 0.15 mg/dl. A 2-hour "window" for testing between 9 and 11 A.M. or between 2 and 4 P.M. does not add much "noise" from circadian variation; however, testing children across the workday hours (e.g., 9 A.M. to 5 P.M.) may make it difficult to separate individual differences in levels from circadian changes. Furthermore, low and often nonsignificant correlations between baseline cortisol and clock time in between-subject analyses cannot be used to argue that subjects tested across the workday hours can be included in the same analysis. The standard deviation in salivary cortisol is typically around 0.15 to 0.25 mg/dl for baseline samples obtained during the workday hours. Even using the smaller value, it is easy to see how individual variation overwhelms circadian variation in between-subject analyses, despite being a significant factor when more sensitive within-subject analyses are used.

As an example of this point, Gunnar, Broderson, Krueger, and Rigatuso (1996a) calculated the cross-age correlations in cortisol for infants tested longitudinally at 4 and 6 months of age. The correlation with clock time at each age was negligible even though samples were collected over the morning hours (8:30 A.M. to 11:30 A.M.). Despite this, as shown in Table 9.1, the cross-age correlation increased as the researchers narrowed the window of time difference allowed between 4 and 6 months. Thus, although the correlation with clock time was low, individual patterns of circadian variation were clearly influencing the assessment of baseline or pretest cortisol. In adults, there is also an increase in cortisol that occurs about 45 minutes after the noon and the evening meals (postprandial surge). The increase following the noon meal has also been observed in infants and toddlers 9 to 18 months of age (Ward et al., 1995). Whether younger infants, with their smaller and more closely spaced feedings, also exhibit increases in cortisol within the hour following a meal is not known. Feeding is a significant concern additionally because cortisol is present in breast milk and in milk-based formulas (Magnano, Diamond, & Gardner, 1989). Thus, if milk gets into the saliva sample, a spuriously high reading may be obtained. Swabbing with extra cotton that is discarded or rinsing the mouth with water prior to sampling is an effective method for clearing milk. Of course, if the infant's mouth has been rinsed, or if the infant has a water or juice feeding prior to sampling, re-

TABLE 9.1. Cross-Age Correlations between 4 and 6 Months of Age for Pretest and Cortisol Response T Scores at Similar or Different Test Times

	Cortisol	
	Pretest (4 months)	Response T score (6 months)
Total Sample N = 80	.27*	.21
Greater than 1 hr test time difference N = 32	−.05	.12
Less than 1 hr test time difference N = 48	.49**	.28**
Less than 30 min test time difference N = 31	.56**	.38**

Note. From Gunnar, Broderson, Krueger, and Rigatuso (1996a). Copyright 1996 by the Society for Research in Child Development. Reprinted by permission.

* p <. 05;   ** p < .01

searchers need to be certain that the saliva is not diluted as this will yield spuriously low cortisol readings.

Another caution regarding infant sampling is to screen the breastfeeding mother's history carefully for smoking, coffee consumption, or medications that may influence breast milk. Nicotine and caffeine can stimulate the HPA axis and are known to be present in breast milk (Nehlig & Debry, 1994; Stepans & Wilkerson, 1993). Likewise, fluoxetine hydrochloride (Prozac) has been identified in breast milk (Lester et al., 1991). Although the effects of this medication, and others similar to it, such as sertraline (Zoloft), on the infant's HPA axis are currently unknown, researchers would be wise to document these potential mediators of individual differences in cortisol concentrations in breastfed infants.

Sleep is associated with many changes in HPA activity (e.g., Spangler, 1991). The onset of nighttime sleep in adults typically occurs close to the nadir in cortisol and falling deeper asleep produces a further decrease in HPA activity. Corticoid activity stimulates slow-wave sleep, perhaps affecting a form of conservation–withdrawal. Conversely, the circadian increase in cortisol in the hours prior to morning wakening typically occurs during rapid eye movement sleep in adults. Sleep in the newborn and young infant is not organized as it is in adults (Anders, 1975; Coons & Guillemineault, 1982); nonetheless, sleep still bears an important relationship to HPA activity early in development. In newborns, events that elevate cortisol (e.g., circumcision) will stimulate an increase in quiet sleep at the expense of active sleep (Emde, Harmon, Metcalf, Koenig, & Wagonfeld, 1971). This change in sleep may reflect central effects of cortisol. Furthermore, quiet sleep appears to correspond to periods of rapid clearance of cortisol from circulation (Gunnar, Malone, Vance, & Fisch, 1985). In older infants, napping has been shown to temporarily lower cortisol (Larson, Gunnar, & Hertsgaard, 1991).

The normative fluctuations in cortisol related to time of day, sleeping, and eating provide a solid argument for a careful assessment of the infant's daily schedule and health characteristics when conducting research on this system. Interestingly, and importantly, these daily events do not appear to be as strongly associated with posttest (i.e., response) as they are with pretest (i.e., baseline) cortisol levels (e.g., Gunnar et al., 1996a). This is consistent with evidence suggesting that when a stimulus produces a change in cortisol, pretest and posttest levels are almost never significantly correlated (Kirschbaum, personal communication, September 1995). When difference scores (posttest–pretest) are used, however, these normative fluctuations may affect the magnitude of the response that is estimated for each child.

DEVELOPMENTAL MODEL

There are at least two ways in which measures of cortisol can inform understanding of child development. First, altered or abnormal activity of the system, due to either repeated or chronic stress or constitutional factors, may affect brain development and consequently influence behavior. Second, because psychosocial factors affect activity of the HPA system, measures of salivary cortisol enrich our understanding of the psychobiology of stress in early development. The following presents a brief elaboration of each reason.

Implications of Atypical Cortisol Levels

Cortisol is an intensely potent steroid. It has a broad spectrum of effects, influencing activity of nearly all cells in the body (Munck, Guyre, & Holbrook, 1984). Although the capacity to mount a cortisol response to noxious events is necessary for survival, cortisol can also have negative effects, perhaps particularly for the developing child. High levels of cortisol interact with the growth hormone system, suppressing its activity and contributing to poor physical growth. Further, high levels of cortisol permit activity in excitatory receptors in the brain (N-methyl-D-aspartate, or NMDA, receptors), increasing the risk of cell death in areas such as the hippocampus. High levels of cortisol can also increase the activity of cortisol releasing hormone in other areas, including the amygdala, potentially stimulating a lower threshold for stress reactions of the sympathetic nervous system (Schulkin, McEwen, & Gold, 1994). Finally, elevated levels of cortisol decrease the efficacy of the immune system, thereby increasing disease susceptibility (Sapolsky, 1994).

Given these potentially deleterious effects, it is reasonable to assume that there are safeguard mechanisms to protect the organism from chronic elevations.

Indeed, mechanisms for controlling elevations in cortisol are built into the HPA system itself. Following CRH increases, basal levels of cortisol are reestablished through two negative feedback systems, one a fast rate-sensitive system and the other a delayed proportional control system (Dallman et al., 1992). Chronic or repeated activation of the HPA system can lead to changes in receptors for cortisol that affect negative feedback efficacy (Yehuda, Boisoneau, Mason, & Giller, 1993). In general, an increase in receptor number will increase the efficacy of negative feedback and allow a more rapid termination of stress-induced increases than might be expected with fewer receptors. A decrease in receptor numbers will have the opposite effect. Prolonged increases in cortisol can also alter activity of CRH, ACTH, and cortisol producing cells, affecting the response capabilities of the system. Because these effects on receptors and cell activity can occur in "different directions" (e.g., changes that increase CRH activity may be balanced by changes that reduce ACTH production), prolonged or repeated activation of the system can theoretically result in increases in activity at one level of the system, combined with normal or even decreased activity at other levels.

The impact of chronic or repeated adverse conditions on the HPA system has not been studied fully in human adults (see Rose, 1980, for review), let alone in children. Recently, Yehuda, Resnick, Kahana, and Giller (1993) demonstrated that posttraumatic stress disorder in adults is associated with lower than normal cortisol levels and attenuated cortisol reactions to stressors. Low cortisol levels have also been noted to co-occur in a number of other stress-related disorders in adults (Heim, Ehlert, & Hellhammer, 2000). Whether chronic stress increases or decreases baseline cortisol in young children and infants is presently not known (however, see DeBellis et al., 1994; Gunnar & Vazquez, in press). The bottom line is that both high cortisol levels and greater than normal cortisol responses to stressors and extremely low cortisol levels with attenuated reactions to stressors may reflect stress-related alterations in HPA activity (McEwen, 1998).

Salivary cortisol measures in high-risk infants and children may reflect the effects of chronic or repeated HPA activation. These measures may also offer an estimation of physiological integrity for infants who are at risk for developmental impairment because of histories of prematurity, difficult pregnancies and deliveries, and drug, alcohol, and other teratogen exposures. To date, only a few studies of this nature have been conducted. The results from studies using other plasma measures of cortisol, however, suggest the importance of adequate adrenocortical functioning to survival (Murphy, 1983). The results of several studies suggest that sequelae of prematurity, such as respiratory distress syndrome and chronic lung disease, are associated with inadequate cortisol secretion (Kotre et al., 1996; Watterberg, Scott,

Backstrom, Gifford, & Cook, 2000; Watterberg & Scott, 1995). Moreover, there is evidence that hypotension, which is also common among ill premature infants, may be related to adrenal insufficiency (Helbock, Insoft, & Conte, 1993). Because of the role of cortisol in the stimulation of surfactant, there is a close relationship between adrenocortical activity and respiratory distress syndrome (RDS), a complication of prematurity. The results of several studies suggest that controlling for gestational age, lowered umbilical cord blood cortisol concentrations are associated with developing RDS (Murphy, Joyce, Dyas, & Hughes, 1983). Once RDS has developed, increasingly elevated cortisol concentrations are seen which then stabilize at high concentrations (Hughes et al., 1987; Siamopoulou-Mavridou, Mavridis, Vizandiadis, & Harsoulis, 1986).

In addition to baseline measures, stress reactivity of the HPA system can be studied in premature infants. Baden et al. (1972) found that infants as young as 26 weeks gestational age showed a cortisol response to stressors associated with RDS. At one time, there was a controversy over whether premature infants showed higher or lower cortisol levels than did full-term infants (Murphy, 1983; Rokicki, Forest, Loras, & Bertrand, 1987). This early controversy was based on plasma cortisol data. More recent work using salivary cortisol (Magnano et al., 1992) demonstrated nearly identical basal and response concentrations for healthy premature infants (30–37 weeks gestational age) compared to healthy full-term infants.

There is a large and growing animal literature on prenatal stress and the HPA axis (e.g., Clarke, Wittwer, Abbott, & Schneider, 1994). To date, there are no human studies of prenatal stress effects on postnatal cortisol reactivity unless cocaine exposure and/or alcohol exposure *in utero* can be viewed as a prenatal stress paradigm. Magnano et al. (1992) found what appeared to be a downregulation of the HPA axis in premature infants exposed prenatally to cocaine. Specifically, they found a diminished salivary cortisol response to both invasive and noninvasive stressors in cocaine-exposed premature infants compared to nonexposed controls. Similar findings of atypical physiological responding (enhanced instead of depressed) have been identified in infants who were exposed prenatally to alcohol (Jacobson, Bihun, & Chiodo, 1999). These effects on the HPA axis may reflect more general physiological disturbances in the support mechanisms for modulated state behavior in early infancy. This hypothesis fits nicely with observations of poor behavioral state regulation in infants exposed to cocaine (Coles, Platzman, Smith, James, & Falek, 1992; Gardner, Karmel, & Magnano, 1990; Lester et al., 1991). It is an empirical question whether altered HPA reactivity in these newborns may serve as a physiological marker of later subtle attentional and state regulation problems that have been observed in cocaine-exposed and alcohol-exposed children.

There is also a large animal literature on the effects of postnatal events on the HPA axis. For example, there are a number of studies investigating repeated separations of infant–mother dyads in rodents and primates that suggest long-term consequences on stress reactivity and regulation (Clarke, Kraemer, & Kupfer, 1995; Meaney et al., 1993; Suchecki, Rosenfeld, & Levine, 1993). Similar findings have been obtained in recent research on 2-year-old children reared in deprived orphanage conditions in Romania (Carlson & Earls, 1997). These researchers showed that elevated cortisol concentrations in these children were negatively correlated with the children's measures of cognitive, motor, physical, and social development. Thus, abnormal activity of the HPA axis as revealed in salivary cortisol measures may index biobehavioral dysregulation predictive of nonoptimal behavioral development.

Psychosocial Regulation of Cortisol

In adults, three psychological variables largely determine reactivity of the HPA system to emotionally charged events: (1) the importance of the event to the individual, (2) suspenseful anticipation, and (3) control or the individual's sense of efficacy with regard to managing the threat posed by the event (Kirschbaum & Hellhammer, 1994; Mason, 1968; Rose, 1980). With development, psychological factors begin to regulate the HPA axis in children (Gunnar, 1986; Stansbury & Gunnar, 1994). There is a great deal of interest in using salivary cortisol as a measure of stress-reactive temperament. However, it is important to note that in infants perhaps especially, measures of cortisol reflect both infant characteristics and characteristics of the caregiving environment.

For infants and young children, the most relevant psychological factor in regulating stress is probably the presence of a sensitive and responsive adult (Bowlby, 1969; Compas, 1987). The adult provides the resources the infant needs to cope with and to help control aversive stimulation. A history of sensitive, responsive care also alters the child's threshold for anticipating aversive outcomes (Sroufe, Waters, & Matas, 1974). Over the course of the first year, as specific attachment relationships form, the presence of the attachment figure should be increasingly important in regulating reactivity of the infant's HPA system.

In the newborn period, the HPA system is highly labile and responsive to a variety of perturbations. Events as seemingly mild as undressing, weighing, and measuring the infant provoke two- to threefold increases in cortisol, while highly noxious events such as circumcision without anesthesia will elicit five- to sixfold increases. Giving the newborn a pacifier will reduce crying but does not inhibit the increase in cortisol. This has been shown for events such as circumcision and blood sampling, which involve nocioceptive stimulation, and also for physical exams, which presumably do not (see Gunnar, 1989, for review).

Over the course of the first months of life, the stimulation involved in physical exams (e.g., well-baby checkups) ceases to elicit increases in cortisol for most infants (Gunnar et al., 1996a; Larson et al., 1998; Lewis & Ramsay, 1995a). By the end of the first year, even events such as inoculations fail to elicit increases in cortisol on average (Gunnar et al., 1996a). Separations of up to a half hour or more in strange settings with unfamiliar yet responsive, caregivers elicit elevations in infants of 9 months of age (Gunnar, Mangelsdorf, Larson, & Hertsgaard, 1989), but by a year of age separations of this sort do not elicit increases in cortisol for most infants (Gunnar & Nelson, 1994). Finally, in the second year, events that elicit behavioral inhibition fail to elevate cortisol for most infants (Nachmias, Gunnar, Mangelsdorf, Parritz, & Buss, 1996).

There are a number of reasons to expect that this decrease in reactivity is related to the organization of the caregiver–infant attachment relationship. First, in infant monkeys, the presence of the mother has been shown to be a powerful buffer of cortisol responses to a variety of stressors (Levine & Wiener, 1988). Even when the infant monkey cannot gain physical contact with the mother, being able to see, hear, and smell her presence results in smaller increases in cortisol on separation when compared to conditions in which neither distal or proximal contact is possible (Coe, Wiener, Rosenberg, & Levine, 1985). This difference exists even though seeing the mother in the first condition elicits more protest behavior in the infant monkey than does complete isolation. Furthermore, in species of monkeys where adult females other than the mother carry and "aunt" infants, the presence of an "aunt" during maternal separation has resulted in reduced cortisol response (Coe et al., 1985). In nonhuman primates, procedures that chronically disrupt the mother's social relations with other adult females and produce long-term disturbances in mothering behavior also elicit elevations in cortisol in both mother and infant (Coe, Weiner, & Levine, 1993).

A second line of evidence supporting attachment relationships in HPA regulation is provided by rat studies. Infant rodents exhibit a well-studied period during early development (approximately postnatal Day 4 through Day 14) when the pup's HPA system is relatively nonresponsive to stressors (Rosenfield, Suchecki, & Levine, 1992). This period, called the relative stress hyporesponsive period—or SHRP—is controlled and maintained by maternal stimulation. When the mother is removed for prolonged periods (i.e., 24 hours), the infant's HPA system becomes adult-like in its responsiveness. Low levels of HPA activity can be maintained during maternal separation by providing relevant elements of maternal care. Moreover, procedures that disrupt the mother–infant relationship have long-term effects on HPA reactivity in the rodent. Brief separations that mimic what would naturally occur in the wild tend to result in a well-regulated system in the adult, whereas long separations tend to result in a hyperreactive HPA system (Plotsky & Meaney, 1993). Continuity in mammalian adaptation suggests that the mother would be an important buffer for the human infant as well.

The third reason to argue the importance of attachment relationships in human infant HPA regulation is provided by evidence that attachment security moderates the relations between behavioral inhibition and cortisol response. In insecure, but not secure, attachment relationships, behavioral inhibition is associated with elevations in cortisol to novel events and brief separations (Nachmias et al., 1996). Moreover, even though most toddlers do not show elevations in cortisol to inoculations, those who do tend to be insecurely attached to the person accompanying them to the clinic (Gunnar, 1998). Taken together, the data discussed in this section argue that by the end of the first year, assessment of the HPA system may allow a measure of whether the attachment relationship is functioning effectively as a "stress buffer." Furthermore, it argues that without assessment of the psychosocial buffers of the HPA axis, reactions in this system cannot be used to "index" individual differences in infant emotional reactivity (see also Spangler & Schieche, 1998).

STRUCTURAL AND/OR THEORETICAL CONSTRAINTS/CONTROVERSIES

Although salivary cortisol may be reliably used to index physiological response to external events, the developmental researcher must consider limitations. As discussed in the previous section, cognitive appraisals of what constitutes "stressful situation," emotional competencies, and available resources (e.g., mother) change over time and likely influence an individuals' capacity for responding. Further, HPA activity to environmental events is a normal and adaptive response. What constitutes an optimal versus suboptimal response developmentally is not yet fully understood, although the literature suggests that it is the sustained response in comparison to rebounded baseline levels that may be most salient (Spangler & Schieche, 1998). There is the need for more basic research in this area. Finally, there is some suggestion that although cortisol response is linked to cry behavior in infants, it may not be linked in a linear fashion. For example, a recent study investigating infants with colic found that while the colic infants cried longer and more intensely than did control infants, the two groups did not differ in cortisol responses (White, Gunnar, Larson, Donzella, & Barr, 2000).

There are several common analytic strategies used in cortisol–behavior studies. These strategies are often used because of the complex nature of cortisol measures and the HPA system. First, cortisol distributions are often positively skewed. This problem is particularly acute for salivary cortisol. The pulsitile release of cortisol appears partially responsible for influencing this positive skew. In addition, when a reaction of the HPA system has been elicited it is typical that some, but not all, subjects will respond. Those who respond may produce cortisol levels that begin to exceed available CBG sites. This results in a shift in the ratio of bound to free cortisol and a marked rise in the free fraction that enters the saliva pool (Gunnar, Marvinney, Isensee, & Fisch, 1988). It is not unusual when a marked response is elicited to find some subjects exhibiting salivary cortisol levels that are more than three or more standard deviations above the mean. These values have considerable effects in most parametric analyses. Because of the skew of cortisol distributions, it is common to log transform the data. This helps but does not eliminate problems with extreme outliers. Researchers should be alert to these in their data.

Lewis and Ramsay (1995b) supported correcting cortisol response measures for the law of initial values (LIV). The concern arises in physiological data because changes in the activity of a system may be controlled, in part, by the state of the system prior to stimulation. Typically, a system that is already highly active responds less than one that is at more quiescent levels of activity when a stimulus occurs. However, whether pretest values constrain posttest values is also an empirical issue. It has been argued that data must meet two criteria, at least, before the researcher need be concerned that an initial value constraint is operating (Jin, 1992). First, a significant change in level of response must be observed. Second, pretest and posttest values must be significantly correlated. When these conditions are met, the recommended correction for the LIV is a regression procedure that effectively removes the variance from posttest measures that can be attributed to pretest levels. This allows researchers to analyze their response data without concern that it is "contaminated" with variance due to factors affecting the pretest levels. Evidence that pretest is correlated with delta or change scores (post–pre) is not sufficient to require the correction for LIV. Indeed, unless pretest and posttest measures are significantly correlated, the regression procedures to "correct" for LIV will have no statistical effect.

TRAINING REQUIREMENTS

There are no formal training requirements prior to using this method in research. However, it behooves the researcher to contact someone who is using this method successfully and develop strategies for proceeding at his or her own site.

IMPLICATIONS

Measures of salivary cortisol are likely to become widely used in infant research particularly because these measures promise to afford researchers a noninvasive method of assessing activity of the HPA system. Although we have much to learn about using these measures in infant assessment, several points seem clear to date. First, extremely high or extremely low measures of cortisol responding may be related to suboptimal developmental capacities in the human infant. Failure to mount an adequate cortisol response to aversive stimulation as well as extreme elevations that do not return adaptively to baselines may reflect underlying disturbances in the competencies supporting adaptation. Second, as development progresses in the first year, caregivers emerge as important buffers of stress reactions of the HPA system. Therefore, attempts to understand individual differences in cortisol stress reactivity in relation to child temperament and developmental integrity need to be made in consideration of the quality of the infant's care environment.

Future studies should carefully control factors affecting baseline activity, including, for example, sampling time of day, sleep/nap schedules, feeding schedules, and salient characteristics of routine family life (e.g., car trips). Important aspects of future research should include analyses of the time course of the response to the challenge or stressor that the experimenter has imposed. Time-course analyses should contain both peak response measures and estimates of the duration of the response. Because in many cases parents can obtain saliva samples reliably at home, studies conducted in laboratories or other out-of-home settings can employ home samples taken concurrently with the laboratory assessments to more fully understand responses made from baseline concentrations. These assessments can be critical in understanding responsivity patterns. For example, in a number of studies, Gunnar and colleagues (Larson et al., 1991) found that cortisol levels when infants first arrive at the laboratory for testing are actually lower than levels at the same time of day at home, presumably as a result of the car ride into the laboratory setting. Changes in response to laboratory procedures, thus, may be imposed on an already lowered baseline. This may affect interpretation of findings, as when an elevation to procedures in the laboratory returns levels merely to those that would be seen at home at that time of day. The researcher may wish to question the extent to which this kind of finding should be interpreted as a stress response.

There are a number of populations in which the questions about regulation of the HPA axis may be particularly pertinent. The following, though not exhaustive, presents some suggestions. First, studies of infant and young child behavior as a result of prenatal stress to the mother may provide information about the mechanisms underlying individual response to early stressful challenges as the result of intrauterine experience. Second, there is a need for further research investigating early stress experiences and subsequent neurobiological development in the child that may affect regulation of the HPA system, particularly the potential effects on neural structures involved in negative feedback control of cortisol levels (e.g., events affecting hippocampal development). Third, further research should investigate situations in which social regulation of the stress response system may be disrupted (e.g., attachment disorders). With careful attention to issues such as the foregoing assessment of this system may well provide important insights into psychobiological processes influencing development in infancy and early childhood.

ACKNOWLEDGMENTS

We wish to express thanks to the families and children who participated in the work discussed in this chapter and to the many graduate and undergraduate students without whom the research could not be conducted. Thanks is also due to the members of the Endocrine Laboratory at the University of Minnesota Hospitals for their careful assaying of the salivary cortisol samples. The writing of this chapter was partially supported by research grants and awards from the National Institute of Child Health and Human Development (No. HD16494) and the National Institute of Mental Health (No. MH00946) to Megan R. Gunnar.

REFERENCES

Anders, T. (Ed.). (1975). *Maturation of sleep patterns in the newborn infant.* New York: Spectrum.

Anders, T., Sachar, E., Kream, J., Roffwarg, H., & Hellman, L. (1970). Behavioral state and plasma cortisol response in the human newborn. *Pediatrics, 46*(4), 532–537.

Baden, M., Bauer, C. R., Colle, E., Klein, G., Taeusch, H. W., & Stern, L. (1972). A controlled trial of hydrocortisone therapy in infants with respiratory distress syndrome. *Pediatrics, 50,* 526.

Barnes, C. M., Kenny, F. M., Call, T., & Reinhart, J. B. (1972). Measurement management of anxiety in children for open heart surgery. *Pediatrics, 19*(2), 250–259.

Bowlby, J. (1969). *Attachment and loss* (Vol. 1). New York: Basic Books.

Carlson, M., & Earls, F. (1997). Psychological and neuroendocrinological sequelae of early social deprivation in institutionalized children in Romania. *Annals of the New York Academy of Sciences, 807,* 419–428.

Clarke, A. S., Kraemer. G. W., & Kupfer, D. J. (1995). Effects of rearing condition on HPA axis response to fluoxetine and desipramine treatment over repeated social separations in young rhesus monkeys. *Psychiatry Research, 79*(2), 91–104.

Clarke, A. S., Wittwer, D. J., Abbott, D. H., & Schneider, M. L. (1994). Long-term effects of prenatal stress on HPA axis activity in juvenile rhesus monkeys. *Developmental Psychobiology, 27*(5), 257–269.

Coe, C. L., Weiner, S. G., & Levine, S. (1993). Psychendocrine responses of mother and infant monkeys to disturbance and separation. In L. A. Rosenblum & H. Moltz (Ed.), *Symbiosis in parent–offspring interactions* (pp. 189–214). New York: Plenum Press.

Coe, C. L., Wiener, S. G., Rosenberg, L. T., & Levine, S. (1985). Endocrine and immune responses to separation and maternal loss in nonhuman primates. In M. Reite & T. Fields (Eds.), *The psychobiology of attachment* (pp. 163–199). New York: Academic Press.

Coles, C. D., Platzman, K. A., Smith, I., James, M. E., & Falek, A. (1992). Effects of cocaine and alcohol use in pregnancy on neonatal growth and neurobehavioral status. *Neurotoxicology and Teratology, 14,* 23–33.

Compas, B. E. (1987). Coping with stress during childhood and adolescence. *Psychological Bulletin, 101*(3), 393–403.

Coons, S., & Guilleminault, C. (1982). Development of sleep-wake patterns and non-rapid eye movement sleep stages during the first six months of life in normal infants. *Pediatrics, 69,* 793–798.

Dallman, M. F., Akana, S. F., Scribner, K. A., Bradbury, M. J., Walker, C. D., Strack, A. M., & Cascio, C. S. (1992). Stress, feedback and facilitation in the hypothalamo–pituitary–adrenal axis. *Journal of Neuroendocrinology, 4*(5), 517–526.

Davis, M., & Emory, E. (1995). Sex differences in neonatal stress reactivity. *Child Development, 66*(1), 14–27.

DeBellis, M. D., Chrousos, G. P., Dorn, L. D., Burke, L., Helmers, K., Kling, M. A., Trickett, P., & Putnam, F. W. (1994). Adrenal axis dysregulation in sexually abused girls. *Journal of Clinical Endocrinology and Metabolism, 78,* 249–255.

De Kloet, E. R. (1991). Brain corticosteroid receptor balance and homeostatic control. *Frontiers in Neuroendocrinology, 12*(2), 95–164.

Emde, R. N., Harmon, R. J., Metcalf, D., Koenig, K. L., & Wagonfeld, S. (1971). Stress and neonatal sleep. *Psychosomatic Medicine, 33*(6), 491–496.

Emory, E. K., Konopka, S., Hronsky, S., Tuggey, R., & Dave, R. (1988). Salivary caffeine and neonatal behavior: Assay modification and functional significance. *Psychopharmacology, 94*(1), 64–68.

Flinn, M. V., & England, B. G. (1995). Childhood stress and family environment. *Current Anthropology, 36*(5).

Francis, S. J., Walker, R. F., Riad-Fahamy, D., Hughes, D., Murphy, J. F., & Gray, O. P. (1987). Assessment of adrenocortical activity in term newborn infants using salivary cortisol determinations. *Journal of Pediatrics, 111,* 129–133.

Franks, R. C. (1967). Diurnal variation of plasma 17–Hydroxycorticosteroids in children. *Journal of Clinical Endocrinology, 27,* 75–78.

Gardner, J. M., Karmel, B. Z., & Magnano, C. L. (1990). Neurobehavioral indicators of early brain insult in high-risk infants. *Developmental Psychology, 26,* 563–575.

Gunnar, M. R. (1986). Human developmental psychoendocrinology: A review of research on neuroendocrine responses to challenge and threat in infancy and childhood. In M. Lamb, A. Brown, & B. Rogoff (Ed.), *Advances in developmental psychology* (Vol. 4, pp. 51–103). Hillsdale, NJ: Erlbaum.

Gunnar, M. R. (1989). Studies of the human infant's adrenocortical response to potentially stressful events. In M. Lewis & J. Woroby (Ed.), *Infant stress and coping* (Vol. 45, pp. 3–18). San Francisco: Jossey-Bass.

Gunnar, M. R. (1998). Quality of early care and buffering of neuroendocrine stress reactions: Potential effects on the developing human brain. *Preventive Medicine, 27*(2), 208–211.

Gunnar, M. R., & Barr, R. G. (1998). Stress early brain development, and behavior. *Infants and Young Children, 11*(1), 1–14.

Gunnar, M. R., Broderson, L., Krueger, K., & Rigatuso, J. (1996a). Dampening of adrenocortical responses during infancy: Normative changes and individual differences. *Child Development, 67,* 877–889.

Gunnar, M. R., Broderson, L., Nachmias, M., Buss, K., & Rigatuso, R. (1996b). Stress reactivity and attachment security. *Developmental Psychobiology, 29,* 10–36.

Gunnar, M. R., Malone, S., Vance, G., & Fisch, R. O. (1985). Coping with aversive stimulation in the neonatal period: Quiet sleep and plasma cortisol levels during recovery from circumcision in newborns. *Child Development, 56,* 824–834.

Gunnar, M. R., Mangelsdorf, S., Larson, M., & Hertsgaard, L. (1989). Attachment, temperament and adrenocortical activity in infancy: A study of psychoendocrine regulation. *Developmental Psychology, 25,* 355–363.

Gunnar, M., Marvinney, D., Isensee, J., & Fisch, R. O. (Eds.). (1988). *Coping with uncertainty: New models of the relations between hormonal behavioral and cognitive processes.* Hillsdale, NJ: Erlbaum.

Gunnar, M., & Nelson, C. (1994). Event-related potentials in year-old infants predict negative emotionality and hormonal responses to separation. *Child Development, 65,* 80–94.

Gunnar, M. R., & Vazquez, D. M. (in press). Low cortisol and a flattening of expected daytime rhythm: Potential indices of risk in human development. *Development and Psychopathology.*

Hadjian, A. J., Chedin, M., Cochet, C., & Chambaz, E. M. (1975). Cortisol binding to proteins in plasma in the human neonate and infant. *Pediatric Research, 9,* 40–45.

Hart, J., Gunnar, M., & Cicchetti, D. (1996). Altered neuroendocrine activity in maltreated children related to symptoms of depression. *Development and Psychopathology, 8,* 201–214.

Heim, C., Ehlert, U., & Hellhammer, D. H. (2000). The potential role of hypocortisolism in the pathophysiology of stress-related bodily disorders. *Psychoneuroendocrinology, 25,* 1–35.

Helbock, H. J., Insoft, R. M., & Conte, F. A. (1993). Glucocorticoid responsive hypotension in extremely low birthweight newborns. *Pediatrics, 92,* 715–717.

Hughes, D., Murphy, J. F., Dyas, J., Robinson, J. A., Riad-Fahy, D., & Hughes, I. A. (1987). Blood spot glucocorticoid concentrations in ill preterm infants. *Archives of Disease in Childhood, 62,* 1014–1018.

Jacobson, S. W., Bihun, J. T., & Chiodo, L. M. (1999). Effects of prenatal alcohol and cocaine exposure on infant cortisol levels. *Development and Psychopathology, 11,* 195–208.

Jin, P. (1992). Toward a reconceptualization of the law of initial value. *Psychological Bulletin, 111*(1), 176–184.

Kandel, E., Schwartz, J., & Jessell, T. (1991). *Principles of neural science* (3rd ed.). New York: Elsevier.

Kirschbaum, C., & Hellhammer, D. H. (1989). Salivary cortisol in psychobiological research: An overview. *Neuropsychobiology, 22,* 150–169.

Kirschbaum, C., & Hellhammer, D. H. (1994). Salivary cortisol in psychoneuroendocrine research: Recent developments and applications. *Psychoneuroendocrinology, 19*(4), 313–333.

Kotre, C., Styne, D., Merritt, A. T., Mayes, D., Wertz, A., & Helbock, H. J. (1996). Adrenocortical function in the very low birthweight infants: Improved testing for sensitivity and association with neonatal outcome. *Journal of Pediatrics, 128,* 257–263.

Krieger, D. T. (1979). Regulation of circadian periodicity of plasma corticosteroid concentrations and of body temperature by time of food presentation. In M. Suda, O. Hayaishi, & H. Nakagawa (Eds.), *Biological rhythms and their central mechanism* (pp. 247–255). North Holland, Amsterdam: Elsevier Biomedical Press.

Larson, M., Gunnar, M., & Hertsgaard, L. (1991). The effects of morning naps, car trips, and maternal separation on adrenocortical activity in human infants. *Child Development, 62,* 362–372.

Larson, M. C., White, B. P., Cochran, A., Donzella, B., & Gunnar, M. R. (1998). Dampening of the cortisol response to handling at 3 months in human infants and its relation to sleep, circadian cortisol activity, and behavioral distress. *Developmental Psychobiology, 33*(4), 327–337.

Lester, B. M., Corwin, M. J., Sepkoski, C., Seifer, R., Peucker, M., McLaughlin, S., & Golub, H. L. (1991). Neurobehavioral syndromes in cocaine-exposed newborn infants. *Child Development, 62,* 694–705.

Levine, S., & Wiener, S. G. (1988). Psychoendocrine aspects of mother-infant relationships in nonhuman primates. *Psychoneuroendocrinology, 13*(1 & 2), 143–154.

Lewis, M. (1992). Individual differences in response to stress. *Pediatrics, 90*(3), 487–490.

Lewis, M., & Ramsay, D. S. (1995a). Developmental change in infants' responses to stress. *Child Development, 66,* 657–670.

Lewis, M., & Ramsay, D. S. (1995b). Stability and change in cortisol and behavioral responses to stress during the first 18 months of life. *Developmental Psychobiology, 28*(8), 419–428.

Magnano, C. L., Diamond, E. J., & Gardner, J. M. (1989). Use of salivary cortisol measurements in young infants: A note of caution. *Child Development, 60*(5), 1099–1101.

Magnano, C. L., Gardner, J. M., & Karmel, B. Z. (1992). Differences in salivary cortisol levels in cocaine-exposed and noncocaine-exposed NICU infants. *Developmental Psychobiology, 25*(2), 93–103.

Mason, J. W. (1968). A review of psychoendocrine research on the sympathetic–adrenal medullary system. *Psychosomatic Medicine, 30,* 631–653.

McEwen, B. (1998). Protective and damaging effects of stress mediators. *New England Journal of Medicine, 338,* 171–179.

Meaney, M. J., O'Donnell, D., Viau, V., Bhatnagar, S., Sarrieau, A., Smythe, J., Shanks, N., & Walker, C. D. (1993). Corticosteroid receptors in the rat brain and pituitary during development and hypothalamic–pituitary–adrenal function. In I. Zagon & P. McLaughlin (Eds.), *Receptors in the developing nervous system: Growth factors and hormones* (Vol. 1, pp. 163–201). London: Chapman & Hall.

Montagner, H., Henry, J. C., Lombardot, M., Benedini, M., Burnod, J., & Nicolas, R. M. (1978). Behavioral profiles and corticosteroid excretion rhythms in young children Part 2: Circadian and weekly rhythms in corticosteroid excretion levels of children as indicators of adaptation to social context. In V. Reynolds & N. G. Blurton Jones (Ed.), *Human behavior and adaptation* (pp. 229–265). London: Francis & Taylor.

Moore-Ede, M. C. (1986). Physiology of the circadian timing system: Predictive versus reactive homeostasis. *American Journal of Physiology, 250,* 735–752.

Munck, A., Guyre, P. M., & Holbrook, N. J. (1984). Physiological functions of glucocorticoids in stress and their relation to pharmacological actions. *Endocrine Review, 4*(1), 25–67.

Murphy, B. E. P. (1983). Human fetal serum cortisol levels at delivery: A review. *Endocrine Reviews, 4*(2), 150–154.

Murphy, J. F., Joyce, B. G., Dyas, J., & Hughes, I. A. (1983). Plasma 17–hydroxy-progesterone concentrations in ill newborn infants. *Archives of Disease in Childhood, 58,* 532–534.

Nachmias, M., Gunnar, M., Mangelsdorf, S., Parritz, R., & Buss, K. (1996). Behavioral inhibition and stress reactivity: Moderating role of attachment security. *Child Development, 67,* 508–522.

Nehlig, A., & Debry, G. (1994). Consequences on the newborn of chronic maternal consumption of coffee during gestation and lactation: A review. *Journal of the American College of Nutrition, 13*(1), 6–21.

Plotsky, P. M., & Meaney, M. J. (1993). Early, postnatal experiences alters hypothalamic corticotropin-releasing factor (CRF) MRNA, median eminence CRF. Content and stress-induced release in adult rats. *Brain Research. Molecular Brain Research, 18*(3), 195–200.

Price, D. A., Close, G. C., & Fielding, B. A. (1983). Age of appearance of circadian rhythm in salivary cortisol values in infancy. *Archives of Disease in Childhood, 58,* 454–456.

Ramsay, D. S., & Lewis, M. (1994). Developmental changes in infant cortisol and behavioral stress response to inoculation. *Child Development, 65*(5), 1491–1502.

Riad-Fahmy, D., Read, G., & Hughes, I. A. (1979). Corticosteroids. In C. H. Gray & V. H. T. James (Ed.), *Hormones in blood* (Vol. 3, pp. 179–262). New York: Academic Press.

Riad-Fahmy, D., Read, G. F., Joyce, B. G., & Walker, R. F. (1981). Steroid immunoassays in endocrinology. In A. Vollar, A. Bartlett, & J. D. Bidwell (Eds.), *Immunoassays for the 80's.* Baltimore: Maryland: University Park Press.

Rokicki, W., Forest, M., Loras, B., & Bertrand, J. (Eds.). (1987). *Physiologic foundations of perinatal care* (Vol. 2). New York: Elsevier.

Rose, R. M. (1980). Endocrine responses to stressful psychological events. *Psychiatric Clinics of North America, 3*(2), 251–275.

Rosenfield, P., Suchecki, D., & Levine, S. (1992). Multifactorial regulation of the hypothalamic–pituitary–adrenal axis during development. *Neuroscience and Biobehavioral Reviews, 16,* 553–568.

Sapolsky, R. (1994). *Immunity, stress, and disease, Why zebras don't get ulcers: A guide to stress, stress related diseases and coping.* New York: Freeman.

Schulkin, J., McEwen, B. S., & Gold, P. S. (1994). Allostasis, amygdala, and anticipatory angst. *Neuroscience and Behavioral Reviews, 18*(3), 385–396.

Schwartz, E. B., Granger, D. A., Susman, E. J., Gunnar, M. R., & Laird, B. (1998). Assessing salivary cortisol in studies of child development. *Child Development, 69*(6), 1503–1513.

Siamopoulou-Mavridou, A., Mavridis, A. K., Vizandiadis, A., & Harsoulis, P. (1986). Free urinary cortisol immunoreactive levels in premature and full term infants. *Acta Pediatrica Scandinavica, 75,* 919–922.

Spangler, G. (1991). The emergence of adrenocortical circadian function in newborns and infants and its relationship to sleep, feeding, and maternal adrenocortical activity. *Early Human Development, 25*(3), 197–208.

Spangler, G., & Scheubeck, R. (1993). Behavioral organization in newborns and its relation to adrenocortical and cardiac activity. *Child Development, 64*(2), 622–633.

Spangler, G., & Schieche, M. (1998). Emotional and adrenocortical responses of infants to the strange situation: The differential function of emotional expression. *International Journal of Behavioral Development, 22*(4), 681–670.

Sroufe, L. A., Waters, E., & Matas, L. (Eds.). (1974). *Contextual determinants of infant affective response.* New York: Wiley.

Stansbury, K., & Gunnar, M. R. (1994). Adrenocortical activity and emotion regulation. In Fox, N. (Ed.), Emotion regulation in infancy and childhood. *Monographs of the Society for Research in Child Development, 59*(2–3), 108–134.

Stepans, M. B., & Wilkerson, N. (1993). Physiologic effects of maternal smoking on breast-feeding infants. *Journal of the American Academy of Nurse Practitioners, 5*(3), 105–113.

Suchecki, D., Rosenfeld, P., & Levine, S. (1993). Maternal regulation of the hypothalamic–pituitary–adrenal axis in the rat: The roles of feeding and stroking. *Developmental Brain Research, 75*(2), 185–192.

Tennes, K., & Carter, D. (1973). Plasma cortisol levels and behavioral states in early infancy. *Psychosomatic Medicine, 35*(2), 121–128.

Tennes, K., Downey, K., & Vernadakis, A. (1977). Urinary cortisol excretion rates and anxiety in normal 1-year-old infants. *Psychosomatic Medicine, 39*(3), 178–186.

Tepperman, J., & Tepperman, H. M. (1987). *Metabolic and endocrine physiology: An introductory text* (5th ed.). Chicago: Year Book Medical Publishers.

Van Cauter, E. (1990). Diurnal and ultradian rhythms in human endocrine function: A mini-review. *Hormone Research, 34*, 45–53.

Ward, M. J., Brathwaite, J., Maloney, H. A., Lee, S., Polan, H. J., & Lipper, E. G. (1995, March 31). *Time course of adrenocortical activity: Associations with maternal behavior, calorie intake, and mother–infant attachment.* Poster session presented at the biennial meeting of the Society-for Research in Child Development, Indianapolis, IN.

Watterberg, K. L., & Scott, S. M. (1995). Evidence of early adrenal insufficiency in babies who develop bronchopulmonary dysplasia. *Pediatrics, 95*, 120–125.

Watterberg, K. L., Scott, S. M., Backstrom, C., Gifford, K. L., & Cook, K. L. (2000). Links between early adrenal function and respiratory outcome in preterm infants: Airway inflammation and patent ductus arteriosus. *Pediatrics, 105*, 320–324.

White, B. P., Gunnar, M. R., Larson, M. C., Donzella, B., & Barr, R. G. (2000). Behavioral and physiological responsivity and patterns of sleep and daily salivary cortisol in infants with and without colic. *Child Development, 71*(4), 862–877.

Yehuda, R., Boisoneau, D., Mason, J. W., & Giller, E. L. (1993). Glucocorticoid receptor number and cortisol excretion in mood, anxiety, and psychotic disorders. *Biological Psychiatry, 34*, 18–25.

Yehuda, R., Resnick, H., Kahana, B., & Giller, E. L. (1993). Long-lasting hormonal alterations to extreme stress in humans: Normative or maladaptive? *Psychosomatic Medicine, 55*, 287–297.

10

Assessment of Temperament in Early Development

MARY K. ROTHBART
KEAN H. CHEW
MARIA AMY GARTSTEIN

HISTORY

Temperament has been defined as constitutionally based individual differences in reactivity and self-regulation, influenced over time by heredity, maturation, and experience (Rothbart & Derryberry, 1981). Temperament represents the core of the developing personality, but the processes constituting temperament themselves undergo development, especially during the early years of life (Rothbart & Bates, 1998).

In the Western intellectual tradition, the concept of temperament extends to the fourfold typology of Greco-Roman physicians developed over 2,000 years ago (Diamond, 1974). Even in those times, temperament was seen as constitutionally based and linked to individual physiology. The term "temperamentum" referred to a "proportionate mixture" or *balance* of body humors and their related behavioral tendencies. The melancholic individual, tending to sad and negative affect, was thought to have a predominance of black bile; the sanguine person, positive and outgoing, a predominance of blood; the choleric individual, prone to anger, a predominance of yellow bile; and the phlegmatic person, slow in rising to alertness, emotion, and action, a predominance of phlegm. There has been considerable historical continuity in the attempt to link body structure and behavior, and the idea of a balance among internally regulated tendencies. The fourfold typology persisted into the Middle Ages, and more recently was linked to the models of Burt (1935, 1937) and Eysenck (1947, 1967). The structure–behavior links and ideas about balance have also persisted (see reviews by Rothbart, 1989; Rothbart, Derryberry, & Posner, 1994).

The great normative studies of the 1920s and 1930s identified infant temperament as an important domain of study, even though the term was not always used. Mary Shirley initially set out to study motor development, designing an intensive longitudinal study of the first 2 years of infants' lives. Her observations of a "personality nucleus" led her to devote a full volume to reporting infants' temperament and personality characteristics (Shirley, 1933). Gesell (as cited in Kessen, 1965) and Washburn (1929) also noted early individual differences in affect and irritability.

EARLY ASSESSMENT OF TEMPERAMENT

More recently, systematic temperament assessments of infants were begun, including observational and caregiver report measures. Observational measures of newborns and young infants included assessments of reactivity to multiple modes of stimulation (Birns, 1965; Escalona, 1968; Korner, 1964) and contributed to development of structured laboratory observations (Garcia-Coll, Halpern, Vohr, Seifer, & Oh, 1992; Kochanska, Coy, Tjebkes, & Husarek, 1998; Riese, 1987; Stifter & Braungart, 1995).

The most influential contribution to caregiver report research on infant temperament resulted from the detailed parent interviews in Chess and Thomas's New York Longitudinal Study (NYLS; Thomas, Chess, Birch, Hertzig, & Korn, 1963). Birch carried out a content analysis of 22 young infants' reactions to daily events, which resulted in nine dimensions of temperament that guided subsequent research: Activity Level, Approach/Withdrawal, Threshold, Mood, Intensity, Rhythmicity, Adaptability, Distractibility, and Attention Span/Persistence.

The NYLS, however, did not include newborns and initially focused on infants 2 to 6 months of age. The dimensions derived from the NYLS must therefore be constrained by the developmental characteristics of the subjects. The major goals of the NYLS were also clinical; attempts were made to identify patterns of early behavior that might influence the development of behavior disorders. One result of this approach was the emergence of the idea of "goodness of fit," the concept that child developmental outcomes will relate to the extent to which child characteristics fit with parents' demands and expectations (Thomas, Chess, & Birch, 1968). There was no initial attempt to establish conceptual or empirical independence of the scales measuring the nine temperament dimensions. Later questionnaire measures of the dimensions, including the Revised Infant Temperament Questionnaire (RITQ; Carey & McDevitt, 1978), have also not attempted to satisfy these criteria.

In the NYLS sample, approximately 10% of infants were identified as difficult (Thomas et al., 1968), characterized as showing low rhythmicity, high withdrawal, slow adaptation to change, high frequency of negative mood, and intense reactions. Infants at the opposite poles were described as "easy." A "slow-to-warm-up" group was also described, showing low-intensity negative reactions to new stimuli or situations but tending to adapt after repeated experiences.

In adaptations of the "difficultness" construct, such as the RITQ, five attributes from the NYLS have often been used to derive a "difficulty" measure (i.e., nonadaptability, tendency to withdraw, negative mood, intense reactions, and rhythmicity). Other studies have failed to find rhythmicity to be part of a cluster of infant "difficult" behaviors. Thus, measures of "difficulty" sometimes, but not always, include a rhythmicity measure, creating some confusion in use of the construct (see Rothbart & Bates, 1998).

Additional problems have persisted in the "difficulty" construct. When applied to an individual child, its use may lead parents to look for problems in their children of which they would otherwise have been unaware. Behavior seen as difficult in one situation, or at one age, may not be in another; for example, a more distractible child may be both more easily soothed (often seen as a positive characteristic) and less persistent (often seen as a negative characteristic). A more distractible infant may be seen as "easier," but a more distractible grade-school child may have problems completing home and school tasks. Given the ubiquity of the difficultness construct, however, current reviews of the literature must often rely on measures of difficulty in order to carry out an adequate sampling of studies (e.g., Rothbart & Bates, 1998; Putnam, Sanson, & Rothbart, in press). In these cases, it is important that reviews be clear about how the difficulty construct is operationalized in a given piece of research.

"Difficulty" might also be given a consistent substantive referent. Bates (1987), for example, suggested that difficultness can be seen as the perceived demandingness of the child that often accompanies irritability. This set of characteristics, as well as the young child's distress to novelty, have proven predictive of later behavioral problems (Bates & Bayles, 1988). Using a descriptive name for this construct without adding the term "difficulty" might be just as helpful, however; it would also avoid further confusion in use of the term.

GENERAL DESCRIPTION

Three major goals have been prominent in the assessment of infant temperament. One goal has been to measure individual differences in reactivity and self-regulation under controlled conditions, typically in the laboratory (e.g., Garcia-Coll et al., 1992; Goldsmith & Rothbart, 1991; Matheny & Wilson,

1981; Riese, 1987). More recently the development of laboratory marker tasks assess variability in behavior associated with the activation of brain regions as demonstrated in imaging studies (Gerardi-Caulton, 2000).

A second goal has been to identify the structure of infant temperament via parent or caregiver reports which allow measurement of individual differences both broadly and narrowly, and take advantage of the caregiver's extensive observations. Recent work on parent-report instruments has yielded a revision of the list of temperament variables originally identified in the NYLS (see reviews by Rothbart & Bates, 1998; Rothbart & Mauro, 1990). Results of item-level factor-analytic studies (e.g., Sanson, Prior, Garino, Oberklaid, & Sewell, 1987) indicate that instead of yielding bipolar scales such as Approach *versus* Withdrawal, Withdrawal items along with items from Adaptability and other fear-related items tend to cluster together in a Fear or Inhibition/Withdrawal factor. Approach items, on the other hand, tend to cluster with positive affect items from the Mood scale to form a Positive Affect/Approach factor. In the assessment of negative affect, Fear also tends to be differentiated from Irritability or Frustration (Rothbart & Mauro, 1990).

Other factors extracted that more closely resemble the NYLS dimensions are Activity level, Persistence or Duration of Orienting, and sometimes a small Rhythmicity factor. Threshold as a factor has been identified in an extremely limited context in one instrument only, and Intensity does not emerge in the factor structure of the instruments, due to its lack of generalizability across response modalities. Dimensions of temperament represented in this revised list thus seem to correspond more to specific affective–motivational processes than to overall styles of behavior, except for the activity-level variable.

A third goal has been to adapt temperament measures to clinical uses (Bates, 1989; Sheeber & Johnson, 1994). These include the informal use of questionnaires or observations. Measures of temperament have also been used in concurrent and longitudinal studies of the development of behavior problems and have been linked with adjustment in adulthood (Newman, Caspi, Moffit, & Silva, 1997; Sanson, Prior, & Smart, 1996; Schmitz et al., 1999). However, temperament measures have not yet achieved the psychometric qualities necessary for predicting future problems for individual infants.

BIOBEHAVIORAL BASIS OF ASSESSMENT

Temperament has been historically related to our understanding of individual physiology. Mental processes have been linked with brain functioning by recent studies in cognitive neuroscience (see Posner & Raichle, 1994). Selective orienting and attentional effortful control have been associated with orienting and executive attentional systems. The posterior orienting network develops first and involves a set of cortical, midbrain, and thalamic areas (Posner & Raichle, 1994). Later development of the anterior or executive attentional system is related to volition and awareness and allows flexible control of reactive tendencies. The anterior cingulate may be an important connection between different aspects of attention (Posner & Rothbart, 1998).

The limbic system has been implicated in the processing of reward-related information. Single-cell recording, lesion, and intracranial self-stimulation studies provide support for this function of limbic circuits, which regulate endocrine, autonomic, and motor activity when activated by rewarding stimuli. The role of these circuits in temperament and personality has been discussed by several theorists. For example, Gray (1987) described the behavioral activation system (BAS), sensitive to reward cues and responsible for approach tendencies. In aversive contexts the BAS can be activated by signals of nonpunishment, and is associated with relief and avoidance. Gray (1987) further proposed that the reactivity of the BAS may underlie the temperamental dimension of impulsivity. Depue and Iacono (1989) proposed a similar model, the behavioral facilitation system (BFS). They suggested that when reward is blocked and avoidance is impossible, the BFS may facilitate aggressive behavior aimed at removing the object of frustration.

Limbic structures, especially the hippocampus and amygdala, have also been linked with fear circuitry, promoting defensive behaviors. Gray (1982) proposed a model of anxiety based on the limbic circuits that constitute the behavior inhibition system (BIS), activated in situations involving novelty, threat, high intensity, or punishment. The BIS inhibits ongoing activity, increases cortical arousal, and enhances analysis of the threatening situation by directing attention to danger-related signals. Individual differences in the reactivity of the BIS underlie differences in the experience of anxiety.

Additional neural pathways have been discussed in connection with irritability and anger. Panksepp (1982) described a "rage" system, on the basis of evidence that lesions of the ventromedial hypothalamus significantly increase aggression. Panksepp (1982) suggested that this region inhibits aggressive behaviors controlled by the midbrain's central gray area. Helpful, trusting, and friendly behaviors are seen when aggressive tendencies are suppressed. Panksepp (1982) also linked prosocial behaviors with the opiate projections from higher limbic regions (e.g., amygdala and cingulate cortex). Brain opiates are thought to promote social bonding, whereas opiate withdrawal is associated with irritability and aggression.

Research on behavioral genetics has indicated considerable heritability of temperamental characteristics. Genetic makeup influences the developing physical structures; subsequently, neural and neurochemical individual differences are reflected in individual variability in temperamental characteristics (Rothbart & Bates, 1998). Research addressing genetic influences on the development of temperament has generated considerable evidence of heritability (Loehlin & Nichols, 1976; Goldsmith, Buss, & Lemery, 1997; Saudino & Eaton, 1991), especially for Extraversion (positive affect, approach) and Neuroticism (anxiety, moodiness, irritability) (Henderson, 1982). An influential report by Tellegen, Lykken, Bouchard, and Wilcox (1988) also found considerable concordance in heritability of Negative Emotionality (neuroticism) and Constraint (fear and effortful control) for twins reared together and apart. Recent work has continued to support genetic influences on temperament, expanding the subejct to include additional behavioral domains, such as activity level (Goldsmith et al., 1997; Saudino & Eaton, 1991).

RELIABILITY AND VALIDITY

Researchers of infant temperament have been concerned about measurement error of both questionnaires (e.g., Kagan, 1994, 1998) and observation measures (Rothbart & Bates, 1998). Sources of error include those related to characteristics of the rater, effects of the measure on child behaviors, and their interactions (Rothbart & Goldsmith, 1985; Rothbart & Bates, 1998). Method factors also exist and are of concern insofar as they affect reliability and validity. Reliability estimates reported vary depending on the approach. Reliability of questionnaires with several subscales is described through estimates of internal consistency and test–retest reliability (Table 10.1). Interrater agreement can be determined for questionnaires and for laboratory observations.

Caregiver report, home observation, and laboratory observation all have considerable strengths as well as considerable and sometimes complementary limitations. It is often helpful to employ more than one approach. Questionnaire respondent biases can be minimized by including a laboratory assessment that yields converging evidence.

DEVELOPMENTAL MODEL

Some of the earliest views of temperament in children were developmental: Gesell (as cited in Kessen, 1965) wrote of both the stability of temperament and of the possibility of multiple trajectories and outcomes for a given initial set of temperamental characteristics. Shirley (1933) noted that the infants' "personality nucleus" demonstrated relative stability in the rank ordering of infants but that this occurred within the context of major developmental change. Thomas and Chess (Thomas et al., 1968) also expected temperament to change with development. Nevertheless, many who have used the nine NYLS dimensions have expected them to apply without revision across broad segments of the lifespan. Buss and Plomin (1975, 1984) have also argued that "temperament" measures must show both early appearance and long-term stability.

Even in the first year of life, however, developmental changes in temperament-related processes occur, and expressions of temperament differ greatly in the newborn, the 3-month-old, and the 12-month-old. If temperament constructs include individual differences in emotional reactivity and self-regulation, while the developmental onset of particular primary emotions and attentional processes varies across the first year, it is not possible to measure all characteristics of infant temperament at all developmental periods. Because some emotions and attentional processes regulate other emotions and actions, the time of onset of control dimensions also has important implications for the assessment of other temperamental characteristics.

During the newborn period, assessments of temperament have chiefly been made using the Brazelton Neonatal Behavioral Assessment Scale (NBAS; Brazelton, 1973) (see Chapter 18, this volume) and laboratory assessments specifically developed to measure newborn temperament (e.g., Riese, 1983). (See also Table 10.1.) Temperament dimensions identified in this period include distress proneness or irritability, soothability, alertness, and activity level. For neonates, activity tends to covary with behavioral distress. Psychophysiological methods measuring heart rate, vagal tone, and cortisol levels are also frequently employed in the assessment of the newborn (see Chapters 6 and 9, this volume). Newborn behavioral measures have shown some predictability to later measures of temperament and attachment (e.g., van den Boom, 1989), with the outcome sometimes depending in part on the culture in which the child is raised (see review by Sanson & Rothbart, 1995). Both behavioral and psychophysiological measures show promise for the assessment of infants in special populations. The newborn period represents the "initial state" of the child for social interaction, and qualities of distress proneness, soothability, and aspects of arousal and alertness are all important characteristics of the newborn to assess (see Chapters 7 and 8, this volume; Barr, Hopkins, & Green, 2000).

1–3 Months

During early infancy, infants often demonstrate obligatory looking, appearing to have difficulty shifting attention from a visual location, a phenomenon likely related to early cortical development (Johnson, Posner, & Rothbart, 1991), and often show a high susceptibility to distress to overstimulation and colic. Stifter (1992) has found, however, that measures of colic during this period are not predictive of later measures of temperament, and measures of distress proneness during this period do not always predict to later measures of negative affectivity (see reviews by Barr & Gunnar, 2000; Rothbart & Bates, 1998). Some evidence suggests that the 1- to 3-month period may not be ideal for assessing temperament characteristics expected to demonstrate longitudinal stability; however, stability between 2 weeks and 2 months, and subsequently 2 and 12 months, was reported for activity level, duration of orienting, and distress to limitations (Worobey & Blajda,

1989). Smiling and laughter emerge as part of a positive affectivity dimension, and motor activity is sometimes linked to infants' positive as well as negative affect. Infants by 2 months also demonstrate anger/frustration (Lewis, Alessandri, & Sullivan, 1990).

4–8 Months

During this period, fear and irritability become differentiated and distress to overstimulation at 4 months becomes predictive of later behavioral inhibition (fear) in older infants (Kagan, 1994). Infants can now reach for and grasp objects; latency to contact objects can be measured. A rapid (short latency) grasp is positively related to smiling and laughter, and early physical approach tendencies can be assessed during this period before behavioral inhibition exercises control over it (Rothbart, 1988; Rothbart, Derryberry, & Hershey, 2000; Schaffer, 1974). At 4 to 6 months, infants tend to be quite tractable and interested in the stimuli presented in the laboratory. Perhaps because of this cooperation, much information on the cognitive capacities of the 4-month-old is available. This period may be especially appropriate for the study of early approach and attention.

9–12 Months

Behavioral inhibition and the fear response develop late in the first year (Schaffer, 1974), modulating infants' approach responses. Frustration reactions are discriminable from fear in the motor movements versus inhibition of the infant. By this time, the novelty of the laboratory often suppresses positive affect and approach. It is important to consider approach tendencies separately from fear responses in assessment of temperament. This can be done by first observing the infants at the earlier period of 4 to 6 months and/or by assessing the infants' reactions under both novel (threatening) and familiar (safe) conditions.

Temperamental characteristics are not all in place at the end of the first year. In particular, development of the executive attention system during the toddler and preschool periods will have important implications for effortful control, planning, and the ability to inhibit or delay action and expression (see reviews by Rothbart & Bates, 1998; Ruff & Rothbart, 1996). Although effortful control can operate in the service of fear, it also provides the opportunity for more flexible control of emotion and action.

SPECIAL POPULATIONS

In another review, we have discussed specific implications of temperamental variability for special populations and for infants' social development (Rothbart, 1996). Two important approaches to developmental disabilities address (1) whether specific sets of temperamental characteristics are associated with particular conditions or disabilities, and (2) the extent of variability of temperament within a special population and implications of that variability for the development and treatment of infants in special populations. Continuing application of temperament measures to special populations will be both theoretically and practically important to the field.

WIDELY USED INSTRUMENTS FOR ASSESSMENT
OF INFANT TEMPERAMENT

It is important to recognize that measures of infant temperament were developed to assess particular variables for particular age groups. Thus all measures of temperament are not interchangeable. Careful study of the particular dimensions assessed, their operational definitions, and lists of items used to assess them are essential to this purpose. Table 10.1 lists some widely used infant temperament measures, with information about the specific constructs assessed, ages to which the measures apply, and information on internal homogeneity of the scales (coefficient alpha).

INTEROBSERVER RELIABILITY

Interobserver reliability estimates for the Infant Behavior Questionnaire (IBQ; Rothbart, 1981) range from .45 (Duration of Orienting) to .69 (Activity Level), and for the Infant Characteristic Questionnaire (ICQ; Bates, Freeland, & Lounsbury, 1979), from .29 (Unpredictable) to .58 (Fussy/Difficult) (Wolk, Zeanah, Garcia-Coll, & Carr, 1992); for the different dimensions of the Laboratory Assessment of Infant Temperament (LTS), from .65 (Orientation to Staff) to .92 (Emotional Tone) (Wilson & Matheny, 1983); for trained raters using the NBAS (Brazelton, 1973) from .85 to 1.00 (Hubert, Wachs, Peters-Martin, & Gandour, 1982); and for the RITQ, from .00 (Persistence) to .59 (Rhythmicity). Garcia-Coll et al. (1992) reported interobserver agreement exceeding 85% for scales retained in their final analyses.

ADDITIONAL APPROACHES
TO THE MEASUREMENT OF TEMPERAMENT

Physiological measures such as the assessment of vagal tone, cortisol levels, hemispheric asymmetries, and other related methods are yielding results of great interest in their relation to caregiver reports and direct observations of children's temperament-related behavior (see Chapters 7 and 9, this volume). The use of these methods with other temperament assessments may

TABLE 10.1. Summary and Description of Widely Used Instruments Assessing Infant Temperament

Name of instrument (ages to which it applies)	Constructs assessed	Description 1. Number of items 2. Response options 3. Respondent(s)	Internal consistency as measured with Cronbach's alpha
BBQ (3–10 mo)	7 orthogonal factors Intensity/Activity, Regularity, Approach–Withdrawal, Sensory Sensitivity, Attentiveness–Manageability, Sensitivity to New Food	1. 54 items 2. 5 response options 3. Caregiver	.51 (Manageability) to .71 (Regularity); mean = .61, *n* = 791 3- to 10-mo-old infants
IBQ (3–12 mo) (2 wk–2 mo)[a]	6 scales: Activity Level, Smiling and Laughter, Fear, Soothability, Distress to Limitations, Duration to Orienting	1. 94 items 2. 7 response options and "Does Not Apply" 3. Caregiver	.72 (Duration of Orienting) to .85 (Smiling and Laughter); mean = .76, *n* = 93 3-mo-old infants .67 (Duration of Orienting) to .81 (Fear); mean = .76, *n* = 63 6-mo-old infants .73 (Soothability, Smiling and Laughter) to .84 (Fear); mean = .77, *n* = 59 9-mo-old infants .72 (Duration of Orienting) to .84 (Activity Level); mean = .80, 12-mo-old infants
ICQ (4–6 mo)	4 orthogonal factors: Fussy-Difficult, Unadaptable, Dull, Unpredictable	1. 24 items 2. 7 response options 3. Caregiver	.39 (Dull) to .79 (Fussy–Difficult); mean = .61, *n* = 196 4- to 6-mo-old infants
IRI (4 mo)	1 factor: Distress to Sensory Stimulation	1. 45 items 2. 7 response options and "Does Not Apply" 3. Caregiver	.91 (for Study 1); *n* = 89 4-mo-old infants .84 (for Study 2); *n* = 89 4-mo-old infants
LAB-TAB (6 mo)	5 dimensions: Activity Level, Fearfulness, Anger Proneness, Interest/Persistence, Joy/Pleasure	1. 20 settings, 4 per dimension 2. Videotape coding by staff	
LTS[b] (3, 6, 9, 12 mo)	Videotaped assessment of Emotional Tone, Attentional Activity, Orientation to Staff. Observations during physical measures of Emotional Tone, Activity, Cooperation	1. Prescribed set of videotaped 2-min vignettes 2. 9 response options 3. Video coding by staff	.80 (Activity) to .91 (Emotional Tone); mean = .86, *n* = 84 12-mo-old infants (for videotaped assessment measures)

(continued)

TABLE 10.1. *(continued)*

Name of instrument (ages to which it applies)	Constructs assessed	Description 1. Number of items 2. Response options 3. Respondent(s)	Internal consistency as measured with Cronbach's alpha
NBAS (1–30 days)	Responses and Orientation of infants in 6 clusters/scales: Orientation, Motor Performance, State Regulation, Range of State, Autonomic Regulation, and Habituation	1. 27 behavioral items, 20 elicited responses 2. 9 response options for behavioral items; 4 response options for elicited responses 3. Trained examiners	
RITQ (4–8 mo)	9 NYLS categories: Activity, Rhythmicity, Approach, Adaptability, Threshold, Mood, Intensity, Persistence Distractibility	1. 95 items and 9 global ratings 2. 6 response options 3. Caregiver	.49 (Distractibility) to .71 (Intensity); mean = .59, $n = 203$
EITQ (1–4 mo)	9 NYLS categories: Activity, Rhythmicity, Approach, Adaptability, Threshold, Mood, Intensity, Persistence Distractibility	1. 76 items and 9 global ratings 2. 6 response options 3. Caregiver	.43 (Intensity) to .76 (Rhythmicity); mean = .62, $n = 404$
SITQ (4–8 mo)	5 factors: Approach, Irritability Rhythmicity, Activity–Reactivity, Cooperation–Manageability	1. 30 items 2. 6 response options 3. Caregiver	.57 (Activity–Reactivity) to .76 (Approach); mean = .66, $n = 2,443$ 4- to 8-mo-old infants
Garcia-Coll et al.[c] (3 and 7 mo)	Activity, Sociability, Irritability, Approach, Inhibition, Soothability, Total positive, Total negative, Total neutral	1. 17 and 14 visual, auditory, and tactile stimuli presented to 3- and 7-mo-old infants, respectively 2. Absolute frequencies and affective quality 3. Staff	.41 (Activity) to .91 (Total Positive); mean = .74, $n = 17$ full-term and $n = 62$ preterm 3-mo-old infants with resampling at 7 mo

Note. BBQ, Baby Behavior Questionnaire (Bohlin, Hagekull, & Lindhagen, 1981); IBQ, Infant Behavior Questionnaire (Rothbart, 1981); ICQ, Infant Characteristic Questionnaire (Bates, Freeland, & Lounsbury, 1979); IRI, Infant Reactions Inventory (O'Boyle & Rothbart, 1996); LAB-TAB, Laboratory Temperament Assessment Battery (Goldsmith & Rothbart, 1991); LTS, Laboratory Assessment of Infant Temperament: Louisville Twin Study (Matheny & Wilson, 1981); NBAS, Brazelton Neonatal Assessment Scale (Brazelton, 1973); RITQ, Revised Infant Temperament Questionnaire (Carey & McDevitt, 1978); EITQ, Early Infancy Temperament Questionnaire (Medoff-Cooper, Carey, & McDevitt, 1993); SITQ, Short-Form Infant Temperament Questionnaire (Sanson, Prior, Garino, Oberklaid, & Sewell, 1987)

[a]Appropriateness of IBQ for the first month has also been examined. Worobey and Blajda (1989) reported that 37 of the 94 IBQ items were appropriate for 2- to 3-week-old infants ($n = 48$). Part–whole correlations of the abbreviated version for the first month sample with the full IBQ for an independent sample of ($n = 48$) 3-month-old infants were .95, .95, .66, and .90 for activity level, distress to limitations, distress to sudden/novel stimuli, and soothability, respectively.

[b]The Laboratory Assessment of Infant Temperament measure is often referred to as the Louisville Twin Study.

[c]Garcia-Coll et al. (1992) did not name their behavioral assessment measures.

validate a given approach and indicate something about the processes involved in temperamental individual differences. We are currently developing a laboratory assessment for toddlers and older children to assess aspects of effortful control that are part of an executive attention system (Gerardi-Caulton, 2000). To measure executive effortful control, we use a conflict task that requires the child to inhibit a dominant response in order to perform a subdominant response. Efficient performance on the related Stroop task (naming an ink color when it spells the name of a different color) and other conflict tasks is associated with frontal activation, in particular the anterior cingulate gyrus and adjacent structures (see reviews by Bush, Luu, & Posner, 2000; Posner & Raichle, 1994).

In our spatial conflict task, children match one of two buttons covered by animal pictures with the picture of an animal presented on a computer screen. The animal on the screen is presented either on the same (spatially compatible) or on the opposite (spatially incompatible) side of the correct button. In 2- to 3-year-olds, children were more accurate and responded more quickly to compatible than incompatible trials, and accuracy improved with age. Children's performance was related to mothers' reports of the children's temperament. Children who were more accurate and/or less slowed during incompatible trials were reported by their mothers as showing higher Attentional Focusing, higher Inhibitory Control, and lower Impulsivity. Anger/Frustration scores were also significantly lower for older children who were more accurate. This kind of model task may prove to be a marker for the development of frontal brain regions linked to attentional effortful control, and we have now developed a touch screen version of this and other conflict tasks (Berger, Jones, Rothbart, & Posner, 2000).

STRUCTURAL AND/OR THEORETICAL
CONSTRAINTS/CONTROVERSIES

In caregiver report, error may occur due to failure in informants' comprehension of items and instructions, lack of knowledge of the infant's behavior and its meaning, or of the behavior of other infants with whom the child is compared, or low accuracy of memory of events involving the infant. These concerns can be partially addressed by careful item pretesting that asks only about recently occurring events and by inquiring about concrete infant behaviors rather than asking the parent to make abstract or comparative judgments (Rothbart & Goldsmith, 1985; Rothbart & Mauro, 1990).

A second set of problems includes the extent to which caregivers' responses are driven by their own state or clinical disorder (e.g., anxiety or depression) or response sets such as social desirability. Maternal characteristics have been assessed and related to their reports of infant temperament. In a review of this research, we concluded that although caregivers' characteristics and their reports about their children are often related at low but significant levels, additional variance in reported children's behavior indicates agreement between caregiver and observer (Rothbart & Bates, 1998). Moreover, maternal characteristics can predict their biological children's behavior in the laboratory directly, raising the issue that correlations between parent and child characteristics as reported by the parent may be in part a function of their shared genetic makeup (Matheny, Wilson, & Thoben, 1987).

For home observations, error associated with observer characteristics is present, although less of a problem. When *in vivo* coding is done, information-processing capacities of the coder can limit the number of behaviors adequately coded at any given time. Coder state also influences accuracy, and social desirability biases may especially affect global ratings, lowering interobserver reliability.

In the laboratory, such concerns are moderated by the use of detailed videotapes, and strict controls on reliability are possible. All approaches have problems in detecting low intensity or ambiguous reactions of the child. A tendency to "overcode" the tapes, resulting in a microanalysis of behavior, is costly of experimenter time and effort yet may yield little in terms of establishing relationships with other variables.

OTHER METHOD FACTORS

In the measurement of temperament, adequate item selection for questionnaires and an adequate selection of codes for *in vivo* and videotape coding is essential. If a relevant behavior is not captured within an item or a coding category, it will be lost. Home observations suffer in that events necessary for the assessment of a disposition may occur rarely or not at all during the window of behavior sampling. Rare events can be directly elicited in the laboratory, but fear states and the inability of the child to exercise usual coping options may constrain the infant's responses.

In the past, we concluded, based on a cost-benefit analysis, that the least satisfactory approach to assessing temperament was direct home observation (Rothbart & Goldsmith, 1985). However, with small video equipment, recording in the home might now be used to capture the child's behavior in a more expectable environment. Nevertheless, adjustment of infant and caregiver to the presence of the camera is necessary, and the problem of varying behavior of different caregivers toward their infants would continue to exist. Careful consideration of child behavior characteristics and child observer interactions is important because these may affect the outcome of an assessment. In the home, especially when the caregiver serves as the observer, the infant's typical behavior is most likely to occur. The presence of an observer, on the other hand, can influence both the caregiver's and the infant's behavior, due in part to the novelty of the visitor. These effects are exacerbated when the child is brought into a strange laboratory. In the home, however, the child's behavior will also be a function of the kind of care the infant is receiving, with the intensity and qualities of care varying from home to home and caregiver to caregiver. Any stability found in caregiver or observer report of home behavior may be as much a function of the parent's treatment of the child as of any endogenous characteristics of the child.

Another limitation is that the child's behavior is often observed over short periods, yielding a limited number of observations and creating problems in getting a reliable picture of the child's behavior. An advantage of caregiver report is that when the caregiver is asked about the relative frequency of occurrence of events (a cognitive judgment that adults can make easily), it is possible to get a measure based on a much larger set of observations than occur during a home visit or a visit to the laboratory (Rothbart, 1981), without the novelty effects of a strange observer and/or a strange laboratory.

In the laboratory, there is more control over stimuli presented, but there are problems of carryover effects where the child's reaction to one set of stimuli or situations influences the child's reaction to subsequent stimuli. This is most clearly seen when the child becomes distressed and never becomes fully soothed as the additional stimuli are presented. In the laboratory, children often cannot use their usual coping strategies, such as crawling away or giving distress signals resulting in caregiver assistance, leading to negative affect. As noted previously, the novelty of the laboratory may also make fear particularly potent, and the fear responses observed at 8 months and beyond can inhibit the expression of other emotions and behavior (Rothbart, 1988; Schaffer, 1974). The laboratory may be an excellent place for the assessment of fear and behavioral inhibition, but these reactions in themselves can raise problems for the assessment of other temperamental characteristics.

TRAINING REQUIREMENTS

Training requirements in the area of assessment of temperament in early development are as diverse as the approaches described in this chapter. No special training, aside from familiarity with the questionnaire, is necessary for administering parent-report measures. Nonetheless, familiarity with the specific measures, and temperament in general, is important for applying questionnaires to appropriate constructs and addressing respondents' questions/concerns. Home observations require considerable training. Home observations are usually based on specific coding systems, and all observers are systematically trained to make reliable observations using the code. This training process is intensive, and sporadic reliability checks must be performed even after training has been completed. Laboratory procedures also require considerable training. First, the examiner must become familiarized with the procedure, repeatedly performing it in a standard manner. Second, training in the technical aspects of laboratory measurement (e.g., administration of a computerized task and preparation for a physiological recording) may be necessary. Third, laboratory observations require training establishing reliable adherence to a coding system.

IMPLICATIONS

The construct of temperament is extremely old. It has been studied in adults for over 60 years, but the major advances in assessment of infant temperament have occurred only in the last 20 years. There have been three major goals in temperament assessment: (1) measurement of individual differences, (2) identifying the structure of infant temperament based on caregiver report, and (3) adapting measures of temperament for clinical use. Not surprisingly, specific measures of temperament may be more appropriate for one of these goals than the others. In all cases, however, issues concerning reliability and validity need to be carefully evaluated when decisions regarding instruments are being made. Different approaches to the measurement of temperament in infancy have different limitations. Generally, the use of multiple approaches minimizes the shortcomings associated with single method.

Temperament is generally described as relatively stable. It is subject to developmental processes, however, which are especially rapid during infancy. Rapid development makes stability estimates vulnerable to systematic maturation effects, contributing to lower levels of test–retest reliability estimates. Recent research has indicated considerable heritability of temperamental characteristics and demonstrated links between aspects of temperament and measures of physiological activity (e.g., heart rate) and brain functioning. Evaluations of biobehavioral mechanisms further contribute to our understanding of processes underlying stability and developmental change in temperament.

Much additional work is needed in improving laboratory, caregiver report, and home observational assessments of infant temperament. Cooperation among researchers in developing the best scales and the best laboratory assays would benefit the field. To the extent that assessments may be used for future diagnosis and prediction, improvements in the reliability and validation of measures will be needed. Finally, basic research on temperament and development in both atypical and typical infants will inform our understanding of temperament and its appropriate assessment throughout the period of infancy.

REFERENCES

Barr, R. G., & Gunnar, M. (2000). Colic: The "transient responsivity" hypothesis. In R. G. Barr, B. Hopkins, & J. A. Green (Eds.), *Crying as a sign, a symptom, and a signal: Clinical emotional and developmental aspects of infant and toddler crying* (pp. 41–66). New York: Cambridge University Press.

Barr, R. G., Hopkins, B., & Green, J. A. (2000). *Crying as a sign, a symptom, and a signal: Clinical emotional and developmental aspects of infant and toddler crying.* New York: Cambridge University Press.

Bates, J. E. (1987). Temperament in infancy. In J. D. Osofsky (Ed.), *Handbook of infant development* (2nd ed., pp. 1101–1149). New York: Wiley.

Bates, J. E. (1989). Applications of temperament concepts. In G. A. Kohnstamm, J. E. Bates, & M. K. Rothbart (Eds.), *Temperament in childhood* (pp. 321–355). Chichester, UK: Wiley.

Bates, J. E., & Bayles, K. (1988). The role of attachment in the development of behavior problems. In J. Belsky & T. Nezworski (Eds.), *Clinical implications of attachment* (pp. 253–299). Hillsdale, NJ: Erlbaum.

Bates, J., Freeland, C. A. B., & Lounsbury, M. L. (1979). Measurement of infant difficultness. *Child Development, 50,* 794–803.

Berger, A., Jones, L., Rothbart, M. K., & Posner, M. I. (2000). Computerized games to study the development of attention in childhood. *Behavior Research Methods, Instruments, and Computers, 32*(2), 297–303.

Birns, B. (1965). Individual differences in human neonates' responses to stimulation. *Child Development, 36,* 249–256.

Bohlin, G., Hagekull, B., & Lindhagen, K. (1981). Dimensions of infant behavior. *Infant Behavior and Development, 4,* 83–96.

Brazelton, T. B. (1973). *Neonatal Behavioral Assessment Scale.* London: Spastics International Medical Publications.

Burt, C. (1935). General and specific factors underlying the primary emotions. *British Association Annual Report, 694,* 6.

Burt, C. (1937). The analysis of temperament. *British Journal of Medical Psychology, 17,* 158–188.

Bush, G., Luu, P., & Posner, M. I. (2000). Cognitive and emotional influences in anterior cingulate cortex. *Trends in Cognitive Sciences, 4*(6), 215–222.

Buss, A. H., & Plomin, R. (1975). *A temperament theory of personality development.* New York: Wiley.

Buss, A. H., & Plomin, R. (1984). *Temperament: Early developing personality traits.* Hillsdale, NJ: Erlbaum.

Carey, W. B., & McDevitt, S. C. (1978). Revision of the infant temperament questionnaire. *Pediatrics, 61,* 735–739.

Depue, R. A., & Iacono, W. G. (1989). Neurobehavioral aspects of affective disorders. In M. R. Rosenzweig & L. Y. Porter (Eds.), *Annual review of psychology* (Vol. 40, pp. 457–492). Palo Alto, CA: Annual Reviews.

Diamond, S. (1974). *The roots of psychology.* New York: Basic Books.

Escalona, S. K. (1968). *The roots of individuality: Normal patterns of development in infancy.* Chicago: Aldine.

Eysenck, H. J. (1947). *Dimensions of personality.* London: Routledge & Kegan Paul.

Eysenck, H. J. (1967). *The biological basis of personality*. Springfield, IL: Thomas.

Garcia-Coll, C. T., Halpern, L. F., Vohr, B. R., Seifer, R., & Oh, W. (1992). Stability and correlates of change of early temperament in preterm and full-term infants. *Infant Behavior and Development, 15*, 137–153.

Gerardi-Caulton, G. (2000). Sensitivity to spatial conflict and the development of self-regulation in children 24–36 months of age. *Developmental Science, 3*(4), 397–404.

Goldsmith, H. H., Buss, K. A., & Lemery, K. S. (1997). Toddler and childhood temperament: Expanded content, stronger genetic evidence, new evidence for the importance of environment. *Developmental Psychology, 33*, 891–905.

Goldsmith, H. H., & Rothbart, M. K. (1991). Contemporary instruments for assessing early temperament by questionnaire and in the laboratory. In J. Strelau & A. Angleitner (Eds.), *Explorations in temperament: International perspectives on theory and measurement* (pp. 249–272). New York: Plenum Press.

Gray, J. A. (1982). *The neuropsychology of anxiety*. London: Oxford University Press.

Gray, J. A. (1987). Perspectives on anxiety and impulsivity: A commentary. *Journal of Research in Personality, 21*, 493–509.

Henderson, N. D. (1982). Human behavior genetics. *Annual Review of Psychology, 33*, 403–440.

Hubert, N. C., Wachs, T. D., Peters-Martin, P., & Gandour, M. J. (1982). The study of early temperament: Measurement and conceptual issues. *Child Development, 53*, 571–600.

Johnson, M. H., Posner, M. I., & Rothbart, M. K. (1991). Components of visual orienting in early infancy: Contingency learning, anticipatory looking and disengaging. *Journal of Cognitive Neuroscience, 3*, 335–344.

Kagan, J. (1994). *Galen's prophecy: Temperament in human nature*. New York: Basic Books.

Kagan, J. (1998). Biology and the child. In W. Damon (Series Ed.) & N. Eisenberg (Vol. Ed.), *Handbook of child psychology: Vol. 3. Social, emotional and personality development* (5th ed., pp. 177–235). New York: Wiley.

Kessen, W. (1965). *The child*. New York: Wiley.

Kochanska, G., Coy, K. C., Tjebkes, T. L., & Husarek, S. J. (1998). Individual differences in emotionality in infancy. *Child Development, 64*, 375–390.

Korner, A. F. (1964). Some hypotheses regarding the significance of individual differences at birth for later development. *The Psychoanalytic Study of the Child, 19*, 58–72.

Lewis, M., Alessandri, S. M., & Sullivan, M. W. (1990). Violation of expectancy, loss of control, and anger expressions in young infants. *Developmental Psychology, 26*, 745–751.

Loehlin, J. C., & Nichols, R. C. (1976). *Heredity, environment, and personality: A study of 850 twins*. Austin: University of Texas Press.

Matheny, A. P., Jr., & Wilson, R. S. (1981). Developmental tasks and rating scales for the laboratory assessment of infant temperament. *JSAS Catalog of Selected Documents in Psychology, 11*, 81–82.

Matheny, A. P., Jr., Wilson, R. S., & Thoben, A. S. (1987). Home and mother: Relations with infant temperament. *Developmental Psychology, 23*, 323–331.

Medoff-Cooper, B., Carey, W. B., & McDevitt, S. (1993). The Early Infancy Temperament Questionnaire. *Developmental and Behavioral Pediatrics, 14*, 230–235.

Newman, D. L., Caspi, A., Moffitt. T. E., & Silva, P. A. (1997). Antecedents of adult interpersonal functioning: Effects of individual differences in age 3 temperament. *Developmental Psychology. 33*, 206–217.

O'Boyle, C. G., & Rothbart, M. K. (1996). Assessment of distress to sensory stimulation in early infancy through parent report. *Journal of Reproductive and Infant Psychology, 14,* 121–132.

Panksepp, J. (1982). Toward a general psychobiological theory of emotions. *Behavioral and Brain Sciences, 5,* 407–467.

Posner, M. I., & Raichle, M. E. (1994). *Images of mind.* New York: Scientific American Library.

Posner, M. I., & Rothbart, M. K. (1998). Attention, self-regulation, and consciousness. *Philosophical Transactions of the Royal Society of London B, 353,* 1915–1927.

Putnam, S. P., Sanson, A. V., & Rothbart, M. K. (in press). Child temperament and parenting. In M. Bornstein (Ed.), *Handbook of parenting* (2nd ed.). Mahwah, NJ: Erlbaum.

Riese, M. L. (1983). Assessment of behavioral patterns in neonates. *Infant Behavior and Development, 6,* 241–246.

Riese, M. L. (1987). Temperament stability between the neonatal period and 24 months. *Developmental Psychology, 23,* 216–222.

Rothbart, M. K. (1981). Measurement of temperament in infancy. *Child Development, 52,* 569–578.

Rothbart, M. K. (1988). Temperament and the development of inhibited approach. *Child Development, 59,* 1241–1250.

Rothbart, M. K. (1989). Biological processes in temperament. In G. A. Kohnstamm, J. E. Bates, & M. K. Rothbart (Eds.), *Temperament in childhood* (pp. 77–110). Chichester, UK: Wiley.

Rothbart, M. K. (1996). Social development. In M. J. Hanson (Ed.), *Atypical infant development* (2nd ed., pp. 273–309). Austin, TX: Pro-Ed.

Rothbart, M. K., & Bates, J. E. (1998). Temperament. In W. Damon (Series Ed.) & N. Eisenberg (Vol. Ed.), *Handbook of child psychology: Vol. 3. Social, emotional and personality development* (5th ed., pp. 105–107). New York: Wiley.

Rothbart, M. K., & Derryberry, D. (1981). Development of individual differences in temperament. In M. E. Lamb & A. L. Brown (Eds.), *Advances in developmental psychology, Vol. 1* (pp. 37–86). Hillsdale, NJ: Erlbaum.

Rothbart, M. K., Derryberry, D., & Hershey, K. (2000). Stability of temperament in childhood: Laboratory infant assessment to parent report at seven years. In V. J. Molfese & D. L. Molfese (Eds.), *Temperament and personality across the life span* (pp. 85–119). Hillsdale, NJ: Erlbaum.

Rothbart, M. K., Derryberry, D., & Posner, M. I. (1994). A psychobiological approach to the development of temperament. In J. E. Bates & T. D. Wachs (Eds.), *Temperament: Individual differences at the interface of biology and behavior* (pp. 83–116). Washington, DC: American Psychological Association.

Rothbart, M. K., & Goldsmith, H. H. (1985). Three approaches to the study of infant temperament. *Developmental Review, 5,* 237–260.

Rothbart, M. K., & Mauro, J. A. (1990). Questionnaire approaches to the study of infant temperament. In J. W. Fagen & J. Colombo (Eds.), *Individual differences in infancy: Reliability, stability and prediction* (pp. 411–429). Hillsdale, NJ: Erlbaum.

Ruff, H. A., & Rothbart, M. K. (1996). *Attention in early development: Themes and variations.* New York: Oxford University Press.

Sanson, A., Prior, M., Garino, E., Oberklaid, F., & Sewell, J. (1987). The structure of infant temperament: Factor analysis of the Revised Infant Temperament Questionnaire. *Infant Behavior and Development, 10,* 97–104.

Sanson, A., Prior, M., & Smart, D. (1996). Reading disabilities with and without behavior problems at 7–8 years: Prediction from longitudinal data from infancy to 6 years. *Journal of Child Psychology and Psychiatry and Allied Disciplines, 37*, 529–541.

Sanson, A., & Rothbart, M. K. (1995). Child temperament and parenting. In M. Bornstein (Ed.), *Parenting* (Vol. 4, pp. 299–321). Hillsdale, NJ: Erlbaum.

Saudino, K. J., & Eaton, W. O. (1991). Infant temperament and genetics: An objective twin study of motor activity level. *Child Development, 62*, 1167–1174.

Schaffer, H. R. (1974). Cognitive components of the infant's response to strangeness. In M. Lewis & L. A. Rosenblum (Eds.), *The origins of fear* (pp. 11–24). New York: Wiley.

Schmitz, S., Fulker, D. W., Plomin, R., Zahn-Waxler, C., Emde, R., & DeFries, J. (1999). Temperament and problem behavior during early childhood. *International Journal of Behavioral Development, 23*, 333–355.

Sheeber, L. B., & Johnson, J. H. (1994). Evaluation of a temperament-focused, parent-training program. *Journal of Clinical Child Psychology, 23*, 249–259.

Shirley, M. M. (1933). *The first two years: A study of 25 babies.* Minneapolis: University of Minnesota Press.

Stifter, C. A. (1992). Infant colic: A transient condition with no apparent effects. *Journal of Applied Developmental Psychology, 13*, 447–462.

Stifter, C. A., & Braungart, J. M. (1995). The regulation of negative reactivity in infancy: Function and development. *Child Development, 31*, 448–455.

Tellegen, A., Lykken, D. T., Bouchard, T. J., & Wilcox, K. J. (1988). Personality similarity in twins reared apart and together. *Journal of Personality and Social Psychology, 54*, 1031–1039.

Thomas, A., Chess, S., & Birch, H. G. (1968). *Temperament and behavior disorders in children.* New York: New York University Press.

Thomas, A., Chess, S., Birch, H. G., Hertzig, M. E., & Korn, S. (1963). *Behavioral individuality in early childhood.* New York: New York University Press.

van den Boom, D. C. (1989). Neonatal irritability and the development of attachment. In G. A. Kohnstamm, J. E. Bates, & M. K. Rothbart (Eds.), *Temperament in childhood* (pp. 299–318). Chichester, UK: Wiley.

Washburn, R. W. (1929). A study of the smiling and laughter of infants in the first year of life. *Genetic Psychology Monographs, 6*, 397–537.

Wilson, R. S., & Matheny, A. P. (1983). Assessment of temperament in infant twins. *Developmental Psychology, 19*, 172–183.

Wolk, S., Zeanah, C. H., Garcia-Coll, C. T., & Carr, S. (1992). Factors affecting parents' perceptions of temperament in early infancy. *American Journal of Orthopsychiatry, 62*, 71–82.

Worobey, J., & Blajda V. M. (1989). Temperament ratings at 2 weeks, 2 months, and 1 year: Differential stability of activity and emotionality. *Developmental Psychology, 25*, 257–263.

11

Attachment Assessment in the Strange Situation

SUSAN GOLDBERG

HISTORY

The concept of attachment and the use of the "Strange Situation" procedure have played important roles in studies of early social development. Although "attachment" is often used as a general term for parent–child relationships, the original construct was used by John Bowlby (1969) to describe a specific aspect of parent–child relationships: that part concerned with the function of protection and the infant's use of a caregiver as a "haven of safety" in stressful situations. Emphasis on this narrow traditional definition led to the design of the assessment procedure.

The most commonly used procedure for assessing individual differences in attachment was developed by Mary Ainsworth and her associates (Ainsworth, Blehar, Waters, & Wall, 1978). Ainsworth's graduate work was completed at University of Toronto with William Blatz who propounded the theory that feelings of security were rooted in experiences within the family. Blatz (1966) used the concept of "secure base," now a central concept in the assessment of attachment. After Ainsworth worked with Bowlby at the Tavistock Clinic on studies of parent–child separation, she subsequently went to Uganda, where she was intrigued by the traditional local custom of sending infants to stay with a relative during weaning. This situation promised to provide an opportunity to study a prolonged but normal separation. However, she soon discovered that this custom was no longer common and changed her plan to examine the early development of infant–mother relationships.

Some of her first ideas about individual differences in attachment emerged during these observations (Ainsworth, 1967), leading to an observational study in Baltimore. In this study, a small group of infants and their mothers were observed at home for several hours every 3 weeks throughout the first year. Separations observed in these Baltimore homes were minimally distressing for the infants. To study potentially more stressful situations, she and a staff member designed a laboratory observation involving a series of separations and reunions from the mother and a female stranger (Ainsworth & Wittig, 1969).

Measures from both home and the laboratory observation session included frequency and duration of specific behaviors as well as more global ratings. There were no direct relations between any of the home and laboratory measures. What was most striking was that there were three distinct patterns of behavior that echoed those she had seen in Uganda and were related to the home observations. The notion that a brief observation period in the laboratory could serve as a reliable marker of many hours of home observation was naturally appealing. To Ainsworth's chagrin (Ainsworth & Marvin, 1995), researchers eagerly adopted the paradigm known as the Strange Situation as an assessment of infant–parent relationships. Over the years, the Strange Situation has been used extensively by dedicated attachment researchers well versed in the theory, many of them students of Ainsworth or her trainees, as well as by researchers with other roots and interests, sometimes with little consideration of the original underlying concepts. Thus, there is a rich and extensive literature examining infant behavior in the Strange Situation in relation to prior, concurrent, and subsequent developmental phenomena. There are also questions and disagreements concerning interpretation of the Strange Situation and what it actually measures.

GENERAL DESCRIPTION

Procedure

The Strange Situation can be conducted with any potential attachment figure including father, mother, or alternative caregiver. Because it is used most often with mothers, the term "mother" or "caregiver" for the attachment figure is used here unless a specific other figure participated. The intent of the Strange Situation is to engage both infant and caregiver in a brief scenario that is close to real-life situations and moderately stressful for the infant. Stress is expected to activate attachment behavior, thus providing opportunities to observe the infant's strategy for using an attachment figure to manage stress and distress.

The procedure consists of eight episodes of up to 3 minutes each (see Table 11.1). In the first episode, an experimenter introduces mother and in-

TABLE 11.1. Episodes of the Strange Situation

Episode	Participants	Duration	Description
1	Mother, baby experimenter	< 1 min	Experimenter brings mother and baby to the room, gives instructions.
2	Mother, baby	3 min	Mother sits in chair and reads, baby explores. Mother responds if approached but does not initiate.
3	Mother, baby, stranger	3 min	Stranger enters, silent (1 min), converses with mother (1 min), approaches baby (1 min).
4	Baby, stranger	3 min[a]	First separation: mother departs, stranger comforts baby if needed, otherwise sits in chair.
5	Mother, baby	3 min	First reunion: mother returns, greets and/or comforts baby, returns to chair and reads.
6	Baby	3 min[a]	Second separation: mother departs, saying "bye-bye."
7	Baby, stranger	3 min[a]	Second separation continues: stranger enters, comforts baby if necessary, otherwise sits in chair.
8	Mother, baby	3 min	Second reunion: mother returns, greets, comforts baby if needed then free to interact as she chooses.

Note. Adapted from Ainsworth, Blehar, Waters, and Wall (1978). Copyright 1978 by Lawrence Erlbaum Associates, Inc. Adapted by permission. Adaptation reprinted from Goldberg (2000). Copyright 2000 by Edward Arnold Publishers. Reprinted by permission.

[a]These episodes are shortened if the baby does not settle within 20–30 seconds.

fant to the laboratory playroom. The mother is instructed to engage the infant with the toys and then sit in a designated chair to read (or pretend to read). Once sitting, she is asked to respond to the infant's overtures but not to initiate activities.

The second episode begins when the infant is settled with the toys and the mother is sitting in her chair. The third episode is marked by the entry of an unfamiliar female who sits quietly for the first minute, chats with the mother for the second minute, and then approaches and tries to engage the infant. At the first separation (Episode 4) the mother leaves her purse on the chair and departs unobtrusively. The "stranger" continues play with the baby but returns to her chair if it is evident that the baby is not overtly distressed. If the baby is distressed, the stranger offers comfort, but if the baby cries hard for more than 20 seconds, the mother is asked to return.

In the first reunion (Episode 5), the mother's instructions are to knock and call the child's name at the door, then enter, pause to allow the child to initiate a greeting, do whatever necessary to resettle the child, and then sit in the chair and read. The stranger leaves unobtrusively when it is clear that the initial reunion has been completed. After 3 minutes, the mother is signaled to depart again to begin Episode 6. This time the child is left alone and the stranger returns (Episode 7) before the mother (Episode 8). As before, Episodes 6 and 7 are curtailed if intense distress continues for more than 20 seconds.

On the mother's second return, her instructions are, as before, to knock, call, and give the child a chance to greet her. Then she is free to do whatever seems appropriate for the remainder of the 3 minutes. This entire scenario is videotaped and scoring is based on careful review of the videotape.

Primary Classifications

The procedure yields an attachment classification which includes one of three patterns (Ainsworth et al., 1978) and a rating for organization/disorganization (Main & Solomon, 1990). The scoring procedures described here are intended for 12- to 18-month-olds and focus on infant behavior. The caregiver's behavior is taken into account primarily as the context for the infant's behavior. Six 7-point rating scales are available to rate behavior in the reunion episodes: proximity seeking, proximity maintaining, avoidance, resistance, search behavior (during the mother's absence, and distance interaction. The latter two scales are not widely used, but the pattern of scores on the first four (along with clinical impressions) is used to arrive at a classification.

In the Baltimore study, Ainsworth described three patterns. The first fit the description of secure base behavior and was called "secure." These babies explored the playroom when the mother was present, reduced exploration in her absence, went to their mothers for comforting at the reunion, and soon returned to play and exploration. On the rating scales, these babies would be rated low for avoidance and resistance and moderate to high on proximity seeking and contact maintaining or high on distance interaction.

The second pattern, "avoidant," was marked by minimal involvement with the mother before separations, little sign of distress in her absence, and snubbing or ignoring her on reunions. These infants would be rated high on the avoidance scale and low on the remaining scales.

The third pattern, "resistant" or "ambivalent," featured preoccupation with the mother at the expense of exploration: limited exploration before separation, intense distress at departures, and strong contact-seeking mingled with anger at the reunions. These babies would be rated high on resistance but also high on proximity seeking or contact maintaining or both.

To indicate that she did not want to make value judgments regarding these patterns, Ainsworth designated letters to represent them: B for the secure pattern, A for the avoidant pattern, and C for the resistant pattern. Much of the literature uses these pattern names and although Ainsworth was careful not to assign A to the pattern she thought optimal, the value judgments she tried to avoid were quickly attached to the letter names with B emerging as "good."

Each primary classification includes subgroups. The secure classification includes four subgroups. B_1 and B_2 babies resemble avoidant babies in showing little upset and less contact seeking during reunions than B_3 and B_4 babies. But they differ from the avoidant group in making clear positive initiations to the mother on her returns. B_3 and B_4 babies resemble the resistant group in being readily upset by separations and engaging in strong contact seeking at reunions. B_4 babies are also slow to settle. But these babies are distinguished from the resistant group in showing little anger and being unambivalent about their desire for contact.

The avoidant and resistant classifications both include two subgroups. A_1 babies are consistently avoidant whereas A_2 babies show mixed behavior: some tendency to greet or approach the mother mixed with marked tendency to move away or look away at reunions. The A_2 baby might approach the mother on her return but then continue past her to the door or veer off toward the toys. In the resistant group, C_1 babies are overtly angry, whereas C_2 babies are passive and helpless, signaling for pickup rather than making active approaches. The C_2 babies are also thought to be angry but to express it passively through pouting and inappropriate helplessness rather than overt protest.

Figure 11.1 shows the full range of attachment patterns along a rough continuum that reflects the threshold for activating attachment behavior. At the far left, the threshold is relatively high for the avoidant infants (attachment behavior is not easily elicited) and it drops as one moves to the right

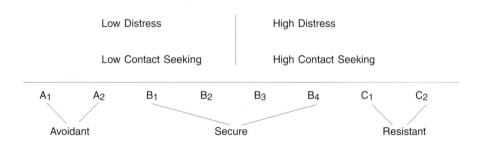

FIGURE 11.1. Scheme for classifying primary (ABC) attachment types. Reprinted from Goldberg (2000). Copyright 2000 by Edward Arnold Publishers. Reprinted by permission.

where the resistant (C) babies have an extremely low threshold for activating attachment behavior.

Disorganization

During the first 10–15 years that the Strange Situation was in use, the majority of children fit the foregoing classifications. In community samples, approximately two-thirds of babies showed the secure pattern, one-fifth the avoidant pattern, and one-ninth the resistant pattern (van IJzendoorn & Kroonenberg, 1988). However, a small percentage of infants (10–14%) did not fit these categories. In reviewing these "unclassifiable" tapes, Main and Solomon (1986) identified a fourth group of babies, those described as primarily disorganized/disoriented (Type D) with respect to attachment.

These babies were distinguished by the presence of odd or unusual behaviors that seemed to reflect fear or confusion regarding the caregiver. Thus, the infant either lacked a strategy or experienced the breakdown of his or her preferred strategy. For this reason, if the most characteristic feature of an infant's attachment behavior is disorganization, this classification is made in conjunction with the best fitting alternative of the three primary strategies (secure, avoidant, resistant). If the alternative (ABC) classification is not evident, the first alternative may be Unclassifiable (U), followed by a "best guess" alternative (e.g., D/U/A2; D = Type D).

The procedures for scoring disorganization (Main & Solomon, 1990) are applicable to infants up to 21 months of age. They are not appropriate for infants with neurological problems as it is difficult to distinguish generally disorganized behavior linked to neurological impairment from disorganization specific to attachment.

There is no inclusive list of disorganized behaviors. Main and Solomon (1990) list seven categories with detailed examples: (1) sequential; or (2) simultaneous displays of contradictory behavior (e.g., strong proximity seeking followed by strong avoidance, avoiding the parent while extremely distressed); (3) undirected, misdirected, incomplete, and interrupted movements and expressions (e.g., crying and attempting to follow the stranger out of the room); (4) stereotypies, asymmetrical movement, and anomalous postures (e.g., falling prone after starting to approach the mother on her return); (5) freezing, stilling, and slowed movements and expressions (e.g., no movement and a dazed expression); (6) direct indices of apprehension of the parent (e.g., fearful expression on pickup); and (7) direct indices of disorganization or disorientation (e.g., flinging hands about or in front of the face in response to the mother's return).

In evaluating a Strange Situation videotape for disorganized behavior, the coder makes detailed notes of behaviors occurring in the parent's presence that fit the foregoing seven categories and indicates the context in which they occur. Behaviors that occur during reunions, particularly in the initial moments, are weighted more heavily than those occurring at other times. There are some behaviors which in and of themselves are sufficient for a disorganized classification (e.g., falling into a huddled prone posture after starting to approach the mother on her return). In the absence of such definitive behaviors, the coder makes a judgment based on the frequency, intensity, and context of the salient behaviors whether or not an infant should be considered disorganized. A rating for disorganization is given on a 9-point scale with 1 representing no disorganized behaviors; 3, presence of some disorganized behaviors but not enough to seriously consider a disorganized classification; 5, moderate indices of disorganization but not clearly sufficient for disorganized classification; 7, definite qualification for disorganization; and 9, definitely disorganized with strong, frequent, and/or intense indicators. When a score of 5 is assigned, the coder decides whether the infant should be assigned to the disorganized group. In normative samples, about 15% of infants are found to be disorganized with respect to attachment. In high-risk and clinical samples, this figure is higher (35–48%; van IJzendoorn, Shuengel, & Bakermans-Kranenburg, 1999).

BIOBEHAVIORAL BASIS OF ASSESSMENT

Evolutionary Significance

Bowlby (1969) argued that affectional ties between children and their caregivers have a biological basis, best understood in an evolutionary context. Because human infants do not survive without adult care, our evolutionary history has selected "prewired" dispositions on the part of both infants and adults to behave in ways that increase the likelihood of infant survival and well-being. Thus, infants are biased to behave in ways that maintain and enhance proximity to caregivers and elicit their care and investment. Conditions that threaten health and survival, such as fatigue, illness, and environmental dangers, serve as triggers to evoke attachment behaviors. Adults are similarly biased to engage in protective behavior in response to infant signals of exhaustion, illness, or perception of danger and to proactively monitor/prevent or alter potentially dangerous situations.

Through repeated experience of parental response when attachment behavior is activated, the infant constructs organized representations of the parent's behavior in the protective role. If, by the end of the first year, the infant is confident of the caregiver's protection, he or she is considered securely attached. If the infant lacks this confidence, he or she is insecurely attached. When an infant is confident of the caregiver's protection he or she is able to freely explore the environment, using the caregiver as "a secure base for exploration." Less confident infants must direct some of their attention to strategies to maintain or ensure the caregiver's attention and therefore explore less freely.

Psychobiology of Attachment

Bowlby also considered the dyadic attachment system to serve as a buffer between stresses impinging on the infant from the external environment and the infant's internal homeostatic mechanisms. Thus, the more effective the attachment system in this buffering function, the less demand is made on the infant's internal regulatory systems. A substantial literature on primate development documents differences in neurobiological organization associated with different rearing conditions (Kraemer, 1992), entailing artificial mother surrogates and peers as well as mother-rearing conditions.

In human infants, individual differences are considered within the broad condition of "mother rearing" because experimental assignment to rearing conditions is not possible. However, a number of studies indicate that the Strange Situation evokes different physiological responses in dyads with different attachment classifications. In secure dyads relative to insecure dyads, both heart rate and salivary cortisol give evidence of less physiological arousal (Donovan & Leavitt, 1985; Hertsgaard, Gunnar, Erickson, & Nachmias, 1995; Sroufe & Waters, 1977; Spangler & Grossmann, 1993; Spangler & Schieche, 1998). Furthermore, two of three studies which used salivary cortisol measures showed that infants in disorganized dyads experience greater increases in cortisol during the Strange Situation than those in all other groups (Hertsgaard et al., 1995; Spangler & Grossmann, 1993). These data are consistent with Bowlby's notion in showing that absence of an organized caregiver-oriented strategy for managing stress is associated with greater impact of environmental stressors on the infant's internal regulatory systems.

RELIABILITY AND VALIDITY

Test–Retest Reliability

In evaluating the Strange Situation, test–retest reliability and coder reliability in making classifications should be considered. Test–retest reliability has proved to be elusive. In Ainsworth's early work, 23 infants were retested within 2 weeks of the first assessment (Ainsworth et al., 1978). Although there were significant correlations from Time 1 to Time 2 for some of the ratings (the strongest being for avoidance: $r = .66$), none was high enough to be a satisfactory reliability coefficient. More important, infants gave evidence of remembering the previous experience and becoming more upset more quickly the second time. Thus, the second Strange Situation is a significantly different experience for the infant.

In this pilot study, 86% of secure babies were classified secure on the second occasion, as were 50% of the resistant babies, but all the initially avoidant babies were classified secure at the second session, giving an overall concordance of 57%. As a result of concerns about interpreting a second Strange Situation close in time to the first, researchers have been advised not to readminister the Strange Situation without an intervening 4- to 6-week gap. Thus, no further reliability data have been produced.

For 12- to 18-month-olds, 4 to 6 weeks is a relatively long time during which it is possible that life circumstances affecting attachment could change. Hence, repeated testings that are separated by 1 month or more are appropriately treated as assessments of stability rather than reliability. Stability of classifications is relevant to developmental questions but not to questions regarding the psychometric properties of this assessment.

Attachment theory emphasizes the propensity for attachment strategies to persist. Initially, this view was supported by studies showing high stability (> 80%) within infancy under stable life conditions (e.g., Connell, 1976; Waters, 1978) coupled with "lawful instability" in less stable households (Egeland & Farber, 1984). Changes from secure to insecure attachment were associated with deterioration in life circumstances whereas changes from insecure to secure were associated with improving conditions. However, more recent data (Belsky, Campbell, Cohn, & Moore, 1996) showed low stability (46–55%) in infancy. In interpreting these last data, the authors suggest that home conditions may have changed considerably since the time of the early stability studies, with, for example, more infants living in dual-wage-earner families and experiencing alternative caregivers. Given these more recent data, it appears that the assumption of stability of attachment in infancy may need to be reassessed on an ongoing basis.

Coder Reliability

Because the Strange Situation was not designed as a routine assessment, there has not been a formal study of coder reliability. Rather, each individual study, of which there are hundreds, includes a reliability report. The majority of published studies utilize the three-category Ainsworth classification scheme, with most published before the criteria for recognizing disorganization were widely available. Because there are so many studies that could not use the disorganized classification, more recent studies often analyze data using both the three- and four-category schemes. Reliability may be reported for the full four-category scheme, or for the three-category scheme with separate information for the D/not-D distinction. In general, trained coders from the same laboratory agree on primary classifications better than 80% of the time.

In preparing a standard reliability videotape, Carlson and Sroufe (1993) found that six expert coders agreed with Ainsworth on three-way classifications 86% of the time; with Sroufe 83%, and 79% overall agreement among coders. Agreement on subgroup classifications was poor (44% overall). Subgroup classifications are rarely analyzed. Agreement on

the disorganized classification or the four-category scheme is more variable but reaches similar levels (> 75%) among well-trained coders (van
IJzendoorn et al., 1999).

In one recent multicenter study (NICHD Early Child Care Network,
1997) three coders jointly coded 1,201 Strange Situations using five categories (A, B, C, D, and U). Each coder also rated the confidence with which
each classification was made on a scale of 1 (extremely difficult to code) to 5
(classic example of the subcategory). Overall agreement across coder pairs
was 83%. When both coders gave confidence ratings of 3 or higher, agreement was 94%; when both coders rated confidence less than 3 (13% of cases),
agreement was only 53%.

Validity

The initial acceptance of the Strange Situation as a valid indicator of attachment was based on evidence that attachment classifications could be predicted from observations of home behavior. In the Baltimore study, maternal
"unresponsiveness" to infant crying, the nature and context of physical contact, and behavior during feeding and emotional expressiveness distinguished secure and insecure dyads and subgroups of these behaviors differentiated avoidant and resistant groups from the others (Ainsworth et al.,
1978, Chap. 8). In line with the theoretical view that infant behavior in the
Strange Situation represents the outcome of maternal responsiveness and
sensitivity to infant behavior in the first year, these observations of maternal
behavior served as the "gold standard" against which Strange Situation
classifications were validated.

In 1987, Goldsmith and Alansky conducted a meta-analysis of 13 studies with similar home/Strange Situation analyses and reported an average
effect size of .30 linking maternal behavior with Strange Situation classifications. Ten years later, De Wolff and van IJzendoorn (1997) could include 66
such studies in their meta-analysis and reported comparable average effect
sizes of .24–.34. In both these statistical reviews the Ainsworth study, with
effect sizes 4–13 times that of other studies, was excluded, partly as a statistical outlier and partly because it represented a small hypothesis-generating
study. The variability of these effect sizes, coupled with their generally low
to moderate size, has raised questions regarding interpretation of behavior
in the Strange Situation.

Why has clear replication of the original validation data been so elusive? The Strange Situation has considerable face validity as an opportunity
to observe secure base behavior under moderately stressful conditions.
Home observation conditions vary considerably in these replication efforts,
yet De Wolff and van IJzendoorn (1997) found that methodological similarity to the original Baltimore study did not account for differences in effect
sizes. Of course, even the most "similar" methods in this review were quite
dissimilar from Ainsworth's original. They also note that in most of these

studies, parental warmth and acceptance are confounded with sensitivity, a distinction made by MacDonald (1992) and underlined by Ainsworth (Ainsworth & Marvin, 1995).

Among the commentaries on this meta-analysis, Thompson (1997) raises the concern that few of the replications focus on attachment-relevant situations (i.e., those that are stressful to the infant), a point also made by Goldberg, Grusec, and Jenkins (1999). Given that these replication studies blur the distinction between attachment and other aspects of the infant–mother relationship, low to moderate effect sizes should perhaps be expected. The dilemma for researchers seeking to sharpen the constructs is that mothers who are sensitive in attachment situations may be the same mothers who are sensitive under other conditions.

When Bell and Ainsworth (1972) examined maternal response to infant crying in the Baltimore study, they noted that mothers who were highly responsive to cries were also responsive to other infant signals, and it was this notion that led to developing the global rating scales used in many of the replication efforts. Some studies do not specifically distinguish attachment and other aspects of infant–mother relationships. Further confounding has arisen because the term "attachment" is widely used in both professional and popular literature as a general term for infant–parent relationships, generating confusion as to what the Strange Situation measures. Is it infant confidence in caregiver protection (i.e., felt security), social reciprocity, emotion regulation, or "good mothering"?

There is a prodigious literature on the predictive validity of the Strange Situation. Several major longitudinal studies followed children from infancy to various stages of later childhood, showing links between infant attachment and aspects of later functioning, such as relations with parents (e.g., Main, Kaplan, & Cassidy, 1985), representations of family (Fury, Carlson, & Sroufe, 1997), peer relations (e.g., Lieberman, 1977; Sroufe, Egeland, & Carlson, 1999), classroom behavior (e.g., Erickson, Sroufe, & Egeland, 1985; Lyons-Ruth, Alpern, & Repacholi, 1993), and behavioral problems (e.g., Goldberg, Gotowiec, & Simmons, 1995; Lewis, Feiring, McGuffog, & Jaskir, 1984; Renken, Egeland, Marvinney, Mangelsdorf, & Sroufe, 1989). In some cases, similar studies failed to find these same relations (e.g., Bates, Maslin, & Frankel, 1985; Goldberg, Corter, Lojkasek, & Minde, 1990; Lewis, Feiring, & Rosenthal, 2000). Thus, there is ongoing discussion concerning the extent to which infant attachment classifications predict later outcomes in social development.

Because these studies touch on such a wide range of later abilities and the literature for any particular later behavior is limited, few comprehensive discursive statistical reviews are available. An exception is a recent meta-analysis by van IJzendoorn, Dijkstra, & Bus (1995) which showed that although attachment was not related to measures of intelligence, secure children were more competent in language skills than were their insecure peers (effect size = .28). However, it is worth noting that links with social competence would be predicted not only for attachment but for other aspects of early caregiver–child relationships. Accordingly, Belsky and Cassidy (1994) suggest the importance of elaborating our developmental models in ways that focus on a more differentiated view of infant–adult relationships and specific sequelae for each component. The most recent review (Thompson, 1999) indicates that the strength of the relation between infant attachment and later outcomes is moderate and "more contingent and provisional than earlier expected." However, thoughtful and well-designed long-term studies have yielded impressively strong predictions from early attachment to later behavior in areas such as peer relations (Sroufe et al., 1999) and psychopathology (Carlson, 1998).

The mechanism linking early attachment to later outcomes is also debated. These findings may represent the effects of early incorporated attachment behavior or representations on later behavior or may also be attributable to continuity of care: Caregivers effective in supporting secure attachment in infancy also provide appropriate support for the acquisition of later developing skills. Some support for this attribution may be found in the results of four recently completed longitudinal studies. In one study, attachment classifications at 12 months of 60 white, middle-class infants who were recontacted 20 years later were remarkably stable with their classifications in early adulthood (Cohen's Kappa = .44, $p < .001$) (Waters, Merrick, Treboux, Crowell, & Albersheim, 2000). In another study, infant attachment classification significantly predicted adolescent classification with 77% stability (Hamilton, 2000). However, Weinfield, Sroufe, and Egeland (2000), in an impoverished, high-risk sample, of 57 young adults, found no continuities in attachment classification from infancy. All three studies, however, found change in attachment security to be meaningfully related to change in the family environment. Similarly, Lewis et al. (2000) found no continuity of attachment classification between 1 and 18 years for a middle-class sample. In contrast to the three aforementioned studies, there was no relationship found between adolescent maladjustment and infant attachment status, but divorce was related to insecure attachment at 18 years and insecurely attached 18-year-olds were more likely to rate themselves as maladjusted.

DEVELOPMENTAL MODEL

The notion that early relationships with caregivers have a major influence on subsequent development is a pervasive one. What originally distinguished attachment theory from other theories of the influence of parent–infant relationships is its emphasis on protective situations as the formative experiences. As the concept of attachment has been implicitly broadened, it has come to include other aspects of caregiver behavior linked with generally "good parenting." According to Bowlby's original notion, infant experiences with caregivers in situations that trigger attachment behavior are preserved and organized in representations that he called "internal working models." As such models become moderators of subsequent behavior, early experiences with caregivers are carried forward to shape later personality and behavior.

Although these models include both cognitive and affective information, conscious and unconscious, and are subject to revision with input from new experiences, there are limits to flexibility and change. First, new information regarding relationships is processed through the filter of the existing model. Second, those aspects of working models which are not accessible to consciousness may be particularly resistant to change. Elements of working models laid down in infancy are likely to be in this category because they were not coded linguistically.

The procedures of the Strange Situation enable the trained coder to identify strategies relevant to secure base behavior. In identifying these strategies and associating them with an attachment classification, the coder is, in fact, making inferences concerning the infant's expectations of the caregiver in a moderately stressful situation, one aspect of early internal working models. It is assumed that all infants experience the separations of the Strange Situation as stressful and the physiological data discussed earlier in "Biobehavioral Basis of Assessment" support this assumption. Even avoidant infants who appear unconcerned show elevated heart rate and cortisol secretion during and after the Strange Situation (Donovan & Leavitt, 1985; Hertsgaard et al., 1995; Spangler & Grossmann, 1993; Sroufe & Waters, 1977).

From the ease with which the secure infant approaches and is comforted by the caregiver, we infer that the child is confident of an appropriate response to expressed needs for comfort. The inability of the avoidant infant to signal his or her distress leads to the inference that the infant expects such signals to be ignored or rejected. From the strong contact seeking and inability to be comforted on the part of the resistant infant, it can be inferred that the infant expects to lose the caregiver's attention when he or she settles. In theory, these three different expectations regarding the caregiver are the foundation for three different kinds of working models that will become increasingly stable as subsequent experience supports them through the child's development.

STRUCTURAL AND/OR THEORETICAL CONSTRAINTS/CONTROVERSIES

Attachment and Temperament: A Dispute

The Strange Situation procedure is considered to measure infant–parent attachment and evidence indicates that caregiver behavior in the home is related to infant behavior in the Strange Situation. However, because the effect size is small to moderate, there are clearly other contributing factors. Theorists who study temperament suggest that the Strange Situation really measures temperamental differences (e.g., Chess & Thomas, 1982; Kagan, 1994), because infants differ in the latency and intensity of expressing distress as well as ability to modulate distress once it occurs. What is observed in the Strange Situation reflects proneness to distress.

"Avoidant" infants do not become distressed in the Strange Situation and therefore do not need to seek contact on reunions. "Resistant" infants readily become extremely distressed and take a long time to settle once their mothers return. Hence they appear to resist comforting and do not easily return to exploring.

It is not clear how temperament theorists explain the secure pattern because secure infants vary considerably in the amount of overt distress they exhibit in the Strange Situation. Indeed, those who focus on temperamental predictors may categorize behavior in the Strange Situation primarily in terms of the amount of distress and contact seeking (see Figure 11.1) rather than criteria relevant to security. The main point made by temperament theorists is that behavior in the Strange Situation is determined primarily by infant characteristics rather than history of caregiving.

The Evidence

It is worth noting that in Ainsworth's early work (Ainsworth et al., 1978, Chap. 7), infant behavior at home in the first and fourth quarter of the year was related to later attachment classifications. In the first quarter, infants who were later considered secure cried less and less often and had more positive responses to being held as well as being put down. In face-to-face interactions with their mothers, smiling and vocalizing did not distinguish attachment groups but infants who were later secure were less likely to ignore their mothers and took more initiative in ending interactions than those who were later insecure.

In the fourth quarter, infants who were later secure cried less at home, took more initiative in making contact, were more compliant to maternal requests, and showed less anger than infants who were later avoidant or resistant. Ainsworth and her colleagues interpreted both sets of data as indicators of infant–mother relationships rather than as measures of infant characteristics. While both sets of data certainly reflect experiences with caregiving, temperament theorists are more likely to consider the first-quarter data as evidence of infant contributions to attachment.

In a meta-analysis of early studies examining home behavior and attachment classifications, Goldsmith and Alansky (1987) found an effect size of .19 of prior infant behavior on attachment classification. Although smaller than the effect size reported for maternal behavior (.30) these figures are not statistically significantly different. The more recent meta-analysis of De Wolff and van IJzendoorn (1997) did not include infant behaviors as predictors. Hence, on the basis of the best meta-analytic evidence we have, infant and caregiver appear to make equal contributions to the formation of attachment. Two relatively recent studies support the notion of a complex relation between attachment and temperament, showing both direct and indirect effects of infant temperament and maternal behavior on behavior in the Strange Situation (Seifer, Schiller, Sameroff, Resnick, & Riordan, 1996; Susman-Stillman, Kalkoske, Egeland, & Waldman, 1996).

Measuring a Trait or a Relationship?

Attachment theorists would say "both." On the one hand, the Strange Situation characterizes the mother–infant relationship (a dyadic characteristic) as inferred from the infant's behavior. But to do so, we assume that the infant has formed an internal representation of the relationship that filters perceptions and regulates behavior (a trait). However, in the dispute between attachment and temperament theorists, attachment theorists emphasize the dyadic view while temperament theorists argue for a trait view.

If attachment is a "trait," then infants should show the same attachment pattern with different caregivers. If attachment is a dyadic characteristic, then infants can have different patterns of attachment with different caregivers. Infants can and do exhibit different patterns of attachment with mothers and fathers (Fox, Kimmerly, & Schafer, 1991; De Wolff & van IJzendoorn, 1997). However, a high degree of concordance between infant patterns of attachment with different caregivers would support the temperament position.

Studies with data on attachment to both mother and father initially failed to find concordance between them. Fox and his colleagues (1991) suggested that this reflected lack of statistical power in single studies. However, concordance for security/insecurity in the aggregated data was significant in one meta-analysis (Fox et al., 1991) but not in a second and larger one (De Wolff & van IJzendoorn, 1997). When data were analyzed according to the high distress/low distress split shown in Figure 11.1, concordance was greater than chance (Fox et al., 1991). That is, if an infant was on the "limited expression," "low distress," "low contact seeking" side of the continuum with one parent, he or she was most likely to be on the same side with the other parent. However, security/insecurity within the split was not concordant: Within the group of high-distress infants, security with one parent did not predict security or insecurity with the other. The same was true within the low-distress group.

A Resolution of the Dispute?

An appealing "empirical rapprochement" between the temperament and attachment views, consistent with the foregoing data was previously suggested by Belsky and Rovine (1987). The basic notion is that the attachment classification system itself incorporates a temperament dimension evident by examining Figure 11.1: attachment patterns characterized by high distress and contact seeking (the right side of the figure) form one temperament group; those characterized by low distress and contact seeking (the left half of the figure) represent another. Each group includes both secure and insecurely attached infants. Belsky and Rovine (1987) suggested that maternal behavior determines security/insecurity whereas temperament (i.e., proneness to distress) determines type of security or insecurity (i.e., high distress/low distress or biased toward limiting or exaggerating expression of attachment needs).

This argument was buttressed with data from three studies showing that temperament measures differentiated infants in these two groups. Attachment classifications on the left side of the figure were associated with easy temperament and those on the right with difficult temperament. Attempts to replicate these findings (e.g., Mangelsdorf, Gunnar, Kertenbaum, Lang, & Andreas, 1990; Neuman & Goldberg, 1990; Susman-Stillman et al., 1996; Vaughn, Lefever, Siefer, & Barglow, 1989; Vaughn et al., 1992) have been mixed. These mixed findings may reflect the "rough approximation" of the continuum along which the attachment groups are shown to lie. For example, C_2 infants are usually not more distressed than C_1 infants. Furthermore, it is unlikely that the B_3 pattern (supposedly both optimal and most common) would be associated with difficult temperament (the least optimal and least common temperament type). Thus, a simple match between attachment subgroups and temperament may not be as plausible as it first seemed.

Because the attachment behavioral system represents a system for regulating infant distress, it is likely that temperamental qualities involving distress (e.g., proneness to distress and intensity of expression) contribute to its development. By the same token, because the function of the caregiver in this system is to protect the infant by responding to distress, the caregiver also makes a contribution. To the extent that the Strange Situation successfully assesses attachment, both infant and caregiver influences are expected. Because caregivers have a wider and more flexible repertoire than does the developing infant, the caregiver can adapt more readily to variations in infant behavior than the infant can compensate for limitations in the caregiver. It may be more useful to focus in future research on how these two contributory factors are related.

Clinical Limitations

The Strange Situation has been used mainly as a research tool. However, a measure of caregiver–infant relationships is naturally of interest to clinicians who have eyed the Strange Situation as a potential clinical tool. In its present form, the Strange Situation is limited in clinical applications. First, the available data are group data, with little attention given to individual clinical utility. Second, it is time-consuming and relatively costly, requiring a minimum of two people to run, a room with appropriate video facilities, and 1–2 hours of a trained coder's time. However, there are numerous outstanding examples of academic clinicians whose research funding allows them to use the Strange Situation with their clinical cases. One promising project has explored classification of attachment based on the standard pediatric examination as an adaptation of the Strange Situation (Berger, 1994). Such adaptations may eventually result in other procedures for clinical use.

TRAINING REQUIREMENTS

The procedures for running the Strange Situation and criteria for identifying the three primary categories are described in Ainsworth et al. (1978), a thorough reading of which is the groundwork for training. The basic information for coding disorganization is found in two chapters by Main and Solomon (1989, 1990). A potential coder should first learn to work with the three primary categories and gain coding experience before trying to code disorganization. Systematic training with an experienced coder is necessary. For many years, Alan Sroufe has taught an annual 1-week course in the basic coding scheme at the Institute of Child Development, University of Minnesota. Recently, a week on coding of disorganization taught by Elizabeth Carlson has also been offered. Occasional institutes in coding disorganized attachment are offered by Mary Main and Erik Hesse of the University of California, Berkeley. Generally, in learning the basic scheme, an individual needs to follow the formal course with practice on 20–40 cases before passing the reliability test (available from the Institute for Child Study).

   For use in research situations, this formal training and standard reliability test are essential. For other uses, formal training is less urgent but advisable. There is considerable disagreement and confusion regarding the constructs and interpretation of the Strange Situation. Increased uniformity in training and usage can make a major contribution to eliminating such confusions.

IMPLICATIONS

The Strange Situation was not designed as a standardized assessment tool but has been widely, and successfully, used in research. To recapture the richer environment in which Ainsworth developed the procedure, two other approaches to assessing attachment have emerged. The first, developed by Waters and Deane (1985), used Q-sort methodology to enable parents or research staff to report infant home behavior. The second, by Pederson and

Moran (1995), establishes classifications based on observations of home behavior. Both methods are at least as labor intensive as the Strange Situation and both relied on the Strange Situation as the gold standard for validation. Neither of these are cost-effective clinical tools in their present form.

Thus, the Strange Situation, whatever its limitations, remains the most widely used, accepted, and best validated method of assessing infant attachment. Because of its immense value as a heuristic tool, it captured the imagination of many researchers and gave rise to an impressive body of research. The approach of examining organization of behavior rather than specific behaviors or outcomes marked a general shift in the study of behavioral development.

The controversies surrounding the Strange Situation are, to a great extent, those surrounding attachment theory itself. Those who work within the conceptual framework of attachment theory generally endorse the Strange Situation; critics of attachment theory are also critical of the Strange Situation. These controversies have enriched the field of child development as debates and disagreements pressed researchers to sharpen and refine their constructs and to conduct increasingly sophisticated studies to reach definitive answers.

REFERENCES

Ainsworth, M. D. S. (1967). *Infancy in Uganda: Child care and the growth of love*. Baltimore: Johns Hopkins University Press.

Ainsworth, M. D. S., Blehar, M. C., Waters, E., & Wall, S. (1978). *Patterns of attachment*. Hillsdale, NJ: Erlbaum.

Ainsworth, M. D. S., & Marvin, R. S. (1995). On the shaping of attachment theory and research: An interview with Mary D. S. Ainsworth. In E. Waters, B. E. Vaughn, G. Posada, & K. Kondo-Ikemura (Eds.), Caregiving, cultural and cognitive perspectives on secure-base behavior and working models. *Monographs of the Society for Research in Child Development, 60*(Serial No. 244), 3–24.

Ainsworth, M. D. S., & Wittig, B. A. (1969). Attachment and exploratory behavior of one-year-olds in a Strange Situation. In B. M. Foss (Ed.), *Determinants of infant behavior IV*. London: Methuen.

Bates, J. E., Maslin, C. A., & Frankel, K. A. (1985). Attachment security, mother–child interaction and temperament as predictors of behavior problems at age three years. In I. Bretherton & E. Waters (Eds.), Growing points of attachment theory and research. *Monographs of the Society for Research in Child Development, 50*(1–2, Serial No. 209), 67–193.

Bell, S. M., & Ainsworth, M. D. S. (1972). Infant crying and maternal responsiveness. *Child Development, 43*, 1171–1190.

Belsky, J., Campbell, S. B., Cohn, J. F., & Moore, G. (1996). Instability of infant–parent attachment security. *Developmental Psychology, 32*, 921–924.

Belsky, J., & Cassidy, J. (1994). Attachment: Theory and evidence. In M. Ratter, D. Hay, & S.

Baron-Cohen (Eds.), *Developmental principles and clinical issues in psychology and psychiatry* (pp. 373–402). Oxford: Blackwell.

Belsky, J., & Rovine, M. J. (1987). Temperament and attachment security in the Strange Situation: An empirical rapprochement. *Child Development, 58,* 787–795.

Berger, S. (1994, September). *Applying an attachment framework to psychosocial screening of infants in primary care pediatrics.* Paper presented at the meeting of the Society for Behavioral Pediatrics, Minneapolis, MN.

Blatz, W. E. (1966). *Human security: Some reflections.* Toronto: University of Toronto Press.

Bowlby, J. (1969). *Attachment and loss* (Vol. 1). New York: Basic Books.

Carlson, E. A. (1998). A prospective longitudinal study of attachment disorganization/disorientation. *Child Development, 69,* 1107–1129.

Carlson, E. A., & Sroufe, L. A. (1993, Spring). Reliability in attachment classification. *SRCD Newsletter,* p. 4.

Chess, S., & Thomas, A. (1982). Infant bonding: Mystique and reality. *American Journal of Orthopsychiatry, 52,* 213–222.

Connell, D. B. (1976). *Individual differences in attachment: An investigation into stability, implications, and relationships to structure of early language development.* Unpublished doctoral dissertation, Syracuse University.

De Wolff, M. S., & van IJzendoorn, M. H. (1997). Sensitivity and attachment: A meta-analysis on parental antecedents of infant attachment. *Child Development, 68,* 571–591.

Donovan, W., & Leavitt, L. (1985). Physiologic assessment of mother–infant attachment. *Journal of the American Academy of Child Psychiatry, 24,* 65–70.

Egeland, B., & Farber, E. (1984). Infant–mother attachment: Factors related to its development and changes over time. *Child Development, 55,* 753–771.

Erickson, M. F., Sroufe, L. A., & Egeland, B. (1985). The relationship between quality of attachment and behavior problems in a preschool high-risk sample. In I. Bretherton & E. Waters (Eds.), Growing points of attachment theory and research. *Monographs of the Society for Research in Child Development, 50*(1–2, Serial No. 209), 147–166.

Fox, N. A., Kimmerly, N. L., & Schafer, W. D. (1991). Attachment to mother, attachment to father: A meta-analysis. *Child Development, 62,* 210–225.

Fury, G., Carlson, E. A., & Sroufe, L. A. (1997). Children's representations of attachment relationships in family drawings. *Child Development, 68,* 1154–1164.

Goldberg, S. (2000). *Attachment and development.* London: Edward Arnold.

Goldberg, S., Corter, C., Lojkasek, M., & Minde,K. (1990). Prediction of behaviour problems in four-year-olds born prematurely. *Development and Psychopathology, 2,* 15–30.

Goldberg, S., Gotowiec, A., & Simmons, R. J. (1995). Infant–mother attachment and behavior problems in healthy and chronically ill preschoolers. *Development and Psychopathology, 7,* 267–282.

Goldberg, S., Grusec, J., & Jenkins, J. (1999). Confidence in protection: Another look at attachment and other components intimate relationships. *Journal of Family Psychology, 13,* 475–483.

Goldsmith, H. H., & Alansky, J. A. (1987). Maternal and infant temperamental predictors of attachment: A meta-analytic review. *Journal of Consulting and Clinical Psychology, 55,* 805–816.

Hamilton, C. E. (2000). Continuity and discontinuity of attachment from infancy through adolescence. *Child Development, 71,* 690–764.

Hertsgaard, L., Gunnar, M., Erickson, M. F., & Nachmias, M. (1995). Adrenocortical responses to the Strange Situation in infants with disorganized/disoriented attachment relationships. *Child Development, 66,* 1100–1106.

Kagan, J. (1994). *Galen's prophecy.* New York: Basic Books.

Kraemer, G. W. (1992). A psychobiological theory of attachment. *Brain and Behavior Sciences, 15,* 493–541.

Lewis, M., Feiring, C., McGuffog, C., & Jaskir, J. (1984). Predicting psychopathology in six-year-olds from early social relations. *Child Development, 55,* 123–136.

Lewis, M., Feiring C., & Rosenthal, S. (2000). Attachment over time. *Child Development, 71,* 707–720.

Lieberman, A. F. (1977). Preschoolers' competence with a peer: Relations with attachment and peer experience. *Child Development, 48,* 1277–1287.

Lyons-Ruth, K., Alpern, L., & Repacholi, B. (1993). Disorganized infant attachment classification and maternal psychosocial problems as predictors of hostile–aggressive behavior in the preschool classroom. *Child Development, 64,* 572–585.

MacDonald, K. (1992). Warmth as a developmental construct: An evolutionary analysis. *Child Development, 63,* 753–773.

Main, M., Kaplan, N., & Cassidy, J. (1985). Security in infancy, childhood and adulthood: A move to the level of representation. In I. Bretherton & E. Waters (Eds.), Growing points of attachment theory and research. *Monographs of the Society for Research in Child Development, 50*(Serial No. 209), 66–104.

Main, M., & Solomon, J. (1986). Discovery of a new,insecure-disorganized/disoriented attachment pattern. In T. B. Brazelton & M. Yogman (Eds.), *Affective development in infancy* (pp. 95–124). Norwood, NJ: Ablex.

Main, M., & Solomon, J. (1990). Procedures for identifying infants as disorganized/disoriented during the Ainsworth Strange Situation. In M. T. Greenberg, D. Cicchetti, & E. M. Cummings (Eds.), *Attachment in the preschool years* (pp. 121–160). Chicago: University of Chicago Press.

Mangelsdorf, S., Gunnar, M., Kertenbaum, R., Lang, S., & Andreas, D. (1990). Infant proneness to distress, temperament, and maternal personality and mother–infant attachment. *Child Development, 68,* 820–831.

Neuman, J., & Goldberg, S. (1990, April 1). *Temperament and attachment: Health and illness.* Presented at the International Conference on Infant Studies, Montreal.

NICHD Early Child Care Network. (1997). The effects of early child care on infant–mother security: Results of the NICHD Study of Early Child Care. *Child Development, 68,* 860–879.

Pederson, D. R., & Moran, G. (1995). A categorical description of infant–mother relationships in the home and its relation to Q-sort measures of infant–mother interaction. In E. Waters, B. Vaughn, G. Posada, & K. Kondo-Ikemura (Eds.), Caregiving, cultural and cognitive perspectives on secure-base behavior and working models. *Monographs of the Society for Research in Child Development, 60*(2–3, Serial No. 244), 111–133.

Renken, B., Egeland, B., Marvinney, D., Mangelsdorf, S., & Sroufe, L. A. (1989) Early childhood antecedents of aggression and passive-withdrawal in early elementary school. *Journal of Personality, 57,* 257–281.

Seifer, R., Schiller, M, Sameroff, A. J., Resnick, S., & Riordan, K. (1996). Attachment, maternal sensitivity and temperament during the first year of life. *Developmental Psychology, 32,* 12–25.

Spangler, G., & Grossmann, K. E. (1993). Biobehavioral organization in securely and insecurely attached infants. *Child Development, 64,* 1439–1450.

Spangler, G., & Schieche, M. (1998). Emotional and adrenocortical responses of infants to the Strange Situation: The differential function of emotional expression. *International Journal of Behavioural Development, 22,* 681–706.

Sroufe, L. A., Egeland, B., & Carlson, E. A. (1999). One social world: The integrated development of parent–child and peer relationships. In W. A. Collin & B. Laursen (Eds.), *Relationships as developmental contexts: Minnesota Symposium on Child Psychology* (Vol. 30, pp. 241–261). Hillsdale, NJ: Erlbaum.

Sroufe, L. A., & Waters, E. (1977). Heart rate as a convergent measure in clinical and developmental research. *Merrill–Palmer Quarterly, 23,* 3–27.

Susman-Stillman, A., Kalkoske, M., Egeland, B., & Waldman, I. (1996). Infant temperament and maternal sensitivity as predictors of attachment security. *Infant Behavior and Development, 19,* 33–47.

Thompson, R. A. (1997). Sensitivity and security: Questions to ponder. *Child Development, 68,* 595–597.

Thompson, R. A. (1999). Early attachment and later development. In J. Cassidy & P. R. Shaver (Eds.), *Handbook of attachment* (pp. 265–286). New York: Guilford Press.

van IJzendoorn, M. H., Dijkstra, J., & Bus, A. G. (1995). Attachment, intelligence, and language: A meta-analysis. *Social Development, 4,* 115–128.

van IJzendoorn, M. H., & Kroonenberg, P. (1988). Cross-cultural patterns of attachment: A meta-analysis of the Strange Situation. *Child Development, 58,* 147–156.

van IJzendoorn, M. H., Schuengel, C., & Bakermans-Kranenburg, M. J. (1999). Disorganized attachment in early childhood: Meta-analysis of precursors, concomitants and sequelae. *Development and Psychopathology, 11,* 225–249.

Vaughn, B. E., Lefever, G. B., Siefer, R., & Barglow, P. (1989). Attachment behavior, attachment security and temperament during infancy. *Child Development, 60,* 728–737.

Vaughn, B. E., Stevenson-Hinde, J., Waters, E., Kotsaftis, A., Lefever, G. B., Sdhouldice, A., Trudel, M., & Belsky, J. (1992). Attachment security and temperament in infancy and childhood: Some conceptual clarifications. *Developmental Psychology, 28,* 463–473.

Waters, E. (1978). The reliability and stability of individual differences in infant–mother attachment. *Child Development, 49,* 483–494.

Waters, E., & Deane, K. E. (1985). Defining and assessing individual differences in attachment relationships: Q-methodology and the organization of behavior in infancy and early childhood. In I. Bretherton & E. Waters (Eds.), Growing points of attachment theory and research. *Monographs of the Society for Research in Child Development, 50*(1–2, Serial No. 209), 41–64.

Waters, E., Merrick, S., Treboux, D., Crowell, J., & Albersheim, L. (2000). Attachment security in infancy and early adulthood: A twenty year longitudinal study. *Child Development, 71,* 684–689.

Weinfield, N. S., Sroufe, L. A., & Egeland, B. (2000). Attachment from infancy to early adulthood in a high risk sample: Continuity, discontinuity, and their correlates. *Child Development, 71,* 695–702.

IV

Learning and Attention

12

Learning and Memory in Infancy

Habituation, Instrumental Conditioning,
and Expectancy Formation

JEFFREY W. FAGEN
PHYLLIS S. OHR

As every student of psychology knows, *learning* can be defined as a relatively permanent change in behavior which occurs as a result of practice or experience (Kimble, 1961). The process part of learning involves the acquisition of *information* which helps the organism adapt to his or her environment (Flaherty, 1985). When an organism responds in an adaptive way to a stimulus, *information processing* has occurred. Thus, "we can define learning as a potential change in behavior resulting from experience in processing information" (Walker, 1996, p. 4).

Although learning forms an integral part of cognitive and intellectual development, its exact role remains unclear, and researchers do not always agree on what behaviors of the neonate and young infant fit accepted definitions of the phenomenon. In this chapter, we review theory and research in three areas of assessment of infant learning: habituation, expectancy formation, and instrumental conditioning. These areas hold the most promise for assisting researchers and clinicians in assessing the biobehavioral integrity of the newborn and young infant. Individual differences in these areas are not simply "error variance" but relate to individual differences in underlying processes important to an optimal developmental outcome.

The chapter begins with a detailed look at habituation, focusing on the process of habituation, some of the variables which account for individual differences in habituation, and the relation between infant habituation and later intelligence. Missing from this section is an analysis of the infant's behavior to novel stimuli following habituation. As will become clear in that section, although the recovery of responding following habituation may be meaningful (but see Colombo, 1993, p. 104), we believe that this phenomenon has little if anything to do with learning. Expectancy formation, the newest area of research, appears to occur in both habituation and instrumental conditioning, although for opposite adaptive reasons for the infant. Thus, this section forms a natural bridge between studies of habituation and studies of instrumental conditioning. It appears that a major reason why both infant habituation and expectancy formation are predictive of later intellectual development is that they both tap individual differences in the speed with which the infant can process information. Infants' ability to retrieve expectancies is also related to their later intellectual development and together, speed of processing and memory may be the threads that tie habituation, learned expectancies, and instrumental conditioning together as indices of cognitive development.

HABITUATION

History

Habituation refers to the decrease in a response due to the repeated or continuous presentation of the stimulus that *elicits* the response. The utility of habituation as a procedure for studying infant development is directly tied to the theoretical accounts used to explain it. Several explanations of habituation exist, but a complete review is beyond the scope of this chapter. However, two prominent explanations deserve discussion: Sokolov's (1963) neuronal model and Groves and Thompson's (1970) dual-process theory.

Sokolov (1963) proposed that a perceived stimulus will elicit an orienting response which can be defined as "a generalized system of responses which includes central, motor and ANS [autonomic nervous system] components that enhance stimulus reception" (Graham, 1973, p. 166). Repeated presentation of the same stimulus in the same context leads to the construction of an internal representation of the stimulus (a neuronal template or engram) to which subsequent stimulus encounters are compared. This comparison process continues until a match occurs between the incoming stimulus information and the internal template. Once the match is complete, habituation occurs and attention is directed elsewhere. As noted by Colombo (1993), Sokolov's model was unclear regarding why an infant would ever stop orienting to a stimulus prior to the completion of the engram-forming process. To clarify this problem, several investigators of infant habituation (e.g., Jeffrey & Cohen, 1971; Olson, 1976) have proposed that infants process only a small amount of stimulus information during any given orienting response with more salient aspects of the stimulus encoded first.

Sokolov's model assumes that the comparison process that occurs between the current and prior representations of the stimulus is based on some memory process. This has led directly to tests of infant "recognition memory" based on the renewal of the habituated response when the infant is presented with a novel stimulus. Fagen and Rovee-Collier (1982) have argued, however, that procedures that rely on altered attention are more parsimoniously explained via conceptualizations than those based on memory processing. For example, Spear (1973) proposed that orienting toward novel cues distracts the organism's attention away from familiar cues in the environment that may potentially serve to cue the retrieval of stored memories. With infants, Jeffrey (1976) proposed that the infant's response to a novel stimulus is a simple, perceptual processing strategy with no memorial implications. Rovee-Collier and Hayne (1987) have also pointed out that Sokolov's explanation of habituation as involving the formation of an engram of the repeatedly presented stimulus makes no sense from a functional point of view. "What is the point of encoding and storing information about an event that will not be attended to again until it is forgotten?" (Rovee-Collier & Hayne, 1987, p. 187).

A non-memory-based theory of habituation has been proposed by Groves and Thompson (1970). This "dual-process theory" assumes that novel stimuli have two distinctly different effects on an organism, each of which occurs in a separate biological system. On the one hand, a stimulus elicits a specific response through a stimulus–response (S-R) reflex arc. This "habituation" pathway is a direct route through the nervous system from the stimulus to the response which leads to a decrease in responsiveness with repeated or prolonged stimulus presentations. On the other hand, a stimulus also has a generalized arousing or sensitizing effect through its action on the part of the central nervous system that modulates the organism's state. This "sensitization" process has the opposite effect from the habituation process in that it leads to an increase in general arousal, making the organism more responsive to any stimulus that is perceived while in this heightened state. The behavioral changes seen across repeated trials of stimulus presentations reflect the transaction of the hypothetical processes of habituation and sensitization.

To explain why the habituation and sensitization processes do not simply cancel each other out, Groves and Thompson (1970) proposed that the sensitization process is short-lived compared to the habituation process. Furthermore, sensitization, but not habituation, is presumed to be highly dependent on the strength of the stimulus. Early in the habituation sequence, especially with a strong stimulus, sensitization will be greater than habituation. This difference will result in an increase in responsiveness over the first few stimulus presentations in spite of the fact that the habituation process is also taking place. As sensitization rapidly wanes, the habituation process becomes dominant and responding decreases.

General Description

One way to appreciate the utility of studying habituation in infants is by briefly discussing what habituation is not. Habituation does not refer to *any* loss of responding due to repeated stimulus presentations. Were an infant to stop responding to a repeatedly presented stimulus due to fatigue or either the sensory inputs responsible for perceiving the stimulus or the effector outputs necessary for the infant to respond, it would be of little interest to psychologists. Although overtly the change in behavior produced by sensory or effector fatigue may look identical to the change resulting from habituation, clearly it is unrelated to learning. Also, it is important to keep in mind that habituation refers to the diminution of a specific response. Several years ago, for example, Brackbill (1973) demonstrated that continuous auditory, visual, proprioceptive–tactile, and temperature stimulation produced reductions in 1-month-olds' heart rate, respiratory irregularity, and motor activity as well as an increase in the percentage of time the infants spent in various sleep states. Such global changes in behavior reflect the infant's attempt to deal effectively with the "overload" of stimulation on the nervous system rather than any learning.

Following habituation, an organism will once again respond to the stimulus if sufficient time has elapsed since habituation occurred. Such "spontaneous recovery" is of little interest because it does not rule out fatigue as an explanation for the original decline in behavior. There are, however, procedures for doing this. Presenting a novel stimulus prior to presenting the habituation stimulus will lead to a renewal of the habituated response. This *dishabituation* is central to understanding habituation as a simple form of learning because it clearly rules out sensory or effector fatigue as a plausible explanation for the change in behavior. Why dishabituation occurs, however, is poorly understood. From the perspective of dual-process theory, dishabituation may not result from the renewal of habituation per se but may, instead, reflect the recovery of responsiveness due to the renewal of sensitization (Thompson & Glanzman, 1976). This view leads directly to the conclusion that studies of infants that use the recovery of the habituated response to a novel stimulus as an indication that the infant is somehow comparing the novel stimulus with an engram of the familiar one are, in actuality, measuring the sensitization elicited by the novel stimulus (see also Bieber, Kaplan, Rosier, & Werner, 1997). A second way of ruling out fatigue is to change an aspect of the stimulus to which the infant has habituated. The recovery of the habituated response in this instance is of special interest to infant researchers because it can be used to measure the infant's ability to discriminate small changes in the details of a stimulus. A third technique that has not been widely used with either human infants or other organisms produces a recovery in the habituated response by changing the context in which the stimulus has been presented while not changing the details of the eliciting stimulus itself (cf. Marlin & Miller, 1981). With recent research showing that infants are sensitive to changes in the context in which events take place (see, e.g., Rovee-Collier & Shyi, 1992), the study of the effects of contextual changes on infant habituation seems warranted.

Biobehavioral Basis of Assessment

What does habituation to a repeatedly presented visual stimulus tell us about the biobehavioral integrity of the infant? We begin with the assumption that the habituation process reflects the infant's attempt to process the information contained in a stimulus and to learn from it. What the infant learns is that the stimulus has no current ecological significance. This allows the infant to be ready to process additional stimuli that may, by their associations with biologically or socially important events, have meaning (Kaplan, Werner, & Rudy, 1990). Normally developing infants are "built" to cease responding to *irrelevant stimuli*. The extent to which an infant cannot successfully accomplish this rudimentary task may be a general measure of the infant's risk status as well as put the infant at risk for developmental failures. Thus, the infant who perseverates too long on a stimulus may not be ready to process when an important stimulus appears. On the other hand, the infant who habituates without processing all the information in a stimulus may miss something meaningful in that stimulus.

Reliability and Validity

Several reviews of the literature on infant habituation exist (e.g., Bornstein, 1985; Colombo, 1993; Colombo & Mitchell, 1990; Malcuit, Pomerleau, & Lamarre, 1988; Olson & Sherman, 1983; Rovee-Collier, 1987), almost all of which have focused on the infant's habituation to visual stimuli.

Which aspect of visual habituation to use as a predictor of risk has been the focus of much debate (see, e.g., Bornstein, 1985; Colombo, 1993; Colombo & Mitchell, 1990; McCall, 1994; McCall & Mash, 1995). The debate is complicated by the fact that some studies of habituation present the infant with a fixed number of habituation trials whereas others keep presenting the stimulus to the infant until his or her responding meets a criterion of attentional decline. The latter has been defined by either the absolute duration of one or more fixations (e.g., two trials ≤ 4 seconds each) or the duration of one or more fixations relative to the duration of the initial fixations (e.g., two consecutive fixations < 50% of the first two fixations). In general, early studies of infant habituation were of the fixed-trial type, whereas in more recent studies, each trial is fixed by the experimenter or determined by how long the infant keeps looking at the stimulus. Similarly, the intertrial interval has sometimes been fixed by the experimenter or else determined

by when the infant looks back toward the place where the habituation stimulus is presented. (For more detailed discussion of these procedural issues,
see reviews by Bornstein, 1985; Colombo, 1993; Colombo & Mitchell, 1990;
Horowitz, Paden, Bhana, & Self, 1972; Olson & Sherman, 1983.)

In general, investigators have used quantitative dependent measures
based on either the number of trials to achieve a habituation criterion or the
duration of attention (e.g., the duration of initial fixations on or toward the
stimulus, the duration of the longest look(s), the total looking time during
habituation). Qualitative measures designed to describe the shape or pattern
of the habituation function have also been used.

Given the theoretical accounts of habituation presented previously, it
would seem that *habituation rate* should serve well as a simple and straightforward measure of the progress of the engram forming or habituation processes.
The usefulness of this measure for assessing the influence of sensitization is,
however, questionable (Kaplan & Werner, 1991). The assumption behind the
utility of measures of habituation rate has generally been that with respect to
individual infants, faster or greater is better. Investigators of habituation rate
have typically either used an infant's actual number of trials to criterion as
their dependent measure or, when a fixed number of trials have been used, the
magnitude of response decrement across trials. Regardless of how rate has
been operationalized, the end result has generally been to classify infants into
groups such as "nonhabituators," "slow habituators," or "fast habituators."

Part of the logic behind using habituation rate as a dependent measure
of the underlying habituation process rests on the assumption that older infants should habituate faster than younger infants. However, Colombo and
Mitchell (1990) have reported that older infants actually required more trials
to achieve a 50% decrement criterion than did younger infants (cf. Lewis,
1969). In addition, the slope of the habituation function, which theoretically
should become steeper with age, actually showed the reverse trend (see also
Bornstein & Benasich, 1986; McCall, 1979). On the other hand, Colombo and
Mitchell found that several measures of *fixation duration* (e.g., total looking
time across trials and the duration of the longest fixation) all showed the expected decline with age. Furthermore, this decline was more rapid in infants
whose mothers were more highly educated. These findings led Colombo
(1993; Colombo & Mitchell, 1990) to propose that fixation duration is the
preferred metric with which to assess individual differences in infants'
habituability.

Using fixation duration as a method of quantifying the infant visual habituation function leads to classifications of infants as either "long lookers"
or "short lookers." Colombo (1993) has also pointed out the not so obvious
fact that differences in habituation rate with criterion-based procedures are
largely attributable to differences in duration measures.

A third method of measuring infant habituation does not rely on quantitative measures such as rate or duration but instead attempts to capture the

habituation pattern. McCall (1979) identified 44% of infants exhibiting a linear, monotonically decreasing pattern, but 44% exhibited peak fixations on later trials, which then declined (see Figure 12.1). McCall (1979) pointed out that based on measures of rate of habituation typically employed with fixed trial procedures, infants in these latter clusters would have erroneously been classified as nonhabituators because there was no difference in their fixation durations between the first and last trials. It should also be noted that the habituation patterns of infants in these clusters fit nicely with the non-monotonic function predicted by two-process theory.

Although McCall (1979) used a fixed number of habituation trials, his results are relevant to interpretations of data from criterion-based experiments. Because all three clusters showed identical declines in attention following their longest fixation, it can be assumed that the rate of habituation per se did not differ among them. What did differ, however, was the number of short-duration fixations that preceded the infants' longest fixation. Bornstein and Benasich (1986) obtained similar results using a criterion-based habituation procedure with 5-month-old infants. Participants were tested in two sessions, 10 days apart. They found that they were able to classify each infant's habituation pattern into one of three categories: approximately 60% were labeled "exponential decrease" (looking declined monotonically from its initial level to the criterion), approximately 10% were labeled "increase–decrease" (looking increased from its initial level before decreasing to the criterion), and approximately 30% were labeled "fluctuating" (looking that showed at least two reversals of direction and at least one fixation higher than baseline and/or lower than criterion). Furthermore, 66% of the participants had their habituation patterns classified into the same category across the two experimental sessions.

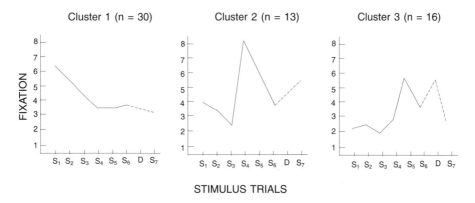

FIGURE 12.1. Patterns of habituation in 5-month-old infants. From McCall (1979). Copyright 1979 by the American Psychological Association. Reprinted by permission.

It is becoming increasingly clear that individual differences in infant habituation are moderately related to individual differences in cognitive performance in later childhood (see Bornstein & Sigman, 1986; Colombo, 1993;
Colombo & Mitchell, 1990; McCall & Carriger, 1993; McCall & Mash, 1995;
Slater, 1995; for review). For example, McCall and Carriger (1993) reported
an average correlation of .39 between various measures of infant habituation
and childhood cognition obtained in 10 studies. Similarly, Colombo (1993)
reported an average correlation of .48 between measures of fixation duration
during infant habituation tasks and various standardized measures of childhood cognition obtained in 11 studies. The magnitude of the correlations obtained in these studies did not change as a function of either the age during
infancy when the habituation task was administered or the age during childhood when the cognitive assessment was made.

The reliability of the measures of infant habituation is far below what
would typically be acceptable for an assessment instrument. Bornstein and
Benasich (1986), for example, reported the mean test–retest reliability of habituation aggregated over six sets of conditions in five separate studies to be
only .44. Similarly, data summarized by Colombo (1993) revealed an average
within-session test–retest correlation of .53 for six studies which compared
various measures of fixation duration during habituation in 3- to 4-month-
old infants. Five other studies summarized by Colombo (1993) yielded an
average between-session (1 week) test–retest correlation of .46 for infants
ranging in age from 3 to 7 months. These reliability coefficients are too small
to permit the accurate diagnosis of an individual infant based solely on his
or her habituation performance. If, however, the test–retest reliability of infant habituation could be increased to the .80–.90 level typical of the standardized childhood tests, the predictive correlation to childhood IQ could
easily rise to .70–.80, making habituation a useful diagnostic tool. As McCall
(1994) concluded:

> These results [the infancy to childhood correlations] are more important
> theoretically than practically. From a practical standpoint, the level of cor-
> relation is still too modest for the diagnosis of individuals, and the correla-
> tion is not higher than for parental socioeconomic status (SES), which is
> much easier to assess (McCall & Carriger, 1993). Theoretically, however,
> this research represents one of the first replicable, relatively substantial
> predictions from specific behaviors assessed on infants, and therefore, it
> may reveal an underlying and stable process that mediates mental devel-
> opment. (pp. 107–108)

Developmental Model

Two key questions of concern to infant researchers have been the following:
(1) Are newborns capable of habituation? and (2) How does habituability
change in the months from birth? In one of the earliest studies with new-

borns, Haith (1966) attempted to demonstrate habituation of the "Bronstein effect" (the suppression of nonnutritive sucking in response to stimulation). No habituation was found after 12, 10-second trials with a set of lights illuminated in a series to give the impression (at least to adults) of movement. This and similar findings led Jeffrey and Cohen (1971) to conclude the following: "Habituation is not readily obtained in the neonate. . . . By 2 to 3 months of age, however, habituation of orienting behavior is clearly observable" (p. 92). However, research by Friedman and colleagues (Friedman, 1975; Friedman, Bruno, & Vietze, 1974) and Slater, Morrison, and Rose (1982, 1984) indicates that this conclusion, which was based primarily on studies using a fixed number of habituation trials, was premature. Evidence of the ability of newborn infants to habituate also comes from an ingenious study of habituation to repeated tactile stimulation in human fetuses who were between 28 and 37 weeks gestational age (Madison et al., 1986).

There has been surprisingly little research on the question of how habituation changes with age. A notable exception has been the research by Colombo and colleagues (see Colombo & Mitchell, 1990) that included a group of infants tested longitudinally at 3, 4, 7, and 9 months of age as well as separate cross-sectional groups tested at these same ages. As noted earlier, this study found that the number of trials to reach the 50% habituation criterion increased with age and the slope of the infants' habituation function became shallower. What did decrease with age, however, was the duration of fixation time. Because the criterion of habituation is based on the duration of the infant's earliest fixations, Colombo and Mitchell (1990) concluded that the age-related increase in the number of trials to criterion as well as the flattening of the habituation function were due to the decline in fixation duration. In other words, it is "easier" for an infant with initially long fixations to meet the criterion, and this infant's habituation function is likely to be quite steep.

Given the theoretical accounts that habituation is related to central nervous system integrity (Groves & Thompson, 1970; Sokolov, 1963; Thompson & Spencer, 1966) it is not surprising to find that researchers have investigated the efficacy of using the habituation paradigm for possible diagnostic and predictive purposes (see Lewis & Brooks-Gunn, 1984; Mayes, Bornstein, Chawarska, & Granger, 1995; Zelazo, Weiss, Papageorgiou, & Laplante, 1989).

At-Risk Infants

The bulk of the research investigating the habituation performance of high-risk infants has used the preterm population, a readily identifiable group of infants at risk for developmental delay. A common assertion is the pre- and perinatal complications accompanying prematurity may account for neurologically based differences in responsivity that, in turn, affect habituation performance. Preterm infants may display either a hyposensitivity or a hypersensitivity to novel stimuli depending on the different levels of maturity in various sensory or response systems (Field, Dempsey, Hatch, Ting, & Clifton, 1979).

Many studies comparing the responses of preterm and full-term infants during habituation have determined that given sufficient trials, preterm infants can reliably reach a habituation criterion. Regarding various other aspects of habituation, however, no consistent patterns of responding have been obtained, with strong indications that performance may vary in complex and interacting ways as a function of socioeconomic status (e.g., Cohen, 1981), complexity of the habituation stimuli (e.g., Field et al., 1979), and concomitant medical complications (e.g., Fox & Lewis, 1983; Landry, Leslie, Fletcher, & Francis, 1985; Vervloed, 1995).

Field et al. (1979) proposed that difficulties demonstrated by preterm infants during habituation may reflect a lack of integration between cardiac and behavioral response systems. They presented healthy full-term and high-risk preterm newborns with both auditory (buzzer, rattle) and tactile (plastic filament) stimuli. Both groups demonstrated behavioral and cardiac increases, but only the full-term infants reliably demonstrated both cardiac and behavioral decrements during habituation. The preterms showed behavioral response decrements but not cardiac decrements. Field et al. (1979) concluded that as task complexity increases, the preterm infant is less able to integrate different response systems, possibly due to immaturity. In support of this, clear differences regarding preterm and full-term performance during habituation have been obtained with increases in task complexity (see, e.g., Rose & Orlian, Chapter 13, this volume; Rose, Feldman, McCarton, & Wolfson, 1988a; Rose, Feldman, & Wallace, 1988b; Rose, Feldman, Wallace, & McCarton, 1989).

Only a handful of studies have examined habituation in other neurologically compromised groups. Whereas prematurity is a clearly identifiable risk condition, other neurologically at-risk conditions may not be recognizable as soon after birth. One exception is Down syndrome, a disorder with clear evidence of neurological insult which affects current and subsequent cognitive functioning. Most of the research has used habituation procedures with complex stimuli or paired-comparison techniques in order to demonstrate differences in "visual information processing" (e.g., Fantz, Fagan, & Miranda, 1975; Miranda & Fantz, 1973, 1974).

Cohen (1981) used a simple visual habituation paradigm to detect differences between infants with Down syndrome and normally developing infants at 19, 23, and 28 weeks. The infants with Down syndrome differed from the normally developing infants in two ways (i.e., in all three age groups the infants with Down syndrome had significantly longer fixation times and the pattern of habituation and dishabituation differed). At 19 weeks their fixation time decreased temporarily to meet the habituation criterion but increased again during posthabituation trials. Only at 28 weeks did the infants with Down syndrome show both habituation and response recovery to a novel stimulus. Cohen concluded that the habituation paradigm can differentiate between normally developing infants and those with Down syndrome.

Lewis and Brooks-Gunn (1984) also investigated habituation in a group of neurologically compromised 3- to 7-month-old infants diagnosed with Down syndrome. They found that in general, response decrement did not occur in the majority of infants in this age group and initial fixation times were quite low. Lewis and Brooks-Gunn further determined that regardless of diagnosis, infants with higher mental functioning showed more rapid habituation than those with lower mental functioning.

The impaired motor ability of infants with cerebral palsy makes traditional, motor-oriented assessment of cognitive functioning less than appropriate. McDonough and Cohen (1982) found that infants with cerebral palsy demonstrated habituation and discrimination of novel from familiar faces comparable to normally developing infants. Motor difficulties appeared, however, to contribute to considerably longer latencies to initial looking (cf. Vervloed, 1995). They found that infants with cerebral palsy took longer to orient their attention to the task but did not differ regarding how long they looked at the stimuli.

There has been some recent activity regarding the assessment of cognitive functioning of prenatally cocaine-exposed newborns and young infants. It has been suggested that early information processing may be compromised by disturbances in neurotransmitter regulation and fetal brain development believed to be associated with prenatal cocaine exposure (Mayes et al., 1995). In support of this, both Eisen et al. (1990) and Mayes, Granger, Frank, Schottenfield, and Bornstein (1993) found depressed habituation performance in cocaine-exposed neonates but not in 3-month-old, cocaine-exposed infants (Mayes et al., 1995). Interestingly, significantly more cocaine-exposed infants failed initially to attend to the habituation stimulus, a finding characteristic of other neurologically compromised groups of infants including preterms (e.g., Landry et al., 1985; Vervloed, 1995) and infants with cerebral palsy (e.g., Lewis & Brooks-Gunn, 1984; McDonough & Cohen, 1982).

In spite of the numerous studies examining habituation in preterms and the fewer studies using other groups of neurologically impaired infants, few conclusive statements can be made. Overall, the habituation performance of infants born preterm, drug exposed, or with cerebral palsy or Down syndrome differed within the same diagnostic group, between diagnostic groups, and from normally developing infants but did not show any consistent patterns of response deficit that would distinguish these compromised groups from normally developing infants. As suggested by several researchers who use a simple habituation paradigm to detect differences, more complex stimuli and procedures are necessary in order for the habituation procedure to be sensitive to differences. Interestingly, somewhat repeated findings of problems with recruiting attention across most diagnostic groups may have implications for later development, not in terms of overall cognitive functioning but in attention regulation.

Structural and/or Theoretical Constraints/Controversies

As previously discussed, research from several laboratories indicates that measures of infant habituation share a small but significant amount of variance with measures of childhood cognition. Why this is so, however, remains a mystery. In addressing this issue, Bornstein and Sigman (1986) suggested three possible models: continuity of identical behavior, continuity of developmental status, and continuity of underlying processes. The behaviors measured during habituation and those tapped by the standardized childhood tests (intelligence or verbal proficiency) are different; therefore, the first model cannot account for the obtained continuity. Continuity of developmental status implies that habituation and childhood cognition are based on different processes but there is continuity in the rate or level of development of these processes across age. Although possible, and hard to disprove, this explanation seems unlikely. Bornstein and Sigman (1986) claim that the repeated failure to obtain correlations between standardized tests of infant development such as the Bayley scales and childhood intelligence tests argues against this model.

There are several candidates for developmental processes that could be shared by both infant habituation and childhood cognition. These candidates include such things as general intelligence; the ability to initiate, sustain, and/or inhibit attention; motivation to explore novel or interesting events; and the speed or level of information processing. The latter explanation has been favored by most infant researchers (e.g., Bornstein, 1985; Colombo, 1993; Colombo & Mitchell, 1990).

Colombo (1993; Colombo & Mitchell, 1990) has been on the forefront of proposing that infant and later cognition are linked via individual differences in an underlying information-processing ability. Colombo's proposition rests on the fact that infants classified as "short lookers" based on their fixation times during habituation are more likely to score higher on childhood tests than are infants classified as "long lookers." Colombo assumes that the two types of infants do not differ in the *level or amount* of stimulus information processed; rather, they differ in their *speed* of processing. These differences may arise either as a result of "hardware" differences in the nervous system (e.g., neural conduction speed) or "software" differences (e.g., strategies for information intake).

McCall (1994; McCall & Mash, 1995) argues that rate of information processing may not be the underlying process that shares variance with later cognitive test scores. McCall bases his argument on the assumption that habituation itself (i.e., the processing of the information contained in the repeatedly presented stimulus) occurs quite rapidly, perhaps on a single trial or within a few seconds on an infant-controlled trial (see also Richards,

1988). What may be important about habituation is what the infant is doing before he or she takes a "long, hard look" at the stimulus and, what process is involved in causing the infant to shift attention to it. McCall makes a cogent argument that this process involves the ability to inhibit attention to, or to disengage from, stimuli in the surrounding environment which are presumably less salient than the habituation stimulus.

Training Requirements

The recently released second edition of the Bayley Scales of Infant Development (Bayley, 1993) contains two items that purportedly assess the infants' ability to habituate. On item 7, "Habituates to Rattle," the examiner presents the infant with five 10-second trials of a shaking rattle. Credit is given if the infant exhibits a decrease in an "alerting response." For item 26, "Habituates to a Visual Stimulus," the infant views two cross-shaped stimuli for 30 seconds. To receive credit on this item, the infant must display a decrease in attention. On neither item, however, is any attempt made to rule out fatigue as an explanation for the change in the infant's behavior; thus, it is questionable whether these items are tapping the infant's ability to habituate. Interestingly, if the infant "passes" item 26, the examiner immediately administers item 27, "Discriminates Novel Visual Pattern," in which the previously seen cross-shaped stimulus is paired with a circle. Credit is given for this item if the infant looks longer at the novel stimulus (the circle) during two 10-second trials. Consistent with our earlier discussion regarding separating habituation from fatigue, credit for item 26 should probably be given only if the infant also receives credit for item 27.

The amount of training required to study infant habituation to a visual stimulus depends on the dependent measure employed. The question to be answered is whether the infant is looking at the stimulus being presented. The simplest way to answer this question is to observe whether the infant's head and eyes are oriented in the general direction of the stimulus. This response is what the Bayley scales use. This "gross" measure of attention requires very little training. Most investigators, however, rely on the fact that the reflection of the stimulus can easily be seen by looking directly into the infant's eyes usually from a peephole located behind the stimulus (or the screen onto which the stimulus is being projected). This "corneal reflection technique" is easily learned with minimal practice. Investigators who are interested in exactly where on a stimulus an infant is fixating have incorporated infrared corneal reflection photography (e.g., Salapatek & Kessen, 1966) into the basic corneal reflection process (interrater reliability).

Implications

As we have seen, measures of habituation are predictive of current and future cognitive functioning. A better understanding of why this is so will only come when we have a better understanding of the underlying basis of habituation. Although most infant researchers base their interest in habituation on a Sokolovian model of engram formation, this may be a mistake: A more fruitful explanation may come from the Groves and Thompson two-process model. Data in support of the two-process model of infant habituation have been summarized by Kaplan et al. (1990) and Kaplan and Werner (1991). Kaplan et al. (1990) also pointed out that this model fits well with the extensive research conducted by Kandel and his associates that has investigated the biological underpinnings of habituation (see Kandel, 1991, for review). Using the sea slug *Aplysia*, Kandel has demonstrated that habituation and sensitization involve distinct neural mechanisms leading to decreases (habituation) and increases (sensitization) in different neurotransmitters. This commonality in the behavioral and biological approaches to our understanding of habituation holds much promise for using habituation as a tool for assessing the biobehavioral integrity of the young infant.

McCall's focus on the early part of the habituation function also shares important parallels with the two-process theory of habituation that proposes that sensitization, which occurs on early trials, must be suppressed or inhibited before the habituation process can take over. Conceivably, the different patterns of habituation noted by McCall, that again reflected individual differences in the number of trials prior to the infants' peak fixation, resulted from differences in sensitization. By this account, the presentation of a novel stimulus results in a change in the infant's state (sensitization) such that the infant shifts to a heightened state of arousal. Once in this state, the infant seeks out biologically or socially relevant information in the environment. Infants differ in the time it takes them to focus their attention on the stimulus being presented by the experimenter which is typically the only silent stimulus. Once attention shifts to the habituation stimulus, habituation rapidly occurs because the infant quickly learns that the stimulus lacks relevance or meaning. Thus, what may be important about the individual differences seen in infant habituation, at least with respect to their relation to later cognitive functioning, is that this procedure is tapping into differences in state- and attention-control processes. Presumably, these differences are developmentally stable and related, to some degree, to information intake and cognitive competence in childhood.

LEARNED EXPECTANCIES

What else might the infant learn in the typical habituation study apart from the fact that the repeatedly presented stimulus is of no consequence and thus attention should be directed elsewhere? One possibility is that over trials, the infant learns that a particular stimulus will disappear and reappear at a particular location. Furthermore, the infant may come to *anticipate* the occurrence of this event and may therefore form an *expectation* for it. Habituation studies, as currently conducted, do not allow for the direct assessment of the acquisition of learned expectancies by young infants. Studies of operant conditioning can be used for this purpose (see Fagen, 1993) and these are discussed in the next section.

History

The concept of expectancy has a long tradition in the psychology of learning (e.g., Tolman, 1932). Furthermore, expectancy plays a major role in modern theories of learning (e.g., Bolles, 1972, 1979; Dickinson, 1980; Rescorla, 1988) and has even been invoked to explain habituation (e.g., Wagner, 1976, 1979). Piaget's theory of sensorimotor development emphasized the roles of expectancy formation for accomplishing the cognitive tasks of early (e.g., circular reactions) and later (e.g., object permanence) infancy (Piaget, 1952).

General Description

In this section, we briefly review the pioneering work of Haith and his colleagues (e.g., Canfield & Haith, 1991; Haith, 1993, 1994; Haith, Wentworth, & Canfield, 1993) using what he calls the visual expectation paradigm (VExP). Studies of expectancy formation in early infancy can provide a window on the development of a basic component of cognitive functioning and also hold promise as an early means of predicting individual differences in later cognition.

The logic behind the VExP is straightforward. It is based on the infant's ability to learn a spatiotemporal pattern. The infant views a series of multicolored stimuli presented to the left or right of the center of the visual field. The stimuli can be presented to the infant in a regular (left–right–left–right, etc.) sequence with a constant interstimulus interval (ISI) or an irregular sequence with a variable ISI. The acquisition of an expectancy is inferred from the infant's behavior during the regular sequence where, presumably, the infant gradually realizes that the stimuli appear in a predictable pattern and can therefore anticipate the appearance of the stimuli. Typically, there are 30 to 70 repetitions of stimuli in a particular sequence (complete sequences can include over 120 stimulus presentations). The procedure is always videotaped for later coding. It takes between 3 to 4 minutes to complete. The task is done in a small, dark, quiet laboratory room with the parent present. Young infants (i.e., 2- to 3-month-olds) are typically tested while lying supine, whereas older infants are seated in either an infant seat or a parent's lap.

Two dependent measures of expectancy formation are typically scored from the videotapes. One is based on the infant's *anticipation*, that is, looking at the location where the stimulus should appear prior to its actual appearance (i.e., during the ISI). A second is used when the infant fails to anticipate the stimulus. This measure, *facilitation*, reflects the infant's rapid looking (fast reaction time) at the stimulus after it appears. Typically, facilitation is assessed by comparing the infant's *reaction time* (RT) during predictable conditions versus unpredictable ones (e.g., baseline).

Biobehavioral Basis of Assessment

Expectations are representations in memory formed from past experiences that guide future behaviors. Learned expectancies may be among the earliest forms of future-oriented processes to occur in infancy (Haith et al., 1993).

The ability to detect regularities in the environment, to form expectations based on those regularities, and to modulate activity based on those expectations provides the infant with important cognitive advantages. Rovee-Collier and Hayne (1987) have argued that memories are metabolically costly and that a storehouse for information about the past is not useful in and of itself. Rather, the utility of memories of the past lies in their potential for informing behavioral decisions regarding events that lie in the future (see also Fagen & Rovee-Collier, 1982).

Reliability and Validity

The measures of expectation used in the VExP, namely anticipations and reaction times, appear to possess a moderate amount of reliability and stability. Haith and McCarthy (1990) reported a median split-half correlation of .58 for reaction times (postbaseline) and .52 for anticipations for 3-month-olds given 60 trials across two sessions separated by an average of 4.3 days. Across sessions, the correlations for reaction times and anticipations were .48 and .34, respectively. Canfield, Wilken, Schmerl, and Smith (1995) investigated whether reaction times and anticipations were stable over a 2-month period (4 to 6 months). In addition to replicating the reliability data of Haith and McCarthy (1990), Canfield et al. (1995) obtained cross-age stability for both baseline ($r = .56$) and postbaseline ($r = .82$) reaction times. Individual differences in percent anticipation, however, were not stable across the 2-month period ($r = -.12$).

Three recent studies have found measures of infants' mastery of the VExP task to be related to later intellectual performance. DiLilla et al. (1990) obtained a significant negative correlation ($r = -.46$) between reaction time during the VExP at 8 months of age and the Stanford–Binet Intelligence Test administered at 3 years. The percent anticipation measure, however, was not predictive ($r = .04$). Benson, Cherny, Haith, and Fulker (1993) found that infants' reaction times were correlated with the average of their parents' IQ scores ($r = .47$). This midparent IQ score was considered to be a proxy for each infant's later IQ. Doughtery and Haith (1997) obtained correlations of

–.44 and .43 between reaction times and percent anticipations, respectively, at 3.5 months and 4-year full-scale IQ as measured by the Wechsler Preschool and Primary Scales of Intelligence (Revised). Together, reaction times and anticipations accounted for 28% of the variance ($R = .53$) in IQ. Infant reaction times were also correlated with childhood visual reaction times ($r = .51$). This latter finding suggests that there is a common and stable cognitive process akin to speed of information processing that is stable from infancy to the preschool years. Recall that Colombo (1993) proposed that speed of information processing is the mechanism underlying the finding that infants classified as "short lookers" in habituation studies tend to have higher IQs as children.

Developmental Model

The initial use of the VExP (Haith, Hazan, & Goodman, 1988) involved 3.5-month-old infants' ability to acquire an expectancy for a simple left–right spatiotemporal sequence. Each infant was exposed to a predictable sequence of 30 pictures consisting of schematic faces, bull's-eyes, checkerboards, diagonal stripes, and diamond shapes. Each picture appeared for 700 msec to the left or right of midline with an ISI of 1,100 msec. The infants were also exposed to 30 trials of the same stimulus in an irregular sequence (randomly determined left–right sequence) with ISIs varying among 900, 1,100, and 1,300 msec. The entire experiment lasted less than 2 minutes. As shown in Table 12.1, the median reaction times decreased from baseline during the alternating condition but not during the irregular condition. Furthermore, the percent anticipations were nearly twice as high during the alternating condition as compared to the irregular condition. Thus, both measures converged to indicate that the infants formed an expectation during the alternating condition.

In a later study, Canfield and Haith (1991) found that 3-month-olds, but not 2-month-olds, were capable of acquiring an expectation for a more complicated 2/1 sequence in which two pictures on the left were followed by one picture on the right (or vice versa). Both age groups successfully acquired a simple 1/1 (left–right) sequence similar to the one used by Haith et al. (1988). The 3-month-olds provided equivocal evidence, however, for the acquisition of a 3/1 series (left–left–left–right or vice versa); although their reaction times failed to decrease from baseline, and the percentages of anticipations did not differ during regular versus irregular conditions, the infants did show a higher likelihood of shifting their fixations after the third picture in the series as compared to the second or the first. Clear evidence of the ability of 3-month-olds to form expectancies for as many as four pictures in a series was obtained using a double-alternation (left–left–right–right or vice versa) sequence (Lanthier & Haith, 1993). Finally, the expectancies that infants acquire from simple left–right sequences appear to be transferable to

TABLE 12.1. Median Reaction Times and Percent
of Anticipations

Measure	Sequence	
	Alternating	Irregular
Reaction time		
Baseline	475 msec	462 msec
Postbaseline	391 msec	462 msec
Anticipations	22.1%	11.1%

Note. From Haith, Hazan, and Goodman (1988). Copyright
1988 by the Society for Research in Child Development.
Reprinted by permission.

other stimulus sets and motor acts (i.e., up–down sequences), at least by 3.5
months of age (Bihun, Hanebuth, & Haith, 1993). This last finding is important because it indicates that infants' expectations are based on simple rules
that govern their behavior in similar situations.

In a recent monograph, Canfield, Smith, Breznyak, and Snow (1997) reported the results of a longitudinal investigation in which 13 infants were
tested monthly with the VExP from 2 to 9 months of age and again when they
were 12 months of age to describe the developmental function for the age
changes in reaction times and anticipations. The study also addressed the important issue of the minimum latency required for an infant to initiate an eye
movement in the direction of a stimulus. This latency defines the cutoff between when an infant is reacting to the appearance of a stimulus versus his or
her anticipation of the appearance of the stimulus. Briefly, they found this latency to be 133 msec; substantially lower than the 200 msec used in previous
studies. This finding was based on an analysis of the infants' latency distributions, anticipation errors, and corrective eye movements. In addition, the minimum reaction time did not change significantly from 2 to 12 months of age.
The analysis of the developmental changes in mean reaction times indicated
that there was little change from 3 to 4 months of age, a period of rapid change
between 4 and 8 months, and a slowing of the rate of change until 12 months.
Overall, mean reaction time decreased monotonically from a mean of 440
msec at 2 months to 285 msec at 12 months. Variability in reaction time also declined with age. This decline was independent of that seen in the mean reaction time, suggesting that variability in performance is a separate measure
that may be worth a more detailed investigation. In the period from 2 to 5
months there was little age-to-age stability in reaction times when the span of
time between assessments was greater than 1 month. However, this picture
changed in the 6- to 12-month period when the median correlation for
nonadjacent months rose to .70. Virtually no stability was obtained for the
variability measure. This must be qualified, however, by the limited power in
this study that, as mentioned previously, contained only 13 infants. Most disappointing was the finding that anticipatory responses that are theoretically

expectancy driven showed a predicted increase over the early portion of the age span studied, but then declined sharply between the 9- and 12-month assessments. This is probably not the result of a decline in infants' abilities to anticipate the stimulus sequence, but rather of motivational changes in how interesting the infants found the task to be. When the 12-month data were removed from the analysis, there was virtually no evidence of any age-related change in anticipatory responses. In addition, there was little evidence of any stability, especially in the first 6 months.

Structural and/or Theoretical Constraints/Controversies

As with measures of infant habituation, young infants' abilities to form visual expectancies are related to their later IQ, but the reasons for this relation are unclear. Speed of information processing, which develops in a lawful manner during the first year (Canfield et al., 1997), appears to be a likely candidate; however, this variable may only explain part of the prediction. For one thing, the infant measures of reaction times and percent anticipations obtained by Dougherty and Haith (1997) were only weakly correlated ($r = -.35$). Also, Dougherty and Haith found that the infants' reaction times correlated better with performance IQ than with verbal IQ ($-.47$ vs. $-.29$) whereas the reverse was true for percent anticipations ($.24$ vs. $.53$). Percent anticipations, therefore, probably reflect something other than speed of information processing, something that is related to later verbal IQ. Dougherty and Haith proposed that percent anticipations tap stable individual differences in infants' memory abilities that will later be relevant to the acquisition of the types of knowledge (e.g., vocabulary) assessed by the subscales comprising the verbal component of IQ. Thus, two factors, speed of information processing and memory, may underlie the value of tasks such as habituation and VExP for assessing the biobehavioral integrity of the young infant (see also Colombo, 1993; Jacobson et al., 1992).

Training Requirements

The use of the VExP requires sophisticated equipment and extensive training. Anyone wishing to use this procedure would be wise to contact Dr. Marshall Haith at the University of Denver or one of his former students (e.g., Richard Canfield at Cornell University). Scoring of the videotapes is done on a frame-by-frame basis and is greatly facilitated by the use of one of two computer programs designed specifically for this purpose (Coder 2 or Super Kluge). Scoring does not rely on assessing the exact location of the infant's fixations, which is procedurally difficult; rather, only the latency and direction of the infant's eye movements need to be scored. Stimulus position, onset, and offset are known, and coders make judgments about whether and at what time pupils move to the location where the next stimulus should be, move to a different stimulus location while waiting for onset of stimulus (false anticipation), or do not move. It takes approximately 6 to 10 weeks to become a proficient coder who can obtain high interobserver reliability.

Implications

The question of how infants classified as "at risk" perform in the VExP has barely begun to be addressed. One recent report indicated that cocaine- and non-cocaine-exposed 6-month-old infants did not differ (Chawarska, Mayes, Reznick, & Miranda, 1997). Interestingly, drug-exposed infants were more likely to fail to complete the procedure.

The VExP is quite new and many basic issues need to be resolved. As Canfield et al. (1997) noted:

> The major problem seems to be that % ANT [percent anticipations] is not being measured with acceptable reliability. A possible way to increase the reliability would be to increase the absolute number of anticipations produced. As currently implemented, anticipations in the VExP are rare events. One likely reason is that the stimuli are not highly rewarding and there is little cost associated with not anticipating. The infant's rate of anticipation may reflect a personal cost/benefit analysis, the elements of which vary dramatically from one day to the next. Attempts to increase the reward value of the stimuli and make the reward contingent on anticipatory responses may increase the rate of anticipation and at the same time amplify individual and age differences in the ability to detect the contingencies. (pp. 125–126)

INSTRUMENTAL CONDITIONING

History

Like habituation, the study of instrumental conditioning has a long history in psychology. Instrumental as well as classical conditioning is dependent on the organism's detection of the contingency between environmental events. Specifically, instrumental conditioning involves the acquisition of information regarding a predictive relation between the organism's behavior and a stimulus, typically a reward.

Bolles (1972, 1979) has provided a useful theoretical framework for understanding instrumental conditioning. According to Bolles, when learning occurs, an organism acquires a direct appreciation of the new environment contingencies. What is learned is that certain cues (S) predict other consequences (S), S–S*. Organisms not only encounter stimulus contingencies but also contingencies between their behavior and its consequences. In other words, there may be a predictive relation between the organism's behavior

(R) and the consequences of responding (S*), an R–S* expectancy. Organisms can learn R–S* expectancies that represent and correspond to the R–S* contingencies in their environment. Finally, Bolles proposed a "law of performance" in which two expectancies of the form S–S* and R–S* are combined (S–R–S*) so that in the presence of cue S, the organism is likely to make response R because of the expectation of S*.

General Description

Habituation and expectancy formation aid the infant in organizing the environment and creating a simple knowledge base of the recurring yet unimportant stimuli around them. In both paradigms, however, the infant is a passive recipient of stimulation over which there is no direct control.

Instrumental conditioning tasks also provide a *direct* means of assessing infant memory. Although investigators have attempted to use habituation tasks for this purpose, as discussed earlier tasks such as habituation, which rely on novelty preference, are, at best, *indirect* assessments of memory (see also Fagen & Rovee-Collier, 1982; Jeffrey, 1976). On the other hand, a conditioning approach to the study of infant memory allows determination of the extent to which infants can use what they have learned. It is modeled after studies of animal memory in which the focus has been on the factors that affect retrieval. Infants can be trained to perform a distinctive response in a particular setting and can then be returned to that setting after a delay. Memory is evident when, following the delay, the infant once again performs the instrumental response above its pretraining level.

Biobehavioral Basis of Assessment

Earlier, we argued the instrumental conditioning involves the learning of expectancies. To illustrate this point, consider a study by Fagen, Morrongiello, Rovee-Collier, and Gekoski (1984) in which 3-month-old infants learned to move an overhead crib mobile by kicking one of their feet (mobile conjugate reinforcement; see Rovee & Rovee, 1969). Infants received four (Experiment 1) or three (Experiment 2) daily conditioning sessions. Each session contained a 9-minute period during which the infants' kicks moved the mobile. This period was sandwiched between 3-minute periods during which the infant could see the mobile but could not move it. These "nonreinforcement" periods established the infants' baseline rate of kicking (outset of Session 1) and, once learning occurred, were used to determine whether the infants persisted in making the operant response (kicking) in the absence of reinforcement (mobile movement). Fagen et al. (1984) randomly assigned infants to three (Experiment 1) or four (Experiment 2) groups defined by the mobile they received during each daily session. As shown in Figure 12.2, infants trained with the same mobile (Groups AAAA and AAA) or a different mobile (Groups ABCD and ABC) in each session exhibited increasing response rates at the outset of each session. However, infants exposed to a violation of the serial pattern of mobiles (Group ABCA, ABA) reduced their response rate when reexposed to the familiar Session 1 mobile (A) after being trained to expect a new reinforcer each day. Similarly, infants trained for 2 days to expect similarity (Group AAB) also reacted with reduced responding when a novel mobile was used. These data indicate that very young infants are capable of extracting a rule of consistency defined by the serial pattern with which events occur and furthermore, that this rule governs their expectancies. Fagen et al. (1984) concluded that such a rule must be a higher-order attribute, which served as a retrieval cue in the test session. In other words, when the rule was violated, the infants failed to show response transfer between sessions. Furthermore, the data from Experiment 2 indicate that as few as two encounters with an invariant or varying stimulus provides the infant with sufficient information to develop a reward expectancy. Consistent with Haith's work cited earlier, it appears that, like adults, infants attempt to find consistency in their world whenever possible and use the minimum amount of information to do so.

Reliability and Validity

There have been relatively few longitudinal studies of instrumental conditioning in infants. One study examined contingency acquisition and retention in 3-, 7-, and 11-month-old infants (Fagen & Ohr, 1990). At 3 months, infants were trained in the same mobile conjugate reinforcement task used by Fagen et al. (1984). At 7 months the infant was placed in a high chair and learned to activate a musical toy and a bank of 10 lights via an arm-pull response. At 11 months, a bar-press response activated this toy in a different enclosure containing a red and a green light. A different conditioning task was used at each age to accommodate the developing infant's motoric maturity and the fact that the effectiveness of various reinforcers used in infant conditioning studies changes with the age of the infants. The temporal parameters at each age, however, were similar. Specifically, the infants were trained on 2 consecutive days and each daily session consisted of a brief nonreinforcement period, a period of reinforced practice, and a final nonreinforcement period. Acquisition speed, or how fast the infant learned the contingency, was defined as the number of minutes necessary for the infant to achieve a level of responding greater than or equal to 150% of his or her baseline response rate. Following training, the infants received a retention test, 1, 7, or 14 days later. The procedure for the retention test was the same as during the two training sessions. Retention was measured at each age by calculating two scores for each infant (see Fagen & Rovee-Collier, 1982; Rovee-Collier, 1996). The first, the baseline ratio, indexed the percentage of the baseline response rate that the infants continued to exhibit during the

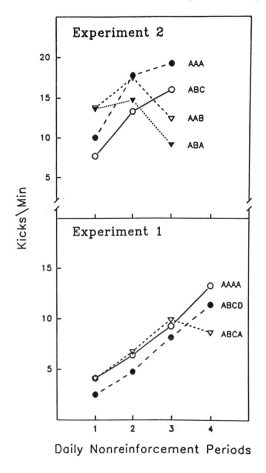

FIGURE 12.2. Changes in response rate of three (Experiment 1) and four (Experiment 2) groups of infants over successive 3-minute nonreinforcement periods given at the outset of three (Experiment 2) or four (Experiment 1) daily conditioning sessions. The letters designating the groups represent the mobile seen on each day. Adapted from Fagen, Morrongiello, Rovee-Collier, and Gekoski (1984). Copyright 1984 by the Society for Research in Child Development. Adapted by permission.

nonreinforcement phase at the outset of the retention test session. This is an all-or-none measure of retention; ratios greater than 1 indicate that responding following the retention interval continues to exceed baseline (i.e., retention) whereas ratios not greater than 1 reflect no retention. The second measure, the retention ratio, reflected the proportional change in responding between the nonreinforcement phases given at the end of the second session and the beginning of the third. As shown in Table 12.2, across age there was stability in the retention measures but not in the acquisition speed. Fagen and Ohr (1990) argued that the lack of stability in the acquisition speed measure was an artifact of the fact that the conditioning tasks used at each age were specifically chosen because they were "easy" and therefore there was little variability in this measure. Thus, the question of the utility of using acquisition speed as a measure of the infant's biobehavioral integrity remains open (see also Table 12.3).

Measures derived from instrumental conditioning tasks, especially those assessing long-term memory, have also been found to be predictive of intellectual performance in later childhood. Fagen and Ohr (1990) followed a group of children who had participated in their conditioning tasks at 3, 7, and 11 months of age (details of these tasks were discussed in the previous section). At 2 years of age, participants received a first administration of the Stanford–Binet Intelligence Scale. At 3 years of age, the Stanford–Binet was again administered along with the Kaufman Assessment Battery for Children (K-ABC) and the Peabody Picture Vocabulary Test (PPVT-R). The K-ABC and PPVT-R were administered again at 5 years of age.

The results of this study revealed that the rapidity with which the infants acquired the conditioning tasks (acquisition speed) was not correlated with the measures of preschool intelligence. On the other hand, the retention measures were consistently correlated with the various preschool intelligence measures (see Table 12.3). Average correlations between the infant memory measures (baseline and retention ratios) and the 2-, 3-, and 5-year assessments were .45, .40, and .38, respectively. These correlations are higher than those obtained between the Bayley Mental Development Index (MDI) at 3, 7, and 11 months and the preschool IQ scores. Specifically, the average MDI/IQ correlations were .35 at 2 years, .31 at 3 years, and .20 at 5 years. More important than the differences in the magnitudes of these correlations were the findings that our retention measures were uncorrelated with concurrent Bayley MDI scores ($r = .09$), indicating that the amount of shared variance between the MDI and memory measures and the preschool tests was unique.

TABLE 12.2. Stability Correlations

Measure	Ages (months)		
	3 to 7	7 to 11	3 to 11
Acquisition speed	.09	.18	−.07
Retention ratio	.31**	.39**	.10
Baseline ratio	.42**	.46**	.29*

Note. From Fagen and Ohr (1990). Copyright 1990 by Lawrence Erlbaum Associates, Inc. Reprinted by permission. Correlations for retention and baseline ratios are pooled within-cell correlations adjusted for retention interval.

*$p < .05$; **$p < .01$; two-tailed.

TABLE 12.3. Mean Correlations between Infant Memory Measures at 3, 7, and 11 Months and Intelligence Test Scores at 2, 3, and 5 Years

Intelligence test	Memory measure	
	Baseline ratio	Retention ratio
2 years		
Stanford–Binet	.41**	.49**
3 years		
Stanford–Binet	.37**	.42**
Kaufman	.34**	.40**
Peabody	.40**	.44*
5 years		
Kaufman	.31*	.38*
Peabody	.39**	.42**

Note. Correlations are pooled within-cell correlations adjusted for retention interval during infancy (1, 7, or 14 days).

$*p < .05; **p < .01$; two-tailed.

Developmental Model

Because the behavioral repertoire of the newborn is limited, researchers studying instrumental conditioning have capitalized on modifying responses associated with feeding (e.g., headturning and sucking). Furthermore, conditioning in the newborn is most successful when the operant is a low-energy response that does not habituate (Rovee-Collier & Lipsitt, 1982). Effective reinforcers, that is, what the newborn will "work" for, have not been similarly limited. For example, acoustic stimuli such as speech or music appear to be as effective as nutritive stimuli in reinforcing the behavior of the newborn. Furthermore, although older infants condition faster than younger ones, as discussed in the next section, speed of conditioning does not appear to be a stable or predictive measure of infant functioning.

Research by DeCasper and colleagues illustrates how adept newborn infants are at detecting the contingency between their behavior and the environment and at forming expectations (e.g., DeCasper & Fifer, 1980; DeCasper & Spence, 1986; see DeCasper & Spence, 1991, for review). This research capitalizes on the fact that when newborn infants suck on a nipple, their sucking occurs in groups or bursts that are separated from each other by distinct pauses (interburst interval [IBI]). DeCasper and colleagues differentially reinforce bursts of sucking that are immediately preceded by specific IBIs (see later). Awake newborns are fitted with earphones and a nonnutritive nipple is placed in their mouth. A baseline period of sucking is obtained to determine each infant's characteristic burst–pause pattern of sucking. During contingency training, infants can be assigned to groups which receive auditory reinforcement (e.g., a woman singing) for sucking bursts that occur after "long" or "short" IBIs (e.g., longer than the 70th percentile of an infant's baseline IBI distribution or shorter than the 30th percentile). Under these conditions, newborns not only appropriately modify their sucking pattern to match the contingency but maintain the modified pattern (i.e., remember) 20 hours after *in the absence of reinforcement* (DeCasper & Spence, 1991). They are also capable of successfully demonstrating a preference for one reinforcer (e.g., the mother's voice) for bursts following long IBIs and a different reinforcer (e.g., a strange women's voice) for bursts following short IBIs (DeCasper & Fifer, 1980; see Figure 12.3).

The IBI preference procedure has also been used to demonstrate that third-trimester human fetuses experience their mothers' speech sounds and remember the details of what they hear. DeCasper and Spence (1986) had pregnant women read a children's story out loud each day during the last 6 weeks of pregnancy. Following birth, sucking bursts above or below each infant's median baseline IBI were reinforced with a strange woman reciting either the familiar story or a novel story. The results revealed a clear preference for the story that the infants had heard *in utero*.

Newborn infants are also extremely sensitive to changes in the schedule of reinforcement. Kobre and Lipsitt (1972), for example, reinforced new-

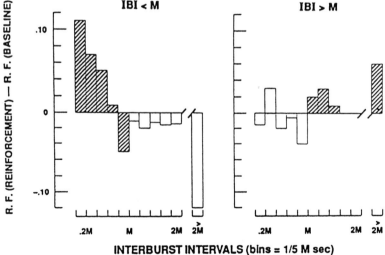

MOTHER VS. OTHER

FIGURE 12.3. Mean of the differences between the relative frequencies of interburst intervals (IBIs) occurring during baseline and reinforcement with the maternal (shaded bars) and nonmaternal (unshaded bars) voices. From DeCasper and Spence (1991). Copyright 1991 by Ablex Publishing Corporation. Reprinted by permission.

borns' sucking with alteration periods of water and 15% sucrose. The rate of sucking during water periods was lower than that seen in a control group reinforced only with water. The negative contrast effect reflects the "devaluation" of the water reward as a function of the fact that the infants had had prior experience with sucrose.

Temperament

Several recent studies have found that temperament shares a small amount of variance with measures of conditioning and memory. Three studies, for example, have investigated relations between parental reports of infant temperament and the performance of 1- to 3-month-old infants trained in the mobile conjugate reinforcement task discussed previously. Dunst and Lingerfelt (1985) failed to find any significant correlations between infants' rates of kicking and any of the nine temperament dimensions of the Carey and McDevitt Revised Infant Temperament Questionnaire (activity, rhythmicity, approach, adaptability, intensity, mood, persistence, distractibility, and threshold). Rhythmicity and persistence were, however, correlated with the rate of learning (rate of response during conditioning minus the rate during baseline) (average $r = .44$). Thus, faster conditioning occurred in infants rated by their mothers as (1) more predictable in terms of their daily sleeping and feeding patterns and (2) having longer "attention spans." In a similar study, Worobey and Butler (1988) also found that duration of orienting, as measured by Rothbart's Infant Behavior Questionnaire (IBQ) (see also Chapter 10, Rothbart, Chew, & Gartstein, this volume), was related to speed of conditioning (the number of minutes necessary to achieve a level of responding greater than or equal to 150% of an infant's baseline response rate) ($r = .23$). Speed of conditioning was also positively correlated with fear ($r = .30$) and negatively correlated with smiling and laughter ($r = -.25$). Fagen and Ohr (1990), however, failed to obtain significant correlations between speed of conditioning in the mobile conjugate reinforcement task and these, or any other, IBQ dimension (activity level, distress to limitations, soothability, and duration of orienting).

Worobey and Butler (1988) used a second conditioning session which allowed them to investigate relations between temperament and memory for the contingency. However, none of the correlations between the infants' baseline or retention ratios and the six IBQ temperament dimensions (activity level, smiling and laughter, fear, distress to limitations, soothability, and duration of orienting) was significant. In a similar study, Fagen and Ohr (1990) found only a single significant correlation: activity level correlated .23 with the retention ratio.

Other research from our laboratory has examined the relation between infant temperament, as measured by the IBQ, and crying during instrumental conditioning. In our first study (Fagen & Ohr, 1985), infants were trained with the mobile conjugate reinforcement task to produce movement in an overhead crib mobile containing 10 components and were subsequently shifted to a mobile containing only two of these components during a third daily conditioning session. This change in mobile reinforcers led to crying in 55% of the infants. Comparisons of the maternal ratings on the six IBQ scales indicated that the criers were rated as more active and fearful than the noncriers. A stepwise discriminant function analysis revealed that these two measures of temperament, plus the duration of orienting and the number of reinforced footkicks, reliably predicted membership in these two groups ($R = .42$). Fagen, Ohr, Singer, and Fleckenstein (1987) examined the relation between temperament and the failure to complete the 2-day training phase of the mobile conjugate reinforcement task because of continuous crying. A discriminant function analysis revealed that female infants who cried could be discriminated from those who did not based on IBQ scores for duration of orienting and fear ($R = .36$). No reliable discriminant function was obtained for males.

The picture that emerges from the foregoing studies is far from clear. The obtained correlations seem to be fleeting and inconsistent. On the other hand, it would be wrong to conclude that individual differences in temperament have no relation to instrumental conditioning performance. There is a small amount of variance in contingency acquisition and retention that can be accounted for by various aspects of individual differences in infant temperament.

At-Risk Infants

As with habituation, the majority of the research on instrumental conditioning in at-risk infants has focused on preterm infants and infants with Down syndrome. One of the first studies to be done with either group was by Solkoff and Cotton (1975). These investigators used a modified version of the mobile conjugate reinforcement task with preterm neonates. Although the authors reported that there was some evidence of conditioning, no data or statistics were presented. Rovee-Collier and Lipsitt (1982) have pointed out that the general negative results obtained by Solkoff and Cotton are not too surprising in light of the response chosen as the operant. As discussed earlier, Rovee-Collier and Lipsitt concluded that high-energy responses such as kicking typically are not conditionable during the neonatal period. It is not until after the first month of life, when the infant achieves psychological control over body temperature, that these responses are appropriate. Support for the hypothesis that young preterm infants can be successfully conditioned, provided that a low-energy response is chosen as the operant, comes from a study by Werner and Sequeland (1978) in which the illumination of a visual stimulus was contingent upon nonnutritive, high-amplitude sucking.

A study by Thoman and Ingersoll (1993) indicates that certain non-low-energy but high-frequency responses in the preterm neonate can be instrumentally conditioned. Experimental infants at 33 weeks conceptional age learned to approach and achieve contact with a "breathing" teddy bear placed inside their isolettes. Unlike the experimental infants, control infants for whom the bear did not "breathe" showed no change in either the total contact time with the stimulus or the latency to contact the bear following intervention by a caregiver. This study is also notable because the contingency was in place throughout a 2 week period. In most instrumental conditioning studies with both nonrisk and at-risk infants, the infants are only tested for a few minutes usually on only 1 day.

Although the studies by Solkoff and Cotton (1975), Werner and Sequeland (1978), and Thoman and Ingersoll (1993) used preterm infants, none contrasted the preterms' performance with that of full-term infants. Gekoski, Fagen, and Pearlman (1984) used the mobile conjugate reinforcement task to compare conditioning and retention in preterm infants who were 3 months of age (corrected for prematurity, i.e., the infants' conceptional age was 53 weeks) with that of 3-month-old full-term infants. As shown in Figure 12.4, the full-term infants demonstrated a response increase from pretraining baseline during the first daily conditioning session whereas the preterms did not achieve this criterion until the second session. The full-term infants also had superior 1-week retention; their baseline ratio averaged 1.73 compared with 1.02 for the preterms (recall that a baseline ratio of 1.00 reflects a return to operant level). Measures of pre- and perinatal complications indicated that regardless of term, retention was related to perinatal risk ($r = .40$). Fagen and Ohr (1990) conducted a multiple regression analysis of the Gekoski et al. data, entering the term variable first followed by the two Littman and Parmelee scale scores. By itself, the categorization of preterm/full-term accounted for 19% of the variance in the 1-week baseline ratios; adding the additional information concerning pregnancy and neonatal status increased the R^2 to .41. The importance of information regarding perinatal risk is emphasized by the findings of a recent study by Vervloed (1995) who reported that low-risk but not high-risk preterm infants successfully acquired the footkick/mobile-movement contingency in a single 10-minute reinforcement period.

In an extension of the Gekoski et al. (1984) study, Ribarich (1990) examined conditioning in 7-month-old (corrected) preterm and full-term infants using the Fagen and Ohr (1990) panel-press apparatus previously described. The preterms in this study were all generally healthy (e.g., no intraventricular hemorrhages). They had gestational ages between 28 and 36 weeks and birthweights between 1,000 and 2,500 grams. Unlike Gekoski et al., Ribarich found that as a group, the 7-month-old preterm infants' response rate never reliably exceeded its operant level. An examination of the individual preterm infants' data did reveal, however, that 11 of the 20

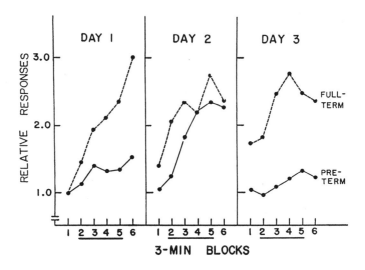

FIGURE 12.4. Mean relative response scores per minute over successive 3-minute blocks during training (Days 1 and 2) and a 7-day long-term retention session (Day 3) for 3-month-old preterm and full-term infants. Blocks 1 and 6 on each day are nonreinforcement periods; Blocks 2–5 on each day represent reinforcement. From Gekoski, Fagen, and Pearlman (1984). Copyright 1984 by Elsevier Science. Reprinted by permission.

preterm infants achieved a standard learning criterion of a response rate during acquisition that was at least 150% of the infant's baseline response rate. Furthermore, these infants had a mean 1-week baseline ratio of 1.98. Although this value was significantly above a theoretical ratio of 1.00 (a return in responding to baseline), it was far below that of the full-term infants, whose mean was 6.20. Finally, a multiple regression analysis, with term entered first, indicated that the term perinatal and complications variables accounted for 30% of the variance in the increase in responding above baseline.

The findings of Gekoski et al. (1984), Vervloed (1995), and Ribarich (1990) suggest that the health of the preterm at birth, not prematurity per se, is important in determining both the acquisition and retention of instrumental contingencies. This conclusion is supported by the findings from recent studies by Millar, Weir, and Supramaniam (1992). Millar et al. divided a sample of predominantly preterm infants into low- and high-risk groups based on the intensity and duration of neonatal respiratory interventions. These infants were tested at an average corrected chronological age of 35.6 weeks and their performance was compared to a group of full-term infants (gestational ages ranging from 37 to 42 weeks) tested at an average corrected chronological age of 32.5 weeks. In addition to its careful delineation of risk status, the Millar et al. study is notable because (1) it contained both contingent and noncontingent groups, and (2) "easy" and "difficult" conditioning tasks. The easy task consisted of the infant being rewarded with audiovisual stimulation emanating from the location of the manipulandum, a 10-cm-tall canister. In the difficult task, the stimulation was displaced 35 cm from the manipulandum and rotated 60 degrees about the vertical axis. This task is more difficult because the infant cannot simultaneously attend to both the manipulandum and the reinforcer (see Millar & Schaffer, 1972, for more details). The results of this study indicated that both the full-term and low-risk groups, but not the high-risk group, successfully acquired the "easy" contingency between touching the canister and the reinforcement. None of the groups acquired the contingency under the displaced reinforcement condition. Unfortunately, acquisition in this study lasted only 3 minutes so it is not known if any or all of the groups in the displaced reinforcement condition or the high-risk group in the nondisplaced reinforcement conditioning would have learned with additional training.

Infants with Down syndrome are a second group of compromised infants who have been studied with instrumental conditioning tasks (e.g., Brinker & Lewis, 1982; Poulson, 1988; Vietze, McCarthy, McQuiston, MacTurk, & Yarrow, 1983). In our laboratory, we have used the mobile conjugate reinforcement task to compare the learning and retention of 3-month-old infants with Down syndrome to that of infants without any identifiable disabilities (Ohr & Fagen, 1991). Both groups of infants successfully acquired this contingency; furthermore, there was no difference in the speed of acquisition. The infants without Down syndrome did, however, produce more movement in the overhead mobile. In addition, there were large individual differences in acquisition response rates for the infants with Down syndrome that were related to maternal ratings of the infants' activity level (Ohr & Fagen, 1993). These findings suggest that the increase in operant responding seen in instrumental conditioning tasks may be more subtle in infants with Down syndrome than in other infant groups. Furthermore, the reactivity of the young infant with Down syndrome in response to external stimulation is related to his or her learning performance. Turning to memory, both groups showed equivalent 1-week retention as measured by both their baseline and retention ratios.

We have also recently investigated the contingency learning in older infants with Down syndrome using the arm-pull apparatus previously described. Ohr and Fagen (1994) found that as a group, 10, 9-month-old infants with Down syndrome failed to show any increase in either their actual or relative response rate during two 8-minute conditioning sessions. An examination of the infants' individual conditioning curves did, however, reveal that 3 of the 10 infants with Down syndrome achieved a conservative learning criterion of a relative response score of at least 2.0 for any 2 of 3 minutes of reinforcement, whereas 5 did so when the criterion was lowered to 1.5 times operant level, the criterion used in our earlier study (Ohr & Fagen,

1991). Furthermore, the relative response rates of the infants with Down syndrome during the two daily reinforcement phases were correlated with their Mental Development scores on the Bayley Scales of Infant Development. Ohr and Fagen (1994) concluded that the lack of conditioning in the 9-month-old infants with Down syndrome as compared to 3-month-old infants with Down syndrome reflected a decline in conditionability with age. This maturational explanation is consistent with the developmental declines in infants with Down syndrome reported by other investigators (e.g., Carr, 1988; Dicks-Mireaux, 1972) during the second half of the first year. This conclusion was also supported by the findings that many of the infants with Down syndrome did acquire the contingency and their conditioning performance was positively correlated with the Mental Development scores.

Finally, Alessandri, Sullivan, Imaizumi, and Lewis (1993) conducted a study of instrumental conditioning in cocaine-exposed infants. Four-, 6-, and 8-month-old infants' arm pulls activated a slide of an infant's smiling face accompanied by a recording of children singing. Both cocaine-exposed and nonexposed infants reliably increased their response rate during a brief (3 minutes) contingency period. However, the nonexposed infants also increased their response rate during a 2-minute extinction phase whereas the cocaine-exposed infants did not. During a 3-minute reacquisition phase, the responding of the cocaine-exposed infants, but not the nonexposed infants, dipped below its acquisition rate. Over the entire conditioning procedure, the cocaine-exposed infants had a lower response rate. Allesandri et al. (1993) concluded the following:

> [The] arousal level of the cocaine infants was incompatible with the demands of the procedure, a finding further supported by a decline in arm pulling when control over the stimulus was reinstated in the final phase of the experiment [reacquisition]. Thus, the cocaine-exposed infants were less engaged in the contingency initially and were unexcited by re-exposure to it. (p. 995)

This conclusion was further supported by data on the infants' emotional expressions. Specifically, the cocaine-exposed infants evidenced fewer expressions of interest and joy during contingency training and also had fewer anger expressions during extinction. Thus, they appeared to be less involved with the learning part of the task and less bothered by the loss of control.

Structural and/or Theoretical Constraints/Controversies

One unanswered question is whether the differences observed between at-risk and nonrisk infants are related solely to the instrumental conditioning procedures used or indicative of more global information-processing difficulties. It is well-known that both infants born prematurely and those with

Down syndrome suffer lags in their motor development. This, coupled with Siqueland's success with the High Amplitude Sucking (HAS) technique, suggests that comparisons between infant groups based on high-energy operants such as kicking or panel/canister pressing may be inappropriate. On the other hand, these and other motor behaviors (e.g., motility; see Thoman & Ingersoll, 1993) occur with equal or greater frequency in preterms as compared to full-terms; thus, they should be modifiable. Furthermore, it is routine in instrumental conditioning studies to assess changes in response rate during acquisition training to each infants' baseline response rate. We would conclude, therefore, that performance differences do reflect underlying differences in information processing abilities.

The results from our laboratory using various age-appropriate operant tasks indicate that a cognitive ability, memory, accounts for a fair amount of the variance in future intellectual functioning. These tasks appear to measure skills during the first year of life that are different from those measured by the Bayley scales. By using the same basic operant conditioning procedure at each age, we have successfully overcome a major problem in previous attempts to assess infant intellectual functioning; namely, that the infant's behavioral repertoire changes during the first year. Our tasks permit us to adapt to the developing infant while focusing on the same cognitive processes at each age. By placing infants in settings in which they *produce* changes in the environment, we have been able to measure how well an infant learns a task and how long and under what conditions he or she retains it. This instrumental conditioning approach to early assessment has the added advantage of going beyond the measurement of basic cognitive competencies to bridge the gap between cognitive and motivational factors in early development.

Training Requirements

The training requirements necessary to use conditioning procedures are highly task specific. Many conditioning tasks used by infant researchers are highly automated with computers controlling both the definition of a response and the presentation of the reinforcer. Others, such as Rovee-Collier's highly successful mobile conjugate reinforcement task, are not automated and require some training in the definition of the operant response.

Implications

The studies of instrumental learning reviewed point to the potential diagnostic value of conditioning procedures as a means of detecting current and future deficits in infants' information processing systems. As discussed in previous sections, studies using other learning paradigms, such as visual habituation of Haith's visual expectation procedure, also provide a window onto this system. Instrumental conditioning tasks, however, offer one additional advantage; namely, they tap into the infant's mastery–motivational system (see also Ulvund, 1980; Watson, 1972; White, 1963). We believe that a detailed understanding of infant cognition can be accomplished only by using paradigms that permit the observation of infants who are both motivated to solve the "problem" presented by the experimenter and are allowed to do so. "Competence implies action, changing the environment as well as adapting to the environment" (Connolly & Bruner, 1974, p. 3). Studies based on visual habituation and visual expectation can only tell us that the infant *knows that* a stimulus repeatedly occurs either in the same location or in a changing but predictable location. Studies of instrumental conditioning tell us that the infant *knows how* to use the information he or she has acquired, both immediately and after a delay.

SUMMARY AND CONCLUSIONS

In this chapter, we have attempted to show how early measures of infant learning and memory can provide important diagnostic information about infants' current and future cognitive functioning. The three paradigms reviewed—habituation, learned expectancies, and instrumental conditioning—all reliably tap areas of cognitive development which are a cause for concern when they are developing atypically due to biological (e.g., preterm birth and chromosomal abnormality) or environmental (e.g., cocaine exposure) insult. Just how much explanatory variance is shared by these three paradigms remains to be determined (cf. Colombo, 1993; Gekoski, 1977; Vervloed, 1995).

The important task for the future is to determine the specific processes underlying the individual differences in habituation, expectancy formation, and instrumental conditioning, and their unique and overlapping relations to later intellectual functioning. Such research not only has theoretical value in explicating the constructs responsible for the obtained data but should also help to create targeted intervention strategies as well (see, e.g., Sullivan & Lewis, 1993).

Recent advances in our understanding of the most likely candidates for the relevant underlying cognitive processes have been made by Colombo (1993; Colombo & Mitchell, 1990) and McCall (1994; McCall & Mash, 1995). In general, the hypothesized processes include (1) information processing, especially the speed with which it is carried out; (2) memory, especially the retrieval of stored information; and (3) attention, including selection, engagement, and especially, disengagement and inhibition. Efficient habituation and fast reaction times to expected events are both indices of rapid information processing (Jacobson et al., 1992; Rose & Feldman, 1997) and, as discussed earlier, they are related to later performance on standardized intelligence tests. The research reviewed from our laboratory also indicates that individual differences in the retrieval of memories for acquired contingencies (another form of learned expectancy) correlates with later IQ measures.

The differential deployment of attentional processes by individual infants probably does not, by itself, account for the obtained infant–child relations. Rather, it may prove to be a critical component of both information-processing speed and memory. That is, the capacity to inhibit attention to stimuli that are redundant or low in salience allows the infant to get on with the business of discovering biologically or socially relevant information in the environment. On the other hand, the efficient engagement of attentional processes permits both the selection and storage of attributes corresponding to important events and associations in the infant's world as well as the later selection of stimuli in the environment that correspond to these stored attributes. This renoticing of stimuli in the environment that correspond to the stored attributes representing previous learning or knowledge permit retrieval to occur. As Tennessee Williams wrote in *The Milk Train Doesn't Stop Here Anymore* (1964, p. 44): "Life is all memory except for the one present moment that goes by so quick you hardly catch it going." Perhaps infants, like baseball players, need to be good catchers.

ACKNOWLEDGMENT

We thank Dr. Joyce Prigot for her invaluable input into the section on "Learned Expectancies."

REFERENCES

Alessandri, S. M., Sullivan, M. S., Imaizumi, S., & Lewis, M. (1993). Learning and emotional responsivity in cocaine-exposed infants. *Developmental Psychology, 29*, 989–997.

Bayley, N. (1993). *Bayley Scales of Infant Development* (2nd ed.). San Antonio, TX: Psychological Corporation.

Benson, J. B., Cherny, S. S., Haith, M. M., & Fulker, D. W. (1993). Rapid assessment of infant predictors of adult IQ: The midtwin–midparent approach. *Developmental Psychology, 29*, 434–447.

Bieber, M. L., Kaplan, P. S., Rosier, E., & Werner, J. S. (1997). Sensitizing properties of spectral lights in 4–month-old human infants. *Developmental Psychobiology, 30*, 275–287.

Bihun, J., Haneburth, E., & Haith, M. M. (1993, March). *Evidence for rule transfer with 20–week-old infants in the visual expectation paradigm.* Paper presented at the meeting of the Society for Research in Child Development, New Orleans.

Bolles, R. C. (1972). Reinforcement, expectancy, and learning. *Psychological Review, 79*, 394–409.

Bolles, R. C. (1979). *Learning theory* (2nd ed.). New York: Holt, Rinehart & Winston.

Bornstein, M. H. (1985). Habituation of attention as a measure of information processing in human infants: Summary, systematization, and synthesis. In G. Gottlieb & N. A. Krasnegor (Eds.), *Measurement of vision and audition in the first year of life* (pp. 253–301). Norwood, NJ: Ablex.

Bornstein, M. H., & Benasich, A. A. (1986). Infant habituation: Assessments of individual differences and short-term reliability at five months. *Child Development, 57,* 87–99.

Bornstein, M. H., & Sigman, M. D. (1986). Continuity in mental development from infancy. *Child Development, 57,* 251–274.

Brackbill, Y. (1973). Continuous stimulation reduces arousal level: Stability of the effect over time. *Child Development, 44,* 43–46.

Brinker, R. P., & Lewis, M. (1982). Contingency intervention in infancy. In J. Anderson & J. Cox (Eds.), *Curriculum materials for high risk and handicapped infants* (pp. 37–41). Chapel Hill, NC: Technical Assistance Development Systems.

Canfield, R. L., & Haith, M. M. (1991). Young infants' visual expectations for symmetric and asymmetric stimulus sequences. *Developmental Psychology, 27,* 198–209.

Canfield, R. L., Smith, E. G., Breznyak, M. P., & Snow, K. L. (1997). Information processing through the first year of life: A longitudinal study using the visual expectation paradigm. *Monographs of the Society for Research in Child Development, 62*(2, Serial No. 250).

Canfield, R. L., Wilkin, J., Schmerl, L., & Smith, E. G. (1995). Age-related change and stability of individual differences in infant saccade reaction time. *Infant Behavior and Development, 18,* 351–358.

Carr, J. (1988). Six weeks to twenty-one years old: A longitudinal study of children with Down's syndrome and their families. *Journal of Child Psychology and Psychiatry, 29,* 407–431.

Chawarska, K. H., Mayes, L. C., Reznick, J. S., & Miranda, R. (1997, April). *Visual expectations in cocaine and non-cocaine exposed 6–month-old infants.* Paper presented at the meeting for the Society for Research in Child Development, Washington, DC.

Cohen, L. B. (1981). Examination of habituation as a measure of aberrant infant development. In S. L. Friedman & M. Sigman (Eds.), *Preterm birth and psychological development* (pp. 241–253). New York: Academic Press.

Colombo, J. (1993). *Infant cognition: Predicting later intellectual functioning.* Newbury Park, CA: Sage.

Colombo, J., & Mitchell, D. W. (1990). Individual differences in early visual attention: Fixation time and information processing. In J. Colombo & J. W. Fagen (Eds.), *Individual differences in infancy: Reliability, stability, and prediction* (pp. 193–227). Hillsdale, NJ: Erlbaum.

Connolly, K. J., & Bruner, J. S. (1974). Competence: Its nature and nurture. In K. J. Connolly & J. S. Bruner (Eds.), *The growth of competence* (pp. 3–7). London: Wiley.

DeCasper, A. J., & Fifer, W. P. (1980). Of human bonding: Newborns prefer their mothers' voice. *Science, 208,* 1174–1176.

DeCasper, A. J., & Spence, M. J. (1986). Prenatal maternal speech influences newborns' perception of sounds. *Infant Behavior and Development, 9,* 133–150.

DeCasper, A. J., & Spence, M. J. (1991). Auditorily mediated behavior during the perinatal period: A cognitive view. In M. J. S. Weiss & P. R. Zelazo (Eds.), *Newborn attention: Biological constraints and the influence of experience* (pp. 142–176). Norwood, NJ: Ablex.

Dickinson, A. (1980). *Contemporary animal learning theory.* New York: Cambridge University Press.

Dicks-Mireaux, M. J. (1972). Mental development of infants with Down's syndrome. *American Journal of Mental Deficiency, 77,* 26–32.

DiLilla, L. F., Thompson, L. A., Plomin, R., Phillips, K., Fagan, J. F. III, Haith, M. M., Cyphers, L. H., & Fulker, D. W. (1990). Infant predictors of preschool and adult IQ: A study of infant twins and their parents. *Developmental Psychology, 26*, 759–769.

Dougherty, T. M., & Haith, M. M. (1997). Infant expectations and reaction times as predictors of childhood speed of processing and IQ. *Developmental Psychology, 33*, 146–155.

Dunst, C. J., & Lingerfelt, B. (1985). Maternal ratings of temperament and operant learning in two to three-month-old infants. *Child Development, 56*, 555–563.

Eisen, L. N., Field, T. M., Bandstra, E. S., Roberts, J. P., Morrow, C., Larson, S. K., & Steele, B. M. (1990). Perinatal cocaine effects on neonatal behavior and performance on the Brazelton Scale. *Pediatrics, 88*, 477–480.

Fagen, J. W. (1993). Reinforcement is not enough: Learned expectancies and infant behavior. *American Psychologist, 48*, 1153–1155.

Fagen, J. W., Morrongiello, B. A., Rovee-Collier, C., & Gekoski, M. J. (1984). Expectancies and memory retrieval in three-month-old infants. *Child Development, 55*, 936–943.

Fagen, J. W., & Ohr, P. S. (1985). Temperament and crying in response to the violation of a learned expectancy in early infancy. *Infant Behavior and Development, 8*, 157–166.

Fagen, J. W., & Ohr, P. S. (1990). Individual differences in infant conditioning and memory. In J. Colombo & J. W. Fagen (Eds.), *Individual differences in infancy: Reliability, stability, and prediction* (pp. 157–191). Hillsdale, NJ: Erlbaum.

Fagen, J. W., Ohr, P. S., Singer, J. M., & Fleckenstein, L. K. (1987). Infant temperament and subject loss due to crying during operant conditioning. *Child Development, 58*, 497–504.

Fagen, J. W., & Rovee-Collier, C. K. (1982). A conditioning analysis of infant memory: How do we know they know what we know they knew? In R. L. Isaacson & N. E. Spear (Eds.), *The expression of knowledge: Neurobehavioral transformations of information into action* (pp. 67–111). New York: Plenum.

Fantz, R. L., Fagan, J. F., & Miranda, S. B. (1975). Early visual selectivity. In L. Cohen & P. Salapatek (Eds.), *Infant perception: From sensation to cognition* (Vol. 1, pp. 249–346). New York: Academic Press.

Field, T. M., Dempsey, J. R., Hatch, J., Ting, G., & Clifton, R. K. (1979). Cardiac and behavioral responses to repeated tactile and auditory stimulation by preterm and term neonates. *Developmental Psychology, 15*, 406–416.

Flaherty, C. F. (1985). *Animal learning and cognition.* New York: Knopf.

Fox, N., & Lewis, M. (1983). Cardiac response to speech sounds in preterm infants: Effects of illness at three months. *Psychophysiology, 20*, 481–488.

Friedman, S. (1975). Infant habituation: Process, problems, and possibilities. In N. R. Ellis (Ed.), *Aberrant development in infancy: Human and animal studies* (pp. 217–239). Hillsdale, NJ: Erlbaum.

Friedman, S., Bruno, L. A., & Vietze, P. (1974). Newborn habituation to visual stimuli: A sex difference in novelty detection. *Journal of Experimental Child Psychology, 18*, 242–251.

Gekoski, M. J., Fagen, J. W., & Pearlman, M. A. (1984). Early learning and memory in the preterm infant. *Infant Behavior and Development, 7*, 267–276.

Gekoski, M. M. (1977). Visual attention and operant conditioning in infancy: A second look. *Dissertation Abstracts International, 38*, 875b. (University Microfilms No. 77–17, 533)

Graham, F. K. (1973). Habituation and dishabituation of responses innervated by the autonomic nervous system. In H. V. S. Peeke & M. J. Herz (Eds.), *Habituation. Volume 1: Behavioral Studies* (pp. 163–218). New York: Academic Press.

Groves, P. M., & Thompson, R. F. (1970). Habituation: A dual-process theory. *Psychological Review, 77,* 419–450.

Haith, M. M. (1966). The response of the human newborn to visual movement. *Journal of Experimental Child Psychology, 3,* 235–243.

Haith, M. M. (1993). Future-oriented processes in infancy: The case of visual expectations. In C. Granrud (Ed.), *Visual perception and cognition in infancy* (pp. 235–264). Hillsdale, NJ: Erlbaum.

Haith, M. M. (1994). Visual expectation as the first step toward the development of future-oriented processes. In M. M. Haith, J. B. Benson, R. J. Roberts, & B. F. Pennington (Eds.), *The development of future-oriented processes* (pp. 11–38). Chicago: University of Chicago Press.

Haith, M. M., Hazan, C., & Goodman, G. S. (1988). Expectation and anticipation of dynamic visual events by 3.5-month-old babies. *Child Development, 59,* 467–479.

Haith, M. M., & McCarthy, M. E. (1990). Stability of visual expectations at 3. 0 months of age. *Developmental Psychology, 26,* 68–74.

Haith, M. M., Wentworth, N., & Canfield, R. L. (1993). The formation of expectations in early infancy. In C. Rovee-Collier & L. Lipsitt (Eds.), *Advances in infancy research* (Vol. 8, pp. 251–297). Norwood, NJ: Ablex.

Horowitz, F. D., Paden, L. Y., Bhana, K., & Self, P. A. (1972). An infant control procedure for the study of infant visual fixations. *Developmental Psychology, 7,* 90.

Jacobson, S. W., Jacobson, J. J., O'Neill, J. M., Padgett, R. J., Frankowski, J. J., & Bihun, J. T. (1992). Visual expectation and dimensions of infant information processing. *Child Development, 63,* 711–724.

Jeffrey, W. E. (1976). Habituation as a mechanism for perceptual development. In T. J. Tighe & R. N. Leaton (Eds.), *Habituation: Perspectives from child development, animal behavior, and neurophysiology* (pp. 279–296). Hillsdale, NJ: Erlbaum.

Jeffrey, W. E., & Cohen, L. B. (1971). Habituation in the human infant. In H. W. Reese (Ed.), *Advances in child development and behavior* (Vol. 6, pp. 63–97). New York: Academic Press.

Kandel, E. R. (1991). Cellular mechanisms of learning and the biological basis of individuality. In E. R. Kandel, J. H. Schwartz, & T. M. Jessell (Eds.), *Principles of neural science* (pp. 1009–1031). New York: Elsevier.

Kaplan, P. S., & Werner, J. S. (1991). Implications of a sensitization process for the analysis of infant visual attention. In M. J. S. Weiss & P. R. Zelazo (Eds.), *Newborn attention: Biological constraints and the influence of experience* (pp. 278–307). Norwood, NJ: Ablex.

Kaplan, P. S., Werner, J. S., & Rudy, J. W. (1990). Habituation, sensitization, and infant visual attention. In C. Rovee-Collier & L. P. Lipsitt (Eds.), *Advances in infancy research* (Vol. 6, pp. 61–109). Norwood, NJ: Ablex.

Kimble, G. A. (1961). *Hilgard and Marquis' conditioning and learning.* New York: Appleton-Century-Crofts.

Kobre, K. R., & Lipsitt, L. P. (1972). A negative contrast effect in newborns. *Journal of Experimental Child Psychology, 14,* 81–91.

Landry, S. H., Leslie, N. A., Fletcher, J. M., & Francis, D. J. (1985). Visual attention skills of premature infants with and without intraventricular hemorrhage. *Infant Behavior and Development, 8,* 309–321.

Lanthier, E. C., & Haith, M. M. (1993, March). Infant's performance in a double- or triple-alternating sequence in the visual expectation paradigm. In M. M. Haith (Chair),

Variations on a theme of visual expectations. Poster symposium conducted at the meeting of the Society for Research in Child Development, New Orleans.

Lewis, M. (1969). A developmental study of information processing within the first three years of life: Response decrement to a redundant signal. *Monographs of the Society for Research in Child Development*, *34*(9, Whole No. 133).

Lewis, M., & Brooks-Gunn, J. (1984). Age and handicapped group differences in infant visual attention. *Child Development*, *55*, 858–868.

Madison, L. S., Adubato, S. A., Madison, J. K., Nelson, R. M., Anderson, J. C., Erickson, J., Kuss, L. M., & Goodlin, R. C. (1986). Fetal response decrement: True habituation? *Journal of Developmental and Behavioral Pediatrics*, *7*, 14–20.

Malcuit, G., Pomerleau, A., & Lamarre, G. (1988). Habituation, visual fixation, and cognitive activity in infants: A critical analysis and attempt at a new formulation. *European Bulletin of Cognitive Psychology*, *8*, 415–440.

Marlin, N. A., & Miller, R. R. (1981). Associations to contextual stimuli as a determinant of long-term habituation. *Journal of Experimental Psychology: Animal Behavior Processes*, *7*, 313–333.

Mayes, L. C., Bornstein, M. H., Chawarska, K., & Granger, R. H. (1995). Information processing and developmental assessments in 3–month-old infants exposed prenatally to cocaine. *Pediatrics*, *95*, 539–545.

Mayes, L. C., Granger, R. H., Frank, M. A., Schottenfeld, R., & Bornstein, M. (1993). Neurobehavioral profiles of infants exposed to cocaine prenatally. *Pediatrics*, *91*, 778–783.

McCall, R. B. (1979). Individual differences in the pattern of habituation at 5 and 10 months of age. *Developmental Psychology*, *15*, 559–569.

McCall, R. B. (1994). What process mediates predictions of childhood IQ from infant habituation and recognition memory? Specifications of the roles of inhibition and rate of information processing. *Intelligence*, *18*, 107–125.

McCall, R. B., & Carriger, R. B. (1993). A meta-analysis of infant habituation and recognition memory performance as predictors of later IQ. *Child Development*, *64*, 57–79.

McCall, R. B., & Mash, C. W. (1995). Infant cognition and its relation to mature intelligence. *Annals of Child Development*, *10*, 27–56.

McDonough, S. C., & Cohen, L. B. (1982). Attention and memory in cerebral palsied infants. *Infant Behavior and Development*, *5*, 347–353.

Millar, W. S., & Schaffer, H. R. (1972). The influence of spatially displaced feedback on infant operant conditioning. *Journal of Experimental Child Psychology*, *14*, 442–453.

Millar, W. S., Weir, C. G., & Supramaniam, G. (1992). The influence of perinatal risk status on contingency learning in six- to thirteen-month-old infants. *Child Development*, *63*, 304–313.

Miranda, S. B., & Fantz, R. L. (1973). Visual preferences of Down's syndrome and normal infants. *Child Development*, *44*, 555–561.

Miranda, S. B., & Fantz, R. L. (1974). Recognition memory in Down's syndrome and normal infants. *Child Development*, *45*, 651–660.

Ohr, P. S., & Fagen, J. W. (1991). Conditioning and long-term memory in three-month-old infants with Down syndrome. *American Journal of Mental Retardation*, *96*, 151–162.

Ohr, P. S., & Fagen, J. W. (1993). Temperament, conditioning, and memory in 3–month-old infants with Down syndrome. *Journal of Applied Developmental Psychology*, *14*, 175–190.

Ohr, P. S., & Fagen, J. W. (1994). Contingency learning in 9–month-old infants with Down syndrome. *American Journal of Mental Retardation, 99*, 74–84.

Olson, G. M. (1976). An information-processing analysis of visual memory and habituation in infants. In T. J. Tighe & R. N. Leaton (Eds.), *Habituation* (pp. 239–277). Hillsdale, NJ: Erlbaum.

Olson, G. M., & Sherman, T. (1983). Attention, learning, and memory in infants. In M. M. Haith & J. J. Campos (Eds.), P. H. Mussen (Series Ed.), *Handbook of child psychology* (Vol. 2, pp. 1001–1080). New York: Wiley.

Piaget, J. (1952). *The origins of intelligence in children*. New York: Norton.

Poulson, C. L. (1988). Operant conditioning of vocalization rate of infants with Down syndrome. *American Journal of Mental Retardation, 93*, 57–63.

Rescorla, R. A. (1988). Pavlovian conditioning: It's not what you think it is. *American Psychologist, 43*, 151–160.

Ribarich, M. T. (1990). *Learning and memory in preterm and full-term infants at 7 and 11 months of age*. Unpublished doctoral dissertation, St. John's University.

Richards, J. E. (1988). Heart rate changes and heart rate rhythms and infant visual sustained attention. In P. H. Ackles, J. R. Jennings, & M. G. H. Coles (Eds.), *Advances in Psychophysiology* (Vol. 3, pp. 189–221). Greenwich, CT: JAI Press.

Rose, S. A., & Feldman, J. F. (1997). Memory and speed: Their role in the relation of infant information processing to later IQ. *Child Development, 68*, 630–641.

Rose, S. A., Feldman, J. F., McCarton, C. M., & Wolfson, J. (1988a). Information processing in seven-month-old infants as a function of risk status. *Child Development, 59*, 589–603.

Rose, S. A., Feldman, J. F., & Wallace, I. F. (1988b). Individual differences in infants' information processing: Reliability, stability, and prediction. *Child Development, 59*, 1177–1197.

Rose, S. A., Feldman, J., Wallace, I., & McCarton, C. (1989). Infant visual attention: Relation to birth status and developmental outcome during the first 5 years. *Developmental Psychology, 25*, 560–576.

Rovee, C. K., & Rovee, D. T. (1969). Conjugate reinforcement of infant exploratory behavior. *Journal of Experimental Child Psychology, 8*, 33–39.

Rovee-Collier, C. (1987). Learning and memory in infancy. In J. D. Osofsky (Ed.), *Handbook of infant development* (2nd ed., pp. 98–148). New York: Wiley.

Rovee-Collier, C. (1996). Measuring infant memory: A critical commentary. *Developmental Review, 16*, 301–310.

Rovee-Collier, C., & Hayne, H. (1987). Reactivation of infant memory: Implications for cognitive development. In H. W. Reese (Ed.), *Advances in child development and behavior* (Vol. 20, pp. 185–238). New York: Academic Press.

Rovee-Collier, C. K., & Lipsitt, L. P. (1982). Learning, adaptation, and memory in the newborn. In P. Stratton (Ed.), *Psychobiology of the human newborn* (pp. 147–190). Chichester: Wiley.

Rovee-Collier, C. K., & Shyi, C. -W. G. (1992). A functional and cognitive analysis of infant long-term retention. In M. L. Howe, C. J. Brainerd, & V. F. Reyna (Eds.), *Development of long-term retention* (pp. 3–55). New York: Springer-Verlag.

Salapatek, P., & Kessen, W. (1966). Visual scanning of triangles by human newborn. *Journal of Experimental Child Psychology, 3*, 155–167.

Slater, A. (1995). Individual differences in infancy and later IQ. *Journal of Child Psychology and Psychiatry, 36*, 69–112.

Slater, A., Morrison, V., & Rose, D. (1982). Visual memory at birth. *British Journal of Psychology, 73,* 519–525.

Slater, A., Morrison, V., & Rose, D. (1984). Habituation in the newborn. *Infant Behavior and Development, 7,* 183–200.

Sokolov, E. N. (1963). *Perception and the conditioned reflex.* New York: MacMillan.

Solkoff, N., & Cotton, C. (1975). Contingency awareness in premature infants. *Perceptual and Motor Skills, 41,* 709–710.

Spear, N. E. (1973). Retrieval of memory in animals. *Psychological Review, 80,* 163–194.

Sullivan, M. W., & Lewis, M. (1993). Contingency, means-end skills, and the use of technology in infant intervention. *Infants and Young Children, 5,* 58–77.

Thoman, E. B., & Ingersoll, E. W. (1993). Learning in premature infants. *Developmental Psychology, 29,* 692–700.

Thompson, R. F., & Glanzman, D. L. (1976). Neural and behavioral mechanisms of habituation and sensitization. In T. J. Tighe & R. N. Leaton (Eds.), *Habituation: Perspectives from child development, animal behavior, and neurophysiology* (pp. 49–93). Hillsdale, NJ: Erlbaum.

Thompson, R. F., & Spencer, W. A. (1966). Habituation: A model phenomenon for the study of neuronal substrates of behavior. *Psychological Review, 73,* 16–43.

Tolman, E. C. (1932). *Purposive behavior in animals and men.* New York: Century.

Ulvund, S. E. (1980). Cognition and motivation in early infancy. *Human Development, 23,* 17–32.

Vervloed, M. P. J. (1995). *Learning in preterm infants: Habituation, operant conditioning, and their associations with motor development.* Groningen, The Netherlands: University of Groningen.

Vietze, P. M., McCarthy, M., McQuiston, S., Macturk, R., & Yarrow, L. J. (1983). Attention and exploratory behavior in infants with Down's syndrome. In T. Field & A. Sostek (Eds.), *Infants born at risk: Physiological, perceptual, and cognitive processes* (pp. 251–268). New York: Grune & Stratton.

Wagner, A. R. (1976). Priming in STM: An information-processing mechanism for self-generated or retrieval-generated depression in performance. In T. J. Tighe & R. N. Leaton (Eds.), *Habituation: Perspectives from child development, animal behavior, and neurophysiology* (pp. 95–128). Hillsdale, NJ: Erlbaum.

Wagner, A. R. (1979). Habituation and memory. In A. Dickenson & R. A. Boakes (Eds.), *Mechanisms of learning and motivation* (pp. 53–82). Hillsdale, NJ: Erlbaum.

Walker, J. T. (1996). *The psychology of learning.* Upper Saddle River, NJ: Prentice-Hall.

Watson, J. S. (1972). Smiling, cooing, and "the game." *Merrill–Palmer Quarterly, 18,* 323–329.

Werner, J. S., & Siqueland, E. R. (1978). Visual recognition memory in the preterm infant. *Infant Behavior and Development, 1,* 79–94.

White, R. W. (1963). Ego and reality in psychoanalytic theory. *Psychological Issues, 3,* 1–40.

Williams, T. (1964). *The milk train doesn't stop here anymore.* New York: New Directions.

Worobey, J., & Butler, J. (1988, April). *Memory, learning, and temperament in early infancy.* Paper presented at the International Conference on Infant Studies, Washington, DC.

Zelazo, P. R., Weiss, M. J., Papageorgiou, A. N., & Laplante, D. P. (1989). Recovery and dishabituation of sound localization among normal-, moderate-, and high-risk newborns: Discriminant validity. *Infant Behavior and Development, 12,* 321–340.

13

Visual Information Processing

SUSAN A. ROSE

ESTHER K. ORLIAN

HISTORY

In recent years, there has been a resurgence of interest in infant cognition. This interest has resulted in a spate of experimental work showing that some mental abilities can be identified as early as the first year of life and that these early abilities bear some measurable relation to later cognition.

To some extent, this resurgence of interest in infancy harkens back to the work of Binet and his colleagues who, around the turn of the century, developed the first intelligence test (Binet & Simon, 1905). Binet's efforts were undertaken for the purpose of identifying children whose cognitive capacities were so limited as to make them unlikely to benefit from regular schooling. Scores on Binet's test proved to be relatively stable, raising the possibility that even earlier identification of cognitive delays and lags might prove possible.

Between the 1930s and the 1960s, much of the infancy research focused on the development of instruments that might be useful for this purpose. These instruments, which were geared primarily to charting age-related changes in developmental functioning, included the Cattell Infant Scale (Cattell, 1940), the Gesell Developmental Schedule (Gesell & Amatruder, 1954), the California First Year Mental Scale, an early version of the Bayley (Bayley, 1933), and the Bayley Scales of Infant Development (Bayley, 1969). The Bayley became the most widely used of these scales because it was the best standardized and had the highest reliability (see Bendersky & Lewis, Chapter 22, this volume).

However, attempts to relate performance on these early developmental tests to later cognition proved largely disappointing. In 1982, Kopp and McCall reviewed the predictive data that had resulted from 19 separate studies. Each of these studies correlated scores on infant psychometric tests, obtained at various points during the first year of life, with IQ scores obtained in later childhood, when the children were between the ages of 3 and 18. The correlations were surprisingly low—ranging from .06 to .32, with a median of .21. Other reviews reported similarly poor cross-age relations (e.g., Fagan & Singer, 1983).

The proper interpretation of this failure to find a clear relation between measures of infant performance and performance in later childhood remains unclear. *On the one hand*, it may point to a discontinuity in development, indicating that mental abilities in infancy differ in some fundamental way from later mental abilities. Indeed, this had long been the prevalent view. It was thought that intellectual development underwent a fundamental shift with the advent of language and the emergence of other symbolic capacities. *On the other hand*, the failure to find evidence of continuity may reflect a limitation of the early instruments, with the poor correlations between infancy measures and later IQ simply reflecting important differences in the measures used at the two ages rather than any real discontinuity in cognitive development. Indeed, a close look reveals that the infant tests are heavily weighted with sensorimotor items, with many items relying on motor development, fine motor control, imitation, and affective responsivity. Although such skills reflect highly important aspects of infant functioning, they bear no obvious relation to cognition, certainly not to the tasks of attention, discrimination, memory, reasoning, and the like that characterize the intelligence tests commonly used at older ages.

What is different about the newer work in infant cognition is precisely the fact that it taps aspects of development that seem, on the face of it, more akin to the cognitive processes tapped by later tests. Much of this work, which has grown apace since the early 1970s, centers on infants' distribution of attention and the changes in attention that appear as new information is introduced. The experimental work in these areas offers measures for assessing infant ability to acquire, store, and retrieve information—skills which seem quite different from those forming the core of existing infant tests.

This newer work, with measures based on visual attention, has figured prominently in recent studies of cognitive continuity. There is now compelling evidence that many such measures tap aspects of information processing in infancy and that these early processes have some measurable relation to later cognition. In this chapter, we describe some of these new measures of visual attention, particularly those related to visual recognition memory, present evidence which supports the cognitive nature of such measures, review some of the studies showing the relation of infant visual attention to later cognition, and offer some thoughts as to the potential clinical utility of these new measures.

DESCRIPTION OF ASSESSMENT

The measures of attention that have played the most prominent role in recent studies of infant cognition come from the paired-comparison paradigm and the habituation paradigm (see also Fagen & Ohr, Chapter 12, this volume). Although the two paradigms have some similarities, the habituation paradigm focuses on the developmental course and speed with which attention wanes to a repeated stimulus, whereas the paired-comparison paradigm is chiefly concerned with the infant's visual recognition memory, as reflected in differential responsivity to familiar and novel stimuli. Such responsivity is assessed after an initial exposure to the familiar stimulus which is considerably briefer than that afforded the infant in the habituation paradigm.

The paired-comparison procedure has a familiarization and a test phase. In familiarization, a single picture, or two identical pictures, are presented to the infant. Typically the pictures are presented on a pivoting stage and the observer, looking through a small (0.64 cm) peephole, views corneal reflections of the target(s). For each problem, the familiarization phase generally lasts anywhere from 5 to 60 seconds, depending on the age of the infant and the complexity of the stimulus (less familiarization is needed for older infants and simpler stimuli). Not only is familiarization relatively brief, but the target remains exposed until the infant has studied it for the specified, predetermined, time. In this way, it is assured that all infants have the same familiarity with the initial stimulus. An interval of about 4 or 5 seconds separates the familiarization from the succeeding test phase. During this break, the stage is pivoted back and, outside the infant's view, the targets are changed; the test phase starts by pivoting the stage forward again. On test, the previously seen picture (familiar stimulus) is paired with a novel picture; the two are presented simultaneously for a fixed interval, with right–left positions of the paired targets switched midway to control for side preferences. Timing of the familiarization and test phases begins with the first look to either target.

Because infants typically spend more time looking at the novel member of the pair, the primary index of performance on test is a "novelty score," defined as the percentage of looking during test that is directed to the novel target (e.g., Fagan, 1974; Rose & Feldman, 1990). Novelty scores are calculated by dividing the amount of looking during test directed to the novel picture by the total looking to both stimuli (novel plus familiar) and multiplying the resulting proportion by 100. Generally, the novelty scores from several different problems are averaged to yield an overall score. It should be noted that preferences for the familiar stimulus occasionally emerge during the early stages of stimulus processing, but these tend to be supplanted by a novelty response when processing is complete (e.g., Rose, Gottfried, Melloy-Carminar, & Bridger, 1982; Wagner & Sakovits, 1986).

Because the proper interpretation of novelty scores rests on the assumption that stimulus preferences are attributable to the relative familiarity/novelty of the stimuli, several controls are used to rule out the possibility that other factors play a role. First, preliminary testing is generally done to ensure that at the outset, members of each pair are approximately equivalent in attractiveness. This is done by presenting the paired-test stimuli without any prior familiarization; equivalence in attractiveness dictates that for the group as a whole, attention to each member of the pair be roughly equal. Second, although the familiar stimuli are generally invariant when individual differences are of principal interest, in preliminary studies the stimuli serving as familiar and novel are counterbalanced; that is, each member of the pair serves as familiar and novel equally often across infants in a group. In this way, it is possible to determine the relative difficulty of processing each member of the pair and to ascertain the relative difficulty of different problems. Finally, as noted previously, position preferences are controlled by reversing the right–left placement of familiar and novel stimuli midway through the test.

An example of a typical paired-comparison procedure is that used in our most recent longitudinal study, in which we followed a group of infants born of very low birthweight (< 1,500 grams) and their full-term counterparts (about 100 infants) from infancy to 11 years. In this study, we used a battery of nine problems to assess visual recognition memory at 7 months (Rose, Feldman, McCarton, & Wolfson, 1988a). The stimuli for these problems were varied abstract patterns, photographs of faces, and three-dimensional geometric forms (three problems of each type). Familiarization times were 5 seconds for patterns, and 20 seconds each for faces and geometric forms. At 1 year, infants were given three problems of visual recognition memory using geometric forms and somewhat less familiarization time—15 seconds instead of 20 seconds—(Rose, Feldman, Wallace, & McCarton, 1989, 1991b). In using the paired-comparison paradigm to probe for individual differences, familiarization times are selected so as to approach the minimum needed for a group of infants of a given age to evidence a significant novelty response. Fagan (see Fagan & Detterman, 1992, for a technical report) used this paradigm to develop a commercially available battery of 10 problems, the Fagan Test of Infant Intelligence.

In addition to novelty scores, several ancillary measures from the paired-comparison paradigm are beginning to be examined as well. These include the duration of individual looks (also obtained in habituation studies), the duration of pauses, the percentage of looks on which the infant shifts between the paired targets (a measure of examining), and exposure time, or the time taken to accrue a given amount of familiarization exposure (a measure of sustained attention). These ancillary measures demonstrate how the infant goes about gathering information, whereas the novelty scores tell more about the end results of that process.

BIOBEHAVIORAL BASIS OF ASSESSMENT

Although there are few studies on the neural substrate for visual recognition memory, there is some recent evidence that (1) structures in the medial temporal lobe, especially the hippocampus, may be critically involved and (2) the visual recognition memory found in nonhuman infant primates has striking developmental parallels to that found in human infants.

Brain Substrate

There is evidence linking infant recognition memory, as assessed with the paired-comparison task, to the same brain substrate that underlies what in adults is called explicit memory. Explicit memory is characterized by the conscious recollection of prior events (see Nelson, 1995) and is the type of memory impaired by amnesia. One line of evidence for such a link comes from studies of infant monkeys with lesions to the medial temporal lobe (Bachevalier, Brickson, & Hagger, 1993; Bachevalier, Brickson, Hagger, & Mishkin, 1990; Malkova, Mishkin, & Bachevalier, 1995). When lesions include the hippocampus, infant monkeys perform poorly on paired-comparison tasks of visual recognition memory and, when they reach adulthood, poorly on "delayed non-match-to-sample" tasks. In the latter, the quintessential task for assessing explicit memory in adult monkeys, a single stimulus is presented and then, following a delay, paired with a new one; to obtain a food reward, the monkey must reach for the new object (the reward is hidden beneath it). Different objects are used on each trial; monkeys are trained until they come to systematically select the new object (nonmatch). Monkeys with lateral medial temporal lesions that include the hippocampus have considerable difficulty learning this task when delays as brief as 8 seconds intervene between familiarization and test, and even when they do learn it, their performance falls off rapidly as delays increase (Zola-Morgan & Squire, 1985). A second major type of memory, implicit memory (which includes the sorts of unconscious and automatic memories involved in classical conditioning, motor memory—like bike riding—and priming), is spared at both ages.

Other evidence comes from studies with adult amnesia patients who have sustained damage to the temporal lobe. When given the same sort of paired-comparison problems used for infants, these patients perform at only chance levels with delays of only 2 minutes between familiarization and test (McKee & Squire, 1993).

Both lines of evidence give weight to the notion that the paired-comparison task assesses explicit memory and may depend on temporal lobe or hippocampal function.

Primate Parallels

Virginia Gunderson and her colleagues, who adapted paradigms used in studies of human infants for use with infant monkeys, has shown striking similarities between macaque and human infants in the development of visual recognition memory and other adaptations of the paired-comparison paradigm, such as cross-modal transfer (e.g., visual recognition of information obtained tactually). In particular, older members of both species show evidence of recognition memory with shorter familiarization times than do their younger counterparts, and the effects of risk on infant cognition are quite similar across species: monkey infants, like human infants, show deficits associated with severe birth trauma, exposure to teratogens (subclinical levels of methylmercury), and low birthweight (e.g., Gunderson, Grant-Webster, & Fagan, 1987; Gunderson, Grant-Webster, & Sackett, 1989; Gunderson, Rose, & Grant-Webster, 1990). The similarities in human and monkey performance suggest similarities in the processes underlying normative and deviant development in both species. If this turns out to be the case, a macaque model could be valuable in elucidating brain–behavior correlates of both normal information processing and the impairments found in high-risk infants. In effect, then, the parallels between the young of both species hold promise for providing insights into the neural basis for infant cognition and for modeling the effects of biobehavioral adversity.

RELIABILITY AND VALIDITY

Infant measures of visual recognition memory were originally used in experimental studies of group differences. In adapting these measures to the study of individual differences, issues concerning their psychometric soundness, specifically, reliability, stability, and validity, assume considerable importance.

Reliability and Stability

Reliability of novelty scores obtained with the paired comparison paradigm is higher when assessed by test–retest methods than by measures of internal consistency (Rose & Feldman, 1987; Rose, Feldman, & Wallace, 1988b). Even then, the data, while surprisingly sparse, point to only moderate test–retest reliability and stability.

In one study, Colombo, Mitchell, and Horowitz (1988) assessed reliabil-

ity for visual recognition at 4 and 7 months. Novelty scores, averaged over
five problems at each age, showed week-to-week reliabilities of .40 and .51
at 5 and 7 months, respectively; stability over the 2-month period was .34.
Similar stability coefficients were obtained by Rose and Feldman (1987) for
groupings of six and nine problems of visual recognition memory given to
infants at 6, 7, and 8 months of age ($r = .30$ to .50 across the 1- and 2-month
period).

Despite the reasonable test–retest reliability for visual recognition memory, it should be noted that interitem correlations are surprisingly low. For
example, at 7 months, the age common to the works of Colombo, Mitchell,
O'Brien, and Horowitz (1987) and Rose and Feldman (1987), interitem correlations averaged only .24 and .21, respectively. It may be that low interitem
correlations are endemic to this task. Because each problem samples such a
small fraction of infant behavior (test periods last only 10–20 seconds),
moment-to-moment fluctuations in attention can carry considerable weight.
If the vagaries in infant attention could be better controlled, or their effects
removed, error variance might be reduced and the percentage of shared
variance increased (see Cattell, 1982).

It is worth noting that test–retest reliability is similarly modest for measures of habituation. For infants 3, 4, 7, and 9 months of age, Colombo et al.
(1987) found that week-to-week reliabilities for measures of peak fixation,
first fixation, mean fixation, and response decrement varied from $r = .30$ to
.50, with the higher values found at the two older ages.

Concurrent Validity

There is now a substantial literature indicating that poorer performance on
tests of visual recognition memory (and slower habituation) are associated
with "risk" for cognitive delay or lags. Among the groups studied are infants with Down syndrome, prenatal exposure to chemical teratogens,
malnourishment, and prematurity.

A study by Miranda and Fantz (1974) is typical of findings in this area.
They compared the performance of infants with Down syndrome with that
of normal infants on problems of visual recognition memory at each of three
ages—3, 5, and 8 months—using three types of stimuli: abstract patterns,
patterns formed by placing the same component elements in different ar-
rangements, and photographs of faces. For each type of stimuli the normal
infants showed a novelty preference several weeks earlier than the infants
with Down syndrome. Similarly, Cohen (1981) found slower habituation
and dishabituation in infants with Down syndrome at 4, 5, and 6 months
compared with normal infants of the same ages.

Evidence that chemical teratogens impair visual recognition memory
was reported by Jacobson, Fein, Jacobson, Schwartz, and Dowler (1985),
using a large sample of 123 7-month-olds exposed prenatally to polychlorinated biphenyls (PCBs). They found that novelty scores decreased sys-

tematically, in dose-dependent fashion, as exposure to PCBs increased. More recently, heavy prenatal cocaine exposure was found to be associated with poorer visual recognition memory (Jacobson, Jacobson, Sokol, Martier, & Chiodo, 1996) in that a large sample of cocaine-exposed infants had lower percent novelty scores than nonexposed children neonatally and over the first year of life (Singer et al., 1998, 1999).

Evidence that nutritional insult may disrupt infant performance comes from a study from our own laboratory (Rose, 1994). We tested a sample of 123 5- to 12-month-olds from India. Weight and length, two anthropometric measures commonly used to index nutritional status in developing countries, were related to both visual recognition memory and cross-modal transfer. Underweight infants not only performed relatively poorly on both cognitive tasks but also failed to show the clear age-related improvements found among the heavier infants. These effects held even after controlling for birthweight, previous illness, and parental education (for related findings in a small group of failure-to-thrive infants, see Singer & Fagan, 1984).

The largest number of studies of infants at risk involve those born preterm. Even though preterms are generally tested at "corrected age" (i.e., age from the expected date of birth), the weight of evidence indicates that they perform poorly, relative to full-term controls. Sigman and Parmelee (1974) found that unlike full-terms, 4-month-old preterms gave no evidence of recognizing a previously exposed checkerboard when it was paired with novel stimuli. Further, when shown a series of complex patterns, such as schematic faces, 3- to 6-month-old preterms attended only to individual elements and failed to recognize the configurational structure created by the elements (Caron & Caron, 1981).

In our own laboratory, we also have found poor performance in preterms in various studies of visual recognition memory and cross-modal transfer, using the paired-comparison paradigm (Rose, 1980, 1983). In one such study (Rose, 1983), both 6- and 12-month-old preterms required considerably longer familiarization than full-terms before they showed significant novelty preferences, suggesting that preterms are slower in processing information and that differences in this very fundamental aspect of cognition persist throughout at least the first year of life. In a more recent longitudinal study, where the sample of preterms was restricted to those of very low birthweight (infants weighing < 1,500 grams at birth), preterms not only had lower novelty scores than full-terms but also took longer to accrue the required amounts of looking at the familiarization stimulus and showed less active comparison of the stimuli (Rose et al., 1988a). Among preterms, performance on both measures was especially depressed in infants at increased medical risk, particularly those with respiratory distress syndrome.

In summary, there is now substantial evidence that groups of infants at risk for impaired cognitive outcomes often show poorer visual recognition memory in infancy.

Predictive Validity

Although the corpus of longitudinal studies is still relatively small, and many of the studies that exist are based on small sample sizes, there is growing evidence that measures of recognition memory (and habituation) have substantial predictive validity. Infants who have higher novelty scores (and habituate quickly) tend to perform well on traditional assessments of cognitive competence in later childhood. Psychometric IQ tests have been the major outcome measure for children ages 3 years and up (and the Bayley Mental Developmental Index for younger children), although other indices of cognition, particularly language proficiency, have also been used with some frequency. Reviews of this literature can be found in Bornstein and Sigman (1986) and Fagan and Singer (1983) and a recent meta-analysis by McCall and Carriger (1993). Overall, the median predictive correlations are comparable for both habituation and visual recognition memory and these tend to be around $r = .45$.

One of the first studies to show a relation between visual recognition memory and later cognition was by Fagan and McGrath (1981). These investigators presented follow-up data for four samples of children who had participated some years earlier in experimental studies on visual recognition memory (ns ranged from 19 to 35). In the earlier studies, each subject had received two or three problems somewhere between the ages of 4 and 7 months. The infant scores correlated .33 to .66 with performance on the Peabody Picture Vocabulary Test and/or other vocabulary scales administered when the children were between the ages of 4 and 7 years. These findings were confirmed in a later study (Fagan, 1984). Two more recent studies, both using paired-comparison problems from the Fagan Test of Infant Intelligence, have reported predictive relations between infancy and 3-year IQ. In one, DiLalla et al. (1990) found that visual recognition memory at 7 months (but not at 9 months) correlated .29 with 3-year IQ ($n = 208$ twin pairs). In the other, Thompson, Fagan, and Fulker (1991) found that the scores obtained by averaging over administrations at 5 and 7 months correlated .25 with 3-year IQ and .30 with 3-year language proficiency ($n = 113$).

In two initial studies from our own laboratory, we also found measures of visual attention related to later IQ. Both studies had relatively small samples, made up largely of preterms who, as infants, had participated in experimental studies. In one (Rose & Wallace, 1985a), we found correlations of .53 to .66 between scores of visual recognition memory obtained at 6 months and outcomes consisting of 2-year Bayley scores and 3-, 4-, and 6-year IQ ($n = 14$ to 35); in the second (Rose & Wallace, 1985b), 1-year measures of visual recognition memory and cross-modal transfer showed similar correlations with these same outcomes ($n = 19$ to 26).

Encouraged by these early findings, we initiated a prospective, longitudinal study to investigate the relation between infant information processing, biological risk, and later cognition ($n = 109$). The participants in this study consist of high-risk preterms (born weighing < 1,500 grams) and a socioeconomically matched group of full-terms. The initial target age was 7 months, but some infants were also seen at 6 and/or 8 months; infants were then seen semiannually through age 3, annually through age 6, and then again at 11 years.

For both groups, preterms and full-terms, we found that visual recognition memory at 7 months (as well as 6 and 8 months) and 1-year cross-modal transfer predicted Bayley scores at 2 years, and IQ at 3, 4, 5, 6, and 11 years (Rose & Feldman, 1995; Rose et al., 1988b; Rose, Feldman, & Wallace, 1992; Rose, Feldman, Wallace, & McCarton, 1989, 1991b). These same 7-month scores also predicted receptive and expressive language at 2.5, 3, 4, and 6 years (Rose, Feldman, Wallace, & Cohen, 1991a; Rose et al., 1992). Correlations of infancy scores with the various outcomes were similar for both groups and ranged from .37 to .65. Visual recognition memory and cross-modal transfer also correlated with several specific abilities at 11 years, including speed of information processing, memory, verbal abilities, and spatial abilities (Rose & Feldman, 1995, 1996, 1997; Rose, Feldman, Futterweit, & Jakowski, 1997, 1998). Infants' ability to sustain attention at 7 months, as measured by exposure time (the time taken to accrue the preset looking during familiarization) was also related to later outcome, but not as strongly as the original novelty scores indexing visual recognition memory and cross-modal transfer.

For the most part, visual recognition memory and cross-modal transfer were related to later intelligence independently of socioeconomic status, maternal education, concurrent 7-month or 1-year Bayley, and medical risk. Moreover, when taken together in multiple regressions, the two infant measures consistently made larger independent contributions to prediction than did any of these more traditional predictors (i.e., socioeconomic status, maternal education, or concurrent Bayley scores). It should be noted that visual recognition memory and cross-modal transfer predicted independently of one another suggests that different infant measures may tap different facets of infant cognition.

Overall, the results of studies in this area contribute to a growing body of evidence indicating that differences in visual attention reflect cognitive abilities that can be assessed in infancy and that individual differences in these abilities are related to later cognition.

DEVELOPMENTAL MODEL

It has been posited that recognition memory taps fundamental aspects of infant information processing. On an *a priori* basis, it is clear that successful performance on paired-comparison problems provides evidence that the infant encoded information about the stimulus during familiarization, stored that information, retrieved it on test, and successfully discriminated the familiar stimulus from the novel one (often when differences are quite subtle). Because research in this area is still relatively new, no formal model yet exists either to explain the developmental trajectory of recognition memory or to outline how genetic and environmental factors may enhance or impede development. Instead, much of the initial work in the area has been concerned with learning more about the nature of infant cognition. Aside from the evidence already discussed on concurrent and predictive validity, developmental evidence that speaks to the cognitive nature of recognition memory has been largely concerned with the following: the role of age in performance, the effect of stimulus complexity, and the representational abilities revealed.

Age-Related Changes

One would expect older infants to process information faster and more efficiently than do younger infants. Indeed, such developmental increases in speed of processing have been considered the *sine qua non* of cognitive growth (see Hale, 1990; Kail, 1986, 1988). The data support this expectation: Older infants need less exposure to a stimulus before they demonstrate novelty preferences than do younger infants, and they also habituate faster and have shorter fixations. For example, in studies of recognition memory, Fagan (1974) found developmental changes from 2½ to 6 months in the familiarization time infants needed to process abstract patterns, rearrangements of the component elements of patterns, and photographs of faces; similarly, Rose (1983) found that 6-month-olds needed twice as much familiarization time as did 1-year-olds to recognize simple three-dimensional shapes. Comparable results were reported for habituation by Bornstein, Pecheux, and Lecuyer (1988) for 3- and 5-month-olds and for infants tested weekly from 2 to 7 months of age: Older infants required less exposure to the stimulus than younger infants to reach the same habituation criterion and total looking time declined systematically across the weekly intervals.

Stimulus Complexity

One would also expect that within a given age, infants might show better recognition memory and more rapid habituation the simpler the stimuli. Indeed, that is exactly what happens. In a classic study in this area, Caron and Caron (1969) assessed habituation of 3.5-month-olds to 2×2, 12×12, and 24×24 checkerboard patterns; habituation was faster the simpler the checkerboard. Similarly, infants who habituated to a single form required fewer trials than did infants who habituated to multiple ones (Ruff, 1978).

Representational Abilities

The fact that infants show recognition memory when they categorize stimuli, transfer information cross-modally, or integrate information in a spatial–temporal manner speaks to the cognitive nature of the abilities detected with recognition memory. By varying the nature of the stimuli, it has been possible to show the presence of fairly abstract perceptual and cognitive abilities in infants.

Categorization

To form categories it is necessary to recognize similarities shared by stimuli that also differ in many ways. Studies in this area generally begin by exposing infants to multiple exemplars from one category. Then, on test, the infants are shown new exemplars from the familiar category as well as exemplars from a totally different category. Despite the fact that neither test stimulus has been seen previously, the stimuli from the novel category tend to elicit more attention than those from the familiar category. A systematic preference of this sort presupposes that the infant categorized the exemplars presented during familiarization and recognized the category membership of the new exemplar from the old category.

A series of studies by Quinn and his colleagues (see Quinn, Eimas, & Rosenkrantz, 1993) is a good case in point. Using a variant of the paired-comparison design, infants were initially given a series of six 15-second familiarization trials. On each trial, colored photographs of two different cats were shown, leading to exposure to 12 cats, all different from one another. On test, infants viewed a novel cat (new exemplar, familiar category) alongside a bird, horse, dog, tiger, or lion (new exemplar, novel category). Infants devoted more attention to the exemplar from the new category, again, a preference that could have come about only if they had categorized the exemplars shown during familiarization. Other studies of visual recognition show that the basis for categorization changes with age, with older infants categorizing objects more on the basis of internal structure and less on specific features or overall global configuration (Fagan & Singer, 1983; Younger, 1993).

Cross-Modal Transfer

Infants show visual recognition even when the initial information is obtained in another modality. In studies of tactual–visual cross-modal transfer, infants obtain information tactually, by feeling a shape that they cannot see, and are then tested for visual recognition. That is, familiarization occurs in one modality and test in another. Transfer is considered to have occurred when infants show a systematic preference on test. The accomplishment of cross-modal transfer has special significance for mental representation, because the information in the test modality must be compared against a representation stored in a different modality. Cross-modal transfer of shape from touch to vision can be accomplished, at least in rudimentary form, by 6 months of age. Infants of this age who are habituated or familiarized to a shape tactually (i.e., where they palpate and manipulate, but do not see, the object) then show evidence of being able to recognize it visually. That is, when the tactually familiar object is subsequently presented visually, along with an object never before handled (or seen), infants show a preference for the novel, just as they do when there is no change in modality (e.g., Rose, Gottfried, & Bridger, 1983). Somewhat older infants accomplish such transfer with greater facility and generality (Bushnell & Weinberger, 1987) and need less exposure to the familiar to achieve the same end (Rose, Gottfried, & Bridger, 1978, 1981).

Integration over Space and Time

Infants show recognition memory for stimuli even when they have to integrate the information over space and time. In studies of aperture viewing (Arterberry, 1993) and point light tracings (Rose, 1988; Skouteris, McKenzie, & Day, 1992) the stimuli are exposed piecemeal during familiarization, either by moving a figure behind a thin slit (aperture) or by tracing it with a point source of light. In both cases, only small portions are revealed at any one time; there are no spatially extended contours. Nonetheless, by 1 year of age, infants show recognition memory when the completed object is presented on test, something they could do only by constructing a representation from the information initially presented piecemeal, over time. That is, infants show evidence that they have synthesized the successive views of the moving point of light into a representation of the entire form.

Taken together, then, the data clearly indicate that infants show recognition memory even when the familiar stimulus has been transformed in ways that are quite complex and the infant must understand principles of categorization, cross-modal equivalence, and spatial–temporal integration.

THEORETICAL AND PRACTICAL CONSTRAINTS

Measures of visual recognition memory clearly hold promise for the early detection of mental retardation, the evaluation of medical and obstetric interventions, and the establishment of primate models of early cognition. Nonetheless, it must be kept in mind that some of the psychometric aspects are less than optimal and that prediction at the individual level is still only modest.

Mental Retardation

Although the correlations between infant abilities and later cognition are only modest, there are some indications that the infant measures may be adequate to help screen for mental retardation. Fagan has developed a screening instrument made up of a series of 10 paired-comparison problems (Fagan & Shepherd, 1987). This test, designed for infants ages 6, 7, 9, and 12 months, uses the same problems at all ages (faces) but decreases the length of the familiarization and test periods as age increases. Early versions of this test (Fagan, Singer, Montie, & Shepherd, 1986) showed good sensitivity (accurate detection of children with retardation) and specificity (accurate detection of normal children). In a recent report, Fagan and his colleagues combined data from three different studies to create a sample of 389 children, all of whom had been tested between 6 and 12 months on problems of visual recognition memory and then retested at 3 years on IQ (Fagan & Haikan-Vasen, 1997). Although the base rate of retardation was relatively low (6.6%), a mean novelty score of 53% or less correctly identified 22 of the 26 children (85%) who later obtained IQ scores of 70 or below; a mean novelty score of 54% or greater correctly identified 336 of the 363 children (93%) whose later IQ scores were normal. Thus, the infant scores showed good sensitivity and specificity.

In a smaller sample ($n = 67$), with a higher base rate of retardation at 3 years (16.4%), Rose, Feldman, and Wallace (1988b) found that mean novelty preference scores of less than 54% correctly identified 8 of the 11 children (73%) with 3-year IQ scores below 70; mean scores above this cutoff correctly identified 42 of the 45 children (75%) with IQ scores equal to or greater than 70. In this latter study, sensitivity and specificity were somewhat better using a cut point of 85, a value which separates those with below-average IQ from those with average IQ (the base rate of below-average IQs was high—46.2%—at this age). Here, sensitivity was 74% and specificity was 83%.

The results of both studies raise the possibility that measures of visual recognition may have clinical utility for the detection of retardation and/or below-average IQ. However, the empirical support for this possibility is still quite sparse, and interpretation is complicated by the fact that overall levels of IQ in the Rose et al. (1988b) sample increased after 3 years.

To improve prediction at the individual level, it will be necessary to increase the reliability of measures. Indeed, given the modest reliability of the infant measures, the correlations between the infant and child measures that have been obtained are quite impressive. Nonetheless, for the assessment of

288 LEARNING AND ATTENTION

clinical risk and the monitoring of clinical interventions reliability needs to be improved.

TRAINING REQUIREMENTS

The administration of tasks of visual recognition memory is actually relatively simple, as is the monitoring of infant looks. Some practice is needed in changing targets, so that the procedure runs smoothly and efficiently, but this can be accomplished quite rapidly.

Looks to the right or left are relatively easy to judge after a little practice. In our lab, we use a four-step procedure to train observers. First, an adult plays the role of infant and tells the observer where she is directing her looks. This is particularly helpful for observers to learn when looks are just off target. Second, the observer verbally indicates where the adult's looks are directed and the adult playing "baby" corrects the observer if he or she errs. Third, the observer records the adult looks by pressing one of two computer keys for the duration of each look. Fourth, the observer practices recording looks from a variety of infants.

For training, several infants are videotaped. Observers score these infants and interrater reliability is calculated by Pearson correlation coefficients. The data entries for the correlations are the total duration of looking to the right and left on each trial. Correlations between observers typically runs better than $r = .95$. Reliability is checked periodically and observers are given refresher training if needed.

IMPLICATIONS

Overall, it is clear that studies of visual attention have led to major advances on two fronts. First, they have indicated that cognitive difficulties can be identified in infants whose development is at risk because of obstetric factors, medical difficulties, and/or environmental insult. Second, they have provided a clear demonstration of the possibility of predicting later cognition from infant behaviors. These two advances by themselves have profound theoretical implications for the issue of cognitive continuity as well as practical implications for early identification of cognitive risk.

Aside from efforts to improve the reliability of measures of visual recognition memory, future work should be directed toward understanding which types of recognition problems best predict which outcomes and why, how attentional factors during familiarization relate to novelty scores and to later cognition, and what processes underlie these links.

ACKNOWLEDGMENTS

This research was supported in part by a Social and Behavioral Sciences Research Grant from the March of Dimes Birth Defects Foundation, by Grant Nos. HD 13810 and HD 01799 from the National Institutes of Health, and by a National Institute of Child Health and Human Development Postdoctoral National Research Service Award (No. HD 07384) to Esther K. Orlian. We are grateful to Judith F. Feldman, Frances Goldenberg, and our many collaborators from the Kennedy Center for their contributions to various facets of this work.

REFERENCES

Arterberry, M. E. (1993). Development of spatial temporal integration in infancy. *Infant Behavior and Development, 16,* 343–364.

Bachevalier, J., Brickson, M., & Hagger, C. (1993). Limbic-dependent recognition memory in monkeys develops early in infancy. *NeuroReport, 4,* 77–80.

Bachevalier, J., Brickson, M., Hagger, C., & Mishkin, M. (1990). Age and sex differences in the effects of selective temporal lesion on the formation of visual discrimination habits in rhesus monkeys (Macaca mulatta). *Behavioral Neuroseience, 104,* 885–899.

Bayley, N. (1933). *The California First Year Mental Scale.* Berkeley: University of California Press.

Bayley, N. (1969). *Bayley Scales of Infant Development.* San Antonio, TX: Psychological Corporation.

Binet, A., & Simon, T. (1905). Methodes nouvelles pour le diagnostic du niveau intellectuel des anormaux. *L' Annee Psychologique, 11,* 191–244.

Bornstein, M. H., Pecheux, M.-G., & Lecuyer, R. (1988). Visual habituation in human infants: Development and rearing circumstances. *Psychological Research, 50,* 130–133.

Bornstein, M. H., & Sigman, M. D. (1986). Continuity in mental development from infancy. *Child Development, 57,* 251–274.

Bushnell, E., & Weinberger, N. (1987). Infants' detection of visual–tactual discrepancies: Asymmetries that indicate a directive role of visual information. *Journal of Experimental Psychology: Human Perception and Performance, 13,* 601–608.

Caron, A. J., & Caron, R. F. (1981). Processing of relational information as an index of infant risk. In S. L. Friedman & M. Sigman (Eds.), *Preterm birth and psychological development* (pp. 219–240). New York: Academic Press.

Caron, R. F., & Caron, A. J. (1969). The effects of repeated exposure and stimulus complexity on visual fixation in infants. *Psychonomic Science, 10,* 207–208.

Cattell, P. (1940). *The measurement of intelligence of infants and young children.* New York: Psychological Corporation.

Cattell, R. B. (1982). *The inheritance of personality and ability.* New York: Academic Press.

Cohen, L. B. (1981). Examination of habituation as a measure of aberrant infant development. In S. L. Friedman & M. Sigman (Eds.), *Preterm birth and psychological development* (pp. 240–254). New York: Academic Press.

Colombo, J., Mitchell, D. W., & Horowitz, F. D. (1988). Infant visual behavior in the paired-comparison paradigm: Test–retest and attention–performance relations. *Child Development, 58,* 1198–1210.

Colombo, J., Mitchell, D. W., O'Brien, M., & Horowitz, F. D. (1987). The stability of visual habituation during the first year of life. *Child Development, 57,* 474–488.

DiLalla, L. F., Thompson, L. A., Plomin, R., Phillips, K., Fagan, J. F., Haith, M. M., Cyphers, L. H., & Fulker, D. W. (1990). Infant predictors of preschool and adult IQ: A study of infant twins and their parents. *Developmental Psychology, 26,* 759–769.

Fagan, J. F. (1974). Infant's recognition memory: The effects of length of familiarization and type of discrimination task. *Child Development, 45,* 351–356.

Fagan, J. F. (1984). The relationship of novelty preference during infancy to later intelligence and later recognition memory. *Intelligence, 8,* 339–346.

Fagan, J. F., & Detterman, D. (1992). The Fagan Test of Infant Intelligence: A technical report. *Journal of Applied Developmental Psychology, 13,* 153–157.

Fagan, J. F., & McGrath, S. K. (1981). Infant recognition memory and later intelligence. *Intelligence, 5,* 121–130.

Fagan, J. F., & Shepherd, P. A. (1987). *The Fagan Test of Infant Intelligence training manual, Vol. 4.* Cleveland: Infantest.

Fagan, J. F., & Singer, L. T. (1983). Infant recognition memory as a measure of intelligence. In L. P. Lipsitt (Ed.), *Advances in infancy research* (Vol. 2, pp. 31–78). Norwood, NJ: Ablex.

Fagan, J. F., Singer, L. T., Montie, J. E., & Shepherd, P. A. (1986). Selective screening device for the early detection of normal or delayed cognitive development in infants at risk for later mental retardation. *Pediatrics, 78,* 1021–1026.

Fagan, J. F., & Haikan-Vasen, J. H. (1997). Selective attention to novelty as a measure of information processing across the life span. In J. A. Burack & J. T. Enns (Eds.), *Attention, development, and psychopathology* (pp. 55–73). New York: Guilford Press.

Gesell, A., & Amatruda, C. (1954). *Developmental diagnosis.* New York: Holber.

Gunderson, V. M., Grant-Webster, K. S., & Fagan, J. F. (1987). Visual recognition memory in high- and low-risk infant pigtailed macaques (*Macaca nemestrina*). *Developmental Psychology, 23,* 671–675.

Gunderson, V. M., Grant-Webster, K. S., & Sackett, G. P. (1989). Deficits in visual recognition memory in low birth weight infant pigtailed monkeys (*Macaca nemestrina*). *Child Development, 60,* 119–127.

Gunderson, V. M., Rose, S. A., & Grant-Webster, K. S. (1990). Cross-modal transfer in high- and low-risk infant pigtailed macaque monkeys. *Developmental Psychology, 26,* 576–581.

Hale, S. (1990). A global developmental trend in cognitive processing speed. *Child Development, 61,* 653–663.

Jacobson, S. W., Fein, G. G., Jacobson, J. L., Schwartz, P. M., & Dowler, J. K. (1985). The effect of intrauterine PCB exposure of visual recognition memory. *Child Development, 56,* 853–860.

Jacobson, S. W., Jacobson, J. L., Sokol, R. J., Martier, S. S., & Chiodo, L. M. (1996). New evidence for neurobehavioral effects of *in utero* cocaine exposure. *Journal of Pediatrics, 129,* 581–590.

Kail, R. (1986). Sources of age differences in speed of processing. *Child Development, 57,* 969–987.

Kail, R. (1988). Developmental functions for speeds of cognitive processing. *Journal of Experimental Child Psychology, 45,* 339–364.

Kopp, C. B., & McCall, R. B. (1982). Predicting later mental performance for normal, at-risk, and handicapped infants. In P. B. Bates & O. G. Brim (Eds.), *Life span development and behavior* (Vol. 4, pp. 33–61). New York: Academic Press.

Malkova, L., Mishkin, M., & Bachevalier, J. (1995). Long-term effects of selective neonatal temporal lobe lesions on learning and memory in monkeys. *Behavioral Neuroscience, 109,* 397–404.

McCall, R. B., & Carriger, M. S. (1993). A meta-analysis of infant habituation and recognition memory performance as predictors of later IQ. *Child Development, 64,* 57–79.

McKee, R. D., & Squire, L. R. (1993). On the development of declarative memory. *Journal of Experimental Psychology: Learning, Memory, and Cognition, 19,* 397–404.

Miranda, S. B., & Fantz, R. L. (1974). Recognition memory in Down's syndrome and normal infants. *Child Development, 48,* 651–660.

Nelson, C. A. (1995). The ontogeny of human memory: A cognitive neuroscience perspective. *Developmental Psychology, 31,* 723–738.

Quinn, P. C., Eimas P. D., & Rosenkrantz, S. L. (1993). Evidence for representations of perceptually similar natural categories by 3–month-old and 4–month-old infants. *Perception, 22,* 463–475.

Rose, S. A. (1980). Enhancing visual recognition memory in preterm infants. *Developmental Psychology, 16,* 85–92.

Rose, S. A. (1983). Differential rates of visual information processing in fullterm and preterm infants. *Child Development, 54,* 1189–1198.

Rose, S. A. (1988). Shape retention in infancy: Visual integration of sequential information. *Child Development, 56,* 1161–1176.

Rose, S. A. (1994). Relation between physical growth and information processing in infants born in India. *Child Development, 65,* 889–902.

Rose, S. A., & Feldman, J. F. (1987). Infant visual attention: Stability of individual differences from 6 to 8 months. *Developmental Psychology, 23,* 490–498.

Rose, S. A., & Feldman, J. F. (1990). Infant cognition: Individual differences and developmental continuities. In J. Colombo & J. W. Fagen (Eds.), *Individual differences in infancy* (pp. 229–245). Hillsdale, NJ: Erlbaum.

Rose, S. A., & Feldman, J. F. (1995). Prediction of IQ and specific cognitive abilities at 11 years from infancy measures. *Developmental Psychology, 31,* 685–696.

Rose, S. A., & Feldman, J. F. (1996). Memory and processing speed in preterm children at eleven years: A comparison with full-terms. *Child Development, 67,* 2005–2021.

Rose, S. A., & Feldman, J. F. (1997). Memory and speed: Their role in the relation of infant information processing to later IQ. *Child development, 68,* 630–641.

Rose, S. A., Feldman, J. F., Futterweit, L. R., & Jankowski, J. J. (1997). Continuity in visual recognition memory: Infancy to 11 years. *Intelligence, 24,* 381–392.

Rose, S. A., Feldman, J. F., Futterweit, L. R., & Jankowski, J. J. (1998). Continuity in tactual-visual cross-modal transfer: Infancy to 11 years. *Developmental Psychology, 34,* 435–440.

Rose, S. A., Feldman, J. F., McCarton, C. M., & Wolfson, J. (1988a). Information processing in seven-month-old infants as a function of risk status. *Child Development, 59,* 589–603.

Rose, S. A., Feldman, J. F., & Wallace, I. F. (1988b). Individual differences in infant information processing: Reliability, stability, and prediction. *Child Development, 59,* 1177–1197.

Rose, S. A., Feldman, J. F., & Wallace, I. F. (1992). Infant information processing in relation to six-year cognitive outcomes. *Child Development, 63,* 1126–1141.

Rose, S. A., Feldman, J. F., Wallace, I. F., & Cohen, P. (1991a). Language: A partial link between infant attention and later intelligence. *Developmental Psychology, 27,* 798–805.

Rose, S. A., Feldman, J. F., Wallace, I. F., & McCarton, C. M. (1989). Infant visual attention: Relation to birth status and developmental outcome during the first 5 years. *Developmental Psychology, 25,* 560–575.

Rose, S. A., Feldman, J. F., Wallace, I. F., & McCarton, C. (1991b). Information processing at 1 year: Relation to birth status and developmental outcome during the first five years. *Developmental Psychology, 27,* 723–737.

Rose, S. A., Gottfried, A. W., & Bridger, W. H. (1978). Cross-modal transfer in infants: Relationship to prematurity and socioeconomic background. *Developmental Psychology, 14,* 643–652.

Rose, S. A., Gottfried, A. W., & Bridger, W. H. (1981). Cross-modal transfer in 6–month-old infants. *Developmental Psychology, 17,* 661–669.

Rose, S. A., Gottfried, A. W., & Bridger, W. H. (1983). Infant's cross-modal transfer from solid objects to their graphic representations. *Child Development, 54,* 686–694.

Rose, S. A., Gottfried, A. W., Melloy-Carminar, P. M., & Bridger, W. H. (1982). Familiarity and novelty preferences in infant recognition memory: Implications for information processing. *Developmental Psychology, 18,* 704–713.

Rose, S. A., & Wallace, I. F. (1985a). Cross-modal and intra-modal transfer as predictors of mental development in fullterm and preterm infants. *Developmental Psychology, 21,* 949–962.

Rose, S. A., & Wallace, I. F. (1985b). Visual recognition memory: A predictor of later cognitive functioning in preterms. *Child Development, 56,* 843–852.

Ruff, H. A. (1978). Infant recognition of the invariant form of objects. *Child Development, 49,* 293–306.

Sigman, M., & Parmelee, A. H. (1974). Visual preferences of four-month-old premature and full-term infants. *Child Development, 45,* 959–965.

Singer, L. T., Arendt, R. A., Fagan, J. F., Minnes, S., Salvator, A., Bolek, T., & Becker, M. (1999). Neonatal visual information processing in cocaine-exposed and non-exposed infants. *Infant Behavior and Development, 22(1),* 1–15.

Singer, L. T., Arendt, R., Minnes, S., Salvator, A., Robinson, J., & Weigand, K. (1998). One year language and developmental outcomes of cocaine-exposed infants. *Pediatric Research, 43,* 228A.

Singer, L. T., & Fagan, J. F. (1984). The cognitive development of the failure-to-thrive infant: A three-year longitudinal study. *Journal of Pediatric Psychology, 9,* 363–384.

Skouteris, H., McKenzie, B. E., & Day, R. H. (1992). Integration of sequential information for shape perception by infants: A developmental study. *Child Development, 63,* 1164–1196.

Thompson, L. A., Fagan, J. F., & Fulker, D. W. (1991). Longitudinal prediction of specific cognitive abilities from infant novelty preference. *Child Development, 67,* 530–538.

Wagner, S. H., & Sakovits, L. J. (1986). A process analysis of infant visual and cross-modal recognition memory: Implications for an amodal code. In L. P. Lipsitt & C. K. Rovee-Collier (Eds.), *Advances in infancy research* (Vol. 4, pp. 195–217). Norwood, NJ: Ablex.

Younger, B. A. (1993). Understanding category members as "the same sort of thing": Explicit categorization in ten-month-old infants. *Child Development, 64,* 309–320.

Zola-Morgan, S., & Squire, L. R. (1985). Amnesia in monkeys following lesions of the mediodorsal nucleus of the thalamus. *Annals of Neurology, 17,* 558–564.

14

Focused Attention
Assessing a Fundamental Cognitive
Process in Infancy

KATHARINE R. LAWSON
HOLLY A. RUFF

Although attention is fundamental to behavior at all ages, behaviors reflecting attention are of particular importance in infancy. Attentional behaviors are especially important in clinical work and research with infants because they are so prominent in the infant's limited behavioral repertoire. Attentional behaviors are also important for strategic reasons because they are one of the few means available to index less visible processes such as learning and memory. Within the general realm of attention, periods of focused attention reflect active uptake of information. That is, when the infant is intently examining targets with eyes and hands, the infant is also actively learning about the target. We think that measures of focused attention would add unique and useful information to developmental assessments of infants, particularly those who are at high risk. Measures of focused attention provide information about the infant's current behavioral style and quality; in addition, several studies from our laboratory indicate that measures of early focused attention provide predictive information for later cognitive status (Ruff & Dubiner, 1987; Ruff, Lawson, Parrinello, & Weissberg, 1990; Lawson & Ruff, 2001).

HISTORY

Focused attention is an important process in perceptual, cognitive, and social functioning. "Focused attention," as the term is used here, refers to both the selective and intensive aspects of attention. It involves selective concentration, with an associated increase in energy or effort devoted to processing information about particular targets and actions on the target. William James (1890/1950) alluded to these selective and intensive processes over a century ago when he wrote:

> Everyone knows what attention is. It is the taking possession by the mind, in clear and vivid form, of one out of what seem several simultaneously possible objects or trains of thought. . . . It implies withdrawal from some things in order to deal effectively with others, and is a condition which has a real opposite in the confused, dazed, scatterbrained state. (pp. 403–404)

In our laboratory, we have been interested in the focused attention shown during active, "hands-on" exploration of objects, which has traditionally been regarded as basic to early cognitive development. This active exploration and play with objects figures prominently in the behavior of the infant in the second half of the first year and throughout the second year. It has been theoretically linked to learning and cognition by a variety of theorists (e.g., Berlyne, 1960; Gibson, 1988; Hunt, 1961; Piaget, 1952; Uzgiris & Hunt, 1975; White, 1959).

Piaget (1952) laid the foundation for the view that the infant's exploration and play with objects is basic to cognitive development. He viewed the processes of exploration and play with objects as fundamental to the development of sensorimotor intelligence (e.g., the development of the object concept, concepts of causality, and imitative learning). Considering intent exploration of objects, Hutt (1970) viewed "specific exploration" as behaviors "essential for the survival of the organism in that they most effectively obtain information for the animal from its particular habitat" (p. 168). Weisler and McCall (1976) describe exploration as a means of reducing "subjective uncertainty," which is related to the "information potential" of the object being explored, the characteristics of the object, and characteristics of the explorer, such as age and rearing conditions. McCall (1974) presented early work on some parameters of exploration in the second half of the first year. He measured duration of mouthing, manipulation with visual regard, length of play session, number of appropriate activities, number of secondary and tertiary circular reactions, frequency of parallel play with two objects, and average duration of interaction with any one object. Among other results, he found that many of the 9.5-month-olds studied could be clustered into groups, with one group characterized by sustained interaction with individual objects.

The component of infants' and young children's exploratory play with an object captured in periods of focused attention—periods when the infant or young child is clearly examining object properties or concentrating on what can be done with the object—is related to information acquisition. For several months after the beginning of independent manipulation of objects, focused attention is seen primarily in careful and deliberate examination of object properties by eyes and fingers. Toward the end of the first year, the behavioral arena expands somewhat to include concentration during other object-related activity. Active object exploration can access physical qualities of objects (e.g., size, shape, weight, rigidity, and texture). Active exploration can also access functional properties and relational information.

A variety of empirical findings indicate that measures of focused attention index an aspect of cognitive processing, as do measures of recovery of looking (see Rose & Orlian, Chapter 13, this volume). Work in our laboratory and others has indicated that the periods of focused attention are more likely than casual attention to be involved in learning. The distinction is supported, for example, by the priority of focused attention over other behaviors when the infant is presented a novel object; that is, the infant is more likely to examine an object, with deliberate visual and haptic exploitation of object properties, before engaging in less attentive behaviors such as mouthing or repetitive banging, shaking, and pushing (Ruff, 1986b). Focused attention increases with the presentation of a novel object, declines as the object becomes more familiar, and then increases when another novel object is introduced (Ruff, Saltarelli, Capozzoli, & Dubiner, 1992). More casual looking or "diversive" exploration does not show these systematic changes in relation to novelty (Hutt, 1970; Oakes, Madole, & Cohen, 1991; Ruff et al., 1992). Infants are also less distractible when focusing on objects than when more casually engaged, suggesting a redistribution of energy with increased energy directed toward exploiting the target object and some buffering against competing stimuli. For example, the infant is less likely to turn, and the latency to turn is longer, to the distracting displays when engaged in focused attention than when engaged in other visual attention (Oakes & Tellinghuisen, 1994; Ruff, Capozzoli, & Saltarelli, 1996; Saltarelli, Ruff, & Capozzoli, 1990).

Several studies from our laboratory (Ruff & Dubiner, 1987; Ruff et al., 1990) indicate that early focused attention, but not casual attention, is predictive of later cognitive status. That is, duration of focused attention by 7-month-old (Lawson & Ruff, 2001) and 9-month-old (Ruff, 1988) very-low-birthweight (VLBW) infants was significantly and positively correlated with later IQ. In neither study was early cognitive index (Bayley Mental Development Index [MDI]) related to later IQ, suggesting that the focused attention measure and the early MDI measure were reflecting different processes. When casual looking and focused attention were entered together to predict later cognitive status, focused attention made a significant unique positive contribution to MDI at 2 years and IQ at 3 years, but casual looking made no contribution (Lawson & Ruff, 1998). Similarly, for infants with Down syndrome (Vietze, McCarthy, McQuiston, MacTurk, & Yarrow, 1983), active attempts to focus on objects and master them were correlated with concurrent MDI whereas simple looking at the object was not. For high-risk preterms (Landry & Chapieski, 1988), the number of shifts of attention and the number of toys noticed at 6 months, regarded by the authors as indexing higher-level attention, were correlated with 1- and 2-year MDI, but simple looking was not.

Our work on the nature and development of focused attention, in conjunction with our work on the development of the low-birthweight infant, led us to explore the possibility of using attention measures as clinical tools. Because attention underlies cognitive, perceptual, and social functioning, the quality and quantity of attention are considered implicitly in all developmental assessments. Assessors monitor quality and amount of attention shown spontaneously and in response to various elicitors to make inferences about the child's behavioral integrity. However, for the low-birthweight, preterm (LBW-PT) children who are of most concern to us, explicit consideration of attention may be of particular significance. Reductions in, or disruptions of, attention have been reported for high-risk infants across testing paradigms (see later). In addition, the findings of several follow-up programs for LBW-PT children have indicated an increased incidence of various forms of attentional difficulties in the preschool and school years (e.g., Hack et al., 1992; Robson & Pederson, 1997; Sykes et al., 1997; Szatmari, Saigal, Rosenbaum, Campbell, & King, 1990; Weisglas-Kuperus, Koot, Baerts, Fetter, & Sauer, 1993; but see also Teplin, Burchinal, Johnson-Martin, Humphry, & Kraybill, 1991). The Low-birthweight Infant Follow-up and Evaluation (LIFE) program at Albert Einstein College of Medicine was such a follow-up program for infants born preterm ($\leq$ 37 weeks estimated gestational age) and of VLBW ($\leq$ 1,500 grams) and was the context for our development of measures of focused attention as a clinical tool. Infants in this program were evaluated at regular intervals to assess functional status. One measure was the Bayley Scales of Infant Development (Bayley, 1969/1993), which is widely used and generally agreed to provide useful information about the infant's current function relative to that of other infants of the same age. However, clinicians and researchers have been concerned about limits to the information provided by the Bayley—the nature of the behavior assessed, its significance for cognition and learning, and its predictive value (e.g., Kopp & McCall, 1982; Bendersky & Lewis, Chapter 22, this volume). This concern has led to the search for alternative procedures that assess dynamic processes underlying cognitive development, such as attention and learning. For example, a large literature (see, e.g., Bornstein, 1989; Bornstein & Sigman, 1986; Colombo, 1993; McCall & Carriger, 1993; Rose, Feldman, Wallace, & McCarton, 1989) supports the usefulness of measures of familiarization or habituation and recovery of looking as an index of learning and memory and as predictive of later function; at least one version of these procedures is currently marketed as an assessment tool (Fagan Test of Infant Intelligence, or FTII, Fagan & Shephard, 1987; see also Fagen & Ohr, Chapter 12, and Rose & Orlian, Chapter 13, this volume).

GENERAL DESCRIPTION

Because of the unique information potentially provided by an understanding of focused attention, we incorporated into our clinical follow-up a measure of focused attention for infants at 7 and 12 months of age. To do this, we had to select measures appropriate to a clinical context and define and monitor assessment and scoring procedures. The development of these measures was based on our laboratory research experience. We decided to use ratings rather than quantitative measures of duration, frequency, and/or latency for several reasons. Ratings seemed more feasible for a clinical setting because they are more readily generated than are quantitative measures, which require specialized recording equipment and considerable time, neither of which is typically available in a clinical follow-up program. In addition, global ratings may also capture several relevant variables in a single score. And, importantly, our previous research with full-term and preterm children had indicated that global ratings of attention could be reliably obtained and were related to concurrent quantitative measures based on the same episodes of play; the ratings were also predictive of later measures of attention and other aspects of behavior (Ruff et al., 1990).

Global ratings, however, imply a reference point for judging the child, and that reference point can vary with the rater's experience and expectations. Therefore, the ratings had to be standardized as much as possible. To help provide consistent anchors, we developed written guidelines and videotapes of play episodes with recommended ratings and explanations and urged the raters to review the guidelines and videotapes frequently.

The global ratings are based in large part on the same aspects of behavior as our quantitative measures of focused attention: steadiness of gaze, facial expression and affect, position of toys relative to eyes, self-consciousness, amount of extraneous movement, speed of object-related movement, and presence of vocalizing. A child who looks steadily at the toys with a serious and intent expression, reduces the distance between toy and self for better inspection, quiets other body movement, and seems to lose awareness of self with no vocalizing and no social bids would be rated highly for focused attention. A child who holds the toy at arm's length, looks away from it frequently, shows a relaxed facial expression, and moves around and vocalizes a great deal would be rated much lower.

Whereas we have previously employed a 3-point rating for research purposes, the raters for the clinical program felt that a 5-point scale would provide more information, particularly in distinguishing low from very low levels of attention, distinctions of potential clinical importance. Therefore, we developed a 5-point rating scale. The ratings range from 1 (relatively little engagement and no signs of concentration) to 5 (an exceptionally high level of object engagement, with clear and prolonged periods of absorption in the object). Specific details of the guidelines for assigning ratings were tailored to the ages at which infants were assessed (in particular, longer durations of focused attention are expected with increasing age), but Table 14.1 presents general working guidelines. The rating of 1 is designed to reflect little or no investment of energy in object exploration and play; trials assigned a 1 can include a fair amount of toy orientation, but looking is not specific to object properties and appears to be related to more general aspects of the toy situation (e.g., movement as the child bangs). A rating of 2 is designed to reflect the possibility of investment in objects without clear evidence for it; episodes of focused attention are marginal and brief or infrequent, with no clear starting and ending points. A rating of 3 is designed to reflect clear demonstration of ability and inclination to invest energy in exploration of object properties and play; even at 7 months, trials should include at least a few clear examples of concentration. Ratings of 4 and 5 are designed to reflect increasing levels of sustained and concentrated attention, with increasing proportions of the trials devoted to well-defined episodes of object-related focused attention.

Although attention can, in principle, be rated at the time of the evaluation, the tester may not be able to adequately monitor the child's concentration due to distractions, for example, picking up and re-presenting toys and interacting with the caretaker of the infant. We have been exploring the feasibility and reliability of more direct ratings. Though testers were requested to attempt direct ratings for most infants, only a few were rated at 7 months, suggesting that the testers were substantially distracted from the task during testing and/or did not feel their ratings were reliable. We currently videotape all sessions and recommend this procedure if it is possible. Videotaped sessions can be rated by several different people, and they can also be scored for quantitative measures, if these are desired.

PROCEDURES

Standard contexts and procedures for free play permit clearer comparisons among children. Our assessment rooms present minimal distractions and our procedures are routinized. The child sits on the lap of a familiar caretaker (usually the mother) and toys are presented at a table at midline and within easy reach. Uniform instructions ask the caretaker to allow the child to play independently in any way with the toys. At 7 months, each of three

TABLE 14.1. Working Guidelines for Rating Focused Attention in Infants

Rating of 1

These trials include no clear evidence for investment in the object(s). There is little visual engagement and looking is primarily to facilitate grasping/mouthing/transfer or to watch movement of toy, as in repetitive behaviors such as banging or waving. Behavior may be unorganized. The infant may look at but does not focus on the properties of specific object (i.e., another toy could be substituted with little or no change in behaviors). Trial may include many extraneous behaviors (e.g., fussing, mouthing, repetitive behaviors such as banging for younger infants and vocalizing, rapid shifting across objects/activities, extraneous motor behaviors for older infants). An inexperienced observer should have little difficulty scoring 0 for duration of focused attention to the object(s).

Rating of 2

These trials suggest that the infant can invest energy in object exploration without providing clear evidence for this investment. Trials can include marginal and poorly defined attention to objects and action on objects. They can include brief to moderate durations of looking, but focused attention is marginal in quality; episodes do not have clear starting and ending points and are characterized by overall lack of effort and organization. An inexperienced rater might have difficulty scoring duration of focused attention for these infants.

Rating of 3

These trials provide clear demonstration of the ability and inclination to attend to objects during object exploration and other actions on objects. Trials include at least a few clear examples of focused attention, with durations of focused attention being relatively short to moderate in length; trials may also include many actions accompanied by casual attention, but even these are somewhat organized and purposeful.

Rating of 4

A greater proportion of the available time is devoted to focused attention toward the object(s) and actions on the objects and extraneous behaviors (non-object-related movements, social bids, vocalizing) are rare. Individual focused attention episodes should be longer and clear-cut, with starting and ending points easily determined. The infant remains oriented to the object(s) for much of the available time in both casual and focused attention episodes.

Rating of 5

Trials include longer periods of absorption in the object(s) and actions on the objects, with focused attention episodes long and clear-cut and extraneous behaviors reduced still further or nonexistent. Level of object-oriented attention is clearly exceptionally high. An inexperienced rater would have no difficulty in scoring duration of focused attention.

Distributions of ratings obtained so far for our VLBW, PT infants at 7 months: all 3 trials, 1 or 1.5, 30%; at least one rating of 2 and none > 2.5, 42%; at least one rating of 3 and none > 3.5, 17%; at least one rating of 4 and none > 4.5, 8%; at least one rating of 5, 3%. Distributions of ratings for our VLBW infants at 12 months: both trials 1 or 1.5, 20%; one rating of 2 or 2.5 and none > 2.5, 22%; at least one rating of 3 and none > 3.5, 35%; at least one rating of 4 and none > 4.5, 14%; at least one rating of 5, 8%.

toys is presented one at a time for 90 seconds each, in a fixed order; toys are presented singly because of infants' limited ability at this age to maintain organized attention and behavior in the face of many toys. At 12 months, a single toy and then a tray of multiple toys in specified layout are presented, each for 2 minutes; both contexts are provided because children at this age vary in their ability to shift attention and to concentrate in the face of competing targets. Every effort is made to have the child complete the prescribed time. However, the session is terminated early if the child is clearly upset and cannot be soothed or if there are three consecutive drops or throws of the toy with no intervening attention or regard to any element of the toy. Toys used for measuring focused attention should be age-appropriate toys of moderate interest; toys that are generally fascinating or boring would generate too limited a range of attention to provide a useful base for comparison across infants.

BIOBEHAVIORAL BASIS OF ASSESSMENT

Physiological measures, and specifically alterations in heart rate, have helped to differentiate attentional responses of infants, particularly in distinguishing orienting and defensive reactions, as proposed by Graham and Clifton (1966). Using characteristics of heart rate change in infants, Porges (e.g., 1984, 1992) differentiates between reactive and sustained attention. Porges described the reactive process as the immediate and short-lived orienting response related to changes in stimulation; it involves both parasympathetic and sympathetic responses leading to an immediate deceleration in heart rate followed by a longer latency heart rate response with direction related to signal value of the stimulus. The sustained process is viewed as a relatively long-term alteration in state related to qualitative aspects of the stimulus—a parasympathetic response with tonic physiological changes such as reduction of heart rate and heart rate variability and generalized inhibition of motor activity and respiration. Richards and Casey (1992) also discuss cardiac and behavioral characteristics underlying stimulus orienting and sustained attention. Richards and Casey describe orienting further as the phase when the infant "evaluates stimulus novelty, processes preliminary stimulus information, and decides whether to allocate further mental resources" (p. 32). Sustained attention, in contrast, is the phase of voluntary, active cognitive processing of detailed stimulus information. We assume that our focused attention measures reflect the period referred to by these investigators as the sustained, cognitively active phase of attention. In fact, evidence suggests that there is temporal overlap between behavioral measures of focused attention and heart rate measures of attention (Lansink & Richards, 1997).

RELIABILITY AND VALIDITY

Various types of evidence suggest that measures of focused attention are reliable and valid, both predictively and concurrently. Reliability is indicated by significant and moderate to high internal consistency, as indexed by intercorrelations among trials in a test session (Ruff, 1995). High/moderate test–retest reliability across 2-week spans has also been reported (Ruff, 1988; Ruff & Dubiner, 1987). Interobserver reliability has also been high. In our laboratory, even when no specific criteria have been defined, interobserver correlations for both frequency and duration of focused attention episodes have usually been greater than .90.

Validity is indicated by the fact that measures of focused attention discriminate among samples of infants according to risk, with higher-risk status associated with lower levels and possibly disordered focused attention. For example, at 7 months, full-terms examined objects more than did preterms, and for full-terms, but not for preterms, examination declined over time. Full-terms' behaviors were consistently ordered, with focused examining having priority, but preterms' behaviors were not consistently ordered (Ruff, 1986a). The discrimination of risk samples by focused attention measures is supported by parallel cardiac changes—relative to normal full-terms, preterms show less pronounced cardiac rhythmic variation (respiratory sinus arrhythmia) at baseline and a reduction in the changes in cardiac rate and variability that are associated with attention (Richards & Casey, 1992). Focused attention measures also differentiate high-risk and low-risk preterms, with higher risk associated with delayed and reduced focused attention (e.g., Ruff, 1988; Ruff et al., 1990; Ruff, McCarton, Kurtzberg, & Vaughan, 1984). Other investigators have reported similar differentiations in attention to objects according to risk (e.g., Landry & Chapieski, 1988; Sigman, 1976).

Preliminary Results for Reliability and Validity of Ratings for VLBW-PT Infants

Since implementing focused attention rating measures in our clinical procedures, we have collected ratings and quantitative measures (duration and number of focused attention episodes) for 71 VLBW-PT infants at 7 months corrected age and 62 VLBW-PT infants at 12 months ($n = 49$ children seen at both ages). Birthweights ranged from 525 to 1,470 g; estimated gestational age ranged from 24 to 36 weeks. Developmental assessments of these children included the Bayley-II Mental and Motor Scales, the Bayley-II Behavior Record Scale (BRS), the Fagan Test of Infant Intelligence (FTII), and a free-play period on which measures of focused attention are based. For the BRS of the Bayley-II, the tester rated specific aspects of behavior and individual items are combined to form general categories for which percentile scores are available; for the ages included here, the relevant general categories are orientation/engagement (indexing "energy level, interest and enthusiasm, initiative and exploration"; Bayley, 1969/1993, p. 209) and emotional regulation (indexing "aspects of temperament including activity level, frustration tolerance, and adaptation to change"; Bayley, 1969/1993, p. 209). Testers also globally rated these two categories and attention on a 5-point scale.

Reliability for Ratings at 7 Months

Two observers viewed the videotapes for the first 48 7-month-old infants; with three trials for each child, reliability was based on 144 trials. Raters had perfect agreement on 65% of the trials, disagreement by 1 point on 34% of the trials, and disagreement by 2 points on only 1% of the trials. For the final scores, we resolved disagreements of 1 point by using the mean rating; disagreements of more than 1 point led to a rerating by the same viewers or a rating by a third viewer.

Concurrent Validity for Ratings at 7 Months

Concurrent validity of the ratings was indicated by high correlations with quantitative measures of focused attention also coded from the videotapes. Summing over the three objects, the ratings were highly correlated with duration of focused attention and number of episodes, r's = .83 and .79, p's < .001. The ratings were also correlated across objects, r's = .42 to .61, p < .01.

Concurrent validity in a broader sense was also supported. The global ratings of attention were related in various ways to other indices of cognitive/perceptual and psychomotor functioning. The global rating at 7 months was significantly correlated to the age-corrected Bayley-II MDI-7, r = .39, p = .001, and PDI-7, r = .47, p < .001, n = 75, indicating some overlap with these measures of attention and learning and psychomotor function. The 7-month global rating was also correlated with the Bayley-II tester's rating for attention/arousal, r = .31, p < .01, and for orientation/engagement as per the BRS percentile score, r = .24, p < .05. The ratings completed by the Bayley tester as part of the administration of the Bayley were independent of the global ratings of focused attention; they were usually completed by a different person, based on a different sample of behavior, and completed at a different time. Thus, the agreement between the global ratings of focused attention and the Bayley tester's ratings supports the validity of the global rating in capturing both attention specifically and engagement/interest/energy somewhat more generally.

The 7-month global rating was marginally related to measures drawn from the Fagan Test of Infant Intelligence (FTII) at 7 months. The correlation with the mean preference for novelty, r = .22, p < .10, n = 61, an independent assessment of cognitive status, again suggests that the global rating of focused attention taps cognitive status in some way.

Reliability for Ratings at 12 Months

At 12 months, the single-object and multiple-object episodes were scored separately because they can elicit quite different types of behavior. Reliability was calculated for the first 40 children. For the single-object episode, raters had perfect agreement on 50% of the trials, disagreement by 1 point on 40% of the trials, and disagreement by ≥ 2 points on 10% of the trials. For the multiple-object episode, the comparable values were 72%, 18%, and 10%.

Concurrent Validity for Ratings at 12 Months

Validity of the global ratings was again supported by their strong relationship with quantitative measures. For the single-object episode, the global ratings were highly correlated with the duration and number of focused attention episodes, $r = .77$ and $.65$, p's $< .001$. The ratings for the multiple object periods were also correlated with the duration of focused attention and number of episodes for this period, $r = .54$ and $.53$, p's $< .001$. The ratings were moderately correlated across the single and multiple object episodes, $r = .30$, $p < .02$. A summary global rating (summed over single- and multiple-object episodes) was correlated with comparable summary duration and number measures, r's $= .71$ and $.66$, p's $< .001$.

The global rating of focused attention at 12 months was only marginally related to concurrent measures of other behaviors. The lack of relationships between the focused attention rating and concurrent measures suggests that by 12 months, focused attention may reflect functions that are somewhat different from those indexed at an earlier age and different from the other components of the developmental assessment.

Predictive Validity of the Global Ratings at 7 Months

Preliminary examination of potential predictive relationships indicates that the 7-month global rating was significantly related to the 12-month global rating, $r = .33$, $p < .02$, $n = 49$, suggesting some stability across this age span for attentiveness. The 7-month global rating was also significantly related to the Bayley MDI at 12 months, $r = .28$, $p < .05$, $n = 55$.

Conclusions

In general, the results of these analyses indicate that the global ratings were reliable and valid, in terms of both their relation to quantitative measures and their consistency across different objects. These results support the usefulness of the rating as a measure of focused attention at 7 and at 12 months. In addition, the global rating at 7 months was related to concurrent measures of other behaviors and to ratings and overall cognitive level at 12 months, suggesting that ratings at this age may be especially useful in tapping important underlying processes.

DEVELOPMENTAL MODEL

The constructs and results we have presented here need to be considered in the context of development—what it is that develops in focused attention. As a starting point, focused attention has been hypothesized to be part of two visual attention systems that develop within the first few years of life (see Ruff & Rothbart, 1996, for a detailed discussion). The first is a system that underlies orienting to and investigating of events and objects. The orienting/investigative system seems to be supported by two neural networks. One contributes to orienting toward important locations in the surrounding environment and functions well by 3 to 4 months of age (Clohessy, Posner, Rothbart, & Vecera, 1991; Johnson, Posner, & Rothbart, 1991); it involves the parietal cortex, subcortical areas, such as the superior colliculus, and the frontal eye fields (Johnson, 1990). The other network contributes to object recognition and functions well by 5 to 6 months (Ruff & Rothbart, 1996); it involves the inferior temporal cortex (Ungerleider & Mishkin, 1982). The operation of this first system of visual attention is strongly motivated by the novelty of objects and events and is therefore very susceptible to habituation.

Toward the end of the first year, a second attention system begins to emerge, which can be seen as the development of higher-level control (Ruff & Rothbart, 1996). The second attention system is governed by plans and instructions, and it plays a role in controlling complex sequences of action (Allport, 1987). The emergence of this system is heralded both by the beginnings of inhibitory control (Diamond, 1991) around 9 months and by an increasing complexity of action. The second system of attention is supported by developmental changes in the frontal cortex and, for this reason, continues to develop for several years (Welsh & Pennington, 1988).

The first system of attention governs focused attention from the emergence of manipulative play with toys at about 5 months. As discussed previously, focused exploration of objects involves orientation to and recognition of objects and high sensitivity to novelty and familiarity—hallmarks of behavior involving the first visual system. Individual differences in degree and duration of focused attention, however, are quite marked. To the extent that these individual differences are related to other aspects of concurrent functioning and predict later cognitive functioning, they may be predictive for the same reason that novelty preference in familiarization and habituation procedures is predictive. That is, infants who are strongly motivated and able to focus attention and explore novel objects and situations may acquire more general information about the world and be more adept at mastering cognitive skills as they develop.

By 12 months of age, although attention is still strongly governed by the first system, the second system is an emerging influence on behavior. Because the period from 12 to 18 months represents a transition period in the control of attention, there may be increased variability and inconsistency in quantity and quality of attention. Infants' focused attention habituates to novelty more rapidly than it does in younger infants. As a result, periods of focused attention to single objects may sometimes be shorter than they were earlier. However, periods of focused attention to multiple objects are likely to be variable and inconsistent, depending on the infant's tendency to use the objects in different ways, such as examining them, relating them to each other, and incorporating them in social bids (Ruff & Lawson, 1990). That is, focused attention may be limited because the infant tends to become distracted in the presence of more than one novel object and does not yet have a strong capacity to tune out nearby distractors; it may be variable, because the infant's ability to integrate discrete elements into a larger whole as a focus of attention is just emerging. Thus, until attention is firmly supported by a more developed second system, focused attention based on episodes of complex, planned activity may be more variable than episodes seen in younger or older children.

According to our preliminary results, the 12-month global ratings were less reliable and less well related to concurrent and subsequent measures than were the 7-month global ratings. Thus, measures of focused attention at 7 months may be particularly informative about current and later function because, around 6 to 9 months of age, focused attention in the exploration of objects represents a qualitative advance in infant capacity (see, e.g., McCall, Eichorn, & Hogarty, 1977). Measures of focused attention at 12 months may be affected by the transitions in attention and other processes occurring at this age (Ruff & Rothbart, 1996).

STRUCTURAL AND/OR THEORETICAL CONSTRAINTS/CONTROVERSIES

The results of a wide range of studies, as noted earlier, indicate that focused attention reflects information processing and learning. Focused attention specifically, rather than more general looking or casual attention, is associated with these cognitive processes. In this sense, focused attention procedures are similar to measures of habituation/recovery of function. However, measures of focused attention have the added advantage that they provide an opportunity to observe the manner in which infants spontaneously organize behavior during independent play. They are also advantageous because almost all infants will engage in play with objects readily and persistently, so that some information can be gained from almost all infants. They have the limitation that they are not so useful with children who are either so immature or so impaired motorically that they cannot grasp and manipulate objects. It also requires a fair amount of training to distinguish focused from more casual attention.

One of the major reasons for regular developmental assessments of VLBW children is to determine which children are most at risk for poor cognitive development. The standardization norms of the Bayley make it possible to establish cutoffs below which a child can be considered abnormal relative to other children of the same age. The measure of focused attention could be used in the same way. Although there are no norms available, we have reported ranges of focused attention for normal infants at different ages based on different studies using a variety of objects (Ruff & Lawson, 1991). Marked changes in context and duration of session may alter these expectations; for example, infants would be expected to show less focus in highly distracting contexts and lower percentages of time focusing given extended exposure to the same toys due to learning effects. However, given contexts and times similar to those used here, infants at 7 months should spend about 11% of available time in focused attention and a percentage less than 2% might be regarded as abnormal (e.g., a range of 2 to 24% of available time in focused attention has been shown by 7-month-old infants given 90-second exposure to each of a variety of toys). Of the 71 infants seen at 7 months in our clinical setting, 19 (27%) were given the lowest mean rating of 1 and, of these, 16 (84%) had durations of focused attention less than 2%. This high concordance between a rating of 1 and very low duration of focused attention suggests that a rating of 1 indeed reflects abnormally low attention.

In the current study, at 7 months, the 71 VLBW-PT infants showed a mean of 5.0 seconds of focused attention per minute (SD = 5.7 seconds, median = 2.4); the mean rating was 1.71 (SD = .63, median = 1.67). At 12 months, the 62 VLBW-PT infants showed a mean of 8.5 seconds per minute (SD = 6.0, median = 7.3) and the mean rating was 2.33 (SD = .86, median = 2.5). Data on duration were available for 38 infants at both ages; they showed significantly more focused attention at 12 than at 7 months, t = 2.49, $p < .02$, and were assigned a significantly higher global rating, t = 5.19, $p < .001$. Thus, these high-risk infants typically engaged in relatively little focused attention at 7 months but typically showed more focused attention 5 months later, as reflected in both the durations and global ratings.

The distributions of the ratings were skewed, as was expected on the basis of previous data for duration, with more infants on the low than the high end of the distribution. At 7 months, when the ratings for all three play trials for individual children were examined, 30% of the infants had a global rating of 1 or 1.5 for all three and no infant had a rating of 4 or 5 for all three; the median total rating (summed over the three trials) was a 5, most typically consisting of two ratings of 2 and one rating of 1. At 12 months, when the ratings for the single- and multiple-object episodes for individual children were examined, 20% had a global rating of 1 or 1.5 for both and 2% had a rating of 4 or 5 for both; the median total rating was again 5, most typically consisting of one rating of 2 and one of 3.

TRAINING REQUIREMENTS

We developed specific written guidelines and videotapes to aid in training individuals who were to rate focused attention. These aids differ in some ways in relation to the specific ages of the infants to be rated—that is, there are some systematic shifts in quality and amount of attention that would be expected at different ages. These aids were based in part on previous experience in scoring focused attention. Although the defining characteristics (described previously) almost constitute an operational definition, it is likely that someone rating focused attention needs to be well acquainted with what focused attention "looks like." Development of the guidelines and videotapes was also based on discussion by the program's raters, who helped to identify factors that made rating particular children difficult or that contributed to disagreements between raters. Raters in our program are instructed to review the guidelines and demonstration tapes frequently to facilitate consistency in approach. We have found that omission of this step can result in fluctuation of the rater's frame of reference.

IMPLICATIONS

We have presented evidence that measures of focused attention provide unique information about the functional integrity of young infants in the second half of the first year. Exploration and play with objects figure prominently in the normal behavior of infants during the second half of the first year, and the infants' concentration promotes selective intake of information and permits learning. The results in general indicate predictive and concurrent validity for measures of focused attention. They suggest that higher risk is associated with delayed, less efficient, and possibly disordered focused attention toward objects. Slower or reduced learning has similarly been indicated by studies based on recognition memory (Rose, 1983). In addition, it is possible that high-risk preterms may be less reactive to stimulation in the sense that they are less likely to be aware of the "information potential" of objects and actions and so less ready to recognize the need to gather information.

We therefore developed a global rating of focused attention during object-related free play, which was incorporated into our clinical follow-up program for preterm VLBW infants. The number of children whose evaluations included this procedure is small, and results obtained to date are only suggestive. The results seem to be in agreement with those obtained in various research contexts; the ratings are reasonably reliable and valid, and the ratings at 7 months are related to a variety of concurrent measures of other behaviors. It will be necessary to collect further data to assess whether the ratings obtained in our clinical setting are predictive of aspects of later function of these high-risk infants, as the duration of focused attention has been for previous research cohorts. While precautions must be taken to ensure that such ratings are reliable, the procedures should be easy to implement, and the ratings should provide important information about individual children that is different from the information provided by standard assessments.

As these procedures are implemented in a wider variety of contexts, it will be important to compare the information obtained from these ratings with other information about attention and learning in the infant. Of particular interest to us is the issue of individual differences in attentional control and how these might be shown in different contexts and across time. For example, we plan further exploration of the extent to which the different types of attention that have been studied in infants reflect a unitary phenomenon as opposed to multiple processes. Infants' sustained attention has been studied in a wide variety of situations: observation of static and moving objects and events, exploration and play with objects, activity in goal-oriented situations, searching for hidden objects, and simply waiting for expected events. The different findings in these studies point to the possible existence of multiple processes underlying sustained attention. We ourselves have found differential relationships concurrently and predictively between different measures of attention (see, e.g., Ruff & Lawson, 1990). The systematic study of effects of different objects, different circumstances, and different demands on infants' attention, in relation to measures of behavior in entirely different contexts, will enlarge our understanding of attention and the usefulness of the attention ratings as a clinical tool.

ACKNOWLEDGMENTS

We would like to acknowledge the support of the March of Dimes Birth Defects Foundation for the writing of this chapter and for the collection and analysis of the data reported in it. The work was also facilitated by a grant from the National Institute of Child Health and Human Development to the Rose F. Kennedy Center for Research in Mental Retardation and Human Development (No. HD 01799); it was carried out as part of the Low-birthweight Infant Follow-up and Evaluation program, directed by Dr. Cecelia McCarton. We thank Katherine Bennett-Jankowski, Amy Damast, Marlene Spector, Lisandra Villalba, and Christine Williams for their help with the ratings. We are particularly grateful to Mary Capozzoli for her contributions to both clinical and laboratory programs.

REFERENCES

Allport, A. (1987). Selection for action: Some behavioral and neurophysiological considerations of attention and action. In H. Heuer & A. F. Sanders (Eds.), *Perspectives on perception and action* (pp. 395–419). Hillsdale, NJ: Erlbaum.

Bayley, N. (1969). *Bayley Scales of Infant Development*. New York: Psychological Corporation. (1993, restandardized)

Berlyne, O. E. (1960). *Conflict, arousal and curiosity*. New York: McGraw-Hill.

Bornstein, M. H. (1989). Stability in early mental development: from attention and information processing in infancy to language and cognition in childhood. In M. H. Bornstein & N. A. Krasnegor (Eds.), *Stability and continuity in mental development* (pp. 147–170). Hillsdale, NJ: Erlbaum.

Bornstein, M. H., & Sigman, M. D. (1986). Continuity in mental development from infancy. *Child Development, 57*, 251–274.

Clohessy, A. B., Posner, M. I., Rothbart, M. K., & Vecera, S. P. (1991). The development of inhibition of return in early infancy. *Journal of Cognitive Neuroscience, 3*, 345–350.

Colombo, J. (1993). *Infant cognition: Predicting later intellectual functioning*. Newbury Park, CA: Sage.

Diamond, A. (1991). Frontal lobe involvement in cognitive changes during the first year of life. In K. R. Gibson & A. C. Petersen (Eds.), *Brain maturation and cognitive development* (pp. 127–180). New York: Aldine de Gruyter.

Fagan, J. F., & Shepherd, P. A. (Eds.). (1987). *The Fagan test of infant intelligence training manual* (Vol. 4). Cleveland: Infantest Corp.

Gibson, E. J. (1988). Exploratory behavior in the development of perceiving, acting, and the acquiring of knowledge. *Annual Review of Psychology, 39*, 1–41.

Graham, F. K., & Clifton, R. K. (1966). Heart rate change as a component of the orienting response. *Psychological Bulletin, 65*, 305–320.

Hack, M., Breslau, N., Aram, D., Weissman, B., Klein, N., & Borawski-Clark, E. (1992). The effect of very low birth weight and social risk on neurocognitive abilities at school age. *Developmental and Behavioral Pediatrics, 13*, 412–420.

Hunt, J. (1961). *Intelligence and experience*. New York: Ronald Press.

Hutt, C. (1970). Specific and diverse exploration. In H. W. Reese & L. P. Lipsitt (Eds.), *Advances in child development and behavior* (Vol. 5, pp. 119–180). New York: Academic Press.

James, W. (1950). *The principles of psychology*. New York: Dover. (Original work published 1890)

Johnson, M. H. (1990). Cortical maturation and the development of visual attention in early infancy. *Journal of Cognitive Neuroscience, 2*, 81–95.

Johnson, M. H., Posner, M. I., & Rothbart, M. K. (1991). Components of visual orienting in early infancy: Contingency learning, anticipatory looking, and disengaging. *Journal of Cognitive Neuroscience, 3*, 335–344.

Kopp, C. B., & McCall, R. B. (1982). Predicting later mental performance for normal, at-risk and handicapped infants. In P. B. Baltes & O. G. Brim (Eds.), *Life span development and behavior* (Vol. 4, pp. 33–61). New York: Academic Press.

Landry, S. H., & Chapieski, M. L. (1988). Visual attention during toy exploration in preterm infants: Effects of medical risk and maternal interactions. *Infant Behavior and Development, 11,* 187–204.

Lansink, J. M., & Richards, J. E. (1997). Heart rate and behavioral measures of attention in six-, nine-, and twelve-month-old infants during object exploration. *Child Development, 68,* 610–620.

Lawson, K. R., & Ruff, H. A. (1998). *Prediction of cognitive function by early measures of attention.* Unpublished data.

Lawson, K. R., & Ruff, H. A. (2001). *Early attention and emotionality predict later behavioral and cognitive function.* Manuscript submitted for publication.

McCall, R. B. (1974). Exploratory manipulation and play in the human infant. *Monographs of the Society for Research in Child Development, 39*(2, Serial No. 155).

McCall, R. B., & Carriger, M. S. (1993). A meta-analysis of infant habituation and recognition memory performance as predictors of IQ. *Child Development, 64,* 57–79.

McCall, R. B., Eichorn, D. H., & Hogarty, P. S. (1977). Transitions in early mental development. *Monographs of the Society for Research in Child Development, 42*(3, Serial No. 171).

Oakes, L. M., Madole, K. L., & Cohen, L. B. (1991). Infant object examining: Habituation and categorization. *Cognitive Development, 6,* 377–392.

Oakes, L. M., & Tellinghuisen, D. J. (1994). Examining in infancy: Does it reflect active processing? *Developmental Psychology, 30,* 748–756.

Piaget, J. (1952). *The origins of intelligence in children.* New York: International Universities Press.

Porges, S. W. (1984). Physiologic correlates of attention: A core process underlying learning disorders. *Pediatric Clinics of North America, 31,* 371–385.

Porges, S. W. (1992). Autonomic regulation and attention. In B. A. Campbell, H. Hayne, & R. Richardson (Eds.), *Attention and information processing in infants and adults* (pp. 201–223). Hillsdale, NJ: Erlbaum.

Richards, J. E., & Casey, B. J. (1992). Development of sustained visual attention in the human infant. In B. Campbell, H. Hayne, & R. Richardson (Eds.), *Attention and information processing in infants and adults* (pp. 30–60). Hillsdale, NJ: Erlbaum.

Robson, A. L., & Pederson, D. R. (1997). Predictors of individual differences in attention among low birthweight children. *Developmental and Behavioral Pediatrics, 18,* 13–21.

Rose, S. A. (1983). Differential rates of visual information processing in fullterm and preterm infants. *Clinics in Developmental Medicine, 54,* 1189–1198.

Rose, S. A., Feldman, J. F., Wallace, I. F., & McCarton, C. (1989). Infant visual attention: Relation to birth status and developmental outcome during the first 5 years. *Developmental Psychology, 25,* 560–576.

Ruff, H. A. (1986a). Attention and organization of behavior in high-risk infants. *Journal of Developmental and Behavioral Pediatrics, 7,* 298–301.

Ruff, H. A. (1986b). Components of attention during infants' manipulative exploration. *Child Development, 57,* 105–114.

Ruff, H. A. (1988). The measurement of attention in high risk infants. In P. Vietze & H. G. Vaughan (Eds.), *Early identification of infants with developmental disabilities* (pp. 282–296). Philadelphia: Grune & Stratton.

Ruff, H. A. (1995). *Internal consistency of focused attention.* Unpublished data.

Ruff, H. A., Capozzoli, M., & Saltarelli, L. M. (1996). Focused visual attention and distractibility in 10–month-old infants. *Infant Behavior and Development, 19*, 281–293.

Ruff, H. A., & Dubiner, K. (1987). Stability of individual differences in infants' manipulation and exploration of objects. *Perceptual and Motor Skills, 64*, 1095–1101.

Ruff, H. A., & Lawson, K. R. (1990). Development of sustained, focused attention in young children during free play. *Developmental Psychology, 26*, 85–93.

Ruff, H. A., & Lawson, K. R. (1991). Assessment of infants' attention during play with objects. In C. E. Schaefer, K. Gitlin, & A. Sandgrund (Eds.), *Play diagnosis and assessment* (pp. 115–129). New York: Wiley.

Ruff, H. A., Lawson, K. R., Parrinello, R., & Weissberg, R. (1990). Long-term stability of individual differences in sustained attention in the early years. *Child Development, 61*, 60–75.

Ruff, H. A., McCarton, C., Kurtzberg, D., & Vaughan, H. G. Jr. (1984). Preterm infants' manipulative exploration of objects. *Child Development, 55*, 1166–1173.

Ruff, H. A., & Rothbart, M. K. (1996). *Attention in early development: Themes and variations.* New York: Oxford University Press.

Ruff, H. A., Saltarelli, L. M., Capozzoli, M., & Dubiner, K. (1992). The differentiation of activity in infants' exploration of objects. *Developmental Psychology, 28*, 851–861.

Saltarelli, L., Ruff, H. A., & Capozzoli, M. (1990). Distractibility during focused attention in infants. *Infant Behavior and Development, 13*, 606.

Sigman, M. (1976). Early development of preterm and full-term infants: Exploratory behavior in eight-month olds. *Child Development, 47*, 606–612.

Sykes, D. H., Hoy, E. A., Bill, J. M., McClure, B. G., Halliday, H. L., & Reid, M. (1997). Behavioral adjustment in school of very low birthweight children. *Journal of Child Psychology and Psychiatry and Allied Disciplines, 38*, 315–325.

Szatmari, P., Saigal, S., Rosenbaum, P., Campbell, D., & King, S. (1990). Psychiatric disorders at five years among children with birthweights < 1000g: A regional perspective. *Developmental Medicine and Child Neurology, 32*, 954–962.

Teplin, S. W., Burchinal, M., Johnson-Martin, N., Humphry, R. A., & Kraybill, E. N. (1991). Neurodevelopmental, health, and growth status at age 6 years of children with birth weights less than 1001 grams. *Journal of Pediatrics, 118*, 768–777.

Ungerleider, L. G., & Mishkin, M. (1982). Two cortical visual systems. In D. J. Ingle, M. A. Goodale, & R. J. Mansfield (Eds.), *Analysis of visual behavior* (pp. 549–550, 578–579). Cambridge, MA: MIT Press.

Uzgiris, I. C., & Hunt, J. (1975). *Assessment in infancy: Ordinal scales of psychological development.* Urbana: University of Illinois Press.

Vietze, P. M., McCarthy, M., McQuiston, S., MacTurk, R., & Yarrow, L. J. (1983). Attention and exploratory behavior in infants with Down's syndrome. In T. Field & A. Sostek (Eds.), *Infants born at risk: Physiological, perceptual and cognitive processes* (pp. 251–268). New York: Grune & Stratton.

Weisglas-Kuperus, N., Koot, H. M., Baerts, W., Fetter, W. P. F., & Sauer, P. J. J. (1993). Behaviour problems of very low-birthweight children. *Developmental Medicine and Child Neurology, 35*, 406–416.

Weisler, A., & McCall, R. B. (1976). Exploration and play. *American Psychologist, 31,* 492–508.

Welsh, M. C., & Pennington, B. F. (1988). Assessing frontal lobe functioning in children: Views from developmental psychology. *Developmental Neuropsychology, 4*, 199–230.

White, R. W. (1959). Motivation reconsidered: The concept of competence. *Psychological Review, 66*, 297–333.

15

The A-Not-B Task

JULIA S. NOLAND

HISTORY

Piaget's (1954) intuitions about children's capacities were so compelling that he was able to describe phenomena that have motivated research in developmental psychology for 50 years. No phenomenon has received more attention than the A-not-B error, which is the tendency for an infant to search for an object in an old location despite seeing it hidden in a new location (see Marcovitch & Zelazo, 1999; Wellman, Cross, & Bartsch, 1986, for reviews).

Piaget's (1954) interpretation of this phenomenon has provoked much research because he suggested that infants' behaviors could offer insight into their understanding of the world. Within Piaget's theory, infants commit the A-not-B error because they do not conceive of fully occluded objects as continuing to exist outside their sensorimotor engagement with them.

For Piaget, the changing search abilities of infants from 6 to 12 months, from the first search for hidden objects through the appearance and disappearance of the A-not-B error, are all stages within the conceptual shift toward object permanence. Piaget's (1954) description of these emerging abilities has been the basis for the standardized assessment of infant development for a quarter century (Uzgiris & Hunt, 1975).

However, since Piaget's proposal, researchers have produced strong empirical evidence to challenge the conceptual-change interpretation of the A-not-B error (see Baillargeon & DeVos, 1991, for review of evidence from the violation of expectation paradigm). Moving away from the Piagetian interpretation has led to an intense debate over the cause of the A-not-B error.

One of the most provocative findings to emerge from this debate is that the time delay between when infants see objects hidden and when they are allowed to search for those objects directly affects the production of the A-not-B error (Harris, 1973). Infants immediately allowed to reach for the occluded object do not perseverate to the old location but do perseverate if there is a delay between hiding and search. This finding is the basis for the representational/memory account of the A-not-B error.

However, a challenge to the memory account soon followed. Harris (1974) found that infants committed the A-not-B error even if the object was visible at the B location. Thus, infants reach to the previously correct location (A) even when the toy is visible behind a transparent cover at the new location (B). Moreover, the mere act of reaching repeatedly to the A location produces a bias toward reaching to that location again. This bias was first demonstrated by Smith, Thelen, Titzer, and McLin (1999) in a version of the A-not-B task in which only the covers are used (i.e., no object is hidden). The infant's attention is drawn to the A lid (the experimenter taps it) and most of the time the infant reaches to the A lid. However, when the experimenter switches and starts tapping the B lid, the infants do not reach for the B lid more than the A lid. With this lids-only task, the lid to which an infant will reach is predicted by the distribution of the previous reaches (Diedrich, Thelen, Smith, & Corbetta, 2000). The current state of this debate on the cause of the A-not-B error is an agreement that both a bias to repeat a previous action and a memory component appear to affect performance (Munakata, 1998; Smith et al., 1999).

A by-product of this debate has been a detailed description of the parameters that influence the production of the A-not-B error. This description provides the empirical background necessary for developing the A-not-B task into a viable assessment tool.

LONGITUDINAL STUDIES

An important finding for the refinement of the A-not-B task is that test age directly affected the time delay between hiding and reaching at which a given infant produces the A-not-B error (Diamond, 1985; Wellman et al., 1986). In a longitudinal study, Diamond (1985) found that between 8 and 12 months of age, there is a steady increase in the delay that infants can tolerate while still succeeding on reversal trials on the A-not-B. At 8 months, most infants in Diamond's cohort were successful only when the delay was less than 1 second. At a 2-second delay, most of the 8-month-old infants perseverated, failing by reaching back to the previously correct location. At 9 months, most of these same infants succeeded at 2 seconds but failed at 5 seconds. Several longitudinal studies have replicated this general pattern of a steady, age-related increase in delay tolerance versions of the A-not-B task (Bell & Fox, 1992; Matthews, Ellis, & Nelson, 1996).

CONVERGENCE WITH NEUROSCIENCE

There is convergent evidence from developmental psychology and neuroscience, reviewed later, that the A-not-B task taps the cognitive capacities of the prefrontal cortex—in particular, working memory. These findings have led to work establishing the delay-tolerance A-not-B tasks as behavioral markers for the functional development of the frontal lobes in human infants (Bell & Fox, 1992, Diamond, Prevor, Callender, & Druin, 1997).

GENERAL DESCRIPTION

In the A-not-B task an infant sees a toy hidden in one of two locations. This first location is called A. After the infant has successfully retrieved the toy from location A on two consecutive trials, it is hidden at location B. It is important that the infant watches as the toy is hidden in the new location, because despite seeing the toy hidden at B, infants between 8 and 12 months of age will often search for it at A. The location (correct vs. incorrect) where the infant reaches on this reversal trial is the central measure of A-not-B performance as it has been used by developmental psychologists (Marcovitch & Zelazo, 1999; Wellman et al., 1986).

Delay-Tolerance A-Not-B Procedures

The distinguishing characteristic of the delay-tolerance versions of the A-not-B tasks is the within-session adjustment of time delay. The adjusted interval is between when the toy is hidden and when the infant is allowed to attempt to retrieve it. This interval is adjusted in order to establish the longest delay the infant can tolerate and still succeed in retrieving the toy on reversal trials. Another important alteration in the delay-tolerance procedure is the inclusion of multiple reversal trials (i.e., alternating the A and B locations between the same two hiding wells). This modification increases the number of responses on which a given infant's performance is assessed. Diamond (1985) was the first to use a delay-tolerance A-not-B task. In doing so she progressed away from the binomial evaluation of the traditional task (correct vs. incorrect) to a continuous measure (i.e., the delay, in seconds, at which an infant failed on two of three reversal trials).

A similar procedure, used by Bell and Fox (1992) in their longitudinal study, differs from the Diamond procedure in several ways. In the Bell procedure, an infant's performance is rated on an ordinal scale. Infants proficient at reversal trials of a given delay receive a score corresponding to that level of delay. Infants not proficient with reversal trials even in the zero delay condition are rated on scaled items similar to the Uzgiris–Hunt Test of Object Permanence.

Looking Versions of the Delay Tolerance A-Not-B Task

A longitudinal study (Matthews et al., 1986) and a cross-sectional study (Bell & Adams, 1999) have found strong parallels in the performance of infants on delay-tolerance A-not-B tasks with an eye-gaze response as compared with the traditional reaching response. This innovation is a particularly exciting development for the use of the A-not-B task as an assessment tool.

BIOBEHAVIORAL BASIS OF ASSESSMENT

There is converging preclinical and clinical evidence that the A-not-B task taps the cognitive functions supported by the prefrontal cortical system. On A-not-B tasks, young human and monkey infants fail by repeating a previously correct action. This tendency increases as the delay period between hiding and when search is allowed increases (Goldman-Rakic, 1987). Diamond and Goldman-Rakic (1989) found that when the prefrontal cortex of young monkeys who no longer made the A-not-B error were lesioned, they regressed to the perseverative, delay-sensitive pattern they demonstrated at younger ages. In contrast, this regression was not true for hippocampal lesions (Diamond, Zola-Morgan, & Squire, 1989).

Electroencephalograph work with human infants also supports the proposal that competence on the A-not-B task depends on the functional development of the prefrontal cortex. This work was first reported by Bell and Fox (1992) and is described in detail in the chapter by Himmelfarb and Fox, Chapter 17, this volume.

There is a third line of evidence based on the selective deficits of early-treated phenylkentoruria (PKU) children, indicating that performance on the delay-tolerance A-not-B task relies on the prefrontal cortex. PKU is the genetic inability to metabolize phenylalanine (Phe), a condition which can severely reduce the brain's supply of dopamine (Diamond, Ciaramitoro, Donner, Djali, & Robinson, 1994). The functioning of the prefrontal cortex and specifically working memory seems to depend directly on the availability of dopamine (Sawaguchi & Goldman-Rakic, 1991). PKU children who are placed on Phe-restricted diets very early in life avoid severe mental retardation secondary to high levels of Phe. Yet, despite their restricted diet, early-treated PKU children show slightly elevated Phe levels. In early childhood (ages 4–12) higher levels of Phe are associated with impaired performance selectively on tests of frontal lobe functioning (Welsh, Pennington, Ozonoff, Rouse, & McCabe, 1990).

Diamond et al. (1997) have published a longitudinal study of infants with early-treated PKU. The infants with high levels of Phe were impaired in overall success on the A-not-B task and showed less delay tolerance compared to their age-matched controls.

Frontal Functions Tapped by the A-Not-B Task

Based on her extensive work with the delayed-response task, Goldman-Rakic (1987) suggests that the specific function of the prefrontal cortex that is tapped by the A-not-B task is the ability to maintain representations that must be updated on a trial-to-trial basis in order to guide behavior correctly. Roberts has elaborated on the working-memory model of frontal lobe functioning by incorporating Baddeley's cognitive model (Roberts, Hager, & Heron, 1994). In this expanded definition, working memory is responsible for "keeping information in mind and performing explicit computations to guide upcoming action" (Roberts et al., 1994, p. 375).

In addition to working-memory functions, it has also been argued that the A-not-B task taps inhibitory control mechanisms of the frontal lobes (Diamond, 1990). The degree to which performance on conflict tasks (like the A-not-B task) is particularly vulnerable to frontal dysfunction has been taken as support for this position. Recently, however, researchers have had success accounting for frontal lobe involvement in other conflict tasks without reference to inhibitory mechanisms (Kimberg & Farah, 1993; Roberts & Pennington, 1996).

RELIABILITY AND VALIDITY

The bulk of empirical work with the A-not-B task has been focused on establishing the cause of the A-not-B error. The breadth of paradigms in which the A-not-B error is reported in this body of work makes clear that the A-not-B task is a robust phenomenon. However, establishing a standardized procedure has not been a priority for most researchers.

Reliability

There is an A-not-B item in the Uzgiris–Hunt Ordinal Scales of Psychological Development (Uzgiris & Hunt, 1975). Uzgiris and Hunt published within session, interobservation agreement ratings (94% agreement) as well as test–retest scores (different examiners, 48-hour interval between test sessions). For the 8- to 11-month-old infants, the lowest stability score was a mean greater than 85%. This test–retest stability might have been higher if the procedure had employed a standardized time delay.

Due to their newness as an assessment tool, not much is known about the reliability of the delay-tolerance A-not-B tasks. Within lab coding, agreements on trial-by-trial decisions are typically high. For instance, the agreement level for videotape recodes from the Bell lab is 95% (Bell & Adams, 1999).

Validity

Performance on the A-not-B task differs between infants with Down syndrome and their controls (Rast & Meltzoff, 1995), autistic children and their controls (Dawson, Meltzoff, Osterling, & Rinaldi, 1998), and toddlers exposed to crack cocaine during gestation and "normative" toddlers of the same age (Espy, Kaufmann, & Glisky, 1999). Delay-tolerance task performance differences have been found between PKU infants and controls (Diamond et al., 1997) as well as between cocaine-exposed infants and socioeconomic matched controls (Noland, Singer, Mehta, & Hoang, 2000).

There have been no demonstrations of predictive validity of the A-not-B task as a measure of individual difference, but there have been follow-up studies of at-risk groups. For instance, infants with early-treated PKU performed more poorly than controls on a delay-tolerance A-not-B task, and when they were tested 4 years later they were still impaired on tests of frontal lobe functioning (Diamond et al., 1997).

DEVELOPMENTAL MODEL

Early experiences have permanent organizational effects on the brain system they employ (Greenough & Wallace, 1987). The importance of early functioning for later organization depends on the process of selective stabilization. Due to its slowly developing neural connections, the frontal lobe may be particularly open to the influence of this selective stabilization. Although all neurons are finished migrating to their appropriate cortical layer at birth, the dendrites of the prefrontal cortex grow more slowly and continue growing for a longer time than those in other cortical regions (Huttenlocher, 1990).

However, what is most unique about the neuronal development of the frontal lobes is the degree of synaptic blooming and pruning it undergoes. In the first postnatal year the human cerebral cortex undergoes a massive overproduction of synapses. In the prefrontal cortex, the maximum number of synapses per neuron (synaptic density) is reached at around one year, and it is roughly 175% of adult synaptic density. A significant decrease in this excessive synaptic density is first noticed around 7 years; adult levels are reached at roughly 16 years of age (Huttenlocher, 1979), a pattern that has been confirmed through a positron emission tomography (PET) scan study of functional development. The metabolic rate as measured by PET is closely linked to synaptic activation (Chugani, Phelps, & Mazziota, 1987). An initial rise in the frontal metabolism occurs around 8 months of age, continues during the first postnatal years, and remains high during childhood, only to decline to adult levels in adolescence.

It has been proposed that the overproduction of synapses allows for anatomical organization of the developing cortex (Huttenlocher, 1984) in the following way: Some of the redundant synaptic connections are stabilized though contact with functioning systems and the others regress. This overproduction and selective stabilization of synapses may allow a more complex system of connections to emerge than could be preprogrammed genetically (Huttenlocher, 1990).

As a result of its relatively protracted development, the frontal lobe may be uniquely affected by selective stabilization. Synaptic blooming and pruning happen more slowly in the frontal lobes than in other cortical areas (Huttenlocher, 1979), and the initial rise of metabolic rate in prefrontal cortex starts later and lasts longer in the frontal lobes as compared with other cortical areas.

Through the process of selective stabilization, functional activity in infancy may permanently affect the organization of the prefrontal cortex. Because of its crucial role in later neural organization, early functioning is likely to be predictive of later functioning. Currently, the delay-tolerance A-not-B task is the best established assessment of this early activity.

THEORETICAL CONSTRAINTS

Given the model of selective stabilization described previously, the predictive power of early frontal functioning lies in the organizational role of that early activity itself. An important constraint on the A-not-B task derives from the interactive aspect of selective stabilization. If the processes by which early functioning predicts later functioning are fundamentally interactive, they must be open to environmental impact on early frontal activity.

There is some correlational evidence that experience affects frontal activity. The work of Kermoian and Campos (1988) suggests that early crawling experience is related to performance on the A-not-B task. (This work is reviewed in detail by Himmelfarb & Fox, Chapter 17, this volume.) Other evidence that experience may affect frontal activity comes from work with preterm infants. When matched with full-term controls for conceptional age, preterm infants were more successful on a delay-tolerance A-not-B task (Matthew et al., 1996). The authors suggest that the increased time out of the womb associated with preterm birth may be responsible for the preterm infants' more developmentally advanced performance. Early environmental impact on frontal activity may also play a role in the significant positive correlation between maternal responsiveness and A-not-B performance (Ayoun, 1998).

If, as this evidence suggests, there is experiential impact on early frontal activity, then early environment may have a role in later functional integrity of the system. The A-not-B task's predictive utility comes hand in hand with its sensitivity to environmental input. If the A-not-B task is used to predict future functioning of at-risk groups, it must be acknowledged that the developmental course predicted is open to both positive and negative environmental influence.

TRAINING REQUIREMENTS

Unlike assessments that measure looking time to mechanically presented stimuli, the A-not-B task requires the infant's active participation. The infant must search for the target on dozens of trials and remain motivated even after repeated failures. Experience working with this age group is important to help the examiner establish a social context in which the trials, failed or passed, are enjoyable play.

There is no established version of the delay tolerance procedure. All published versions have varied from each other (Bell & Fox, 1992; Diamond, 1985; Matthews et al., 1996) and the published method sections are not as extensive as the manuals associated with standardized assessments. Familiarity with the A-not-B literature or consultation on methods would be necessary for minimizing between-subject procedural variations which could potentially affect A-not-B performance. Examples of procedural variations that have been demonstrated to affect the A-not-B error include the location of the ultimate hand motion in the hiding sequence (Diamond, Cruttenden, & Neiderman, 1994), the distance between hiding locations (Horobin & Acredolo, 1986), and the distribution of reaches on warm-up trials (Diedrich et al., 2000).

IMPLICATIONS

The potential of the A-not-B task as an assessment of biobehavioral functioning lies in its newly established incarnation as a marker of prefrontal cortical functioning. The critical evidence for this has come from use of the delay-tolerance versions of the task (Bell & Fox, 1992; Diamond, 1990). There is much work to be done in the development of this assessment: establishing parameters on procedural variations, norms, and predictive validity.

There is even more to be done to develop the A-not-B task as an assessment tool for use with populations of infants at-risk for dysfunction. Single-session versions of the delay-tolerance A-not-B task have been published (Bell & Adams, 1999; Diamond, 1985), but the participants in these studies were, like the infants in the longitudinal studies, from nonrisk samples with middle-class and upper-middle-class backgrounds. Because of this similarity in test populations, the starting delay used in the longitudinal studies could be employed in these cross-sectional studies. But what about high-risk samples? If the initial delay used is significantly different from the optimal delay, the cooperation of the infant may wane significantly over the adjustment process. We have had success in adapting Diamond and Bell's procedures for use in a single test session with a high-risk sample of 11-month-old infants (Noland et al., 2000) but procedures for the whole age range (8–12 months) need to be established for at-risk infants.

In summary, as a biobehavioral assessment, the A-not-B task is new and requires substantial development. However, the potential payoff is great. Pennington (1991) conducted an extensive review of the types of functional deficits exhibited by children with genetic/chromosomal disabilities and postnatal insult. Along with phonological disorders, he identified the attentional/inhibitory functions supported by the prefrontal cortex as the most vulnerable, suggesting that including an A-not-B task in a test battery would significantly increase its sensitivity.

Furthermore, it is clear that frontal lobe functioning is important for the ability to participate in a complex cognitive and social environment. Any appreciable frontal damage in adulthood decreases the patient's ability to motivate action toward internally held goals (Fuster, 1989). Case studies of frontal lobe damage in children suggest that the developmental impact of frontal dysfunction, like adult lesions, is globally debilitating (Gratten & Eslinger, 1991).

The frontal lobes support abilities that underlie goal-directed actions and the A-not-B task has the potential to assess the integrity of this brain system relatively early in life.

ACKNOWLEDGMENTS

Preparation of this chapter was supported by Grant Nos. F32-05904 to Julia S. Noland and R01-07957 to Lynn T. Singer from the National Institute on Drug Abuse, as well as by Grant No. T32-MH19389 from National Institute of Health to Cornell University, Department of Psychology.

REFERENCES

Ayoun, C. (1998). Maternal responsiveness and search for hidden object and contingency learning by infants. *Early Development and Parenting, 7*(2), 61–72.

Baillargeon, R., & Devos, J. (1991). Object permanence in young infants: further evidence. *Child Development, 62,* 1227–1246.

Bell, M. A., & Adams, S. E. (1999). Comparable performance on looking and reaching versions of the A-not-B task at 8 months of age. *Infant Behavior and Development, 22*(2), 221–235.

Bell, M. A., & Fox, N. A. (1992). The relations between frontal brain electrical activity and cognitive development during infancy. *Child Development, 63,* 1142–1163.

Chugani, H. T., Phelps, M. E., & Mazziotta, J. C. (1987). Positron emission tomography study of human brain functional development. *Annals of Neurology, 22*(4), 487–497.

Dawson, G., Meltzoff, A. N., Osterling, J., & Rinaldi, J. (1998). Neuropsychological correlates of early symptoms of autism. *Child Development, 69*(5), 1276–1285.

Diamond, A. (1985). Development of the ability to use recall to guide action, as indicated by infants performance on A not B. *Child Development, 56*, 868–883.

Diamond, A. (1990). The development and neural bases of memory functions as indexed by the A not B and delayed response tasks, in human infants and infant monkeys. In A. Diamond (Ed.), *The development and neural bases of higher cognitive functions* (pp. 276–317). New York: New York Academy of Sciences.

Diamond, A., Ciaramitaro, V., Donner, E., Djali, S., & Robinson, M. B. (1994). An animal model of early-treated PKU. *Journal of Neuroscience, 14*(5), 3072–3082.

Diamond, A., Cruttenden, L., & Neiderman, D. (1994). AB with multiple wells: 1. Why are multiple wells sometimes easier than two wells?; 2. Memory or Memory + Inhibition? *Developmental Psychology, 30*(2), 192–205.

Diamond, A., & Goldman-Rakic, P. S. (1989). Comparison of human infants and rhesus monkeys on Piaget's A-not-B task. Evidence for dependence on dorsolateral prefrontal cortex. *Experimental Brain Research, 74*, 24–40.

Diamond, A., Prevor, M. B., Callender, G., & Druin, D. P. (1997). Prefrontal cortex cognitive deficits in children treated early and continuously for PKU. *Monographs of the Society for Research in Child Development, 62*(4).

Diamond, A., Zola-Morgan, S., & Squire, L. R. (1989). Successful performance by monkeys with lesions of the hippocampal formation on AB and object retrieval, to tasks that mark developmental changes in human infants. *Behavioral Neuroscience, 103*(3), 526–537.

Diedrich, F. J., Thelen, E., Smith, L. B., & Corbetta, D. (2000). Motor memory is a factor in infant perseverative errors. *Developmental Science, 3*(4), 479–494.

Espy, K. A., Kaufmann, P. M., & Glisky, M. L. (1999). Neuropsychologic function in toddlers exposed to cocaine in utero: a preliminary study. *Developmental Neuropsychology, 15*(3), 447–460.

Fuster, J. M. (1989). *The prefrontal cortex* (2nd ed.). New York: Raven Press.

Goldman-Rakic, P. S. (1987). Development of cortical circuitry and cognitive function. *Child Development, 58*, 601–622.

Grattan, L. M., & Eslinger, P. J. (1991). Frontal lobe damage in children and adults: A comparative review. *Developmental Neuropsychology, 7*(3), 283–326.

Greenough, W. T., Black, J. E., & Wallace, C. S. (1987). Experience and brain development. *Child Development, 58*, 539–559.

Harris, P. L. (1973). Perseverative errors in search by young infants. *Child Development, 44*, 28–33.

Harris, P. L. (1974). Perseverative search at a visibly empty place by young infants. *Journal of Experimental Child Psychology, 18*, 535–542.

Horobin, K., & Acredolo, L. (1986). The role of attentiveness, mobility, history, and separation of hiding sites on Stage IV search behavior. *Journal of Experimental Child Psychology, 41*, 114–127.

Huttenlocher, P. R. (1979). Synaptic density in human frontal cortex-developmental changes and effects of aging. *Brain Research, 163*, 195–205.

Huttenlocher, P. R. (1984). Synaptic elimination and plasticity in developing human cerebral cortex. *American Journal of Mental Deficiency, 88*, 488–496.

Huttenlocher, P. R. (1990). Morphometric study of human cerebral cortex development. *Neuropsychologia, 6,* 517–527.

Kermoian, R., & Campos, J. J. (1988). Locomotor experience: A facilitator of spatial cognitive development. *Child Development, 59,* 908–917.

Kimberg, D. Y., & Farah, M. J. (1993). A unified account of cognitive impairments following frontal lobe damage: The role of working memory in complex, organized behavior. *Journal of Experimental Psychology: General, 122*(4), 411–428.

Marcovitch, S., & Zelazo, P. D. (1999). The A-not-B error: Results from a logistic meta-analysis. *Child Development, 70,* 1297–1313.

Matthews, A., Ellis, A. E., & Nelson, C. A. (1996). Development of preterm and full-term infant ability of AB, recall memory, transparent barrier detour, and means–end tasks. *Child Development, 67,* 2658–2676.

Munakata, Y. (1998). Infant perseveration and implications for object permanence theories: A POP model of the AB task. *Developmental Science, 1,* 161–184.

Noland, J. S., Singer, L. B., Mehta, S. K., & Hoang, B. H. (2000). *Delay tolerance on the A-not-B task as a measure of executive functioning in cocaine-exposed infants.* Poster presented at the biannual conference of the ISIS in Brighton, UK.

Pennington, B. F. (1991). *Diagnosing learning disorders: A neuropsychological framework.* New York: Guilford Press.

Piaget, J. (1954). *The construction of reality in the child.* New York: Basic Books.

Rast, M., & Meltzoff, A. N. (1995). Memory and representation in young children with Down syndrome; exploring deferred imitation and object permanence. *Development and Psychopathology, 3,* 137–162.

Roberts, R. J., Hager, L. D., & Heron, C. (1994). Prefrontal cognitive processes: Working memory and inhibition in the antisaccade task. *Journal of Experimental Psychology: General, 123*(4), 374–393.

Roberts, R. J., & Pennington, B. F. (1996). An interactive framework for examining prefrontal cognitive processes. *Developmental Neuropsychology, 12*(1), 105–126.

Sawaguchi, T., & Goldman-Rakic, P. S. (1991). D1 Dopamine receptors in prefrontal cortex: Involvement in working memory. *Science, 251,* 947–950.

Smith, L. B., Thelen, E., Titzer, R, & McLin, D. (1999). Knowing in the context of acting: The task dynamics of the A-not-B error. *Psychological Review, 106*(2), 235–260.

Uzgiris, I. C., & Hunt, J. M. (1975). *Assessment in infancy: Ordinal Scales of Psychological Development.* Urbana: University of Illinois Press.

Wellman, H. M., Cross, D., & Bartsch, K. (1986). Infant search and object permanence: A meta-analysis of the A-not-B error. *Monographs on the Society for Research in Child Development, 51*(3).

Welsh, M. C., Pennington, B. F., Ozonoff, S., Rouse, B., & McCabe, E. R. B. (1990). Neuropsychology of early-treated phenylketonuria: Specific executive function deficits. *Child Development, 61,* 1697–1713.

16

Cortical Electrophysiology and Language Processes in Infancy

DENNIS L. MOLFESE
VICTORIA J. MOLFESE

HISTORY

Attempts to record the brain's electrical activity and relate it to behavior dates back to Richard Caton who, in 1875, recorded evoked potentials from a lead placed directly on the surface of a rabbit's brain. Subsequent attempts were made to use electrodes to record changes in bioelectrical activity from outside the body. In these early attempts, an immersion technique was used that required patients to place each of their limbs in separate buckets of saline solution. The buckets served as "electrodes" to detect electrical signals that were then conveyed via cables to an amplifying system and a chart recorder. By the mid-1920s, however, plate electrodes which were applied directly to the skin were in use. Later, the floater type of electrode that required an electrolyte to be placed in between the skin and the electrode was developed. This type of electrode is similar to the electrodes in common use today. Although this latter approach reduced the electrode movement artifacts that often contaminated or obscured the evoked potential signal obtained from contact or plate electrodes, perplexing problems of finding adequately conductive electrode materials, improving the horrific signal-to-noise ratio, and determining an appropriate means of analyzing the signal precluded rapid advancement in this field. A major improvement occurred in the mid-1940s, when Dawson devised a technique to improve the signal-to-noise ratio through the use of a capacitance-based computer analogue that summed repetitive evoked potentials. By adding together electrical signals recorded on successive trials, Dawson's device built summed potentials that reflected the repetitive information contained in the evoked potential from trial to trial. The nonrepetitive signal which was thought to be irrelevant noise failed to contribute systematically to specific portions of the accumulating sum. The dedicated signal acquisition devices offered by many companies today as well as the more flexible computer routines developed by different laboratories, some of which are commercially available, are logical extensions of Dawson's original idea. An additional issue important to the development and evolution of cortical electrophysiology is the development of analysis techniques useful for evoked potential data. Analysis procedures have developed at an excruciatingly slow pace, as evidenced by the fact that the major methods of data analysis in vogue today have been in use for nearly half a century, with several dating back to the 1920s. Here, as in the case of Dawson's averager, a number of developments have occurred more recently, especially since the development and use of personal computers.

GENERAL DESCRIPTION

The event-related potential (ERP) is a synchronized portion of the ongoing electroencephalographic (EEG) pattern. Evoked potential waveforms are thought to reflect changes in brain activity over time as reflected by changes in the amplitude or height of the wave at different points in its time course. What distinguishes the ERP from the more traditional EEG measure is that the evoked potential is a portion of the ongoing EEG activity of the brain that is time-locked to the onset of some event in the infant's environment. The ongoing EEG activity reflects a wide range of neural activity related to the myriad neural and body self-regulating systems as well as the various sensory and cognitive functions ongoing in the brain at that time. The ERP, on the other hand, because it is time-locked to the onset of an event, enables researchers to evaluate the relationship between this neuroelectrical response and that event (Callaway, Tueting, & Koslow, 1978; Rockstroh, Elbert, Birbaumer, & Lutzenberger, 1982).

ERPs involve the placement of active recording electrodes on the scalp of an individual. The choice of placements is often driven by hypotheses concerning the relationships between the functioning of different brain regions and the cognitive operations or processes assumed to occur in those areas. Unfortunately, the scalp electrode does not simply detect information which originates immediately below that position in the brain. Thus, there are limits as to how far one can speculate about the origins of the scalp-recorded ERP signal.

A variety of strategies have been used to select electrode placement sites. Approximately half the studies use the 10–20 system designed for adults (Jasper, 1958). This technique relies on proportional measures to determine electrode placements and is useful in attempting to replicate placements done across studies using the same technique. Development of a similar system has been attempted with infants (Blume, Buza, & Okazaki, 1974). However, a number of factors, such as a small sample size and the lack of two hemisphere samples from the same infants, limits the usefulness of the Blume et al. approach as a standardized system for electrode placement in infants or children. The 10–20 system in use for electrode placement in adults does not overlay the same cortical regions in young infants. For example, as Blume et al. (1974) note, central leads in infants were found to lay over the postcentral gyrus (sensory) whereas such leads were over the precentral gyrus (motor) in adults. In infants the inferior frontal electrode actually lies inferior to the frontal lobe as opposed to over that area in adults. Additional points of discrepancy between infant and adult placements raise further issues regarding comparability of recordings across infants, children, and adults.

Placement of electrodes on the infant's head is usually driven by hypotheses concerning the relation between functioning of different brain regions and the cognitive processing assumed to underlie the evoking stimulus and to some extent by traditional electrode placements. For example, the brainstem evoked response (BSER), used to screen for sensory processing, involves the placement of only one active electrode over the central processing area (F_z). In investigating more complex cognitive processing, such as language processing, electrodes are typically placed at several sites, including three central sites: F_z, F_L, F_R, and six lateral sites over each side of the head: T_3, T_4, C_3, C_4, P_L, and P_R (see Figure 16.1). These locations are over bilateral frontal, temporal, central, and parietal areas of the brain and are hypothesized to provide information concerning left- versus right-hemisphere responses to the evoking stimuli and information within each hemisphere concerning functioning of different brain areas. Unfortunately, the scalp electrode detects responses from other brain areas than those immediately below the scale location. Responses from the T3, and from other adjacent areas may be detected as well. Thus, caution must be used in attributing ERPs to a single area of the brain thought to be detected by each electrode placement.

In infants, with few exceptions, the number of electrodes placed is smaller than the number used for adults for a number of reasons. Infant tolerance of testing procedures is directly influenced by the time that must be taken to apply electrodes to an infant's scalp. If more are used, the time to apply them necessarily increases. Reliance on the 10–20 system necessitates extended periods to conduct the measurements so that each placement is accurately located. The use of electrode caps has eliminated some of these time demands, although the use of blunted needles to lower impedances by rubbing them through the electrode holes contributes to a level of discomfort

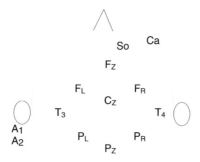

FIGURE 16.1. Schematic representation of the top of a head with scalp electrodes in place at left and right frontal (F_L, F_R), temporal (T_3, T_4), and parietal locations (P_L, P_R), as well as three central leads located at frontal (F_Z), central (C_Z), and parietal (P_Z) sites. Reference electrodes are represented here at the left (A_1) and right ear (A_2), while electrodes to monitor eye movements are indicated at a supraorbital position (So, over the right eye) and to the right of that eye (Ca, at the canthal position).

that some infants do not tolerate well. Another problem relates to a density issue. Because infants' heads are smaller, electrodes must be placed closer together than is possible with adults. If electrodes are within 1.5 cm of each other, however, there is speculation that the electrodes themselves might interfere with the recorded signals creating artifacts.

The ERP scalp activity at different electrode locations is typically referenced to other recording sites such as a calculated average reference or, as in the case of more traditional approaches, a midcentral site (i.e., C_z), mastoids or ears (i.e., A_1, A_2). These referenced recording sites are selected because they are either less electrically active and consequently of less interest(such as the tip of the nose, mastoids, or ear lobes) or are sites that may be characterized by comparable but different levels of electrical activity. These latter sites are chosen so that the investigator can more directly examine the electrical differences between recording sites and other scalp sites. More recent techniques have used a calculated average reference. In addition to scalp and reference electrodes, additional electrodes are usually placed at supraorbital (i.e., above the middle of the eye over the eye brow; labeled as "So" in Figure 16.1) or suborbital (i.e., approximately 2 cm below the eye, on the upper portion of the cheek) and canthal (i.e., to the side away from the eye approximately 2–3 cm; labeled as "Ca" in Figure 16.1) positions in relation to one of the infant's eyes to assist in the detection of artifacts due to horizontal and vertical eye movements.

The ERP recording procedure involves a number of steps. First, the infant's head is measured and positions are marked to indicate where electrodes are to be placed. Next, these positions are cleaned with an abrasive such as pumice paste to lower skin impedances, assuring that the electrodes will be able to conduct a better signal. The abrasive is then removed and a small amount of electrode conducting paste is rubbed onto the scalp. Small disk-shaped electrodes are then filled with the electrode paste and placed on the infant's scalp at these prepared positions. The electrodes are connected via wires to amplifiers that increase the ERP signal by 20,000 to 100,000 times. Given that ERPs are generally very small, on the order of 5 to 10 µV in adults, amplification is needed to provide enough definition of the waveform for further analyses. Amplifiers contain filters that screen out some of the recording system noise and the biological background noise. The output from these amplifiers are connected in turn to a computer which collects the ERPs from each electrode for each stimulus presented. Once the electrodes are in place and connected to the amplifiers and the computer, the stimuli can be presented when the infant is in a reasonably quiet state.

Because of the moment-by-moment variability in the ERP which results from moment-by-moment changes in the physiology of the infant, researchers have a variety of means at their disposal to analyze the collected ERPs. Usually, the ERPs are first recorded to discrete events and then, following artifact rejection, averaged together to build stable waveforms and improve signal-to-noise ratio. The averaged response is thought to be more likely to contain the repetitive activity that reflects the processing of the stimulus from one time to the next. In contrast, non-stimulus-related activity that is not time-locked to the onset of the stimulus is expected to average out or be minimized in the averaged waveform of the ERP. Averages are subjected to a variety of analysis approaches. Traditionally, the technique of choice has involved amplitude measures taken from various peaks in the waveform. These may be made between two adjacent peaks of opposite polarity (e.g., measuring the voltage difference between the most positive peak and the next negative peak), a process referred to as a "peak-to-peak" measure or between the average prestimulus baseline signal and a specific peak amplitude, a process referred to as a baseline-to-peak measure. Subsequent analyses of the ERP are then conducted on the averaged waveforms. These analysis approaches have a range of options including amplitude and latency measures, area measures, discriminant function procedures, and other multivariate approaches including principal-components analysis.

Multivariate analyses of ERP data have been found useful for predicting behavioral outcomes at a later age (e.g., 3) from brain responses at earlier ages (e.g., birth). Principal-components analysis (PCA) has been useful for obtaining information on the location in the brainwave where there is commonality in responsiveness across participants. In these analyses, averaged ERPs from participants across time points are transformed into a covariance matrix and PCA is applied. Factor scores are identified from the variance. The peak for each factor and the area immediately surrounding it in time indicate the region of the brainwave that changed in amplitude or slope across some proportion of the ERPs in the data. The factor scores are used as dependent variables in subsequent analyses. For example, analyses of variance (ANOVA) have been used to determine whether any factors (regions of the ERPs) varied systematically as a function of independent variables (e.g., electrode sites, hemispheres, sex of participant, and stimulus conditions). Factor scores can be used in discriminant function analyses to determine whether scores are useful for discriminating between groups of children based on performance on a specific assessment.

BIOBEHAVIORAL BASIS OF THE ASSESSMENT

The ERP is believed to reflect postsynaptic (dendritic) potentials (Allison, Wood, & McCarthy, 1986). Even so, not all information recorded at the scalp reflects all generated signals originating from all sources. For signals to reach the scalp, they must be produced by extensive sets of activated neurons whose firings must overlap in time. Even so, not all signals reach the scalp. The distance from the cortical regions generating the signal to the scalp may simply be too great relative to the signal's strength detection. Signals that originate within the brain must travel through a variety of tissues of different densities, conductivity, and composition (e.g., neurons, glial cells, fiber tracts, cerebral spinal fluid, bone, and muscle) before they reach the recording electrode. The orientation of the cortical columns where signals originate relative to the scalp may also contribute to whether the signal originating in the brain is seen at the scalp. If these columns are perpendicular to the scalp, the chance of the signal reaching it are better. If the column is parallel or at some other angle, the signal may not project to the scalp or may project to the scalp some distance away from the electrode immediately above it.

The ERP signal finally detected at the scalp is not an exact, completely stable pattern reflecting only those discrete neural events directly related to the evoking stimulus, the task, or the subject's state. Clearly, the ERP is only a by-product of the brain's bioelectrical response to such an event which begins as the stimulus information is transformed by the sensory systems. This signal then progresses through the brainstem into the midbrain and on upward into the higher centers of the brain. Consequently, the final version recorded is a composite of a variety of complex factors, only some of which may relate directly to the variables under manipulation.

STRENGTHS AS AN ASSESSMENT TOOL

The ERP procedure can be applied to all participants regardless of age. Few techniques currently in use can be applied from the newborn through the adulthood period. Consequently, ERPs are useful for direct comparisons between infants and adults to address a variety of developmental questions. Although wave shapes of the ERPs change from infancy to adulthood, one can assess whether brain responses recorded at different ages discriminate reliably between different stimulus, participants, and task conditions obtained concurrently or at different time periods. Moreover, ERP can be used to obtain response information from participants who have difficulty in responding in a normal fashion (as with brain damage) or who cannot respond because of language or maturity factors.

The ERP reflects both general and specific aspects of the evoking stimulus and the person's perceptions and decisions regarding it (Molfese, 1983; Molfese & Betz, 1988; Molfese & Molfese, 1979a, 1979b, 1980, 1985; Nelson & Salapatek, 1986; Ruchkin, Sutton, Munson, & Macar, 1981). ERPs are recognized as providing information concerning between hemisphere differences as well as within hemisphere differences in the brain's electrical activity under specific stimulus conditions. Further, ERP is useful for providing time-related information. It can reveal the onset of one stimulus relative to another and provide information about the different points in time when such information is detected. Because of this excellent temporal resolution and correlations with specific cognitive/linguistic activities, ERP also offers advantages over other brain imaging procedures such as EEG, brainstem evoked responses (BSER), positron emission tomography (PET), and functional magnetic resonance imaging (fMRI). For example, the classic EEG measure, while providing some indication of clinical states such as epileptic seizures, does not resolve cognitive activities to the level offered by the ERP (Callaway et al., 1978). Thus, although frequency analyses of EEG may indicate attentive or inattentive states (as in the case of alpha activity) or an increase in workload (as in the case of beta activity), it is unable to resolve changes in stimulus parameters, decision making, or short-term memory activity. Likewise, although BSER information can reflect initial sensory detection and brainstem response to brief evoking stimuli, the temporal duration of the BSER (approximately 10 msec) precludes studying longer and later occurring cognitive and linguistic decisions regarding the stimulus characteristics or decisions to act on these stimuli. Although both PET and fMRI procedures provide important information concerning metabolic changes throughout the brain during recording that can be associated with cognitive activity (Pugh et al., 1996; Shaywitz et al., 1995), they are unable to resolve the temporal order in which these events occur or the more discrete decisions regarding the processing of this material. Finally, the expense and complexity of setting up an ERP lab are considerably less than that required for the PET and fMRI procedures and may be less formidable to young participants and their parents.

CONSTRAINTS OF THE ASSESSMENT

While offering many advantages, there are limits to the interpretation of the results of ERP studies. ERP studies share the basic limitations indigenous to all experimental approaches—one must make a leap from the data obtained in an experiment to the interpretation of the data. Second, although there may be something seductive in recording electrical currents thought to originate "directly from the brain," the reality is that the specific origins of these currents and the dynamics that lead to their particular presence at the scalp remain beyond our understanding at this time. The measurement-based placement system reflected by the 10–20 system tried to standardize electrode placement across participants so that placements roughly approximate scalp locations to brain regions. However, for reasons already noted, attributing signals from scalp locations to brain regions is fraught with problems. Further, the scalp electrode does not only detect information that originates immediately below that electrode position in the brain. Thus, there are limits as to how far one can speculate about the brain origins of the scalp-recorded ERP signal. In contrast, the linkage between the ERPs and specific behaviors is not accidental and can be effectively exploited in carefully designed and executed experimental paradigms as linked to current and later developing behaviors.

A third limitation concerns our success in comparing ERP waveform characteristics across development. Do similar paradigms used with adult and infant populations tap into the same cognitive or linguistic abilities? Most likely not, given the large cognitive and linguistic differences that exist between these two populations. Although such a question would most likely elicit a resounding "no!" from developmental psycholinguists today, there was a time in the not too distant past when theorists speculated that the holophrastic speech of 1-year-old infants reflected adult-type sentence construction skills that were simply limited by output strategies or abilities for conveying such information. Would we expect that adult paradigms such as the "odd-ball" or P300-type paradigms stimulate structures in young infants that are comparable to those activated when adults engage in such tasks? Based on a host of neuroanatomical studies we know that the brains of infants differ markedly from adults in terms of neurogenesis, dendritic development, and myelination, to mention only a few characteristics. Such differences in neural structure state, as well as in the differential development of brain structures across ages, limit our ability to make developmental comparisons. Thus, the P300 response in adults most likely is not supported by identical structures at comparable levels of functioning in infants or young children. Likewise, just because ERP component latencies are similar in infants and adults, or because the peak polarity and sequence position in the waveform (first peak, third peak, etc.) are the same even though their peak latencies differ, these components do not necessarily reflect similar cognitive or physiological processes. Equally plausible is the alternative explanation that these ERP components tap different cognitive or physiological mechanisms that simply generate such similarities.

DEVELOPMENTAL MODEL

ERPs are among the electrophysiological measures that have been used as the bases for screening techniques and for early measure of brain functioning that can be linked to later cognitive development. Some researchers have used auditory BSER measures to predict developmental outcomes in the first year of life (Barden & Pelzman, 1980; Cox, Hack, & Metz, 1984; Murray, 1988; Murray, Dolby, Nation, & Thomas, 1981). Although the auditory BSER procedure has promise as an effective and relatively low-cost technique for the early identification of hearing impairments, the number of false positives and negatives makes the BSER procedure an ineffective means for identifying infants at risk. Efforts to extend BSER procedures from assessments of hearing impairment into areas of cognitive and language functioning are not well established. Published reports successfully using neonatal BSERs as predictors of later developmental problems are scant. A different result has been obtained through the use of ERPs. ERPs have been shown to reflect general and specific aspects of the evoking stimulus (Molfese, 1980, 1983; Molfese, Buhrke, & Wang, 1985) as well as the individual's perceptions and decisions regarding the stimulus (Molfese, 1989a; Nelson & Salapatek, 1986; Ruchkin et al., 1981). Studies conducted over the past two decades to predict later development based on neonatal ERPs vary in effectiveness. Studies that restricted analyses to a single early peak or peak latency (usually the N_1 component) have achieved some success up to 1 year of age but failed to reveal a long-term relationship (Butler & Engel, 1969; Jensen & Engel, 1971). Butler and Engel (1969) reported the first success in noting correlations between neonatal visual evoked potential latencies and later intelligence measures. They recorded visual evoked potentials from 433 newborn infants in response to a series of photic flashes. Although the correlations between Bayley scores at 8 months and photic latency were significant, the effects were small and accounted for little of the variance. Jensen and Engel (1971) also reported correlations between neonatal photic latencies and later motor skills (age of walking). When they divided the photic latency response into three regions it was found that those infants with the shortest photic latencies were the earliest walkers. Studies that have attempted to extend the period of predictability into the second year of life and beyond have reported little success (Engel & Fay, 1972; Engel & Henderson, 1973; Henderson & Engel, 1974). Engel and Fay (1972) investigated the relationship between neonatal visual evoked responses and later performance on a test of articulation administered at 3- and 4-year Stanford–Binet scores. They found that infants with faster visual evoked response N_1 latencies (less than 146 msec) performed better at 3 years on the articulation task than slow reactors, although no differences were noted on the Stanford–Binet at 4 years. In subsequent studies with older children, Engel and Henderson (1973) and Henderson and Engel (1974) failed to find a relationship between neonatal visual evoked responses and a variety of later IQ and achievement scores. Henderson and Engel (1974) assessed whether the neonatal visual evoked responses predicted total IQ and subtest scores, sensorimotor, perceptual–motor, and achievement test scores at 7 years of age. The photic latency data from 809 infants did not correlate 7 years later with their performance on a variety of IQ tests and subtests.

Although these findings may appear discouraging for using ERPs as predictors of later functioning, recent studies suggest that strong relationships exist (Molfese, 1989b; Molfese & Molfese, 1985; Molfese & Searock, 1986). The differences in success between earlier and more recent studies reflect differences in methodology and design. Molfese and associates analyzed the entire ERP waveform while others typically confine their analysis to one or two points within a single ERP component. Analysis of all data collected instead of one or two selected data points increases the likelihood of finding a relationship between early brain responses and later development. The frequency of the ERPs studied by Molfese includes a lower range (below 2 Hz) than those employed by earlier investigators. Given that brainwave frequencies characterizing ERPs of young infants are concentrated in the frequency range below 3 Hz, this strategy uses more of the neonate's brainwave activity. Molfese also employed language-related speech sounds as the evoking stimuli rather than photic flashes. The relevance of photic flashes to the types of cognitive processing thought to be reflected in cognitive tests is not known. However, it is reasonable to conclude that studies of speech perception (phonetic) abilities are related to auditory language development. Because predictors of successful performance are better if they measure predicted skills, the inclusion of language-relevant sounds as the evoking stimuli should increase the likelihood for predicting later language-related skills. Differences in measures and stimuli across studies may be responsible for the better success found in our studies using auditory ERPs recorded at birth as predictors of later cognitive and language functioning.

It is our contention that phonetic discrimination skills have direct relevance to language development. Infants with difficulty in discriminating phonetic contrasts are at risk for later language disorders. Indeed, studies investigating some types of language-related disabilities, as in reading or learning disabilities, have indicated that these children share a phonological deficit (Lyon, 1994). Research over the past 3 decades indicates that ERPs are sensitive to phonetic variations in auditory stimuli, such as voice onset time (VOT) and place of articulation (POA). Several trends in findings reported from ERP studies must be noted. First, discrimination of different speech cues emerges at different times in early development. Relatively stable and reliable ERP components correlating with consonant POA discrimination have been noted in newborn infants. However, discrimination of VOT does not appear to develop until sometime after birth (Molfese & Molfese, 1979b;

Simos & Molfese, 1997). Second, the scalp distribution for ERP effects in relation to speech sound discrimination change with age. Molfese and Molfese (1979b) noted temporal lateral effects in newborns, while more pronounced frontal effects are noted in 12- to 16-month-old infants (Molfese, 1989a; 1989b) and temporal–parietal effects in children (Molfese & Molfese, 1988) and adults (Molfese, 1980). Different temporal regions of the ERP waveform appear sensitive to phonetic contrasts at different developmental stages. Thus, shortly after birth, speech sound discriminations occur at relatively long latencies (520–920 msec), while they shift forward in the ERP wave to 180–400 msec for preschoolers, and from 50 to 350 msec for elementary school children and adults (Molfese & Hess, 1978; Molfese & Molfese, 1979b, 1988; Simos & Molfese, 1997). Developmental variations in the age of appearance of ERP phonetic-related effects, their scalp distributions, and their latencies within the ERP waveform can influence the effectiveness of the models used to predict different levels of language and cognitive skills across developmental periods. Further, given that the types of tasks measuring language and cognitive skills also change developmentally, developing a predictive model across different developmental periods presents as nearly Herculean. One factor appears evident—attempts to develop accurate static predictive models from infancy to adulthood will be limited. Instead, it appears that any successful model must employ some different predictor variables at different ages to be successful.

VALIDITY AND RELIABILITY

Using this information on phonetic discrimination development and ERPs, Molfese and Molfese (1985, 1988, 1997) and Molfese and Searock (1986) isolated and identified ERP correlates of various speech perception cues across and within a number of developmental periods. In the first study (Molfese & Molfese, 1985), 16 infants were studied longitudinally from birth through 3 years. ERPs were recorded from newborn infants to a series of consonant–vowel speech syllables differing in POA. At 3, children were divided into two groups: with scores above/below the mean on the verbal subscale of the McCarthy Scales of Children's Abilities (McCarthy, 1972). Two regions of ERPs, with one component located between 88 and 240 msec and a second component with a peak latency of 664 msec, reflected differential sensitivity to specific consonant–vowel characteristics and were found to discriminate two groups. In the first ERP component, only ERPs recorded over the left hemisphere of the High group systematically discriminated between the different speech sounds. However, the Low group displayed no lateralized discrimination for the speech sounds. The second component occurred over both hemispheres and, consequently, reflected bilateral activity. This second component did not behave in exactly the same manner as the first. Although the second component discriminated between speech and nonspeech stimuli, discrimination between speech sounds depended on which vowel followed the consonant. A third component of the ERP (peak latency = 450 msec) that varied only across hemispheres failed to discriminate between the two groups.

A stepwise multiple regression model of these data was developed using the Peabody and McCarthy Verbal Index scores as criterion variables and the ERP components obtained at birth that best discriminated the different consonant sounds as the predictor variables. This model accounted for 78% of the total variance in predicting 3-year McCarthy scores from the newborn brain responses and 69% of the variance in predicting 3-year Peabody scores (Molfese & Molfese, 1988). Clearly, early ERP discrimination of speech-related stimuli is strongly related to later language skills.

Molfese and Searock (1986) later noted that this relationship also exists between ERPs recorded at 1 year of age and language skills at 3 years. ERPs were recorded from 16 infants within 2 weeks of their first birthday. A series of three vowel sounds with speech formant structure and three nonspeech tokens containing 1-Hz-wide formants that matched the mean frequencies of the speech sounds were presented to these infants, and their ERPs were recorded in response to each sound. Two regions of the ERPs, one centered between 300 and 400 msec and another centered around 200 msec following stimulus onset, discriminated between the 1-year-old infants who 2 years later would perform better or worse on the McCarthy language tasks. Infants who were able to discriminate between more vowel sounds performed better on the language tasks at 3 years of age.

These findings have been replicated with a different sample of infants (Molfese, 1984), and the predictive range was found to extend to 5 years of age (Molfese & Molfese, 1997). Using two of the three ERP regions identified earlier (Molfese & Molfese, 1985) to predict later language outcomes, Molfese and Molfese (1997) developed three discriminant functions that improved classification accuracy over their earlier work. Seventy-one children were selected for these analyses based on the completeness of their test records and the absence of physical or neurological deficits that would of themselves preclude a normal course of later cognitive/linguistic development. These children were then divided into two groups, one with verbal performance scores on the Stanford–Binet at 5 years of age that were below 100 and the second group with verbal performance scores of 100 or higher. The first discriminant function used three scores obtained from one factor to construct a single discriminant function; a second discriminant function was then developed using six scores derived from two partially overlapping factors; a third discriminant function employed seven scores derived from two factors. All three discriminant functions accurately discriminated Low from High verbal performing children at well above chance levels (50%). As more variables were added, correct classification improved from just below 80% to over 95%. Molfese and Molfese's (1985, 1988) confirmation of their earlier findings regarding the use of neonatal ERPs to predict later language performance outcomes even to 5 years of age are especially intriguing when it is considered that different verbal performance measures were used across these studies. The McCarthy Verbal scores were used by Molfese and Molfese (1985) while Molfese and Molfese (1997) used as target scores the verbal scores derived from the Stanford–Binet. Given this ability to classify children across different performance measures, it appears that ERP factor scores obtained from similar brain regions can effectively discriminate later performance on different standardized tests.

Other consistencies across studies suggest that this phenomenon of later predictability is stable. Molfese and Molfese (1985) used ERPs recorded from only the left and right temporal regions, T_3 and T_4, while Molfese and Molfese (1997) recorded from six scalp electrode sites, two that were identical to those used in the original study. As in the previous study, factor scores derived from the temporal sites were important in discriminating between children with different levels of verbal skills. The discriminative models of Molfese and Molfese (1997) included ERPs recorded primarily from the temporal sites that comprised two of three components in the three-variable model, four of six in the second model, and five of seven in the third model. However, factor scores derived from frontal and parietal leads improved the classification accuracy beyond that produced by the temporal sites alone. Thus, while ERPs recorded from over the temporal regions of the two hemispheres continued to play a prominent role in predicting later developmental outcomes, additional contributions were noted at other electrode sites.

FUTURE IMPLICATIONS

The obvious question that arises is why any type of behavior or brain measure should discriminate developmental outcomes over a large age range with such high accuracy. Are human accomplishments predetermined from birth? Are genetic factors so potent that they all but force certain developmental outcomes? Rather, we hypothesize that these data reflect the state of an underlying perceptual mechanism on which some aspects of later developing and emerging cognitive and language processes are based. As a result of genetic and intrauterine factors, the organism initially develops a set of perceptual abilities responsive to variables in its environment. For most of us, these perceptual abilities are similar and readily enable us to discriminate elements within our environment in quite similar ways. It is these fundamental differences in specific perceptual skills related to phonetic discriminations that set the stage for the early identification of ERP responses that predict later verbal and cognitive performance.

IMPLICATIONS FOR INFANTS AT RISK
FOR NONOPTIMAL DEVELOPMENT

For decades, researchers and practitioners have been interested in developing assessment tools for neonates that can be used to predict cognitive development. Motivating this research has been the belief that early identification can lead to earlier and more effective intervention. However, measures that satisfy all these criteria have proven to be difficult to identify. The most typical approaches to assessment have involved the use of a wide variety of newborn and early infant measures as predictors and a variety of performance measures as the criterion scores. The newborn and early infancy measures used as predictors have included measures of perinatal complications, neurological and behavioral assessments, electrophysiological measures of brain functioning, and measures reflecting attention and tactile abilities. Criterion measures have included scores on scales such as the Bayley Scales of Infant Development (Bayley, 1969, 1993), the Denver Developmental Screening Test (Dunn, 1965), the Stanford–Binet Intelligence Scale (Thorndike, Hagen, & Sattler, 1986), and the McCarthy Scales of Children's Abilities (McCarthy, 1972).

Many attempts have been made to develop systems in which perinatal risk scores reflecting prenatal, intrapartum, and neonatal complications can be used to predict cognitive functioning in infancy and early childhood. Several researchers have shown that perinatal risk scores are predictive of performance scores on developmental tests within the infancy period (Low et al., 1985; Molfese & Thomson, 1985). However, attempts to extend the period to include early childhood have not been as successful, especially when the infants do not possess extreme risk conditions (e.g., very low birthweight and severe types of intraventricular hemorrhage). Researchers report that perinatal risk scores were either not predictive of outcomes in preschool and school-age children (e.g., Cohen & Parmelee, 1983; Crisafi, Driscoll, Rey, & Adler, 1987) or were found to be only weak correlates (e.g., Bee et al., 1982; Largo et al., 1989; Silva, McGee, & Williams, 1984). More successful results have been reported when measures obtained in later infancy and early childhood were used to predict later language and cognitive skills (Molfese & DiLalla, 1995; Molfese, DiLalla, & Lovelace, 1995; Siegel, 1982a, 1982b, 1985; Smith, Flick, Ferris, & Sellman, 1972).

Based on these results that extend earlier reports, it appears that electrophysiological measures obtained at birth involving the auditory ERP can be used successfully to discriminate between infants who 3 to 5 years later will display different levels of verbal skills. More recent studies have tried to link preschool language skills with reading abilities in school-age children. Molfese (2000) used ERP recordings to speech sounds obtained at birth along with reading scores from the Wide Range Achievement Test obtained from the children at 8 years of age. Forty-eight children were grouped as either dyslexic ($n = 17$), poor ($n = 7$), or normal ($n = 24$) readers and discriminant function analyses were used to determine whether the children could be correctly identified using newborn ERP data. The results showed an overall classification accuracy of 81.3%, with 22 of the 24 dyslexic or poor readers correctly identified on the basis of the newborn ERPs. These studies showed that ERPs to speech sounds are related to both different levels of language abilities but also to different levels of subsequently developed reading abilities.

These findings raise exciting possibilities regarding the early identification of children with potential language problems and open up the possibility that successful intervention of language problems could be carried out before these problems become fully manifested in the child's behavior. At present, the identification of children with language, reading, and other cognitive problems occurs relatively late, often occurring in the elementary school years after it is established that the child is performing below grade level. One consequence of this delayed identification strategy is that it occurs so late in the child's overall cognitive and linguistic development. Such late identification may already be pushing the edge of the child's cognitive flexibility and ability to master new skills. Witelson and Swallow (1987) noted that 10 years of age could mark an important transition or major "breaking point" in development because there are marked changes in abilities such as spatial pattern recognition, Braille, and map reading after this time. Others (Curtis, 1977) have shown that the onset of puberty appears to set limits on acquisition of certain language and cognitive skills. Thus, interventions begun at approximately 10 years of age could face ceiling limits placed on their success by the child's developmental level and age. If, however, potential problems in language or cognitive development could be identified much earlier in time, planned interventions could be introduced earlier to the child that could be more successful in remediating the child's emerging language or cognitive problems.

ACKNOWLEDGMENT

Support for this work was provided by the National Science Foundation (Grant Nos. BNS8004429 and BNS 8210846) and the National Institutes of Health (Grant No. R01-HD17860).

REFERENCES

Allison, T., Wood, C. C., & McCarthy, G. M. (1986). The central nervous system. In M. G. H. Coles, E. Donchin, & S. W. Porges (Eds.), *Psychophysiology: Systems, processes, and applications* (pp. 5–25). New York: Guilford Press.
Barden, T., & Pelzman, P. (1980). Newborn brain stem auditory evoked responses and perinatal clinical events. *American Journal of Obstetrics and Gynecology, 136,* 912–919.

Bayley, N. (1969). *Bayley Scales of Infant Development: Birth to two years.* New York: Psychological Corporation.

Bayley, N. (1993). *Bayley Scales of Infant Development: Manual.* San Antonio, TX: Psychological Corporation.

Bee, H., Barnard, K., Eyres, S., Gray, C., Hammond, M., Spietz, A., Snyder, C., & Clark, B. (1982). Prediction of IQ and language skill for perinatal status, child performance, family characteristics and mother–infant interaction. *Child Development, 53,* 1134–1156.

Blume, W. T., Buza, R. C., & Okazaki, H. (1974). Anatomic correlates of the ten–twenty electrode placement system in infants. *Electroencephalography and Clinical Neurophysiology, 36,* 303–307.

Butler, B., & Engel, R. (1969). Mental and motor scores at 8 months in relation to neonatal photic responses. *Developmental Medicine and Child Neurology, 11,* 77–82.

Callaway, C., Tueting, P., & Koslow, S. (1978). *Event-related brain potentials and behavior.* New York: Academic Press.

Caton, R (1875). The electrical currents of the brain. *British Medical Journal, 2,* 278.

Cohen, S., Parmelee, A. (1983). Prediction of five year Stanford-Binet scores in preterm infants. *Child Development, 54,* 1242–1253.

Cox, L., Hack, M., & Metz, D. (1984). Auditory brain stem response abnormalities in the very low birthweight infant: Incidence and risk factors. *Ear and Hearing, 5,* 47–51.

Crisafi, M., Driscoll, J., Rey, H., & Adler, A. (1987, April). *A longitudinal study of intellectual performance of very low birthweight infants in the preschool years.* Paper presented at the Society for Research in Child Development, Baltimore.

Curtis, S. (1977). *Genie: A psycholinguistic study of a modern day "wild child."* New York: Academic Press.

Dunn, L. (1965). *Peabody Picture Vocabulary Test.* Circle Pines, MN: American Guidance Service.

Engel, R., & Fay, W. (1972). Visual evoked responses at birth, verbal scores at three years, and IQ at four years. *Developmental Medicine and Child Neurology, 14,* 283–289.

Engel, R., & Henderson, N. (1973). Visual evoked responses and IQ scores at school age. *Developmental Medicine and Child Neurology, 15,* 136–145.

Henderson, N., & Engel, R. (1974). Neonatal visual evoked potentials as predictors of psychoeducational testing at age seven. *Developmental Psychology, 10,* 269–276.

Jasper, H. H. (1958). The ten–twenty electrode system of the International Federation of Societies for Electroencephalography: Appendix to Report of the Committee on Methods of Clinical Examination in Electroencephalography. *Electroencephalography and Clinical Neurophysiology, 10,* 371–375.

Jensen, D. R., & Engel, R. (1971). Statistical procedures for relating dichotomous responses to maturation and EEG measurements. *Electroencephalography and Clinical Neurophysiology, 30,* 437–443.

Largo, R., Pfister, D., Molinari, L., Kundu, S., Lipp, A., & Duc, G. (1989). Significant of prenatal, perinatal, and postnatal factors on the development of AGA preterm infants at five to seven years. *Developmental Medicine and Child Neurology, 4,* 440–456.

Low, J., Galbraith, R,, Muir, D., Broekhoven, L., Wilkinson, J., & Karchmar, E. (1985). The contribution of fetal-newborn complications to motor and cognitive deficits. *Developmental Medicine and Child Neurology, 27,* 578–587.

Lyon, R. (1994). *Frames of reference for the assessment of learning disabilities: New views on measurement issues.* Baltimore: Brookes.

McCarthy, D. (1972). *Manual for the McCarthy Scales of Children's Abilities*. New York: Psychological Corporation.

Molfese, D. L. (1980). The phoneme and the engram: Electrophysiological evidence for the acoustic invariant in stop consonants. *Brain and Language, 9,* 372–376.

Molfese, D. L. (1983). Event related potentials and language processes. In A. Gaillard & W. Ritter (Eds.), *Tutorials in ERP research—Endogenous components* (pp. 345–368). Holland: Elsevier.

Molfese, D. L. (1984). Left hemisphere sensitivity to consonant sounds not displayed by the right hemisphere: Electrophysiological correlates. *Brain and Language, 22,* 109–127.

Molfese, D. L. (1989a). Electrophysiological correlates of word meanings in 14–month old human infants. *Developmental Neuropsychology, 5,* 79–103.

Molfese, D. L. (1989b). The use of auditory evoked responses recorded from newborns to predict later language skills. In N. Paul (Ed.), *Research in infant assessment* (Vol. 25, pp. 68–81). White Plains: March of Dimes.

Molfese, D. L. (2000). Predicting dyslexia at 8 years of age using neonatal brain responses. *Brain and Language, 67,* 238–245.

Molfese, D. L., Buhrke, R. A., & Wang, S. (1985). The right hemisphere and temporal processing of consonant transition durations: Electrophysiological correlates. *Brain and Language, 26,* 49–62.

Molfese, D. L., & Hess, T. M. (1978). Speech perception in nursery school age children: Sex and hemisphere differences. *Journal of Experimental Child Psychology, 26,* 71–84.

Molfese, D. L. & Molfese, V. J. (1979a). Hemisphere and stimulus differences as reflected in the cortical responses of newborn infants to speech stimuli. *Developmental Psychology, 15*(5), 505–511.

Molfese, D. L., & Molfese, V. J. (1979b). Infant speech perception: Learned or innate. In H. A. Whitaker & H. Whitaker (Eds.), *Advances in neurolinguistics* (Vol. 4, pp. 225–238). New York: Academic Press.

Molfese, D. L., & Molfese, V. J. (1980). Cortical response of preterm infants to phonetic and nonphonetic speech stimuli. *Developmental Psychology, 16*(6), 574–581.

Molfese, D. L. & Molfese, V. J. (1985). Electrophysiological indices of auditory discrimination in newborn infants: The bases for predicting later language development? *Infant Behavior and Development, 8,* 197–211.

Molfese, D. L., & Molfese, V. J. (1988). Right hemisphere responses from preschool children to temporal cues contained in speech and nonspeech materials: Electrophysiological correlates. *Brain and Language, 33,* 245–259.

Molfese, D. L., & Molfese, V. J. (1997). Discrimination of language skills at five years of age using event-related potentials recorded at birth. *Developmental Neuropsychology, 13,* 135–156.

Molfese, D. L., & Searock, K. (1986). The use of auditory evoked responses at one year of age to predict language skills at 3 years. *Australian Journal of Communication Disorders, 14,* 35–46.

Molfese, V. J., & Betz, J (1988). Language and motor development in infancy: Three views with neuropsychological implications. *Developmental Neuropsychology, 3,* 225–274.

Molfese, V. J., & DiLalla, L. (1995). Cost-effective approaches to identifying developmental delay in four to seven-year-olds. *Early Education and Development, 6,* 265–277.

Molfese, V. J., DiLalla, L., & Lovelace, L. (1995). Perinatal, home environment, and infant measures as successful predictors of preschool cognitive and verbal abilities. *International Journal of Behavioral Development, 18,* 103–120.

Molfese, V. J., & Thomson, B. (1985). Optimality versus complications: Assessing predictive values of perinatal scales. *Child Development, 56,* 810–823.

Murray, A. (1988). Newborn auditory brainstem evoked responses (ABRs): Longitudinal correlates in the first year. *Child Development, 59,* 1542–1554.

Murray, A., Dolby, R., Nation, R., & Thomas, D. (1981). Effects of epidermal anesthesia on newborn and their mothers. *Child Development, 52,* 71–82.

Nelson, C., & Salapatek, P. (1986). Electrophysiological correlates of infant recognition memory. *Child Development, 57,* 1483–1497.

Pugh, K. R., Shaywitz, B. A., Shaywitz, S. E., Constable, R. T., Skudlarski, P., Fulbright, R. K., Bronen, R. A., Shankweiler, D. P., Katz, L., Fletcher, J. M., & Gore, J. C. (1996). Cerebral organization of component processes in reading. *Brain, 119,* 1221–1238.

Rockstroh, B., Elbert, T., Birbaumer, N., & Lutzenberger, W. (1982). *Slow brain potentials and behavior.* Baltimore: Urban-Schwarzenberg.

Ruchkin, D., Sutton, S., Munson, R., & Macar, F. (1981). P300 and feedback provided by the absence of the stimuli. *Psychophysiology, 18,* 271–282.

Shaywitz, B. A., Shaywitz, S. E., Pugh, K. R., Constable, R. T., Skudlarski, P., Fulbright, R. K., Bronen, R. A., Fletcher, J. M., Shankweiler, D. P., Katz, L., & Gore, J. C. (1995). Sex differences in the functional organization of the brain for language. *Nature, 373*(6515), 607–609.

Siegel, L. (1982a). Reproductive, perinatal and environmental factors as predictorsx. *Child Development, 53,* 963–973.

Siegel, L. (1982b). Reproductive, perinatal and environmental variables as predictors of development of preterm (grams) and full term infants at 5 years. *Seminars and Perinatology, 6,* 274–279.

Siegel, L. (1985). Biological and environmental variables as predictors of intellectual functioning at 6 years of age. In S. Harel & N. Anastasjow (Eds.) *The at-risk infant: Psychosocial medical aspects.* Baltimore: Brookes.

Silva, P., McGee, R., & Williams, S. (1984). A seven year follow-up study of the cognitive development of children who experienced common perinatal problems. *Australian Pediatric Journal, 20,* 23–28.

Simos, A., & Molfese, D., (1997). Electrophysiological responses from a temporal order continuum in the newborn infant. *Neuropsychologia, 35,* 89–98.

Smith, A., Flick, G., Ferriss, G., & Sellmann, A. (1972). Prediction of developmental outcomes at seven years from prenatal, perinatal and postnatal events. *Child Development, 43,* 495–507.

Thorndike, R., Hagen, E., & Sattler, J. (1986). *Guide for administering and scoring the fourth edition of the Stanford–Binet Intelligence Scale.* Chicago: Riverside.

Witelson, S., & Swallow, J. A. (1987). Neuropsychological study of the development of spatial cognition. In J. Stiles-Davis, M. Kritchevsky, & U. Bellugi (Eds.), *Spatial cognition: Brain bases and development* (pp. 373–409). Hillsdale, NJ: Erlbaum.

17

Electroencephalographic Assessment and Human Brain Maturation

A Window into Emotional and Cognitive Development in Infancy

DALIT HIMMELFARB MARSHALL

NATHAN A. FOX

HISTORY

Developmental theorists have posited that understanding the brain and its developmental growth pattern can provide insight into behavioral changes over time. Not until the last several decades, however, has the role of the developing brain been directly investigated with respect to changes in emotional and cognitive functioning during infancy and early childhood (Byrnes & Fox, 1998; Fox, Schmidt, & Henderson, 2000; Segalowitz, 1994). In recent years, methods within the field have progressed enough to allow validated inferences about the relations between emerging behaviors and brain maturation in a developmental context. The purpose of this chapter is to describe the innovations and utility of electroencephalography (EEG)—a well-used technology in psychophysiological research—and to demonstrate its implications to understanding the development of emotional and cognitive behaviors in infancy.

Brain electrical activity recorded off the scalp was first observed in human subjects by Berger (1929, 1932a, 1932b). Berger identified four typical rhythmic oscillations—alpha, beta, theta, and delta—that could be differentiated from one another in frequency and amplitude. The appearance and pattern of these "wave-like" electrical activities reflected changes in the state of the organism. Increases or decreases in amplitude were associated with changes in specific mental activity. Following Berger's initial description, clinicians and researchers started to use quantitative EEG (qEEG) to study normal and atypical brain development. Because this technique is relatively inexpensive and completely noninvasive, it has rapidly become a common practice in multiple domains of psychophysiological research.

In clinical settings, EEG measures have been used to diagnose neuropathology, by using the electrical signals to localize brain events such as seizures and, in the case of infants, to evaluate gestational age and maturational levels of newborns (Lombroso, 1975; Parmelee et al., 1968). In basic research settings, this assessment technique has been directed toward understanding processes related to brain maturation, such as changes in EEG frequency (Hagne, 1968, 1972; Henry, 1944; Lindsley, 1939; Smith, 1938a, 1938b, 1939, 1941) and intrahemispheric coherence (Thatcher, Krause, & Hrybyk, 1986; Thatcher, Walker, & Giudice, 1987). The increased understanding of brain development has further enabled researchers to study the relations between changes in electrical brain activity and the emergence of particular psychological functions. Examples of the use of qEEG as a probe of psychological function include attempts to relate frontal EEG activation to emotional (Calkins, Fox, & Marshall, 1996; Davidson & Fox, 1989; Fox, Bell, & Jones, 1992) and cognitive (Bell, 1998a, 1998b; Bell & Fox, 1992, 1997) development during the first year of life.

GENERAL DESCRIPTION

The qEEG technology reflects computerized recording as well as signal and statistical analyses of electrical potentials recorded from the surface of the scalp. The purpose of this section is to provide a general description of the procedures involved in recording and analyzing EEG data, as well as to discuss some of the conceptual and methodological issues that influence the interpretation of qEEG data.

Recording the EEG Signal

The EEG signal represents a potential difference between two active sites or between an active site and a computed mathematical reference. An initial assumption in EEG recording technology is that this difference reflects cyclical changes in underlying nerve cell activity. To accurately measure such changes, researchers place individual electrodes on the surface of the scalp according to an accepted international set of placements that defines the major cortical divisions as well as the various sulci of the cortex (i.e., the 10–20 system; Jasper, 1958).

Using this topography, electrical brain activity may be recorded either by fixing individual electrodes on the scalp with an adhesive compound—collodion—or by using a stretch cap, with the electrode array built in. The latter procedure is more common among infant studies mainly because of decreased time for scalp preparation and the potentially aversive nature of individual scalp leads for young infants (Nelson, 1994; Schmidt & Fox, 1998). Following the application of scalp electrodes, the electrical resistance of each electrode is measured to ensure that the impedance is kept below an acceptable limit.

The first step in EEG acquisition is to amplify the weak scalp electrical signals, which are low-voltage analogs of underlying brain activity, convert the signal from analog to digital, and then store the digitized version of this signal on a computer. The device that digitizes the amplified EEG is known as an analog-to-digital converter (ADC). To precisely represent the original analog waveforms, the sampling rate of the ADC has to be set to more than twice the highest frequency found within the EEG, even if its origins are noncerebral (e.g., muscle artifacts; Duffy, 1994).

Another major consideration prior to analyzing the EEG data is related to the detection of artifactual contamination that may affect the signal. Identifying artifacts is of great importance, as researchers may misattribute the source of the signal to specific brain activity even though its actual origin is noncerebral. One source of EEG artifacts is associated with the layers of material that exist between the attached electrodes and the actual electrical impulses elicited by the nerve cells. This interference may be emphasized by the fact that the voltage signal picked up by the EEG electrodes has been conducted from the source through a conductive fluid medium, through the bony structure of the skull, and then through the scalp to the electrode (Hugdahl, 1998).

Electrical signals caused by eye blinks and other motor movements are another major source of EEG artifacts. A typical solution for segregating cortically derived signals from electrical signals from the eyes is to place electrodes around the eyes so as to separately measure eye and motor movements. These electrodes facilitate artifact detection before data are analyzed and may also serve in statistical considerations such as the degree to which outcomes are contaminated by artifacts. In case of consistent disruptions of EEG data by artifact, contaminated epochs should be rejected from further analysis.

EEG Analysis Techniques

The EEG is a time series and as such may be analyzed with techniques suitable for time or frequency domain analysis. Time-domain analysis is used to examine stimulus-locked changes in the EEG. For example, the event-related potential (ERP) is analyzed with time-domain analysis and provides measures of latency and amplitude of response.

Frequency methods include power spectral analysis, coherence analysis, and hemispheric asymmetry analysis. In power spectral analysis, EEG data are submitted to a fast Fourier transformation (FFT; Cooley & Tukey, 1965), which decomposes the EEG signal into its component frequencies. The outcome of this analysis is an estimate of spectral power for each frequency.

Coherence analysis is a technique that computes the degree to which two EEG signals are in or out of phase with each other at a given frequency. The magnitude of the coherence has been interpreted to reflect the degree to which two topographically distinct sites communicate with each other (Nunez, 1981; Thatcher, 1994).

Asymmetry analysis refers to the degree to which a hemisphere or a region within a hemisphere is more or less activated in comparison to the homologous region in the other hemisphere (Davidson, 1988). In laterality studies, asymmetry measures may also provide an index of the dynamic changes in brain electrical activity of both the left and right hemispheres associated with changes in underlying neural activities (Fox, 1994). Traditionally, EEG asymmetry scores are computed by calculating the difference in mean log alpha power between homologous sites. An underlying assumption in asymmetry measures is that alpha power and activation are inversely related, so lower alpha power in one hemisphere, relative to the other hemisphere, reflects greater activity in that hemisphere (Lindsley & Wicke, 1974).

With respect to the asymmetry metric, positive values reflect greater relative right-sided alpha power and denote left-hemisphere asymmetry, whereas negative values reflect greater relative left-sided alpha power and denote right-hemisphere asymmetry (Davidson, 1988). There are at least two ways in which individual or group differences in cerebral asymmetry can be accounted for. Specifically, right EEG asymmetry could result from increased left-hemisphere EEG power, with EEG power in the right hemisphere remaining constant (i.e., left EEG hypoactivation). Alternatively, right asymmetry could be a function of a reduction in right EEG power, with left EEG power remaining constant (i.e., right EEG hyperactivation). Similarly, differences in left-hemisphere asymmetry could be a function of right EEG hypoactivation or left EEG hyperactivation.

Reliability and Stability of EEG Measures

There is moderate test–retest reliability in adult EEG power and asymmetry, suggesting that EEG power and asymmetry are relatively stable. Gasser, Bacher, and Steinberg (1985) found the test–retest reliability of resting alpha power over a 10-month period to be in the .70s, and Wheeler, Davidson, and Tomarken (1993) reported that the test–retest reliability of frontal alpha power asymmetry over a 3-week period was .66. As for within-subject variability in asymmetry measures, it has been proposed that the relations between hemispheric activation and psychological behaviors are more stable for those subjects with stable EEG asymmetry (Wheeler et al., 1993). Referring to frontal electrode sites, these authors defined stable asymmetry as a standardized score in one assessment that is within ± 0.33 standard deviations of the standardized score at another assessment.

To date, there are no data on the stability of asymmetry measures in infants or children. Because the human brain exhibits critical changes over the first years of life, the strong cross-age stability in adult studies do not necessarily generalize to infants. Fox et al. (1992) intended to examine the within-subject stability of EEG measures by testing the same infants across a 6-month period. However, due to small number of subjects and missing data, it was impossible to carry out the test–retest measures adequately.

DEVELOPMENTAL MODEL

The infant brain differs structurally from the adult brain in the number of neurons, degree of myelination, and patterns of connectivity (Goldman-Rakic, 1986; Huttenlocher, 1993; Johnson, 1993). With respect to EEG parameters, differences between adult and infant brain electrical activity are observed in both frequency and amplitude. Infant EEG consists of relatively low-frequency and high-amplitude activity. The dominant frequency of the EEG increases with age and the amplitude of the EEG becomes smaller.

Studies of age-related changes in EEGs are therefore of special interest and may be useful in explaining processes that occur in the human brain during development. Furthermore, if these changes are coincident with emotional and cognitive development, the assessment of brain maturational processes, along with the emergence of emotional and cognitive behaviors, may result in articulating a powerful model of brain–behavior relations. For empirical evidence regarding developmental changes in brain electrical activity over the first years of life, the reader is referred elsewhere (see Bell & Fox, 1994, and Schmidt & Fox, 1998, for reviews).

BIOBEHAVIORAL BASIS OF ASSESSMENT

The Relations between EEG and Emotional Development

Studies examining the relations between EEG activity and emotions have mainly focused on the frontal region of the cortex, as this area of the brain is known to play a key role in the experience, regulation, and expression of emotions. A variety of data have implicated the anterior region of the left cerebral hemisphere in the management and expression of positive, approach-directed emotional responses to attractive stimuli and reward. Activity of the anterior region of the right cerebral hemisphere has been found to be related to processes that facilitate the management and expression of negative, withdrawal-directed emotional responses to aversive stimuli and punishment (Davidson, Ekman, Saron, Senulis, & Friesen, 1990; Davidson & Fox, 1982, 1989; Dawson, 1994; Dawson, Panagiotides, Grofer Klinger, & Hill, 1992c; Fox & Davidson, 1987, 1988).

Frontal EEG Asymmetry and the Expression of Discrete Emotions

Asymmetry measures have been used to demonstrate the presence of differential hemispheric asymmetry during infants' exposure to a variety of elicitors that produce a range of positive or negative emotions (Davidson & Fox, 1982; Fox & Davidson, 1986, 1987). In the initial set of studies, EEG was extracted and analyzed in response to the elicitor itself, and not to the infant's response to the stimuli. For example, Fox and Davidson (1986) presented water, sucrose, and citric acid solutions to newborn infants while recording frontal and parietal brain electrical activity. In this study EEG was not analyzed on the basis of the subject's response to the stimuli but, rather, during the entire stimulus epoch regardless of whether the desired expression (i.e., interest or disgust) was present or absent. Similarly, Fox and Davidson (1987) recorded infants' brain electrical activity during the entire epoch of either approach of mother or approach of stranger. The data derived from this study illustrate changes in frontal asymmetry in response to different environmental conditions. However, precise linkages between facial expressions of affect and EEG activity were not examined.

To specify the precise lateralized changes in infants' EEG associated with discrete emotions, Fox and Davidson (1988) tested 10-month-old infants in the same standard stranger- and mother-approach paradigm and analyzed infants' facial and vocal expressions alongside the corresponding EEG data. Different patterns of EEG asymmetry were found depending on the type of facial and vocal expression of affect observed. Expressions of joy were associated with relative left frontal activation, whereas anger and sadness accompanied greater relative activation in the right. This study demonstrated the linkage among frontal EEG asymmetry and the actual display of discrete emotions in infants.

Frontal EEG Asymmetry and Individual Differences in Social-Emotional Behaviors

The notion that the two frontal hemispheres may be differentially specialized for the expression and control of positive or negative emotions has been extended to include differences in emotional disposition. Specifically, the proposition has been advanced that individuals who differ in tonic activation of either the left or right frontal hemisphere would differ in their predisposition to express either positive or negative affects. Individuals exhibiting relative left frontal activation should be more likely to express positive emotions whereas individuals with relative right frontal activation should be more likely to express negative emotions. These relations have been tested and confirmed in several studies with adults (Tomarken, Davidson, & Henriques, 1990; Wheeler et al., 1993) and with infants and young children (Davidson & Fox, 1989; Fox et al., 1992). To illustrate, Davidson and Fox (1989) reported that a group of 10-month-old infants who cried in response to a brief episode of maternal separation had greater right-sided and less left-sided frontal activation during a preceding baseline period, than did a group of infants who did not cry. These findings were explained in terms of the relations between hyperactivation in the right frontal hemisphere and an inability to regulate negative affect in response to mildly stressful events.

Given the association among specific patterns of EEG asymmetry and early manifestations of negative reactivity, Fox and colleagues suggested that a similar linkage may exist with respect to later characteristics of social behavior. To test their hypothesis, Fox et al. (1995) collected EEG data from 4-year-olds who were also observed in a same-sex quartet play session. Relations among child social behaviors and measures of frontal asymmetry were examined, with the prediction that children showing a high proportion of social reticence and inhibition during a peer playgroup would be distinguishable on patterns of frontal EEG asymmetry. Results indicated greater relative right frontal EEG activation among children who displayed a high proportion of anxiety and wariness in response to unfamiliar peers, compared with children who did not. Further analyses revealed that the right frontal asymmetry exhibited by the highly reticent and inhibited group of children was a function of left hypoactivation (i.e., less activation in the left frontal lead relative to the right frontal lead). This pattern, similar to the one found by Davidson with depressed adults (Henriques & Davidson, 1990), may reflect a tendency toward less positive affect expression in socially reticent children.

A second study, with data from an additional cohort of 4-year-old children (Fox, Schmidt, Calkins, Rubin, & Coplan, 1996), examined whether the interaction between observed social behavior and frontal EEG asymmetry was also related to the occurrence of maladaptive internalizing and externalizing behaviors. It was found that highly inhibited children with a pattern of right frontal asymmetry were more likely to exhibit internalizing problems than were highly inhibited children who displayed a pattern of left frontal asymmetry. Similarly, highly sociable right frontal children were more likely to exhibit externalizing problems than were highly left frontal sociable children. The findings from these two studies suggest that EEG asymmetry may be a marker for inhibition and maladaptive social behavior during the preschool years.

Frontal EEG Asymmetry and the Stability and Instability of Social Behaviors

In addition to being related to specific characteristics of social-emotional behavior, patterns of EEG asymmetry were also found to mediate the relations between early child temperament and later manifestations of social behaviors. Calkins et al. (1996) examined three groups of infants selected at age 4 months on the basis of their frequency of motor activity and on the degree of positive and negative affect displayed in response to novelty. The first group consisted of infants who displayed both high motor activity and negative affect and low positive affect. The second group consisted of infants with both high amounts of motor activity and positive affect and low amounts of negative affect. The third group of infants displayed low motor activity and low positive and negative affect. All infants were seen again in the laboratory at 9, 14, and 24 months of age.

Infants showing high motor activity and negative affect at 4 months of age exhibited greater activation of the right frontal brain at age 9 and 24 months, compared with infants in the other two groups. However, behavioral inhibition in both 14 and 24 months of age was demonstrated only among those infants whose pattern of right frontal activation was stable across the first 2 years of life.

Similar findings were recently reported in a study that compared negatively reactive 4-month-old infants who remained inhibited over a period of 4 years with infants who had the same early temperament characteristics but exhibited changes in patterns of inhibition (Fox, Henderson, Rubin, Calkins, & Schmidt, 2001). The group of infants who remained stable and inhibited exhibited right frontal asymmetry, whereas the other group displayed right frontal asymmetry at 9 months but left frontal asymmetry at later ages.

Of significance from these studies was the finding that patterns of EEG asymmetry predicted change or continuity in emotional and social behaviors during early childhood. This finding illustrates that early temperament characteristics may be associated with the development of specific social behaviors but that this linkage is better understood through the moderating role of frontal brain asymmetry.

Patterns of Frontal EEG in Infants of Depressed Mothers

Studies have indicated a positive relation between maternal depression and a variety of behavioral and emotional difficulties among infants. Infants of mothers with depressive symptoms tend to be more fussy and irritable than infants of nondepressed mothers (Field, 1986; Field et al., 1988) and are more likely to display sad and angry emotional expressions than happy or interest expressions (Cohn, Campbell, Matias, & Hopkins, 1990; Pickens & Field,

1993, 1995). Recent work has investigated a possible relation between maternal depression and differences in infants' patterns of frontal brain electrical activity (Dawson, Frey, Panagiotides, Osterling, & Hessl, 1997a; Dawson, Grofer Klinger, Panagiotides, Hill, & Spieker, 1992a; Dawson, Grofer Klinger, Panagiotides, Spieker, & Frey, 1992b; Field, Fox, Pickens, & Nawrocki, 1995). In these studies, infants of depressed and nondepressed mothers were compared on their EEG patterns during an alert baseline condition or during active play with their mothers. On both occasions, infants of depressed mothers exhibited less frontal EEG activation during baseline than did infants of nondepressed mothers and showed asymmetry with reduced activity in the left (vs. right) hemisphere as early as 3 months of age.

Research has also examined whether these baseline differences are present during the expression of different discrete emotions. Dawson and her co-workers recorded left and right, frontal, and parietal EEG activity in 11- to 17-month-old infants of depressed and nondepressed mothers during the expression of positive, negative, and neutral emotions (Dawson, Panagiotides, Grofer Klinger, & Spieker, 1997b). Infants of depressed mothers, compared with infants of nondepressed mothers, exhibited increased EEG activation in the frontal, but not parietal, region when expressing negative emotions. No differences were found with regard to the expression of positive or neutral emotions. These findings are in line with previous studies illustrating the role of the frontal cortex in the management of negative emotions.

It is possible that increased activation in the frontal lobe, exhibited by this population of infants, reflects a temperamental propensity to express certain emotions in greater frequency and/or intensity, or, alternatively, it may reflect an attempt to mobilize inhibitory or regulatory processes (Dawson, 1994; Fox, 1994). If the atypical patterns of brain activity in infants of depressed mothers reflect a temperamental disposition, one would expect a similar psychophysiological pattern to be present during social situations not involving interactions with the mother. To address this question, EEG was collected in infants of depressed and nondepressed mothers during a baseline condition, interaction with mother, and interaction with a familiar experimenter (Dawson et al., 1999). During all three conditions, infants of depressed mothers exhibited reduced left relative to right frontal activity. These results suggest that the atypical EEG pattern exhibited by infants of depressed mothers generalizes to social interactions with nondepressed adults.

Studies with depressed adults found the same pattern of reduced activation in the left frontal hemisphere (Henriques & Davidson, 1990, 1991). Furthermore, it was demonstrated that the decrease in left frontal activation was also present in recovered depressives, compared to never depressed controls (Henriques & Davidson, 1990). Left frontal hypoactivation among depressed and previously depressed adults has been interpreted as a neural reflection of the decreased capacity for experiencing positive emotions and a decline in goal-related motivation and behavior (Davidson, 1998). This interpretation may also hold for infants of depressed mothers. Interactions between depressed mothers and their infants may lead the infants to mimic the mother's depressive affect (Field et al., 1995) and to exhibit depressive-like affective states, which in turn may be reflected in their atypical left frontal hypoactivation.

The Relations between EEG and Cognitive Development

EEG assessment provides a window into the development of important cognitive functions associated with specific cortical regions. Because changes in EEG during the first year of life may vary as a function of individual differences in brain development, EEG measures may also reflect individual differences in the performance of specific cognitive behaviors.

The relation between infants' enhanced cognitive performance and the development of areas in the cerebral cortex can be illustrated by the emergence of cognition that leads to object permanence over the second half of the first year of life. Several studies by Diamond and coworkers (Diamond, 1990a, 1990b; Diamond & Goldman-Rakic, 1983, 1986, 1989; Diamond, Zola-Morgan, & Squire, 1989) have demonstrated—in intact infant monkeys and in infant and adult monkeys with prefrontal lesions—that the ability to tolerate delay and successfully perform on a Stage IV object permanence task (the A-not-B task; Piaget, 1937/1954) is dependent on maturation or integrity of the dorsolateral prefrontal cortex. In the A-not-B task the infant is required to successfully retrieve an object twice at site A, and then in site B, with either no delay or a timed delay between each search. Diamond has claimed that the underlying abilities essential for solving the A-not-B task include the ability to hold a representation in memory over time (i.e., "recall memory" or "working memory") and the ability to inhibit a motor response that has previously been rewarded (Diamond, 1985, 1988, 1990a, 1990b). Diamond (1990b) showed that rhesus monkeys with lesions of dorsolateral prefrontal cortex could successfully solve tasks that used only one of these skills (recall memory or inhibitory control). Thus, it has been argued that the integration of these two skills is a primary competency of prefrontal cortex.

Bell and Fox (1992) tested this hypothesis in a longitudinal study with 7- to 12-month-old infants. Infants were followed monthly and in each visit baseline EEG was recorded and performance observed on two separated cognitive tasks: the A-not-B task and a novel toy task, which examined response inhibition but not memory. The last task involved presenting different moving novel toys to infants and observing latency to grasp each toy. This study design enabled the assessment of the prediction made by Diamond (1990a, 1990b) regarding the unique function of the prefrontal cortex in the developing ability to solve cognitive tasks that involve the integrative function of inhibiting a motor response and holding a representation in memory over time. It was expected that infant performance on the A-not-B task, but not in the novel toy task, would be related to differences in frontal, but not other regional, EEG development and in coherence development across age.

Results confirmed these expectations. On the A-not-B task, there was high variability in individual infant performance at 10, 11, and 12 months of age, and these individual differences were associated with specific patterns of resting EEG alpha power and coherence. Infants who displayed a long tolerance of delay at 12 months exhibited a decrease in right frontal EEG power between 7 and 8 months of age, as well as the greatest monthly increase in overall frontal EEG power between 9 and 10 months of age. This group of infants also showed greater power in the left occipital lead relative to the right occipital lead across age, and an increase in coherence from 9 to 12 months of age after an initial decrease in coherence between 8 and 9 months. Different results were obtained for infants who displayed a short tolerance of delay at 12 months. For this group of infants, there was only a change in right frontal power between 10 and 11 months of age and no changes at all in coherence.

Performance on the novel toy task also produced individual differences: Some infants displayed an increased latency to grasp each toy between 7 and 12 months of age whereas others displayed a decrease latency across age. Those differences, however, were not related to frontal, parietal, or occipital EEG power or to coherence.

These results indicate the relation between changes in baseline EEG activation and performance on a specific cognitive task. It is now known that the increased ability to successfully solve the A-not-B task with delay is associated with power changes in the frontal region of the cortex, as well as with increased connectivity between frontal and parietal regions and between frontal and occipital regions. Interestingly, the largest monthly increase in power in the frontal leads, exhibited at 10 months of age by the long delay group, occurred simultaneously with the increase in anterior-to-posterior coherence.

Although this initial work has successfully confirmed frontal involvement in cognitive tasks, it is somewhat limited in that it examines cognitive performance on baseline rather than task-related frontal EEG data. Gathering task-related EEG recordings was not useful during the classic reaching version of the A-not-B task because the task demands of reaching and retrieving the object introduce a great deal of artifact into the EEG data. In an attempt to get a task-related account of frontal EEG, Bell (1998a, 1998b) has recently designed a looking version of the A-not-B task that enables infants to indicate the location of the hidden object with only minimal eye movements rather than arm reaches.

A group of 8-month-old infants completed both versions of the A-not-B task in counterbalanced order. Although no significant differences were found in respect to infants' proficiency on each version of the task, analyses of the EEG data in the alpha band revealed differences between baseline and task-related power values. Specifically, infants exhibited higher power values during the looking task than during baseline, which may reflect increased cognitive processing during the looking task. Power values were particularly elevated during the delayed search condition, the most cognitively demanding portion of the task. Keeping in mind that the relation between power and activation is inverse, one may presume that infant EEG power would decrease (and not increase) with mental activity, in resemblance to the alpha suppression tendency found in adults during cognitive processing. These findings suggest that the changes in alpha power exhibited by infants during increased mental activity is more similar to the changes in the adult theta band than to changes in the adult alpha band. To date, more task-related EEG measures are needed to support this speculation. There is no doubt, however, that there are strong relations among the maturation of the prefrontal cortex and successful A-not-B performance.

Other developmental factors may also contribute to the increased successful performance on the A-not-B task. One of these factors is the changes in infants' crawling experience, which was found to be related in itself to maturational changes in EEG. One study with 8-month-old infants showed that resting EEG coherence between intrahemisphereric sites was significantly greater among novice crawlers (1–4 weeks) than among either prelocomotor infants or experienced crawlers, suggesting that the anticipation and onset of locomotion are associated with changes in cortical organization (Bell & Fox, 1996). Several authors have proposed that this developmental motor milestone of hands and knees locomotion is also associated with the increased cognitive performance in object permanence paradigms (Bertenthal, Campos, & Kermoian, 1994; Horobin & Acredolo, 1986; Kermoian & Campos, 1988). They demonstrated that locomotor infants are better than prelocomotor infants at finding hidden objects under variety of experimental conditions. The contribution of hands-and-knees crawling experience and frontal brain maturation to infants' proficiency on the classic Piagetian A-not-B task was examined in an age-held-constant design of 8-month-old infants (Bell & Fox, 1997). Results indicated that locomotor experience and resting frontal EEG power values were both related to enhanced performance on the object permanence task but there was no interaction among the three.

In our view, the results of this study are of special importance to understanding the role of maturation versus experience in cognitive development. Neither brain maturation nor increased experience with the environment can exclusively account for successful cognitive performance. Rather, there are multiple pathways to cognitive development, and each of them plays a significant role. As has been illustrated in the object permanence study, some infants may achieve success via experience and others may do so via brain development. This conclusion highlights the notion that both neurobiological and behavioral influences should be taken into consideration as useful elements in any developmental theory construction.

STRUCTURAL AND THEORETICAL CONSTRAINTS

All the studies described in this chapter have used scalp-recorded brain electrical activity to make inferences about regional brain activation, either during baseline periods or in response to a variety of emotion elicitors and cognitive stimuli. There are several advantages and benefits for the use of this method in studying emotional and cognitive development during infancy. First, the EEG is a noninvasive procedure and does not cause unnecessary discomfort for subjects, which is of special importance in studies with infants and young children. Second, the EEG has a fast time resolution that enables researchers to measure changes in amplitude over time periods in the order of milliseconds. This characteristic is essential for the demanding condition of recording brain electrical activity during the short time interval between the presentation of a stimulus and a behavioral response. Third, EEG data can be accurately synchronized with overt behavioral measures and thus can allow investigators to identify patterns of brain activity that are coincident with overt responses. Fourth, the EEG is relatively inexpensive, which is an important consideration in studies demanding repeated measures and large sample sizes.

In light of these advantages, the recording of EEG has become a common practice for many developmental scholars interested in psychophysiological processes. However, this technique has significant constraints, which include the problems of between-subject variability in the placement of electrodes on the scalp, the choice of reference electrode location, and the problem of muscle and other forms of artifacts. Scalp electrophysiology also has the significant disadvantage of providing ambiguous information about the sources of brain electrical activity (Davidson, 1994; Gevins, 1996). Even when one records electrical activity from a large number of sites, there is a certain degree of uncertainty about the precise cortical locations that are active and the exact behavior of the neurons in this location. Several factors may diminish the spatial resolution of the EEG, including the conductive fluid medium and the skull bone itself. Individual differences in skull thickness and cell densities may obscure the meaning of the output as well. The ratio between measures from individual electrode sites and activity in those regions of cortex underlying the scalp electrode sites is not 1:1.

Despite these considerations, EEG techniques have been developed to aid limited localization of sources of the EEG signal. One development has been the increased application of dense electrode arrays, which consist of as many as 256 electrodes on a specially designed head net. The proposed advantage of the large number of sites is in increasing the precision of spatial localization of the EEG signal, although there are various unanswered questions concerning this technique (Davidson, Jackson, & Larson, 2000). There have also been advances in the spatial modeling techniques that are used to interpret the EEG signal. Most notable among these techniques are brain electrical source analysis (BESA; e.g., Scherg & Von Cramon, 1986) and low-resolution electromagnetic tomography (LORETA; e.g., Pascual-Marqui, Michel, & Lehmann, 1994). Although still not comparable to the spatial resolution of hemodynamic imaging, these techniques have allowed more sophisticated interpretations of EEG findings (e.g., Pizzagalli et al., 2001).

An alternative technique with excellent spatial resolution is functional magnetic resonance imaging (fMRI). This technique is based on the assumption that changes in oxygenated and deoxygenated blood flow in the brain correlate with mental activity. Because oxygenated blood provides a stronger magnetic resonance signal than deoxygenated blood, the fMRI makes use of contrast in the magnetic properties of oxygenated and deoxygenated blood to create accurate images of active areas of the brain (Monnen, 1995).

In contrast to the EEG, magnetic resonance images allow researchers to precisely evaluate the localization of the brain function. Nevertheless, this advanced technique has several disadvantages that should be carefully considered when choosing an adequate psychophysiological tool. First, the decrease in the concentration of deoxygenated blood, on which the magnetic resonance image is based, is associated with a variety of physiological events, and therefore interpretation of fMRI signals is not unequivocal. Until this issue is resolved, changes in fMRI signals in a specific region cannot be attributed in a definite manner to increased neural activity in that region. Second, to identify localized regions of high activity, it is necessary to perform a number of t-tests prior to computing the magnetic resonance image (Casey et al., 1996). The requisite statistical models, which avoid repeated, multiple comparisons, have not yet been developed. Third, the procedure is more expensive than the EEG because of the powerful magnets required for the computation of the signals. And, finally, to date the temporal resolution of the fMRI is still slower than the temporal resolution of the EEG.

Each of the different neuroimaging approaches has strengths and weaknesses. Clearly, the most extensive and defensible approach would involve inferences based on multiple neurophysiological methods that have been used simultaneously in a single study. A combination of fMRI and EEG, for example, may yield powerful inferences regarding both localization and temporal phases of emotional and cognitive brain processes.

TRAINING REQUIREMENTS

It is often the case that researchers who have important questions regarding the interface of behavioral and biological processes wish to employ methods such as qEEG in their research. With current advances in computing and availability of software for analysis, these methods are no longer as esoteric as they once were. However, the methodological issues involved in the recording and analysis of the qEEG remain complex. Appropriate training in the acquisition of such signals should include topics such as electrical circuits, principles of amplification, and analogue-to-digital conversion. As well, researchers should gain some working knowledge of principles involved in the analysis of time-series data. Such knowledge will assist the investigator in the choice of sampling rate for acquisition as well as in the interpretation of the data.

One of the consequences of the increased availability of computers and software for the acquisition and analysis of large data sets such as qEEG is the desire to purchase "black box" systems in which the investigator is not involved in the many technical steps outlined in this chapter. The advantage is the obvious ease. The disadvantages are great and involve an inability in knowing when data are spurious or when they are actually reflecting nervous system processes.

The study of psychophysiological processes may be viewed as only a technical exercise, or it may be viewed as genuinely providing insight into processes by which the nervous system and behavior interact. If researchers are to gain such knowledge about these underlying processes they will have to take the time to undergo the training to understand the technical and methodological issues involved and collecting accurate data.

SUMMARY AND IMPLICATIONS

The information presented throughout this chapter indicates that developmental changes in the brain may be assessed using a noninvasive technology known as the electroencephalogram. Measures derived from the EEG may be associated with emotional and cognitive behaviors in infancy and early childhood. Using advanced psychophysiological techniques such as the quantified EEG, the emergence of emotional and cognitive behaviors may be described in terms of frequency, amplitude, coherence, and asymmetry of brain electrical activity. These parameters are useful not only in describing age-related changes in development but also in explaining individual differences in the rate of arriving at a certain outcome, and in the characteristics of the outcome itself.

REFERENCES

Bell, M. A. (1998a). Frontal lobe function during infancy: Implications for the development of cognition and attention. In J. E. Richards (Ed.), *Cognitive neuroscience of attention: A developmental perspective* (pp. 287–316). Hillsdale, NJ: Erlbaum.

Bell, M. A. (1998b). *A looking version of the A-not-B task: Frontal EEG and infant cognitive functioning*. Paper presented at the International Conference of Infant Study, Atlanta.

Bell, M. A., & Fox, N. A. (1992). The relations between frontal brain electrical activity and cognitive development during infancy. *Child Development, 63,* 1142–1163.

Bell, M. A., & Fox, N. A. (1994). Brain development over the first year of life: Relations between electroencephalographic frequency and coherence and cognitive and affective behaviors. In G. Dawson & K. W. Fischer (Eds.), *Human behavior and the developing brain* (pp. 93–133). New York: Guilford Press.

Bell, M. A., & Fox, N. A. (1996). Crawling experience is related to changes in cortical organization during infancy: Evidence from EEG coherence. *Developmental Psychology, 29,* 551–561.

Bell, M. A., & Fox, N. A. (1997). Individual differences in object permanence performance at 8 months: Locomotor experience and brain electrical activity. *Developmental Psychobiology, 31,* 287–297.

Berger, H. (1929). Über das Elektrenkephalogramm des Menschen: I. *Archiv für Psychiatrie und Nervenkrankheiten, 87,* 527–570.

Berger, H. (1932a). Über das Elektrenkephalogramm des Menschen: IV. *Archiv für Psychiatrie und Nervenkrankheiten, 97,* 6–26.

Berger, H. (1932b). Über das Elektrenkephalogramm des Menschen: V. *Archiv für Psychiatrie und Nervenkrankheiten, 98,* 231–254.

Bertenthal, B. I., Campos, J. J., & Kermoian, R. (1994). An epigenetic perspective on the development of self-produces locomotion and its consequences. *Current Directions in Psychological Science, 3,* 140–145.

Byrnes, J. P., & Fox, N. A. (1998). The educational relevance off research in cognitive neuroscience. *Educational Psychology Review, 10,* 297–342.

Calkins, S. D., Fox, N. A., & Marshall, T. R. (1996). Behavioral and physiological antecedents of inhibited and uninhibited behavior. *Child Development, 67,* 523–540.

Casey, B. J., Cohen, J. D., Noll, D. C., Schneider, W., Giedd, J. N., & Rappaport, J. L. (1996). Functional magnetic resonance imaging: Studies of cognition. In E. D. Bigler (Ed.), *Neuroimaging II: Clinical applications* (pp. 299–330). New York: Plenum Press.

Cohn, J. F., Campbell, S. B., Matias, R., & Hopkins, J. (1990). Face-to-face interactions of postpartum depressed and non-depressed mother-infant pairs at two months. *Developmental Psychology, 26,* 15–23.

Cooley, J. W., & Tukey, J. W. (1965). An algorithm for the machine calculation of Fourier series. *Mathematics of Computation, 19,* 297–301.

Davidson, R. J. (1988). EEG measures of cerebral asymmetry: Conceptual and methodological issues. *International Journal of Neuroscience, 39,* 71–89.

Davidson, R. J. (1994). Temperament, affective style, and frontal lobe asymmetry. In G. Dawson & K. W. Fischer (Eds.), *Human behavior and the developing brain* (pp. 518–536). New York: Guilford Press.

Davidson, R. J. (1998). Affective style and affective disorders: Perspectives from affective neuroscience. *Cognition and Emotion, 12,* 307–330.

Davidson, R. J., Ekman, P., Saron, C., Senulis, R., & Friesen, W. V. (1990). Approach-withdrawal and cerebral asymmetry: Emotional expression and brain physiology I. *Journal of Personality and Social Psychology, 58,* 330–341.

Davidson, R. J., & Fox, N. A. (1982). Asymmetrical brain activity discriminates between positive versus negative affective stimuli in human infants. *Science, 218,* 1235–1237.

Davidson, R. J., & Fox, N. A. (1989). Frontal brain asymmetry predicts infants' response to maternal separation. *Journal of Abnormal Psychology, 98,* 127–131.

Davidson, R. J., Jackson, D. C., & Larson, C. L. (2000). Human electroencephalography. In J. T. Cacioppo, L. G. Tassinary, & G. G. Berntson (Eds.), *Handbook of psychophysiology* (2nd ed., pp. 27–52). New York: Cambridge University Press.

Dawson, G. (1994). Frontal electroencephalographic activity during the expression of emotions: A brain systems perspective. *Monographs of the Society for Research in Child Development, 59*(2–3, Serial No. 240).

Dawson, G., Frey, K., Panagiotides, H., Osterling, J., & Hessl, D. (1997a). Infants of depressed mothers exhibit atypical frontal brain activity: A replication and extension of previous findings. *Journal of child Psychology and Psychiatry, 38,* 179–186.

Dawson, G., Frey, K., Panagiotides, H., Yamada, E., Hessl, D., & Osterling, J. (1999). Infants of depressed mothers exhibit atypical frontal electrical brain activity during interactions with mother and with a familiar, nondepressed adult. *Child Development, 70,* 1058–1066.

Dawson, G., Grofer Klinger, L., Panagiotides, H., Hill, D., & Spieker, S. (1992a). Frontal lobe activity and affective behavior of infants of mothers with depressive symptomes. *Child Development, 63,* 725–737.

Dawson, G., Grofer Klinger, L., Panagiotides, H., Spieker, S., & Frey, K. (1992b). Infants of mothers with depressive symptoms: Electroencephalographic and behavioral findings related to attachment status. *Development and Psychopathology, 4,* 67–80.

Dawson, G., Panagiotides, H., Grofer Klinger, L., & Hill, D. (1992c). The role of frontal lobe functioning in infant self-regulatory behavior. *Brain and Cognition, 20,* 152–175.

Dawson, G., Panagiotides, H., Grofer Klinger, L., & Spieker, S. (1997b). Infants of depressed and non-depressed mothers exhibit differences in frontal brain electrical activity during the expression of negative emotions. *Developmental Psychology, 33,* 650–656.

Diamond, A. (1985). Development of the ability to use recall to guide action, as indicated by infants' performance on AB. *Child Development, 56,* 868–883.

Diamond, A. (1988). Abilities and Neural mechanisms underlying AB performance. *Child Development, 59,* 523–527.

Diamond, A. (1990a). Developmental time course in human infants and infant monkeys, and the neural bases, of inhibitory control in reaching. In A. Diamond (Ed.), The development and neural bases of higher cognitive functions. *Annals of the New York Academy of Sciences, 608,* 637–676.

Diamond, A (1990b). The development and neural bases of memory functions as indexed by the AB and delayed response tasks in human infants and infant monkeys. In A. Diamond (Ed.), The development and neural bases of higher cognitive functions. *Annals of the New York Academy of Sciences, 608,* 267–317.

Diamond, A., & Goldman-Rakic, P. S. (1983). Comparison of performance on a Piagetian object permanence task in human infants and rhesus monkeys: Evidence for involvement of prefrontal cortex. *Society for Neuroscience Abstracts, 9,* 641.

Diamond, A., & Goldman-Rakic, P. S. (1986). Comparative development in human infants and infant rhesus monkeys of cognitive functions that depend on prefrontal cortex. *Society for Neuroscience Abstracts, 12,* 742.

Diamond, A., & Goldman-Rakic, P. S. (1989). Comparison of human infants and rhesus monkeys on Piaget's AB task: Evidence for dependence on dorsolateral prefrontal cortex. *Experimental Brain Research, 74,* 24–40.

Diamond, A., Zola-Morgan, S., & Squire, L. R. (1989). Successful performance by monkeys with lesions of the hippocampal formation on AB and object retrieval, two tasks that mark developmental changes in human infants. *Behavioral Neuroscience, 103*, 526–537.

Duffy, F. H. (1994). The role of quantified electroencephalography in psychological research. In G. Dawson & K. W. Fischer (Eds.), *Human behavior and the developing brain* (pp. 93–133). New York: Guilford Press.

Field, T. (1986). Models for reactive and chronic depression in infancy. In E. Z. Tronick & T. Field (Eds.), *Maternal depression and infant disturbance* (pp. 47–60). San Francisco: Jossey-Bass.

Field, T., Fox, N. A., Pickens, J., & Nawrocki, R. (1995). Relative right frontal EEG activation in 3– to 6–month-old infants of "depressed" mothers. *Developmental Psychology, 31*, 358–363.

Field, T., Healy, B., Goldstein, S., Perry, S., Bendall, D., Schanberg, S., Zimmerman, E., & Kuhn, C. (1988). Infants of depressed mothers show "depressed" behavior even with non-depressed adults. *Child Development, 59*, 1569–1579.

Fox, N. A. (1994). Dynamic cerebral processes underlying emotion regulation. In N. A. Fox (Ed.), The development of emotion regulation: Biological and behavioral considerations. *Monographs of the Society for Research in Child Development, 59*(2–3, Serial No. 240), 152–166.

Fox, N. A., Bell, M. A., & Jones, N. A. (1992). Individual differences in response to stress and cerebral asymmetry. *Developmental Neuropsychology, 8*, 161–184.

Fox, N. A., & Davidson, R. J. (1986). Taste-elicited changes in facial signs of emotion and the asymmetry of brain electrical activity in human newborns. *Neuropsychologia, 24*, 417–422.

Fox, N. A., & Davidson, R. J. (1987). EEG asymmetry in ten-month-old infants in response to approach of a stranger and maternal separation. *Developmental Psychology, 23*, 233–240.

Fox, N. A., & Davidson, R. J. (1988). Patterns of brain electrical activity during the expression of discrete emotions in ten-month-old infants. *Developmental Psychology, 24*, 230–236.

Fox, N. A., Henderson, H. A., Rubin, K. H., Calkins, S. D., & Schmidt, L. A. (2001). Continuity and discontinuity of behavioral inhibition and exuberance: Psychophysiological and behavioral influences across the first four years of life. *Child Development, 72*, 1–21.

Fox, N. A., Rubin, K. H., Calkins, S. D., Marshall, T. R., Coplan, R. J., Porges, S. W., Long, J. M., & Stewart, S. (1995). Frontal activation asymmetry and social competence at four years of age. *Child Development, 66*, 1770–1784.

Fox, N. A., Schmidt, L. A., Calkins, S. D., Rubin, K. H., & Coplan, R. J. (1996). The role of frontal activation in the regulation and dysregulation of social behavior during the preschool years. *Development and Psychopathology, 8*, 89–102.

Fox, N. A., Schmidt, L. A., & Henderson, H. A. (2000). Developmental psychophysiology. In J. T. Cacioppo, L. G. Tassinary, & G. G. Berntson (Eds.), *Handbook of psychophysiology* (2nd ed., pp. 665–686). New York: Cambridge University Press.

Gasser, T., Bacher, P., & Steinberg, H. (1985). Test-retest reliability of spectral parameters of the EEG. *Electroencephalography and Clinical Neurophysiology, 60*, 312–319.

Gevins, A. (1996). Electrophysiological imaging of brain function. In A. W. Toga & J. C.

Mazziotta (Eds.), *Brain mapping: The methods* (pp. 259–274). Orlando, FL: Academic Press.

Goldman-Rakic, P. S. (1986). Setting the stage: Neural development before birth. In S. L. Peterson, K. A. Klivington, & R. W. Peterson (Eds.), *The brain, cognition, and education* (pp. 233–258). New York: Academic Press.

Hagne, I. (1968). Development of the waking EEG in normal infants during the first year of life. In P. Kellaway & I. Peterson (Eds.), *Clinical electroencephalography of children* (pp. 97–118). New York: Grune & Stratton.

Hagne, I. (1972). Development of the EEG in normal infants during the first year of life. *Acta Pediatrica Scandinavica* (Suppl. 232), 25–53.

Henriques, J. B., & Davidson, R. J. (1990). Regional brain electrical asymmetries discriminate between previously depressed subjects and healthy controls. *Journal of Abnormal Psychology, 99,* 22–31.

Henriques, J. B., & Davidson, R. J. (1991). Left frontal hypoactivation in depression. *Journal of Abnormal Psychology, 100,* 535–545.

Henry, J. R. (1944). Electroencephalograms of normal children. *Monographs of the Society for Research in Child Development, 9*(3, Serial No. 39).

Horobin, K., & Acredolo, L. (1986). The role of attentiveness, mobility history, and separation of hiding sites on stage IV search behavior. *Journal of Experimental Child Psychology, 41,* 114–127.

Hugdahl, K. (1998). *Psychophysiology. The mind-body perspective* (pp. 234–265, 309–332). Cambridge: Harvard University Press.

Huttenlocher, P. R. (1993). Morphometric study of human cerebral cortex development. In M. H. Johnson (Ed.), *Brain development and cognition: A reader* (pp. 112–124). Blackwell: Oxford.

Jasper, H. H. (1958). The ten-twenty electrode system of the international Federation. *Electroencephalography and Clinical Neurophysiology, 10,* 371–375.

Johnson, M. H. (1993). Constraints on cortical plasticity. In M. H. Johnson (Ed.), *Brain development and cognition: A reader* (pp. 703–721). Blackwell: Oxford.

Kermoian, R., & Campos, J. J. (1988). Locomotor experience: A facilitator of spatial cognitive development. *Child Development, 59,* 908–917.

Lindsley, D. B. (1939). A longitudinal study of the occipital alpha rhythm in normal children: frequency and amplitude standards. *Journal of Genetic Psychology, 55,* 197–213.

Lindsley, D. B., & Wicke, J. D. (1974). The EEG: Autonomous electrical activity in man and animals. In R. Thompson & M. N. Patterson (Eds.), *Bioelectric recording techniques* (pp. 3–83). New York: Academic Press.

Lombroso, C. T. (1975). Neurophysiological observations in diseased newborns. *Biological Psychiatry, 10,* 527–558.

Monnen, C. T. W. (1995). Imaging of human brain activation with functional MRI. *Biological Psychiatry, 37,* 141–143.

Nelson, C. A. (1994). Neural Correlates of recognition memory in the first postnatal year. In G. Dawson & K. W. Fischer (Eds.), *Human behavior and the developing brain* (pp. 269–313). New York: Guilford Press.

Nunez, P. (1981). *Electrical fields of the brain.* New York: Oxford University Press.

Parmelee, A. H., Schulte, F. J., Akiyama, Y., Wenner, W. H., Schultz, M. A., & Stern, E. (1968). Maturation of EEG activity during sleep in premature infants. *Eletroencephalography and Clinical Neurophysiology, 24,* 319–329.

Pascual-Marqui, R. D., Michel, C. M., & Lehmann, D. (1994). Low resolution electromagnetic tomography: A new method for localizing electrical activity in the brain. *International Journal of Psychophysiology, 18,* 49–65.

Piaget, J. (1954). *The construction of reality in the child.* New York: Basic Books. (Original work published 1937)

Pickens, J., & Field, T. (1993). Facial expressivity in infants of depressed mothers. *Developmental Psychology, 29,* 986–988.

Pickens, J., & Field, T. (1995). Facial expressions and vagal tone in infants of depressed and non-depressed mothers. *Early Development and Parenting, 4,* 83–89.

Pizzagilli, D., Pascual-Marqui, R. D., Nitschke, J. B., Oakes, T. R., Larson, C. L., Abercrombie, H. C., Schaefer, S. M., Koger, J. V., Benca, R. M., & Davidson, R. J. (2001). Anterior cingulate activity as a predictor of degree of treatment response in major depression: Evidence from brain electrical tomography analysis. *American Journal of Psychiatry, 58,* 405–415.

Scherg, M., & Von Cramon, D. (1986). Evoked dipole source potentials of the human auditory cortex. *Electroencephalography and Clinical Neurophysiology, 65,* 344–360.

Schmidt, L. A. & Fox, N. A. (1998). Electrophysiological studies I: Quantitative electroencephalography. In C. E. Coffey & R. A. Brumback (Eds.), *Textbook of pediatric neuropsychiatry: Section II, Neuropsychiatric assessment of the child and adolescent* (pp. 315–329). Washington, DC: American Psychiatric Press.

Segalowitz, S. J. (1994). Developmental psychology and brain development: A historical perspective. In G. Dawson & K. W. Fischer (Eds.), *Human behavior and the developing brain* (pp. 93–133). New York: Guilford Press.

Smith, J. R. (1938a). The electroencephalogram during normal infancy and childhood: I. Rhythmic activities present in the neonate and their subsequent development. *Journal of Genetic Psychology, 53,* 431–453.

Smith, J. R. (1938b). The electroencephalogram during normal infancy and childhood: II. The nature and growth of the alpha waves. *Journal of Genetic Psychology, 53,* 455–469.

Smith, J. R. (1939). The "occipital" and "pre-central" alpha rhythms during the first two years. *Journal of Psychology, 7,* 223–226.

Smith, J. R. (1941). The frequency growth of the human alpha rhythms during normal infancy and childhood. *Journal of Psychology, 11,* 177–198.

Thatcher, R. W. (1994). Cyclic cortical reorganization: Origins of human cognitive development. In G. Dawson & K. W. Fischer (Eds.), *Human behavior and the developing brain* (pp. 232–266). New York: Guilford Press.

Thatcher, R. W., Krause, P. J., & Hrybyk, M. (1986). Cortico–cortical associations and EEG coherence: A two compartmental model. *Electroencephalography and Clinical Neurophysiology, 64,* 123–143.

Thatcher, R. W., Walker, R. A., & Giudice, S. (1987). Human cerebral hemispheres develop at different rates and ages. *Science, 236,* 1110–1113.

Tomarken, A. J., Davidson, R. J., & Henriques, J. B. (1990). Frontal brain asymmetry predicts affective responses to films. *Journal of Personality and Social Psychology, 59,* 791–801.

Wheeler, R. W., Davidson, R. J., & Tomarken, A. J. (1993). Frontal brain asymmetry and emotional reactivity: A biological substrate of affective style. *Psychophysiology, 30,* 82–91.

V

Standard Assessments

18

Behavioral Assessment Scales

The NICU Network Neurobehavioral Scale, the
Neonatal Behavioral Assessment Scale,
and the Assessment of the Preterm Infant's Behavior

BARRY M. LESTER
EDWARD Z. TRONICK

HISTORY

The NICU Network Neurobehavioral Scale (NNNS) was designed for the neurobehavioral assessment of drug-exposed and other high-risk infants. It is based on the Neonatal Behavioral Assessment Scale (Brazelton, 1973). This chapter focuses on the NNNS but also reviews other assessment scales as relevant.

Infant assessment, historically, has been strongly influenced by the current dominant theoretical view of the infant and of the mind or brain. Prior to the turn of the century the infant was viewed as diffusely organized, unstructured, and lacking in sensory capacities and motor abilities. No examinations existed because there was "nothing" to evaluate.

At the turn of the century, infant functioning was associated with the model of reflexes developed by Sherrington (1906). Much of this work was based on studies of the spinal frog and the view that the single neuron was the fundamental unit of the nervous system. This model was elaborated by learning theorists who viewed the reflex, like the neuron, as the building block of behavior. During this period Peiper (1928) began his exploration of the newborn's reflexes, eventually publishing a standard neurological text on newborn neurobehavior. Critical demonstrations of reflexes in anencephalic infants supported the idea that the infant operates only at the spinal level.

Reflex models began to be supplemented by models of more generalized motor functioning. Andre-Thomas (1960) and Saint-Anne Dargassies (1977) developed an examination that focused on the motor tone of the infant in which tone involved passive and active components. They were influenced by models of the brain that were beginning to focus on mass action as enunciated by Lashley (1951) in the United States and those that included inhibitory and excitatory centers, concepts that would not be fully incorporated into thinking about infants for another 25 years. Critically, this idea led to the view that the infant could modulate behavior, not just act in an all-or-none fashion. Concepts of active and passive tone became part of the dominant view of infant assessment and the model started to evolve into one of control or feedback systems, with the thermostat as the mechanical metaphor.

A major advance by Prechtl (Prechtl & Beintema, 1964), was his introduction of the concept of state. Descriptively, states were differentiated, structured organizations of the brain and associated physiology that affected how the infant responded to the same stimulus. The same stimulus resulted in different responses in different states, introducing a substantive change in the view of the infant's neurobehavioral functioning. The brain, not just the spinal cord, was involved in the infant's responses, and more important, the infant's brain was active. When state was considered, the neurobehavioral organization of the infant became more apparent. State, the organization of its components and their sequential organization over time, became "assessable" features of the infant's neurological status. An intact brain was capable of organizing states whereas a damaged brain could not. This advance was derived from early work on sleep and electroencephalograph activity in which it was demonstrated that the brain is not simply quiescent when the organism is asleep but shows differentiated states with different electrical, physiological, and behavioral concomitants. Thus, even when asleep the brain was active. Prechtl's formulation of "state" decimated the reflex model of the infant.

Examination of the infant's neurological status became a feature of standard care. These examinations viewed the infant as active, as in part responsible for generating the responses, and as able to modulate performance. New research demonstrated that even asphyxiated infants and anencephalic infants generated variable reflexes, that healthy infants modulated their responses, and that modulation and state-dependent responsiveness were characteristics of the infant. Simple stimulus–response reflex models were no longer tenable—there was a brain in the baby.

In the 1950s and exploding into the 1960s–1990s, developmental researchers demonstrated highly complex functioning in the infant. Fantz, Fagan, and Miranda (1975) demonstrated preferential gaze and much research followed showing that neonates were capable of complex highly differentiated hand movements (Twitchell, 1965), discrimination of sounds (Eimas, 1975; Eimas & Miller, 1980; Eimas, Siqueland, Jusczyk, & Vigorito, 1971), instrumental conditioning (Papousek, 1967), affective behaviors in response to stimuli (Wolff, 1966), detection of odors (Engen, Lipsitt, & Kaye, 1963), coordination of movement and speech (Condon & Sander, 1974), and different cry patterns (Wolff, 1966; Wasz-Hockert, Lind, Vuorenkoski, Partanen, & Valanne, 1968). The infant also engaged in socially focused activities (Brazelton, Koslowski, & Main, 1974).

As this competent infant arrived on the scene, it was also recognized that the infant had abilities to control (regulate) its own level of arousal and to habituate, a rudimentary form of learning. The recognition of infant functional competence contributed to the development of assessments of more complex forms of behavior. Rosenblith (1961) developed a scale that incorporated qualities of infant orientation, habituation, tone and reflexes. Brazelton and colleagues (Brazelton, 1973) developed the Neonatal Behavioral Assessment Scale (NBAS), which included items focused on the infant's capacity to self-regulate and to interact with animate and inanimate stimuli. Thus, for the first time the infant's social competence was assessed, or at least the infant's competencies in a social context. With these advances and influences from the formulation of the concept of temperament, the field of assessment moved beyond the evaluation of neurological integrity toward assessment of individual differences. The NBAS focused on assessing the infant in a social context and emphasized how the infant's individual differences affected caretaking and development.

NEONATAL BEHAVIORAL ASSESSMENT SCALE

General Description

The NBAS consists of 28 behavioral items scored on a 9-point scale and 18 reflex items scored on a 4-point scale. The reflex items were included to provide some information about neurological status and to manipulate the baby to produce changes in state. The second edition of the NBAS included seven supplementary 9-point rating scales called "qualifiers" designed to summarize the quality of the infant's responsiveness and the amount of input the infant needed from the examiner to elicit the desired responses. The supplementary items were based on scales developed by Horowitz and Linn (1984) in the Kansas version of the NBAS and by Als, Lester, Tronick, and Brazelton (1982) in the Assessment of the Preterm Infant's Behavior, discussed later. The Kansas version is also notable for scoring the infant's "modal" rather than "best" performance, a trademark of the NBAS. The NBAS takes 30–45 minutes to administer in a quiet dimly lighted room. An additional 20–30 minutes is needed to score the exam.

A number of data reduction schemes have been proposed for the NBAS, including factor-analytic solutions. Most studies use the seven clusters of habituation, orientation, motor, range of state, regulation of state, autonomic stability, and reflexes (Lester, Als, & Brazelton, 1982). The clusters are derived by rescoring items so that higher scores represent clinically better performance. However, the direction of some of the items cannot be determined from the cluster score as the original items have to be reexamined. For example, a low score on the motor cluster indicates poor motor performance, but one cannot determine whether the infant is hypertonic or hypotonic without inspecting the individual item scores that comprise the cluster.

Training

The NBAS requires training in handling the infant and scoring the exam. The interactive nature of the exam and the emphasis on eliciting best performance place serious training demands on examiners. Brazelton has established training centers to meet these needs. Certification to perform the exam requires both reliability in administration, based on clinical judgment of the trainer, and reliability in scoring, based on agreement within 1 point on the 9-point rating scales. Training is a several-step process in which trainees are taught the exam, observe several exams, and then practice on their own until ready for a certification test, with periodic consultation of feedback from a certified trainer. Most trainees practice with 20–25 babies before they are ready for certification, although this number is affected by prior experience with handling newborn infants.

Reliability and Validity

Test–retest reliability of the NBAS shows low to moderate correlations, most slightly above or below .30, a finding that has been used as a criticism of the test. However, it has also been suggested that test–retest correlations are appropriate only when the construct measured is expected to be stable (Lester, 1984). A 5-year-old's IQ should be relatively stable from day to day, but the first month of life is a period of rapid change; therefore, behavior may not be stable during this time. Brazelton (1984) has argued that clinically one might worry about infants who show minimal change during the neonatal period. Brazelton suggested that the infant's pattern of change over repeated exams, called recovery curves, might be the best predictor of infant adaptation to the postnatal environment. Most studies have not found evidence for the long-term predictive validity of the NBAS, although some pilot data on the recovery curve idea looked promising (Lester, 1984). Most investigators view the NBAS as a valid description of the contemporary behavior of the infant but not a predictor of long-term development. As a description of current behavior, it is useful to help parents understand the strengths and vulnerabilities of their newborn.

Studies of normal infants raised questions about what might affect the expression of behavior of newborn infants. Brazelton and his colleagues pioneered studies of factors (e.g., obstetric medication) of medical conditions (e.g., low birthweight) that affected the infant's neurobehavioral organization. Thus, with its focus on individual differences and the factors that affect those differences, as well as its conceptualization that these differences affect the caregiver's behavior and infant long term development, the NBAS became the dominant neonatal behavioral assessment in the field. This use of the NBAS confirmed the emerging view that infant development was determined by a complex interactionist perspective. It has been used in several hundred studies focusing on a variety of issues including studies of normal development, at-risk infants, cross-cultural factors, and intervention. As such, the NBAS is the benchmark neurobehavioral examination, the "parent" of the NNNS and several other examinations.

ASSESSMENT OF THE PRETERM INFANT'S BEHAVIOR

The Assessment of the Preterm Infant's Behavior (APIB) was developed by Als et al. (1982) to develop an "ethogram" of the preterm infant's behavioral repertoire. The APIB is based on the NBAS but focuses on the unique characteristics of the preterm infant.

The APIB yields 285 raw scores, most of which are scored on 9-point scales. These are reduced to 32 summary scores organized into five behavioral systems: physiological (e.g., respiratory patterns and skin color), motor (e.g., tonus, posture, and movements), state (level of consciousness, with states also described as diffuse or well defined), attentional–interactive (alertness and ability to attend to social stimuli and inanimate objects), and regulatory (regulatory activity of the infant to maintain itself in a balanced, well-modulated state). The APIB includes ratings of the amount of facilitation by the examiner needed to bring out the infant's best performance. The APIB is administered by organizing the test items of the NBAS into six packages of maneuvers that reflect increasingly challenging and complex interactions: (1) sleep/distal, (2) uncover–supine, (3) low tactile, (4) high tactile, (5) vestibular, (6) attentional–interaction. Time to administer the exam is comparable to the NBAS (30–45 minutes), but because of the number of items, scoring is labor intensive.

The predictive and construct validity for the APIB was reported by Als (1997) on a sample of 160 term and preterm children studied through 9 months of age. The APIB has also been used as an outcome measure to study the effect of intervention in the neonatal intensive care unit (NICU)

(Als, 1994) with a companion NICU intervention based on the same model as the APIB. The APIB requires extensive training. According to Als (1994, 1997), the conceptual basis of the APIB necessitates training in neuro-development and human evolution in addition to training in the assessment itself.

NICU NETWORK NEUROBEHAVIORAL SCALE

General Description

The NNNS was developed as an assessment for the at-risk infant, especially substance exposed, and was meant to have broad applicability. It is a comprehensive assessment of both neurological integrity and behavioral functioning, including withdrawal and general signs of stress.

The NNNS was developed for the National Institutes of Health for the multisite "Maternal Lifestyle" longitudinal study (Lester, 1998) of prenatal drug exposure and child outcome in preterm and term infants. The demands of this project required an examination that evaluated risk status and toxic exposures in a wide range of infants of varying birthweights, which could be reliably used at multiple sites. The exam needed to broadly assess the infant at risk, not just a single group such as preterm infants or only drug-exposed infants for two major reasons. First, most drug-exposed infants are term, not preterm, infants. Second, prenatal drug exposure often occurs in the context of multiple risk factors. These factors may be biological, such as prematurity or intrauterine growth retardation, or social, such as poverty, poor nutrition, and lack of prenatal care, which also have biological consequences for the infant. Therefore, the exam needed to be sensitive to the many risk factors that affect infant neurobehavior and to assess a variety of domains of functional status. Moreover, there was a broader need for an examination that was standardized. The idea was to provide a comprehensive evaluation of the neurobehavioral performance of the high-risk and substance-exposed infant during the perinatal period: neurobehavioral organization, neurological reflexes, motor development, active and passive tone, and signs of stress and withdrawal.

The NNNS draws on prior examinations in addition to the NBAS, including The Neurological Examination of the Full-Term Newborn Infant (Prechtl, 1977), the Neurological Examination of the Maturity of Newborn Infants (Amiel-Tison, 1968), the Neurobehavioral Assessment of the Preterm Infant (Korner & Thom, 1990), and the APIB (Als et al., 1982). Signs of stress and withdrawal observed during a neurobehavioral examination were scored to the Neonatal Abstinence Score (Finnegan, 1986). Use of the examination was not restricted to a particular type of infant (e.g., drug exposed) or to a limited age (e.g., full-terms or preterm); it could be used for a variety of infants and for infants of varying gestational ages.

   The NNNS assesses and scores the full range of infant neurobehavioral performance; assesses infant stress, abstinence and withdrawal, neurological functioning, and some features of gestational age assessment; and specifically and procedurally evaluates behavioral states and frames the assessment of other behaviors within states. It can be used with low- and extremely high-risk infants once they are stable and well out into the postnatal period; has a standardized administrative format that "removes" the examiner from the behavior assessed; evaluates the quality of the examination; was designed to have internal validity and appropriate statistical properties; was designed to generate summary scores for the major domains of neurobehavioral performance, as well as stress and withdrawal; and was designed to be sensitive to the effects of drugs and other risk conditions based on empirical literature.

Description of the NNNS Examination

The exam should be performed on medically stable infants in an open crib/isolette. It is probably not appropriate for infants less than 28 weeks gestational age; the upper age limit may also vary, with a reasonable upper limit of 46 weeks (corrected or conceptional age, i.e., weeks gestational age at birth plus weeks since birth).

Neurological Status

Neurological items were selected to provide a valid assessment of the neurological integrity and maturity of the infant, based on their demonstrated clinical utility and empirical validation, as well as chosen to represent the various "schools" such as the French angles method (Amiel-Tison, 1968) and the primitive reflexes method (Prechtl, 1977). Many items were omitted because they were redundant with other items or because they have shown little utility in research studies. The number of neurological items was limited to balance with the behavioral part of the exam so that it could be completed in less than 30 minutes and would not unduly fatigue or stress the infant. Infant state is specified for each reflex. The NNNS identifies normal or best responses, if applicable, but a wide range of normal is recognized and the best response is meant only as a point of reference. A normal, abnormal, or suspect neurological scoring system is also included.

   A crucial part of the neurological assessment is the assessment of muscle tone, which is assessed under both active and passive conditions. Active tone is assessed while observing spontaneous motor activity, including efforts at self-righting. Passive tone can be assessed during Posture, Scarf Sign, Popliteal Angle, Forearm and Leg Recoil, and Forearm and Leg Resistance. Both may be influenced by infant state, position (i.e., prone, supine, or supported upright), or the effects of postural reflex activity. When assessing muscle tone, both the distribution (proximal vs. distal) and the type of tone (extensor vs. flexor) should be described, as in the developing infant, proximal tone in the neck and trunk may differ from distal tone in the extremities. For example, in the preterm infant, flexor tone develops first in the lower extremities, in contrast to the more mature full-term infant who demonstrates uniform flexion.

Stress/Abstinence Scale

Most work documenting signs of stress in drug-exposed infants involves signs of abstinence or withdrawal, usually in infants of heroin-addicted or methadone-dependent mothers. Less potent opiates have been identified as precipitating a neonatal opiate abstinence syndrome and some nonopiate central nervous system depressants have also been implicated.

In work to date with cocaine-exposed infants, neonatal abstinence symptomatology does not appear to be increased. However, abstinence may occur from the depressants and narcotics used concomitantly with cocaine. Cocaine-exposed infants may show additional signs of stress such as lethargy in which the infant is unable to maintain a quiet awake state or crying during social interaction.

In addition, other signs of stress have been added that have been described in cocaine-exposed, or other high-risk infants, including preterms (Als et al., 1982).

NNNS Procedure

In the NNNS, items are administered in packages with each package beginning with a change in focus or position. The order of administration is relatively invariant. Table 18.1 presents a list of the maneuvers or packages and their respective items in the preferred order of administration.

During the Preexamination Observation the infant is asleep, prone, undressed, and covered. Initial State is scored using the traditional 1–6 criteria described by Prechtl (1974). All other items include criteria for why an item is not administered in addition to criteria for scoring the behavioral response. The Response Decrement items are administered with infant in state 1 or 2 and coded on scales that include criteria for when the infant stops responding ("shutdown") and criteria for when the item is discontinued. During Unwrap and Supine, the infant's posture, skin color, and movement are observed and scored on scales that include, when appropriate, criteria for normal responsivity, hyporesponsivity, and hyperresponsivity. Skin texture is also scored for the presence of specific conditions. The seven Lower Extremity Reflexes, nine Upper Extremity and Facial Reflexes, four Upright and three Infant Prone Responses are administered with the infant in states 3, 4, or 5 and include classic reflexes, measures of tone and angles, scored on

TABLE 18.1. Packages of Neurobehavioral Items in Preferred Order of Administration

Package	Items
Preexamination Observation	Initial state observation
Response Decrement	Response decrement to light; response decrement to rattle; response decrement to bell
Unwrap and Supine	Posture; skin color; skin texture; movement; response decrement to tactile stimulation of foot
Lower Extremity Reflexes	Plantar grasp; babinski; ankle clonus; leg resistance; leg recoil; power of active leg movements; popliteal angle
Upper Extremity and Facial Reflexes	Scarf sign; forearm resistance; forearm recoil; power of active arm movements; rooting; sucking; hand grasp; truncal tone; pull-to-sit
Upright Responses	Placing; stepping; ventral suspension; incurvation
Infant Prone	Crawling; stimulation needed; head raise in prone
Pick Up Infant	Cuddle in arm; cuddle on shoulder
Infant Supine on Examiner's Lap	Orientation (order not determined): animate visual and auditory—animate visual, animate auditory; inanimate visual and auditory—inanimate visual, inanimate auditory
Infant Spin	Tonic deviation of head and eyes; nystagmus
Infant Supine in Crib	Defensive response; asymmetrical tonic neck reflex; foot withdrawal reflex; Moro reflex
Postexamination Observation	Postexamination state observation

scales that also include, where appropriate, criteria for normal responsivity, hyporesponsivity, and hyperresponsivity. The infant, in state 4 or 5, is picked up and cuddled and scored separately for cuddle in arm and shoulder. The six orientation items are then administered with the infant still in state 4 or 5, on the examiner's lap. The types of handling procedures used to keep the infant in a state 4 or 5 during the orientation package are scored along with the orientation responses. The infant is picked up for the Spin items, returned to the crib for the final set of reflexes, and observed for the postexamination period.

Alternatives to this order may be required with some infants. For example, it may be necessary to administer the orientation items after pull-to-sit. This decision is based on whether or not best performance during the orientation would be elicited immediately after pull-to-sit or after the cuddle items. However, the order is not changed simply because the infant is in an alert state after pull-to-sit. Rather, the examiner continues with the standard order and administers the orientation in its proper sequence. For some in-fants, the examiner may need to rearrange the packages but can maintain the preferred sequence within the packages, whereas for others, the items must be administered without regard for the preferred order of either pack-ages or items within packages. The extent of deviation from the standard or-der may provide critical information about the infant's functional status. Finally, although every effort should be made to start with a sleeping infant, this is not always possible and the response decrement items cannot be ad-ministered first.

Table 18.2 shows the items on the Stress/Abstinence Scale divided into organ systems. Each item is scored as present/absent with definitions pro-vided in the manual if the examiner observed the event during the exam.

Inability to Achieve Quiet Awake State (State 4): Data Reduction and Scoring

Missing Data

Specific codes are used to identify reasons an item cannot be scored. Each item contains only codes that are logical outcomes of the specific manipula-

TABLE 18.2. Stress/Abstinence Scale

Organ System	Items
Physiological	Apnea; tachypnea; labored breathing; nasal flaring; bradycardia; tachycardia; desaturation
Autonomic Nervous System	Sweating; spit-up; hiccoughing; sneezing; nasal stuffiness; yawning
Central Nervous System	Abnormal sucking; choreiform movements; athetoid postures and movements; tremors; cogwheel movements; startles; hypertonia; back arching; fisting; cortical thumb; myoclonic jerks; generalized seizures; abnormal posture
Skin	Pallor; mottling; lividity; overall cyanosis; circumoral cyanosis; periocular cyanosis
Visual	Gaze aversion during orientation; pull down during orientation; fuss/cry during orientation; obligatory following during orientation; end-point nystagmus during orientation; sustained spontaneous nystagmus; visual locking; hyperalertness; setting sun sign; roving eye movements; strabismus; tight blinking; other abnormal eye signs
Gastrointestinal	Gagging/choking; loose stools, watery stools; excessive gas, bowel sounds
State	High pitch cry; monotone pitch cry; weak cry; no cry; extreme irritability; abrupt state changes

tion or observation. Codes may indicate that the item was started but discontinued because the infant's response lasted too long (e.g., habituation items), that the item was not administered because the infant did not respond after gentle prodding (e.g., habituation items), that the item was started but discontinued because the infant changed to an inappropriate state, that the item was not administered because the infant was in an inappropriate state or that the item was inadvertently skipped by the examiner.

Asymmetric Reflex Scores

For many reflexes, the left and right sides are evaluated separately. The scoring system is designed to reveal systematic asymmetries across items.

Summary Scores

Summary scores were developed a priori and tested in the Maternal Lifestyles study sample of 1,388 infants. Half the sample was randomly selected and used to test the internal consistency of the summary scores without any information about the characteristics of the infants (i.e., exposure status and birthweight). Alpha coefficients were computed on the summary scores and found to be acceptable. The summary scores were then computed for the entire sample and found to be stable. The summary scores include Habituation, Orientation, Amount of Handling, State, Self-Regulation, Hypotonia, Hypertonia, Quality of Movement, Number of Stress/Abstinence Signs (which can be also computed by organ system), and Number of Nonoptimal Reflexes. Alpha coefficients ranged from .59 to.81 with a median of .71.

Biobehavioral Basis

The term "neurobehavioral" is critical to understanding the NNNS. The term "neurobehavior" was developed to characterize older children and refers to an expanded neurological examination which involves sophisticated observation of higher cortical function and motor output that is often combined with an assessment of the maturation of the central nervous system or a search for minor neurological indicators. Here the term is used broadly to reflect the idea that all human experiences have psychosocial as well as biological or organic contexts. "Neurobehavioral" recognizes bidirectionality—that biological and behavioral systems dynamically influence each other and that the quality of behavioral and physiological processes is dependent on neural feedback. Neurobehavior becomes the interface of behavior and physiology and includes neurophysiological mechanisms that mediate specific behaviors or psychological processes.

These processes are affected by multiple risk factors. Thus, the NNNS was designed to measure processes of biobehavioral organization determined by multiple risk factors. Because much of the biobehavioral organization of the infant is determined by the combination of multiple biological and social risk factors, the exam must be sensitive to the broad range of behaviors that high-risk infants present.

Drug exposure is once such major biological factor and provides a good model for understanding multiple risk factors. Much is known about the mechanism of action of specific drugs and there is concern that illegal (cocaine, opiates, marijuana) and legal (alcohol and tobacco) drugs may act as behavioral teratogens, altering fetal brain development and subsequent function. Typically, the mechanisms of action are construed as individual agents, such as cocaine, on dopaminergic systems or alcohol on inhibitory amino acid systems. However, recent evidence suggests that in addition to these specific effects, there is a mechanism of action common to all drugs of abuse that centers on activation of specific neural pathways that project from the pons and midbrain to more rostral forebrain regions, including the amygdala, medial prefrontal cortex, anterior cingulated cortex, ventral palladium, and nucleus accumbens (Malanga & Kosofsky, 1999). Regardless of the site of initial binding of a drug in the brain, there may be a final common pathway for drug action that affects neurotransmitter systems. The behavioral expression of these effects are not known. This approach also supports the multiple-risk model because it could imply that polydrug exposure acts in a cumulative or synergistic fashion on the same neurotransmitter systems. There is a cumulative effect of risk factors that places increased stress on the nervous system, which in turn affects behavior, and these effects may be different from the effects of the individual risk factor.

Therefore, the NNNS was designed to be generically sensitive to the range of behaviors that at-risk infants display and also attend to the specific dimensions affected by multiple risk factors. Neurological integrity, tone and posture, behavior and signs of stress, and withdrawal were included to assess a variety of functional domains and to be useful for the range of high-risk infants.

Reliability and Validity

Training to reliability criteria, including separate criteria for the administration for scoring, was established for the Maternal Lifestyles study. A training video and manual were developed. Twelve examiners at four sites were initially trained to reliability and periodically rechecked during the 2-year period of data collection. Approximately 1,400 1-month-old infants were given the NNNS providing a database with a cross-section of infants that vary in birthweight, substance exposure, race/ethnicity, social class, and geographical location.

Test–retest reliability was established in two ongoing studies of preterm infants: one in the United States, the other in India, tested at 34, 40, and 44 weeks gestational age. In both studies the NNNS summary scores showed statistically significant correlations ranging from .30 to .44 across the three tests.

Validity of the NNNS was first documented in a study of full-term newborns (Napiorkowski et al., 1996). Infants with cocaine and alcohol exposure were compared with infants with alcohol exposure alone and those without prenatal drug exposure. Differences were found between the cocaine/alcohol and alcohol group as well as between these groups and the unexposed group showing the sensitivity of the NNNS to the effects of cocaine and alcohol. Preliminary analysis from the Maternal Lifestyles study used a multivariate analysis in which the effects of each drug (cocaine, opiates, marijuana, alcohol, and tobacco) and birthweight were tested (covaried) with the effects of all other covariates controlled. Specific independent effects of cocaine, opiates, alcohol, tobacco, and birthweight on the various NNNS summary scores were found (Lester, 1998), demonstrating the NNNS is sensitive to several classes of legal and illegal drugs in term infants and to the effects of prematurity with and without prenatal drug exposure. The sample size of 1,400, approximately half exposed and half comparison infants, is not a standardization sample in the traditional sense but is a large sample relative to those used to standardize most infant tests. The NNNS has also been used in a study of temperament in 150 preterm infants in India and is currently being used in a National Institutes of Health study of very-low-birthweight infants with and without neonatal white matter lesions in the brain.

DEVELOPMENTAL MODEL

Our developmental model of the neonate has certainly come a long way since Sherrington's initial "spinal frog" model and the early reflex models. However, although the NNNS embraces many of the constructs of the competent infant, we are equally impressed with the immaturity, poorly differentiated, and limited nature of the infant. The newborn can only do so much and much of what it can do is affected by the very conditions under study, level of prematurity, effects of pre- and perinatal conditions, and so on.

With the NNNS, we try to portray a comprehensive and integrated picture of the infant without weighting any specific functional domains. This holistic view assumes that an accurate assessment of the infant includes evaluation of classical reflexes, tone, posture, social and self-regulatory competencies, and signs of stress.

The high-risk infant is viewed as struggling to maintain a balance between competing demands. The preterm infant is trying to maintain physiological homeostasis in the face of external stimulation. Internal demands such as maintaining respiratory and metabolic control are competing with external demands—stimulation that increases respiratory and metabolic demands. The drug-exposed infant may be experiencing withdrawal or distur-bances in monoaminergic systems that can result in hyper- or hyporespon-sivity. The assessment of these infants is complex—a simple assessment of reflexes or tone will miss higher-order functioning, regulatory capacities, and coping strategies. Likewise, a focus on social interactive capacities will miss basic neurological function that may determine current and future behavior. In addition, how information is gathered is critical. With the NNNS, some behaviors are observed (e.g., state, posture, and signs of stress), others are elicited (reflexes, motor responses, social interaction) and interpreted in the context of the infant being challenged. Some responses re-quire "scaffolding"; that is, the examiner provides a certain amount of stage setting for the behavior to appear. How much scaffolding or stage setting is necessary to produce a behavior is as important as the actual behavior elic-ited. For example, an infant who is able to track a visual stimulus, who does not need to be swaddled, and who shows minimum respiratory instability and few signs of stress is clearly different than an infant with the same vi-sual tracking ability who requires substantial facilitation by the examiner and shows physiological and behavioral signs of stress.

The concept of state-dependent performance is an important principle of the NNNS. The NNNS requires that items be administered in specific states and that when they are elicited they are only administered a set num-ber of times. This state dependency and the inherent variability of behavior in early infancy require flexibility of administration. However, when an ex-amination is unstructured, a number of problems arise. The primary prob-lem is that different examiners may do the examination differently and elicit different behavioral qualities in the infant. Thus, the scoring may reflect the examiner–infant interaction rather than the infant's performance when faced with a standard challenge.

The NNNS attempts to balance flexibility and structure in several ways. First, state-dependent administration (SDA) is inherently structured and sensitive. Second, the NNNS has a relatively invariant sequence of item ad-ministration in that the specified sequence is one strongly preferred by expe-rienced examiners because most infants can achieve it. Thus individual dif-ferences in examiner style are minimized. The exam allows for modification, but the order of administration and deviations from the standard sequence are recorded.

SDA is facilitated by the use of "packages" of items which allow the ex-aminer to maximize the number of items administered when the infant is an appropriate state.

Finally, the NNNS contains codes for the reason an item was not admin-istered. These reasons include examiner error but more important the failure of the infant to be in an appropriate state. This information is useful for ex-plaining why the preferred order may have been varied. It also provides critical information on the performance of the infant.

SDA helps achieve several critical standardization goals. First, SDA ensures the comparability of how state affects performance. SDA emphasizes the state-dependent features of infant responsiveness. At the same time, it does not fall into the trap of having to do items in a rigid order at all costs. SDA increases the likelihood that the infant's performance is due to the characteristics of the infant per se, rather than the examiner's skills in trying to elicit optimal behavior. SDA facilitates the administration of the examination in the standard order. Finally, SDA also minimizes the time needed to administer the examination because handling procedures aimed at bringing out optimal performance are eliminated, especially the need for time-outs and soothing of the infant.

TRAINING REQUIREMENTS

Use of the NNNS requires certification, and certification procedures have been established that require meeting specified criteria in areas of administration and scoring. Training programs are available in the United States, Europe, South America, and Southeast Asia. There is also a Spanish version of the manual. In general, the recommended training process is for the trainee to practice the exam with intermittent feedback from either a trainer or an already trained examiner until such time as the trainee feels that he or she is ready for the certification test. Through telemedicine, videoconferencing is also being used from remote locations to provide introductory background and didactic material, to observe a "live" exam that includes interaction between the examiner and observers in the remote sites, and to give feedback to trainees as they examine infants in remote sites. The certification test can be arranged by contacting a trainer. Our experience is that the amount of practice that trainees need depends on prior experience and comfort in handling young infants and clinical acumen. A training kit is available that includes the necessary equipment (standard 8" flashlight, red ball, red rattle, bell, foot probe, head supports, manual, and scoring form). Introductory and debriefing scripts as well as scripts appropriate to specific items are provided in the manual. The senior author may be contacted for information on training.

IMPLICATIONS

Information from the NNNS can be used for research and clinical practice. Clinical applications include developing a profile of the infant to write a management plan for the infant while in hospital, evaluation of the infant close to discharge as part of the discharge plan, and transition to home that includes involving the caretakers in the exam. Postdischarge, the exam can be used determine which infants qualify for early-intervention services. The long-term goal is to provide standardized norms for the NNNS at selected gestational ages to be used for the evaluation of at-risk infants prior to and in the few months following hospital discharge. At Women and Infant's Hospital (Providence, Rhode Island) the NNNS is used for the evaluation and behavioral management of infants in the intensive care nursery and for drug-exposed infants.

It is a luxury to be able to choose from a variety of neonatal assessments, reflecting how far the field of neonatal assessment has progressed. The NNNS is appropriate for some uses and not appropriate for others. There are measures for specific purposes, such as the Neurobehavioral Assessment of the Preterm Infant (Korner & Constantinou, Chapter 19, this volume) for assessment of maturity and other procedures that measure aspects of neurological function. Although the NNNS includes these domains, if this were the only interest, there would be no reason to do a full NNNS exam. Similarly, for work with full-term healthy infants, the NBAS should be used, because many of the behaviors measured by the NNNS that would have to be scored will not occur; it would be "overkill." The NNNS is also not appropriate for highly detailed assessments of specific functions. Although the exam includes some classical reflexes, measures of tone and posture, preterm behavior, and stress abstinence, it does not provide the level of detail needed if the focus were only on one of these domains. For example, the exam includes items from the Finnegan scale (Finnegan, 1986) that are used to measure drug withdrawal but does not include all the items or specific cutoffs. Therefore, it would be inappropriate to use the NNNS the way the Finnegan is used to determine drug treatment for addicted infants. Similarly, the NNNS does not provide the detail about preterm behavior that the APIB (Als et al., 1982) provides. The NNNS is best suited for use with infants at risk, term or preterm, when the interest is in providing estimates of a broad range of neurobehavioral function.

REFERENCES

Als, H. (1994). Individualized developmental care for the very low birthweight preterm infant: Medical and neurofunctional effects. *Journal of the American Medical Association, 272,* 853.

Als, H. (1997). Neurobehavioral development of the preterm infant. In A. A. Fanaroff & R. J. Martin (Eds.), *Neonatal–perinatal medicine* (pp. 964–989). St. Louis: Mosby.

Als, H., Lester, B. M., Tronick, E. C., & Brazelton, T. B. (1982). Towards a research instrument for the assessment of preterm infants' behavior (A. P. I. B.). In H. E. Fitzgeral, B. M. Lester, & M. W. Yogman (Eds.), *Theory and research in behavioral pediatrics* (pp. 85–132). New York: Plenum Press.

Amiel-Tison, C. (1968). Neurological evaluation of the maturity of newborn infants. *Archives of Disease in Childhood, 43,* 89–93.

Andre-Thomas, C. Y. (1960). *The neurological examination of the infant: Little Club Clinics in developmental medicine.* London: National Spastics Society.

Brazelton, T. B. (1973). *Neonatal Behavioral Assessment Scale.* (50th ed.). Philadelphia & London: Spastics International Medical Publications; Lippincott.

Brazelton, T. B. (1984). *Neonatal Behavioral Assessment Scale.* Philadelphia: Lippinicott.

Brazelton, T. B., Koslowski, B., & Main, M. (1974). The origins of reciprocity: The early mother–infant interaction. In M. Lewis & M. Rosenblum (Eds.), *The effect of the infant on its caretaker: The origins of behavior* (pp. 49–76). New York: Wiley.

Condon, W., & Sander, L. (1974). Neonate movement is synchronized with adult speech: Interactional participation in language acquisition. *Science, 183,* 99–101.

Eimas, P. D. (1975). Speech perception in early infancy. In L. B. Cohen & P. Salapatek (Eds.), *Infant perception: from sensation to cognition.* New York: Academic.

Eimas, P. D., & Miller, J. L. (1980). Contextual effects in infant speech perception. *Science, 209,* 1140–1141.

Eimas, P. D., Siqueland, E. R., Jusczyk, P., & Vigorito, J. (1971). Speech perception in infants. *Science, 171,* 303–306.

Engen, T., Lipsitt, L. P., & Kaye, H. (1963). Olfactory responses and adaptation in the human neonate. *Journal of Comparative and Physiological Psychology, 56,* 73–77.

Fantz, R. L., Fagan, J. F., & Miranda, S. B. (1975). Early visual selectivity. In L. B. Cohen & P. Salapatek (Eds.), *Infant perception: from sensation to cognition* New York: Basic Visual Processes.

Finnegan, L. P. (1986). Neonatal abstinence syndrome: Assessment and pharmacotherapy. In F. F. Rubatelli & B. Granati (Eds.), *Neonatal therapy and update.* New York: Experta Medica.

Horowitz, F. D., & Linn, P. L. (1984). Use of the NBAS in research. In T. B. Brazelton (Ed.), *Neonatal Behavioral Assessment Scale* (pp. 97–104). Philadelphia: Spastics International Medical Publication.

Korner, A. F., & Thom, V. A. (1990). *Neurobehavioral Assessment of the Preterm Infant.* New York: Psychological Corporation.

Lashley, K. S. (1951). The problem of serial order in behavior. In L. A. Jeffrees (Ed.), *Cerebral mechanisms in behavior—the Hixon Symposium.* New York: Wiley.

Lester, B. M. (1984). Data Analysis and Prediction. In T. B. Brazelton (Ed.), *Neonatal Behavioral Assessment Scale* (pp. 85–96). Philadelphia: Lippincott, Spastics International Medical Publication, Clinics in Developmental Medicine.

Lester, B. M. (1998). The Maternal Lifestyles study. *Annals of the New York Academy of Science, 846,* 296–306.

Lester, B. M., Als, H., & Brazelton, T. B. (1982). Regional obstetric anesthesia and newborn behavior: A reanalysis toward synergistic effects. *Child Development, 53*(3), 687–692.

Malanga, C. J., & Kosofsky, B. E. (1999). Mechanisms of action of drugs of abuse on the developing fetal brain. In B. M. Lester (Ed.), *Clinics in perinatology* (pp. 17–38). Philadelphia: Saunders.

Napiorkowski, B., Lester, B. M., Freier, M. C., Brunner, S., Dietz, L., Nadra, A., & Oh, W. (1996). Effects of in utero substance exposure on infant neurobehavior. *Pediatrics, 98*(1), 71–75.

Papousek, H. (1967). Experimental studies of appetitional behavior in human newborns and infants. In H. W. Stevenson, E. H. Hess, & H. L. Rheingold (Eds.), *Early behavior* (pp. 24–47). New York: Wiley.

Peiper, A. (1928). *Die Hirntatigkeit des Sauglings.* Berlin: Springer.

Prechtl, H. F. R. (1974). The behavioral states of the newborn infant. *Brain Research, 76,* 185–212.

Prechtl, H. F. R. (1977). The neurological examination of the newborn infant (2nd ed.). In *Clinics in developmental medicine, No. 63* (pp. 1–63). London: Lavenham Press.

Prechtl, H., & Beintema, D. (1964). The neurological examination of the newborn infants. In *Clinics in developmental medicine, No. 29* (pp. 1–72). London: Lavenham Press.

Rosenblith, J. F. (1961). The modified Graham behavior test for neotates: Test–retest reliability, normative data and hypotheses for future work. *Biology of the Neonate, 3,* 174–192.

Saint-Anne Dargassies, S. (1977). *Neurological development in the full-term and premature neonate.* New York: Elsevier North Holland.

Sherrington, C. S. (1906). *The integrative action of the nervous system.* New Haven: Yale University Press.

Twitchell, T. E. (1965). The anatomy of the grasping response. *Neuropsychologia, 3,* 247–259.

Wasz-Hockert, O., Lind, J., Vuorenkoski, V., Partanen, T., & Valanne, E. (1968). The infant cry. In *Clinics in developmental medicine, No. 29* (pp. 1–42). London: Lavenham Press.

Wolff, P. H. (1966). The causes, controls and organization or behavior in the neonate. *Psychological Issues, 5*(1), 1–105.

19

The Neurobehavioral Assessment of the Preterm Infant

Reliability and Developmental and Clinical Validity

ANNELIESE F. KORNER
JANET C. CONSTANTINOU

HISTORY

We began a longitudinal intervention study in 1977 in which we asked whether or not gently oscillating waterbeds could enhance the neurobehavioral development of preterm infants as they grew to term. This question was prompted by our prior research with full-term infants and rat pups (Korner & Thoman, 1970, 1972; Gregg, Haffner, & Korner, 1976; Thoman & Korner, 1971) that suggested that vestibular–proprioceptive stimulation may be of fundamental importance for the intactness of early development. To answer our question, we started from the conceptual premise that the most relevant and important goal of any intervention would be to facilitate the normality of the infants' developmental course so that their maturity and ultimate development would not be too discrepant from that of full-term newborns within the normal range (Korner, 1987). Thus, to assess the effects of our intervention, our prime objective was to use an instrument that could measure the differential maturity of functioning of randomly assigned experimental and control groups of preterm infants.

In search for such an instrument, we reviewed the literature on well-established assessments that existed prior to 1977. Commonly used at the time were the Graham Behavior Test (Graham, Matarazzo, & Caldwell, 1956) and Rosenblith's (1961) modification of that test. Although well standardized, these assessments did not include preterm infants. We considered using the Prechtl Neurological Assessment (Prechtl & Beintema, 1964). Although it is a comprehensive examination that was standardized on a large sample of newborn infants, it is primarily a test of neonatal neurological intactness and not one of infant maturity. Again, this test was standardized on full-term infants only. We also considered using the Neonatal Behavioral Assessment Scale (NABS; Brazelton, 1973). But again, the NABS was not ideally suited for our purposes because it was standardized on full-term newborns. The supplemental scales applicable to preterm infants had as yet not been published in 1977 when we needed a suitable procedure for our longitudinal study.

The assessments that came closest to meeting our need to measure differences in the level of the neurobehavioral maturity in preterm infants were those by Saint-Anne Dargassies (1966) and by Amiel-Tison (1968). These French neonatal neurologists systematically assessed and documented the maturational course of neural functions of preterm infants from 28 weeks postconceptional age to term. As neurologists, these investigators were primarily interested in identifying early neurological deficits, but they did this, appropriately, in the context of gathering normative data on preterm infant functioning. They carefully illustrated the age differences in preterm functioning in 2-week increments. Unfortunately, this age differentiation of infant performance was not sufficiently fine-grained for the purposes of assessing the effects of our intervention.

Having reviewed the literature on the major assessments existing in 1977, we decided that we needed to develop our own procedure that could highlight more subtle differences in the maturity of preterm functioning.

FIRST VERSION OF THE NEUROBEHAVIORAL ASSESSMENT OF THE PRETERM INFANT

In developing a procedure that would measure the differential maturity of preterm infants who had been randomly assigned to experimental and control groups in a longitudinal intervention study, we relied most heavily on test items from the Amiel-Tison (1968) examination. Also included were a few items from the Prechtl and Beintema (1964) and the Brazelton (1973) assessments. Because the Amiel-Tison characterizes preterm infants' performance only in 2-week age intervals, and because it was unrealistic to expect that experimental and control groups would differ in the maturity of their functioning by 2 or more weeks, we developed a scoring system that potentially could reveal more subtle differences in performance.

Results from the preliminary version of the Neurobehavioral Assessment of the Preterm Infant (NAPI) revealed that this assessment was sufficiently sensitive to discriminate between the experimental and control groups (Korner, Schneider, & Forrest, 1983; Korner, 1999). Randomly assigned infants raised on gently oscillating waterbeds, examined by a neurologically trained pediatrician who was blinded to the infants' group status, demonstrated significantly more mature motor behavior, were significantly less irritable, were more than twice as often in the visually alert, inactive state and performed significantly better in attending and pursuing visual and auditory stimuli than the control group (Korner et al., 1983). The NAPI also had good test–retest reliability in a number of important functions, and interobserver reliability was adequate. These results prompted us to further develop the NAPI for general use.

To accomplish this task we decided to proceed with a *unique approach that had never been tried before in developing neonatal assessment procedures.* Most often, if the reliability and validity of a procedure were assessed at all, this was done after the development of the test was completed. This after-the-fact approach has frequently led to disappointing results. We chose instead to investigate the reliability and developmental validity of each item and clusters of items before we included them in the final version of the procedure.

PROCESS OF THE NAPI TEST DEVELOPMENT

Conceptual Framework

In revising the preliminary version of the NAPI, we limited our selection of test items to those that promised to show reliable developmental changes over time as suggested by prior studies (e.g., Amiel-Tison, 1968; Brandt, 1979). In line with our goal of developing a maturity assessment, we devised a numerical scoring system in which all item scores ranged from the least to the most mature responses. Also, we made it our first priority to include in the assessment only conceptually and clinically meaningful test items rather than a collection of maneuvers commonly used but whose developmental significance seemed unclear. In addition, we excluded commonly used aversive maneuvers such as the Moro and pinprick and any item that required instrumentation or elaborate equipment. This was done to make sure that the assessment could be used widely in different clinical settings. Once the item selection was completed, the items were grouped into conceptually and statistically cohesive clusters.

Statistical Approach

We next established *a priori* guidelines for all statistical analyses which subsequently were adhered to at all times. These were used to explore the psychometric properties of the procedure. Thus, before incorporating any items or clusters into the procedure, their test–retest reliability, their redundance and their developmental validity were assessed. Any of the test items or clusters failing to have a test–retest reliability of .60 on two consecutive days or were not showing significant developmental changes over several weeks were dropped from the procedure.

In the process of the test development of the NAPI, 179 preterm infants participated on whom 354 examinations were performed (Korner et al., 1987.

REPLICATION AND VALIDATION STUDY

For this study, an independent cohort of 290 preterm infants were recruited on whom 553 examinations were performed. For this sample, the test–retest reliability and the developmental validity were again assessed (Korner, Constantinou, Dimiceli, Brown, & Thom, 1991).

GENERAL DESCRIPTION

Following the methodological and statistical approach described previously, we managed to develop a psychometrically sound assessment procedure to measure the maturity of preterm infants.

SUBJECTS

To recruit as representative a sample of preterm infants as was feasible, infants were picked from both tertiary- and intermediate-care nurseries from four Bay Area hospitals and one nursery in Portland, Oregon. Also, to generate results that would be representative of preterm infants in general, exclusion criteria for the subjects in the two independent cohorts were kept to an absolute minimum. Excluded were infants whose gestational age estimates were discrepant from each other by more than 2 weeks. The four gestational age estimates used were the mother's and obstetrician's dates of confinement (expected date of delivery; EDC); the gestational age assessment by Ballard, Novak, and Driver (1979); the infant's head circumference (Usher & McLean, 1969); and, when available, an ultrasound examination. To further reduce potential errors in gestational age estimates, the most commonly available estimates (EDC and Ballard) of the eligible infants were averaged. The only other infants excluded were those who had diagnoses suggesting central nervous system damage, such as known Grade III and IV intraventricular hemorrhages, persistent seizures, disseminated herpes, or severe asphyxia at birth. Data for the two independent cohorts were collected between 1983 and 1989. Informed consent for the infants' inclusion in the studies was obtained from one or both parents.

THE EXAMINATION

The NAPI is applicable to medically stable infants from 32 weeks post-conceptional age to term, who are on room air and free of intravenous lines and gastric tubes. To obtain a reliable picture of the babies' performance, the examiner should delay testing infants after stressful medical procedures such as circumcision, blood transfusions, or eye examinations. Because both low and high temperatures can be harmful to infants and also adversely affect their performance, they should be examined in an appropriately heated incubator or under an overhead warmer. Scoring is done immediately after each item is presented, lest the examiner forget the exact details of the infants' responses.

Because preterm infants have a relatively small neurobehavioral repertoire, most of the test items in the assessment necessarily overlap with those used in other neurobehavioral examinations. The NAPI differs primarily in the developmental rationale underlying the choice of the test items, in the scoring system, and in the statistical approach to establishing the test's reliability and developmental validity. One of our most important decisions was to use a strictly invariant sequence of item presentation which was designed to bring about the kinds of behavioral states that are most likely to elicit the best possible responses from preterm infants. Although we were keenly aware of the fact that infants' states strongly influence their responses (Korner, 1972), we found empirically that with young preterm infants, the requirement of a predetermined state before administering each item was not feasible. An attempt to achieve the appropriate predetermined state through various rousing and soothing maneuvers would have greatly prolonged the examination, fatigued the infant, or failed altogether. For this reason, we chose to build into the assessment a standard sequence of rousing, soothing, and alerting items that would maximize the chance of testing the various functions in appropriate states and would minimize the need to intervene with some infants more than with others. To illustrate, we try to rouse the infants who, for the most part, are asleep when we begin the examination approximately 45 minutes before they are fed, by administering the scarf sign and the arm and leg recoil. Items such as the popliteal angle, ventral suspension, head lift, and spontaneous crawling can then be administered in more awake states. All infants are then swaddled to calm those who have become irritable. The rotation test is then administered in preparation for modified Brazelton (1973) orientation items, as we had found in earlier studies (Korner & Grobstein, 1966; Korner & Thoman, 1970) that the

TABLE 19.1. NAPI Test Items and the Sequence of Their Presentation

State rating—Remove cover and clothing

State rating—Scarf sign

State rating—Leg resistance and recoil

State rating—Forearm resistance and recoil

State rating—Popliteal angle

State rating—Ventral suspension
  Prone head raising
  Spontaneous crawling

State rating—Dress infant, observe power of active movements

State rating—Swaddle infant

State rating—Rotation test

Response to:
  Inanimate auditory Stimulation
  Inanimate auditory and visual stimulation
  Animate auditory stimulation
  Animate visual and auditory stimulation

State rating—Ratings of quality and duration of visual alertness

Place infant on examining table

State rating—Observe infant's movements for 1 minute

State rating

vestibular–proprioceptive stimulation entailed in moving the infants predictably produced visual alertness. This approach of a standard sequence of item presentation prevents the examination from becoming a different procedure for each infant and guarantees that the examination is comparable from one infant to the next. This strategy also provided the opportunity to systematically study the age changes in the infants' states in response to a standard sequence of identical events (Korner et al., 1988).

Table 19.1 shows the flow of the examination. After completing the examination, summary ratings are made regarding the quality and quantity of the infant's spontaneous movements, irritability and vigor of crying, and quality and duration of alertness during the entire assessment. Also rated is the degree of arousal with which the infant responded to the stimulation of the assessment. All test item scores are then converted to scores ranging from 0 to 100, with 0 representing the least and 100 representing the most mature responses. The process of numerically summing up the test results takes less than 10 minutes.

Our methodological and statistical approach resulted in a relatively brief and gentle instrument consisting of seven reliable and developmentally valid clusters or single-item neurobehavioral dimensions that represent a conceptually and clinically meaningful spectrum of preterm functions (Korner & Thom, 1990). These dimensions, which contain 27 subitems are:

1. Motor development and vigor
2. Scarf sign
3. Popliteal angle
4. Alertness and orientation
5. Irritability
6. Vigor of crying
7. Percent asleep ratings

The test–retest Spearman correlations of the seven neurobehavioral dimensions ranged from .6 to .85 with $p < .001$ for each variable. Testing longitudinally for the developmental validity of the assessment, it was found that the average performance on each of the seven dimensions improved significantly with age, with p values ranging from .01 to .0001 (see Korner et al., 1991). The scores of each variable increased with age except for the percent asleep ratings during the examination, which decreased.

In addition, and in consultation with Prof. Lee Cronbach, we were able to establish normative guidelines for preterm infants between 32 and 38 weeks postconceptional age. As we had hoped, the means and medians of the converted scores for each function showed week-to-week age changes in the expected direction. The normative guidelines also included standard deviations of infant performance in each of the seven neurobehavioral dimensions at each age. This information can then be used to identify consistent lags in performance over time. The normative data also permit developing a profile of the infant's performance at each age, reflecting special strengths and weaknesses of different functions and how these change over time.

Clearly, these normative guidelines must be used judiciously, particularly in clinical contexts. Preterm infants are a heterogeneous group whose performance is readily influenced by variability in state and health status. It is therefore important to use the normative guidelines primarily to identify infants who, on *repeated* examinations, show developmental lags, so that appropriate follow-up and remedial intervention can be instituted.

CLINICAL VALIDITY

Although we had established the test–retest reliability and the developmental validity of the NAPI, we did not as yet know whether this instrument was sufficiently sensitive to detect the impact of adverse perinatal and/or postnatal medical complications on infant performance. To find out, we developed the Neonatal Medical Index (NMI; Korner et al., 1994). Because severe illness usually weakens an organism, we hypothesized that test items requiring infant vigor and strength would be affected by prior medical complications, whereas other functions might be unaffected. Based on the data from 471 infants, the results of this study clearly supported this hypothesis.

Infants' scores in motor development and vigor, irritability, and vigor of crying were significantly reduced in infants with a history of severe illness. The results of this study thus clearly confirming the clinical validity of the NAPI.

The discriminatory power of the NMI was not only seen in this study but was confirmed in a predictive external validation study (Korner et al., 1993). In this study, we had the opportunity to use the preexisting data from the eight-site Infant Health and Development Program (1990). The data from this study indicated that the NMI predicted later Bayley cognitive and motor development, and that in infants born at less than 1,500 grams, the effects of neonatal medical complications persisted at least until the subjects were 3 years old.

Because we had used the NMI for our clinical validity study of the NAPI and for predicting later development in the Infant Health and Development Health Program (1990), other investigators have begun to use the NMI for different purposes. For example, Brown, Bakeman, Cole, Sexton, and Demi (1998) have used it to describe the characteristics of their study population. It also has been used as an outcome measure in an intervention study by Anand et al. (1999). Randomly assigned infants in the experimental group who had not differed in health status at birth from the control group showed significantly better NMIs at hospital discharge after being sedated during ventilatory care. A replication study by these authors is now in progress in 15 different sites.

DESCRIPTION OF THE NMI

In developing the NMI, we sought to produce a simple classification system that, at the time of hospital discharge, would summarize in bold strokes the medical course of preterm infants. The NMI was designed to measure how ill the infants were during their hospital stay rather than give a complete inventory of all the different complications and symptoms the infants had experienced. The few components of the NMI were selected because of their clinical salience and their ready availability on brief chart reviews.

NMI classifications range from I to V, with I describing preterm infants free of significant past medical problems and V characterizing infants with the most serious complications. NMI classification is based on two overarching principles:

1. Infants with birthweights more than 1,000 grams who experienced no major medical complications are assigned NMI classifications of I or II. Infants born at less than 1,000 grams or heavier babies who had experienced major medical complications, receive NMI classifications of III, IV, or V.

2. The need and duration of mechanically assisted ventilation required (ventilatory care or intubation on continuous positive airway pres-

sure [CPAP], or mask or nasal CPAP). The choice of the assisted ventilation classification principle was based on the rationale that, with a few exceptions, the duration of assisted ventilation would be dictated by the length and severity of illness and/or complications.

The following are the criteria for classifying the NMI:

I. Birthweight greater than 1,000 grams; free of respiratory distress and other major medical complications; no oxygen required; absence of apnea or bradycardia; allowable complications are benign heart murmur and need for phototherapy.

II. Birthweight more than 1,000 grams; assisted ventilation for 48 hours or less and/or oxygen required one or more days; no PVH-IVH; allowable complications are occasional apnea and/or bradycardia not requiring theophylline or related drugs; PDA not requiring medication such as indomethacin.

III. Assisted ventilation for 3–14 days and/or any conditions listed under III below.

IV. Assisted ventilation for 15–28 days and/or any conditions listed under IV below.

V. Assisted ventilation 29 days or more and/or any conditions listed under V below.

The following conditions require a classification of III, IV, or V, regardless of length of time on assisted ventilation.

III. Birthweight less than 1,000 grams; PVH-IVH grade I or II; apnea and/or bradycardia requiring theophylline; patent ductus requiring indomethacin; hyperbilirubinemia requiring exchange transfusion.

IV. Resuscitation needed for apnea or bradycardia while on theophylline; major surgery including PDA (exclude hernias, testicular torsion).

V. Meningitis confirmed or suspected; seizures; PVH-IVH grade III or IV; periventricular leukomalacia.

All the above criteria for NMI classifications apply to appropriate, small and large-for-gestational age infants. Figure 19.1 displays the algorithm with a set of instructions to compute the NMI.

BIOBEHAVIORAL BASIS OF THE ASSESSMENT

The NAPI clearly taps into the biological givens of preterm infants as these are expressed in behavioral terms. In addition, the infant's behavioral re-

Step 1.   NMI

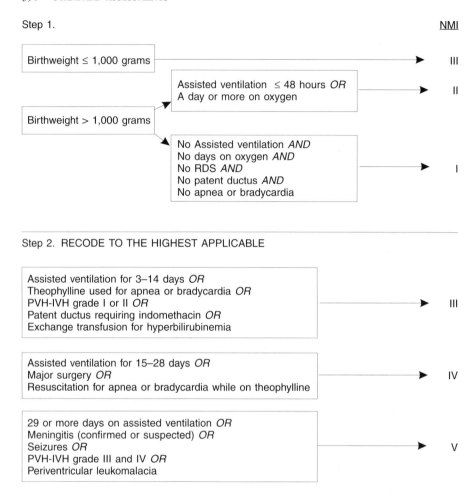

Step 2. RECODE TO THE HIGHEST APPLICABLE

FIGURE 19.1. Instructions for computing the Neonatal Medical Index (screen for criteria in the order listed below). From Korner et al. (1993). Copyright 1993 by Lippincott Williams & Wilkins. Reprinted by permission.

sponses are influenced by their gestational and birth histories, by maternal medical conditions such as toxemia, diabetes or other diseases, maternal drug intake like alcohol, nicotine, cocaine or other drugs, and by the infant's postnatal medical complications. So far, only two areas of influence have been systematically investigated: the effects of infant medical complications on NAPI performance (Korner et al., 1994) and the impact of maternal drug use on the infants' NAPI behavior (Espy, Riese, & Francis, 1995, 1997; Brown et al., 1998).

Another study that speaks directly to the biobehavioral basis of the

NAPI is one that originated from a long-standing interest of the senior author (Korner, 1996). Earlier studies by Korner (1964, 1971) attempted to investigate the biological antecedents of individual differences in temperament, defense mechanisms, and coping styles. These studies were based on the hypothesis that innate individual differences in central nervous system functioning involving sensory thresholds and the quality and strength of the regulatory mechanisms for dealing with stimulation will determine, to a large extent, characteristic individual differences in reaction patterns, which, in turn, would predispose to later temperament.

In her more recent study, Korner (1996) used the longitudinal data from the NAPI that was collected in weekly intervals over three or more assessments to study individual consistencies in responding to the stimulation provided by the examination. Nine rating scales were used to describe the degree to which an infant responded to the procedure with increased activity, tonicity, and crying and with availability to visual and auditory stimuli. Using a regression model that allowed each baby its own slope and intercept over the weeks of observation, it was found that preterm infants between 32 weeks postconceptional age and term already showed high self-consistency over time in their availability to sensory stimuli and their excitability, irritability, and activation. The correlations ranged between .48 and .78, with means of .65 and .63 for the two independent cohorts, respectively.

RELIABILITY AND VALIDITY

As described in the history of the procedure, the test–retest reliability and developmental validity were the cornerstones in developing the NAPI. Its clinical validity also was established. External validation of the NAPI norms at 36 weeks postconceptional age was reported by Dittrichová, Sobotková, Procházková, and Vondrácek (1996). The performance of Czech preterms was almost identical to that of our samples.

Brown et al. (1998) also externally validated our norms. No significant differences were found between the performance of Northern Californian and Oregon babies and black preterm infants in Atlanta, Georgia.

Concurrent Validity

Dittrichová et al. (1996) established concurrent validity between the NAPI and a neurological examination.

Predictive Validity

When we developed the NAPI, our only purpose was to test the differential maturity of preterm infants who had been randomly assigned to experimental and control groups in an intervention study. Although we hoped that the NAPI would identify infants at special risk for developmental delays, we did not expect to find any predictive validity. We held this view because the functions tested at early ages differ from those tested later. Also, we knew that the different socioeconomic and familial circumstances in which children are raised would have a strong impact on their development (e.g., Sameroff & Chandler, 1975; Sameroff, Seifer, Barochas, Zaks, & Greenspan, 1987). We were therefore surprised when a number of investigators using the NAPI discovered both short- and longer-term predictive validity.

Dittrichová et al. (1996) found that NAPI scores at 36 weeks conceptional age correlated significantly with Bayleys and a neurological examination at 3 months corrected age.

Constantinou, Fleisher, Korner, and Stevenson (1997) reported Spearman correlations between the NAPI and 2-year Bayleys ranging from .53 to .75. A longitudinal study with more than 100 infants is now in progress that will test whether or not the predictive validity of the NAPI found in the pilot study can be replicated. Also, Constantinou, Adamson-Macedo, Korner, and Fleisher (2000) predicted to the Bayley Infant Neurodevelopmental Screener from the NAPI administered at 36 weeks postconception.

Newham (1999), in her Australian longitudinal study, predicted cognitive and temperamental characteristics at 1 and 2 years of age from preterm NAPI performance.

Sampers and Caldwell (2000) did a study that identified early predictors of poor motor outcome in extremely premature infants.

Also, DiPietro and her colleagues (2001) are currently preparing an article that attempts to predict later temperament from fetal behavior and NAPI scores.

Our question remains, Why does the NAPI predict to later behavior as early age-specific functions are not necessarily related to those tested at a later time? The only way we could explain the fact that the NAPI did predict to early childhood behavior is that it taps into basic biological factors.

DEVELOPMENTAL MODEL

The underlying developmental model of the NAPI is simple and straightforward: We picked variables that we hypothesized would change with development and the scores of which would significantly increase or decrease with age. We decided *a priori* to drop any dimension that did not meet this criterion. Thus, when we tested the developmental validity of the seven dimensions that represent the core of the assessment, we found that it was highly significant in both independent cohorts.

STRUCTURAL AND/OR THEORETICAL
CONSTRAINTS/CONTROVERSIES

The most important constraint shared by all investigators of developmental processes is the common uncertainty of their subjects' gestational age at birth. Not infrequently, gestational age estimates vary by 3 or more weeks. In our studies we have tried to cope with this problem by excluding all infants whose gestational age estimates varied by more than 2 weeks. This solution resulted in a great loss of eligible subjects.

Another serious constraint also shared by anyone assessing the performance of neonates is that the result from one examination alone may not be fully representative of an infant's capabilities. It is highly desirable, therefore, to assess infants more than once, but this is not always feasible in clinical or research contexts.

Although the NAPI can highlight gross neurological deficits, it is not a neurological assessment. Any suspect evidence from the NAPI should, however, be used to refer an infant for a complete neurological workup.

Even though the NAPI was standardized on preterm infants, several investigators have begun to use it with full-term neonates. It is hoped that normative guidelines will eventually be established for these babies.

TRAINING REQUIREMENTS

Potentially, any professional caring for, or studying preterm infants in an intensive or intermediary-care nursery is eligible to become a NAPI examiner. The training consists of two major and equally important components: achieving reliability of administering the examination and achieving reliability of scoring. Prior experience in handling young preterm infants and knowing about the medical problems and physiological stress reactions commonly seen in preterms are essential.

The NAPI kit contains, among other things, a manual of instructions and a training videotape. To become a qualified examiner, it is essential to repeatedly view the training tape to learn exactly how the examination should be administered. It is especially important to learn the sequence and flow of the examination as well as the standard, slowly paced, gentle method of handling an infant, a method that differs in certain respects from that used in other assessments. Adherence to the standard examination technique is essential, not only to minimize infant stress but also to elicit infant responses within the range of those obtained during the standardization of the assessment. The training period includes practice of administering and scoring the examination of approximately 20 preterm infants of various postconceptional ages, with reviewing the training tape and rereading the manual between assessments as needed. To complete the training, the reliability of administration and scoring should be evaluated by a qualified teacher of the assessment.

More information about training can be obtained on Web site URL http://www-med.stanford.edu/school/pediatrics/NAPI.

IMPLICATIONS

Having established a reliable and a developmentally and clinically valid neonatal assessment procedure, this instrument can and has begun to be used to address a wide variety of research and clinical issues. The following are examples:

1. Assessing the effects of interventions, clinical trials, or changes in medical care (e.g., Korner et al., 1991; Ariagno et al., 1997; Anand et al., 1999).
2. Studying the development of small for gestational age (SGA) babies, and infants of diabetic mothers.
3. Assessing the behavioral differences between addicted babies and controls (e.g., Espy et al., 1995, 1997; Brown et al., 1998).
4. Identifying persistent lags in the development of specific infant functions.
5. Monitoring the developmental progress of individual infants.
6. Generating normative data that describe the gradual unfolding of the behavioral repertoire of preterm infants as they grow to term (e.g., Korner, Brown, Thom, & Constantinou, 2001; Korner & Thom, 1990).
7. Studying basic questions about the development of preterm infants (e.g., Korner et al., 1988).
8. Assessing the stability of individual differences in developmentally changing preterm infants (e.g., Korner et al., 1989).
9. Studying the antecedents of later temperament (e.g., Korner, 1996; Newham, 1999).
10. Showing the NAPI to parents to enhance their understanding of their infant's behavioral cues (e.g., Constantinou & Korner, 1993; Sobotková, Dittrichová, Procházková, & Vondrácek, 1996).
11. Using the NAPI as a therapeutic tool by demonstrating to concerned parents that their infant is making steady progress over weekly examinations.

ACKNOWLEDGMENTS

We thank Helena C. Kraemer whose creative statistical advice was vital to the development of the NAPI. Our research reported in this chapter was supported by Grant No. MH

36884 from the National Institute of Mental Health, Prevention Research Branch, Division of Clinical Research, and by Grant No. RR-81 from the General Clinical Research Center of the Division of Human Resources, National Institute of Health.

REFERENCES

Amiel-Tison, C. (1968). Neurological evaluation of the maturity of newborn infants. *Archives of Diseases of Childhood, 43*, 89–93.

Anand, K. J. S., McIntosh, N., Lagercrantz, H., Pelausa, E., Young, T. E., Vasa, R., & Barton, B. A. (1999, April 1). Analgesia and sedation in ventilated preterm neonates. *Archives of Pediatric and Adolescent Medicine.*

Ariagno, R. L., Thoman, E. B., Boediker, M. A., Krugener, B., Constaninou, J. C., Mirmiran, M., & Baldwin, R. B. (1997, December). Developmental care does not alter sleep and development. *Pediatrics, 100*(6), E91–E97.

Ballard, J. L., Novak, K. K., & Driver, M. (1979). A simplified score for assessment of fetal maturation of newly born infants. *Journal of Pediatrics, 95*(5), 769–774.

Brandt, I. (1979). Patterns of early neurological development. In F. Falkner & J. M. Tanner (Eds.), *Human growth—neurobiology and nutrition* (Vol. 3, pp. 243–304). New York: Plenum Press.

Brazelton, T. B. (1973). *Neonatal Behavioral Assessment Scale.* Philadelphia: Lippincott.

Brown, J. V., Bakeman, R., Cole, C. C., Sexton, R., & Demi, A. S. (1998). Maternal drug use during pregnancy: Are preterm and full-term infants affected differently? *Developmental Psychology, 34*(3), 540–554.

Constantinou, J. C., Adamson-Macedo, E. N., Korner, A. F., & Fleisher, B. E. (2000, July 17). *Prediction of the Neurobehavioral Assessment of the Preterm Infant to the Bayley Infant Neurodevelopmental Screener.* Paper presented at the International Conference of Infant Studies, Brighton, UK.

Constantinou, J. C., Fleisher, B. E., Korner, A. F., & Stevenson, D. K. (1997). Prediction from the Neurobehavioral Assessment of the Preterm Infant to the Bayley II at two years of age. *Journal of Investigative Medicine, 45*, 117A.

Constantinou, J., & Korner, A. F. (1993). Neurobehavioral Assessment of the Preterm Infant as an instrument to enhance parental awareness. *Children's Health Care, 22*(1), 39–46.

DiPietro, J., Costigan, K., Pressman, E., Ruderman, M., Yi, L., & Smith, B. (2001). *From fetus to child: Antenatal origins of individual differences.* Manuscript in preparation.

Dittrichová, J. D., Sobotková, D., Procházková, J., & Vondrácek, J. (1996, August 12–16). *Early development of preterm infants assessed by the NAPI (The Neurobehavioral Assessment of the Preterm Infant).* Paper presented at the 14th biannual SSBD Conference, Quebec City.

Espy, K. A., Riese, M. L., & Francis, D. J. (1995, March 30–April 2). *Neurobehavioral development in preterm infants prenatally exposed to cocaine.* Poster presented at the Society for Research in Child Development, Indianapolis, IN.

Espy, K. A., Riese, M. L., & Francis, D. J. (1997). Neurobehavior in Preterm neonates exposed to cocaine, alcohol and tobacco. *Infant Behavior and Development, 20*(3), 297–309.

Graham, F. K., Matarazzo, R. G., & Caldwell, B. M. (1956). Behavioral differences between normal and traumatized newborns: Standardization, reliability and validity. *Psychology Monograph, 7*(3).

Gregg, C. L., Haffner, M. E., & Korner, A. F. (1976). The relative efficacy of vestibular-proprioceptive stimulation and the upright position in enhancing visual pursuit in neonates. *Child Development, 47,* 309–314.

Infant Health and Development Program. (1990). Enhancing the outcomes of low-birthweight premature infants. *Journal of the American Medical Association, 263,* 3035–3042.

Korner, A. F. (1964). Some hypotheses regarding the significance of individual differences at birth for later development. *The Psychoanalytic Study of the Child, 19,* 58–72.

Korner, A. F. (1971, July). Individual differences at birth: Implications for early experience and later development. *American Journal of Orthopsychiatry, 41*(4), 608–619.

Korner, A. F. (1972). State as variable, as obstacle and as mediator of stimulation in infant research. *Merrill–Palmer Quarterly, 18*(2), 77–94.

Korner, A. F. (1987). Preventive intervention with high-risk newborns: Theoretical, conceptual and methodological perspectives. In J. D. Osofsky (Ed.), *Handbook of infant development* (2nd ed., pp. 1006–1036). New York: Wiley-Interscience.

Korner, A. F. (1996). Reliable individual differences in preterm infants' excitation management. *Child Development, 67,* 1703–1805.

Korner, A. F. (1999). Vestibular stimulation as a neurodevelopmental intervention with preterm infants: Findings and new methods for evaluating intervention effects. In E. Goldson (Ed.), *Nurturing the premature infant: Developmental interventions in the neonatal intensive care nursery* (pp. 111–130). New York: Oxford University Press.

Korner, A. F., Brown, Jr., B. W., Dimiceli, S., Forrest, T., Stevenson, D. K., Lane, N. M., Constantinou, J., & Thom, V. A. (1989). Stable individual differences in developmentally changing preterm infants. *Child Development, 60,* 501–513.

Korner, A. F., Brown, Jr., B. W., Reade, E. P., Stevenson, D. K., Fernback, S., & Thom, V. (1988). State behavior of preterm infants as a function of development, individual and sex differences. *Infant Behavioral Development, 11,* 111–124.

Korner, A. F., Brown, J. V., Thom, V. A., & Constantinou, J. (2001). *The neurobehavioral assessment of the preterm infant* (2nd ed.). Van Nuys, CA: Child Development Media.

Korner, A. F., Constantinou, J., Dimiceli, S., Brown, B. W., & Thom, V. A. (1991). Establishing the reliability and developmental validity of a neurobehavioral assessment for preterm infants: A methodological process. *Child Development, 62*(5), 1200–1208.

Korner, A. F., & Grobstein, R. (1966). Visual alertness as related to soothing in neonates: Implications for maternal stimulation and early deprivation. *Child Development, 37*(4), 867–876.

Korner, A. F., Kraemer, H. C., Reade, E. P., Forrest, T., Dimiceli, S., & Thom, V. A. (1987). A methodological approach to developing an assessment procedure for testing the neurobehavioral maturity of preterm infants. *Child Development, 58,* 1478–1487.

Korner, A. F., Schneider, P., & Forrest, T. (1983). Effects of vestibular–proprioceptive stimulation on the neurobehavioral development of preterm infants: A pilot study. *Neuropediatrics, 14*(3), 170–175.

Korner, A. F., Stevenson, D. K., Forrest, T., Constantinou, J., Dimiceli, S., & Brown, Jr., B. W. (1994). Preterm medical complications differentially affect neurobehavioral functions: Results from a new neonatal medical index. *Infant Behavior and Development, 17*(1), 37–43.

Korner, A. F., Stevenson, D. K., Kraemer, H. C., Spiker, D., Scott, D., Constantinou, J., & Dimiceli, S. (1993, April). Prediction of the development of low birth weight preterm infants by a new neonatal medical index. *Developmental and Behavioral Pediatrics, 14*(2), 106–111.

Korner, A. F., & Thom, V. A. (1990). *Neurobehavioral Assessment of the Preterm Infant.* New York: The Psychological Corporation.

Korner, A. F., & Thoman, E. B. (1970). Visual alertness in neonates as evoked by maternal care. *Journal of Experimental Child Psychology, 10,* 67–78.

Korner, A. F., & Thoman, E. B. (1972). Relative efficacy of contact and vestibular stimulation in soothing neonates. *Child Development, 43*(2), 443–453.

Newham, C. A. (1999). *The prediction of cognitive and temperamental characteristics from neonatal behaviour in preterm infants.* Doctoral dissertation, La Trobe University Bundoor, Victoria, Australia.

Prechtl, H. F. T., & Beintema, D. (1964). *The neurological examination of the full term newborn infant.* London: Heinemann Medical Books.

Rosenblith, J. F. (1961). The Modified Graham Behavior Test for Neonates: Test–retest reliability, normative data and hypotheses for future work. *Biologia Neonatorum, 3,* 174–182.

Saint-Anne Dargassies, S. (1966). Neurological maturation of the premature infant of 28 to 41 weeks gestational age. In F. Falkner (Ed.), *Human development* (pp. 306–325). Philadelphia & London: Saunders.

Samaroff, A., & Chandler, M. (1975). Reproductive risk and the continuum of care-taking casualty. In F. D. Horowitz (Ed.), *A review of child development research* (Vol. 4, pp. 187–244). Chicago: University of Chicago Press.

Samaroff, A. J., Seifer, R., Barochas, R., Zaks, M., & Greenspan, S. (1987). Intelligence quotient scores of 4–year-old children: Social-environmental risk factors *Pediatrics, 79,* 343–350.

Sampers, J., & Caldwell, R. (2000, July 17). *Early predictors of poor motor outcome in extremely premature infants.* Paper presented at the International Conference of Infant Studies, Brighton, UK.

Sobotková, D., Dittrichová, J., Procházková, E., & Vondrácek, J., (1996, August 12–16). *Neurobehavioral Assessment of the Preterm Infant (NAPI) as a technique of early intervention.* Paper presented at the 14th biannual SSBD Conference, Quebec City.

Thoman, E. B., & Korner, A. F. (1971). Effects of vestibular stimulation on the behavior and development of infant rats. *Developmental Psychobiology, 5,* 92–98.

Usher, R., & McLean, F. (1969). Intrauterine growth of live-born Caucasian infants at sea level: Standards obtained from measurements in 7 dimensions of infants born between 25 and 44 weeks of gestation. *Journal of Pediatrics, 74*(6), 900–910.

20

Determining Functional Integrity in Neonates

A Rapid Neurobehavioral Assessment Tool

JUDITH M. GARDNER
BERNARD Z. KARMEL
ROBERT L. FREEDLAND

HISTORY

Survival after an adverse pregnancy or complicated birth has become more common, primarily because of recent medical and technological advances. Significant changes in the nature of the surviving cohorts of infants necessitate adequate assessment of the consequences of these life-altering events on the structure and function of the infants' central nervous system (CNS) and its development. Not surprisingly, as techniques to enhance survival have emerged, there have been corresponding technological advances for diagnosing, monitoring, and intervening. Two significant noninvasive approaches have made it possible to evaluate the newborn infant's CNS status at the bedside. These are the application of neuroradiological techniques to cranial ultrasound (US) measurement to define CNS structural integrity and the application of neurometric analysis of brain electrical activity (John et al., 1977; Karmel, Kaye, & John, 1978) to auditory brainstem evoked responses (ABRs) to evaluate CNS functional integrity (Karmel, Gardner, Zappulla, Magnano, & Brown, 1988). Each provides concurrent criteria against which other information about neurofunction, such as from a neonatal neurobehavioral assessment, can be judged. This chapter concentrates on the neurobehavioral portion of this developmental assessment.

A variety of newborn neurobehavioral assessment procedures currently are available to evaluate the complex nature of early behavioral capabilities and/or their dysfunctions. Efforts have been successful in representing various behavioral functions, involving attention, motoric ability, physiological stability, and their integration, through standardized neurological and neurobehavioral assessment procedures or scales (see Lester & Tronick, Chapter 18; Korner & Constantinou, Chapter 19, this volume). Most of the procedures grew out of an appreciation for the large repertoire of behaviors of the newborn infant. The newborn was realized to be an interactive participant with caregivers and the environment, not just a passive recipient of stimulation or a set of reflexes waiting to mature. The infant's state and arousal modulation as well as other internal characteristics were recognized as important regulators of behavior. The goal of many of these assessments was to understand how all these factors influenced the behaviors involved in normal development, first in healthy term neonates and later in healthy preterm neonates.

In the neonatal intensive care unit (NICU), we needed an efficient clinically useful tool to enable differential decisions about neurobehavioral abnormality associated with known structural and functional injury to the CNS in sick infants who were easily overstressed. Behavioral functions were emphasized that frequently are disrupted by injury to the CNS, such as sensory information processing, motor organization, attention, and arousal. Thus, a procedure was developed with a minimum number of tasks that evaluated behaviors that were likely to differentiate the at-risk population, thereby achieving two goals: accurate assessment of different typology and severity of CNS injury and less stress to the sick infant.

GENERAL DESCRIPTION

Our neurobehavioral assessment is appropriate for use with small, sick infants (who may become overtaxed and cyanotic easily even when they reach term age), can be completed in less than 10 minutes, and was developed to assess those neurofunctional behaviors evident during the neonatal period that differentiate infants at high-risk for brain injury (e.g., as a result of asphyxia, prematurity, and/or prenatal drug exposure). It is appropriate for use between 34 and 48 weeks postconceptional age, and is used most frequently at the time of hospital discharge. It differs from other assessments with respect to the rationale for item selection, presentation methodology, emphasis on including active motor behaviors, and scoring, in addition to its approach to data analysis and emphasis on differential prediction. Tasks cover a range of behaviors but stress attention and active motor systems, as these are the areas consistently shown to have higher probabilities for acute and chronic dysfunction in infants at risk for CNS injury (Allen & Capute, 1989; Dubowitz & Dubowitz, 1981; Graziani et al., 1985; Katona, 1983, 1988; Stewart et al., 1988; Wallace, Rose, McCarton, Kurtzberg, & Vaughan, 1995). The neurobehavioral assessment is a modification of two procedures: (1) the Einstein Neonatal Neurobehavioral Assessment Scale (ENNAS), which consists of passive and active muscle tone items as well as visual and auditory orienting items (Kurtzberg et al., 1979); and (2) the assessment of elicited movement patterns described by Katona (1983, 1988), which has not been incorporated into standardized newborn assessments in the United States. Items selected and modified from the ENNAS have been shown to differentiate preterm from full-term neonates at term age. Items selected from Katona (1983) assess more active motor skills that challenge the infant in order to give additional information about head and trunk control as well as about the amount and quality of extremity movements.

Sensory and motor systems are evaluated using visual and auditory stimuli and both active and passive motor behaviors. Spontaneous behavior or simple reflexes currently are not relied on in the evaluation. Behavioral items were selected based on the types of abnormalities found in the population on which orthogonal sources of information could be established using a minimal number of tasks in a reasonable amount of time. Individual tasks or items are important only to the extent that they enhance judgments of abnormalities by trained observers on categories of behaviors that can cross items. The procedure conforms to a Gutman-like psychophysical decision-making algorithm, and accurate measurement does not require performing every task and every item to make a decision. The infant's performance on the items allows a trained observer to rate categories of behavior as normal or abnormal as described later (see also Gardner, Karmel, Magnano, Norton, & Brown, 1990, Table 1, p. 566), with performance on any one item only relevant to its contribution to category judgments.

Attention

Visual attention is considered abnormal if the infant is unable to fixate differentially an optimal visual pattern (a checkerboard or a bull's-eye) when paired with a blank stimulus (see Figure 20.1a), or is judged to have no (or only transient) tracking of a pattern across midline, as opposed to intermittent good tracking or smooth pursuit. Auditory attention is considered abnormal if the infant is judged unable to consistently turn his or her head from midline to stimuli (a rattle and a voice) presented on the right and left.

Sensory Symmetry

Sensory symmetry is judged abnormal (even if normal in attention) if an infant consistently orients better to one direction than to the other (e.g., tracks

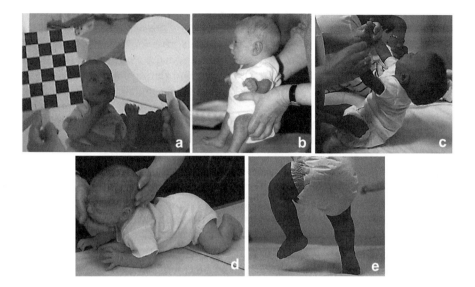

FIGURE 20.1. Selected neurobehavioral assessment items. 1a: Visual fixation; 1b: Sitting in air; 1c: Pull to sit; 1d: Creeping; 1e: Stepping.

the visual pattern with smooth pursuit to the right but tends to lose the pattern to the left, or only turns to sounds when presented on the right but not the left).

Head and Neck Control

Head extension is judged when prone on a horizontal surface, when prone facing upward on an incline, and while sitting in air (verticalization while support given to thighs and hips; see Figure 20.1b). Head flexion (lag) is judged during pull to sit (see Figure 20.1c). Opisthotonia is judged during pull to sit, sitting in air, and when prone facing upward on an incline.

Extremity Movements and Tone

For upper extremities, items judged include arm recoil, grasp, and traction as well as the amount and quality of movement during assisted creeping and crawling while on a horizontal surface and on an incline (see Figure 20.1d). For lower extremities, items judged include popliteal angle and the amount and quality of movement during assisted creeping and crawling, while prone facing downward on an incline, and during stepping (see Figure 20.1e). Generalized hypo- or hypertonicity is judged by an overall impression derived from all these items as well as the head control items.

Motor Symmetry—Lateral and Upper/Lower

All items used to judge extremity movements and tone also are used for judging lateral (left vs. right) and upper/lower (arms vs. legs) motor asymmetry. For example, an infant whose tone or amount or quality of movement is consistently better on one side than the other is judged abnormal in lateral motor symmetry. Similarly, an infant who shows consistent differences in the strength or quality of movement between the arms and legs is judged abnormal in upper/lower motor symmetry.

State Control, Jitteriness, Feeding

The current neurobehavioral assessment contains modifications to the published (Gardner et al., 1990) procedure and includes three additional behavioral categories: state control (alertness, peak excitement), jitteriness, and feeding. Decisions as to alertness and peak excitability are consistent with the modifications made by Dubowitz and Dubowitz (1981) of the Brazelton Neonatal Behavioral Assessment Scale items (Brazelton, 1984). Jitteriness is consistent with neurologists' observations and reflects occurrence of spontaneous or elicited fine or gross tremors. Feeding behavior provides more robust information than related behaviors such as nonnutritive sucking, as more neurological integrity is required to suck and swallow during feeding and its adequacy can be judged directly (e.g., speed and efficiency of swallowing, strength of suck, and/or length of time to feed).

Optional Tasks

In the modified procedure, certain individual items now are considered optional as they provide additional information only in specific situations in which behavior may be questionable in a few infants. These include head turning to a bell, ventral suspension, rotation, and tonic neck reflex.

Consistent with Brazelton (1984), Katona (1988), and Kurtzberg et al. (1979), the sequence of item administration is suggested but not invariant and takes into account the infant's behavior and state. Assessments typically are performed between feedings, but discretion is permitted to ensure alertness and responsivity that varies both within and between infants as a function of environmental conditions characteristic of NICUs and internal conditions inherent to sick or recovering infants. On the rare instances (< 1–2%) when an infant has questionable performance even after modification of the sequence, every attempt is made to retest the infant on those items in question. Because the goal of the assessment is the judgment about the individual infant's areas of functioning, it is more important to obtain an accurate representation of the behavioral repertoire than to compare infants on their ability to cope with or complete the sequence of tasks or to perform any one task. For more complete details on the procedure and findings including items, behavioral categories, population and groupings, and data analyses, see Gardner et al. (1990).

Similarities to and Differences from Other Procedures

When CNS injury occurs, its effects can be both global and local. Our neurobehavioral procedure attempts to discriminate those behaviors that go awry, in contrast to those that remain unaffected. The goal was to include enough diversity in the item repertoire to make accurate decisions with little redundancy and the use of optimal visual, auditory, and vestibular stimulation. High-contrast patterns (e.g., black-and-white checkerboard and bull's-eye patterns of optimal spatial density) are better stimuli for eliciting visual behavior than a red wool ball. With respect to motor behavior, active rather than passive tasks that rely more on self-production and performance and less on maturity or tone are emphasized. Active motor tasks focus on nonreflex-type responses similar to those seen at later ages in subsequent motor organization (see Amiel-Tison & Grenier, 1986; Katona, 1983, 1988). For example, the infant is placed head down on an incline so that crawling-like responses due to vestibular stimulation while righting to gravity can be observed. Such self-produced motor responses can be elicited in neonates through active feedback mechanisms from appropriate sensory input when the infant is in what Amiel-Tison refers to as a "liberated" state. Active motor responses challenge the infant and can be elicited and assessed even if the infant is hyperreflexive or hypertonic.

BIOBEHAVIORAL BASIS OF ASSESSMENT

Both normal and deviant development can be studied from a variety of perspectives with the assumption that subsequent neurofunctional integrity will emerge as a higher-order integration of CNS structure and function with self-produced feedback and environmental experience. The problem of understanding the neurobehavioral consequences of early CNS insult was approached prospectively. We first differentiated the types of brain injuries suffered by risk infants during the perinatal period (to which infants exposed to cocaine *in utero* were added on the basis of its presumed neurotoxicity and effects on development) and then we determined the neurobehavioral correlates to this differentiation. Rather than limit the sample to specific types of pathology or infants (such as intraventricular hemorrhage or preterms), the procedure was designed to evaluate as many neurofunctionally at-risk infants as possible. Cranial US was relied on to identify structural pathology (Levene, Wigglesworth, & Dubowitz, 1981; Papile, Burstein, Burstein, & Koffler, 1978; Rumack & Johnson, 1984; Volpe, 2001),

TABLE 20.1. Neurofunctional Risk Categories

	Normal newborn nursery[a]
Low risk	Too healthy for more than routine clinical evaluation
Environmental risk	Prenatal drug exposure; inadequate prenatal care

	Neonatal intensive care unit
NICU-normal	Normal US, normal ABR
ABR-only	Normal US, abnormal ABR
Slight	GMH alone or with tiny cysts, IVH alone (Papile Grade I–II); prominent choroids; tiny choroid cysts; questionable abnormality
Mild/moderate	IVH (Papile Grade II–III) alone or with cysts; ventriculomegaly ≤ 5 mm
Strong/LM	IVH (Papile Grade III); ventriculomegaly ≤ 10 mm; PV or parenchymal LM, hyperechoic echogenicity, or multiple cysts > 3 mm; subarachnoid hemorrhage; cerebral edema > 48 hours with IVH or LM
Severe	IVH (Papile Grade IV); hydrocephalus > 10 mm; hemorrhage or dilatation of IIIrd or IVth ventricle; large or multiple porencephalic sites, parenchymal hemorrhage or infarct; seizures requiring treatment

Note. NICU, neonatal intensive care unit; ABR, auditory brainstem evoked response; US, cranial ultrasonography; GMH, germinal matrix hemorrhage; IVH, intraventricular hemorrhage; LM, leukomalacia; PV, periventricular.

[a]We estimate no more than 5–7% of infants from this group would be false negatives, that is, might have an abnormal ABR or US. Infants in this group are assigned an additional neurofunctional category if an abnormal ABR or US is obtained.

and the ABR was used to identify functional pathology[1] (Fawer, Dubowitz, Levene, & Dubowitz, 1983; Karmel et al., 1988; Leech & Alvord, 1977; Majnemer, Rosenblatt, & Riley, 1988; Starr, Amlie, Martin, & Sanders, 1977). More complete descriptions of these techniques can be found in Gardner et al. (1990) and Karmel et al. (1988). From these procedures, an ordinal categorical classification for neurofunctional risk (see Table 20.1) was constructed based on the worst-case US and ABR findings that, along with drug exposure, can be reordered to test hypotheses or to establish concurrent validity.

The neonatal neurobehavioral assessment initially was designed to separate infants with different severity and typology of CNS pathology by their patterns of deficits across behavioral categories. As shown later, the assessment also is useful for understanding the process of recovery. By yielding a behavioral profile of the individual infant's strengths and weaknesses on the various categories and their changes with age, it allows for comparisons among different types of infants as well as formulating intervention strategies for targeting a particular area of functioning. The assessment does not reference a normally distributed cumulative scale score, because normality is assumed true for all items in the healthy term infant. Deviation from the low-risk population in this case would not conform to normal distribution assumptions.

In addition, even though some infants are at greater risk for a wide range of developmental problems, not all high-risk infants develop similar problems and, indeed, many such infants develop normally. Thus, although attempts to relate CNS injury to specific outcome measures over the first few years of life have been made, the relationship between CNS injury during the neonatal period and subsequent behavioral consequences still is not clearly determined. If US, ABR, and neurobehavioral assessment are each predictive of outcome and only partially correlated with each other, a combination of information from these and other sources would enhance overall prediction.

One benefit of the current neurobehavioral procedure is that it remains open to further refinement of the tasks and categories, as infant cohorts shift and other areas of functioning may become important for describing and predicting behavior.[2] Another is that the behavioral categories are intuitively easy to comprehend, observe, and demonstrate to parents, thereby facilitating communication and prescription of specific interventions if needed.

RELIABILITY AND VALIDITY

Interobserver Reliability

A description of the original NICU sample (n = 248), neurobehavioral category decisions and reliability measures, and multivariate and logistic regression analyses contrasting at-risk groups can be found in Gardner et al. (1990). In the initial validating sample, interobserver reliability of the categories' forced choice ratings was high, with the average agreement across decisions = 94% and the average Cohen's kappa = .81 when judged on a subset of 32 infants. Training to a reliability criterion can be accomplished by individuals at varying levels of education but is facilitated by experience with handling infants, especially neonates.

Construct Validity, Convergent Validity, and Internal Consistency

The neurobehavioral procedure possesses construct validity in that the items are likely to reflect the same dimensions along which CNS pathology has been distinguished in other procedures, although no other tests of neurofunction to date have been validated against our procedures. High internal consistency has been maintained, and the categories provide relatively nonredundant information as indicated by low correlation coefficients. However, some categories correlate on neurological grounds (such as jitteriness with hypertonic arms; r = .43), and subcategories tend to be related to each other (as long as they are not mutually exclusive, such as having both hypo- and hypertonicity of the arms). Thus, scores on individual test items and subcategories are correlated within behavioral categories (e.g., extremity movements), while correlations among categories are low. In addition, the neurobehavioral procedure has high convergent validity as it correlates with other dimensions of CNS measurement, namely ABRs and US; and, as ABRs and US normalize, so does neurobehavior, although in a somewhat lagged fashion. Furthermore, factors such as postconceptional age at test do not correlate with any of the behavioral categories on the examination given during the newborn period. This effect is consistent with the underlying tenet that abnormality is not defined as a lag in normal growth but reflects an atypicality in development not seen unless CNS damage has occurred.

Because the procedure is criterion-referenced, all normal infants are expected to have perfect scores for all categories, as are all infants who initially have CNS problems that normalize some time during the neonatal period. From a decision–theory perspective, all abnormalities observed would be considered true positives and rate-of-change measures would be viewed as recovery of function rather than unexplained drift. Such measures might yield significant information about individual infants not previously suspect by typical clinical criteria. They might reflect average development in a particular cohort, but not necessarily normal development in the strictest criterion-referenced sense.

The procedure, however, could become norm referenced by establishing the probability of finding abnormality in various categories in some normative group. In this case, theoretically, the degree to which the reference group deviated from the normative group's probability score on individual or combined categories could reflect adverse factors. Alternatively, the probability of errors or abnormalities that were identified could be considered random measurement error and could be used to define a current "basal" standard for a "normative" sample. Several "normal" groups' data are provided (see Tables 20.3 and 20.4) that show estimates in our population as to the probabilities for observed abnormalities in various categories.

Concurrent Validity

Initial Estimate

Concurrent validity is estimated by the ability of the neurobehavioral assessment to differentiate normal from CNS-injured infants and was established using stepwise linear regression. An efficient set of six categories of behavior (visual attention, sensory symmetry, lateral motor symmetry, arms/legs motor symmetry, head/neck control, and hypertonic legs), each contributing independent variance, predicted CNS injury. Although there was a general increase in abnormality with estimates of increasing brain insult across groups, especially in behaviors involving the extremities (e.g., motor asymmetries), the increase was not necessarily linear and did not hold across all categories (e.g., head control and sensory asymmetries). To identify profiles of abnormalities that existed among groups, the choice probabilities of occurrence of abnormal findings for these six predictor categories were entered into logistic regression analysis for categorical data (SYSTAT: LOGIT module). The pattern of abnormalities across categories significantly differentiated the CNS injury groups from the normal group, chi-square ($df = 30$) = 111.70, $p < .001$. For example, infants with abnormal ABRs but normal US (the ABR-only group) showed inadequate visual attention and weak head control but not motor problems whereas infants with leukomalacia (the Strong group) showed visual asymmetry and hypertonic legs.

Intrauterine cocaine exposure presumably is neurotoxic to specific regions in the developing CNS, especially those involving dopaminergic systems. Concurrent validity was demonstrated in contrasting neurobehavioral performance of healthy term cocaine-exposed infants to those who were not exposed. Cocaine-exposed infants are differentiated by jitteriness and hypertonicity in both upper and lower extremities, as well as by state control (peak excitability, alertness) and attention problems (see Table 20.3). Healthy term neonates not exposed to cocaine but with inadequate prenatal care showed jitteriness and hypertonicity, and some increased head lag, but not attention problems. In addition, an additive effect of cocaine exposure and inadequate prenatal care was found on hypertonicity and possibly jitteriness.

Singer, Arendt, Minnes, Farkas, and Salvator (2000) independently assessed cohorts of noncocaine-exposed ($n = 161$), heavily exposed ($n = 82$) and lightly exposed ($n = 76$) infants at 43 weeks corrected ages using our neurobehavioral assessment. Concurrent validity of the assessment was further demonstrated in its differentiation of heavily exposed from lightly and nonexposed infants, with more heavily exposed infants showing more attentional abnormalities, sensory asymmetry, movement and tone abnormalities, and jitteriness. Both maternal self-report measures of drug use and quantification of drug metabolites in meconium also positively related to an increase in abnormalities on various neurobehavioral subcategories.

Replication

Concurrent validity was replicated in our population with an independent sample of NICU infants ($n = 901$). In addition, different cohorts of healthy term infants were tested ($n = 317$; at newborn or 1 month) divided by whether they had prenatal care or were exposed to cocaine *in utero*. Table 20.2 shows the demographic data for the replicate population whereas Table 20.3 shows the proportion of NICU and healthy term infants in the different

TABLE 20.2. Demographic Data by Groups

| | Term nursery | | | | Neonatal intensive care unit[a] | | | | | |
| | No cocaine exposure | | Cocaine exposure | | NICU normal | ABR-only | Slight | Mild/ moderate | Strong | Severe |
	PC	No PC	PC	No PC						
Total ($n = 1,218$)	$n = 131$	$n = 62$	$n = 37$	$n = 87$	$n = 403$	$n = 202$	$n = 96$	$n = 90$	$n = 56$	$n = 54$
BW (g)	3,220	3,196	3,084	2,857	2,575	2,207	1,880	1,570	1,359	2,385
EGA (wk)	39.2	39.0	39.3	38.9	36.7	34.5	33.2	31.1	29.6	35.0
RIUG (z-score)	0.15	0.15	−0.21	−0.69	−0.35	−0.28	−0.51	−0.40	−0.26	−0.11
HC (cm)	33.9	33.6	33.8	32.8	32.2	30.7	29.8	28.4	27.1	31.3
Length (cm)	49.9	49.5	49.4	47.9	46.4	44.1	42.5	39.9	38.8	43.7
Apgar (1 min)	8.7	8.5	8.6	8.7	7.4	6.9	6.7	6.1	5.9	5.1
Apgar (5 min)	9.0	8.9	9.0	9.0	8.4	8.2	8.0	7.5	7.3	6.6
PCA-NB (wk)	40.6	39.7	40.4	39.7	38.6	38.3	38.0	38.4	39.1	40.3
PCA-1 MO (wk)	45.3	45.1	45.3	45.2	44.7	45.0	44.7	45.2	44.7	45.6

Note. NICU, neonatal intensive care unit; ABR, auditory brainstem evoked response; PC, prenatal care; BW, birthweight; EGA, estimated gestational age; RIUG, normalized weight for gestational age; PCA-NB, postconceptional age at newborn test age; PCA-1MO, postconceptional age at 1-month test age.

[a]No cocaine-exposed infants included in this NICU sample.

408

TABLE 20.3. Proportion of Infants with Abnormalities in Neurobehavioral Performance at Newborn Test Age

| | Term nursery | | | | Neonatal intensive care unit[a] | | | | | |
| | No cocaine exposure | | Cocaine exposure | | | | | | | |
	PC	No PC	PC	No PC	NICU normal	ABR-only	Slight	Mild/ moderate	Strong	Severe
Total (n = 1,172)	n = 100	n = 56	n = 33	n = 82	n = 403	n = 202	n = 96	n = 90	n = 56	n = 54
Attention										
Visual	.03	.04	.09	.13	.09	.22	.20	.28	.18	.28
Auditory	.00	.00	.00	.00	.01	.02	.02	.02	.00	.06
Sensory asymmetry	.07	.09	.06	.09	.08	.19	.10	.17	.27	.28
Lateral motor asymmetry	.02	.02	.03	.01	.04	.06	.04	.11	.14	.13
Head/neck control										
Flexion	.15	.25	.03	.22	.27	.37	.39	.39	.46	.69
Extension	.14	.09	.06	.10	.25	.36	.44	.33	.43	.46
Movement/tone										
Hypotonia—arms	.09	.02	.06	.01	.17	.20	.18	.24	.23	.44
Hypotonia—legs	.00	.00	.00	.00	.01	.01	.01	.01	.02	.07
Hypertonia—arms	.24	.50	.45	.61	.11	.12	.15	.21	.20	.24
Hypertonia—legs	.22	.36	.36	.46	.17	.27	.29	.39	.57	.35
Difference	.37	.50	.55	.56	.38	.52	.51	.66	.57	.67
State										
Alertness	.00	.00	.00	.06	.01	.03	.04	.00	.07	.06
Peak excitement	.01	.00	.09	.07	.01	.02	.08	.07	.07	.11
Feeding behavior	.04	.02	.00	.06	.08	.09	.08	.08	.09	.19
Jitteriness	.08	.31	.40	.39	.06	.10	.10	.16	.09	.17

Note. NICU, neonatal intensive care unit; ABR, auditory brainstem evoked response; PC, prenatal care.

[a]No cocaine-exposed infants included in this NICU sample.

risk groups with abnormalities in behavioral categories and subcategories. Analyses selecting only noncocaine-exposed infants from the NICU indicated similar results, but with nine categories efficiently predicting brain injury and a multiple $R = .40$ accounting for 16% of the variance, $F(9, 891) = 18.49$, $p < .001$. Replication of the pattern of abnormalities across different behavioral categories for the various brain injury groups also was quite good. For example, infants with leukomalacia initially were characterized by sensory asymmetries but not visual attention problems and hypertonicity in the lower extremities. In the replicate sample, these infants showed similar problems along with head control problems.

Relation to Other Predictor Variables

When demographic variables (i.e., birthweight, gestational age, head circumference, length, 5-minute Apgar scores) are added to the neurobehavioral categories to predict brain insult, the amount of variance accounted for after adjustment increased from 16% to 40%. Moreover, preliminary multistage discriminant analysis selecting the significant predictors of brain injury from a fuller battery of procedures and birth-related variables used during the newborn period produced a regression equation accounting for 51% of the adjusted variance, $R(150) = .72$.

Comparisons of concurrent validity by grouping infants by maturity at birth, namely, by birthweight or gestational age, accounted for 10–11% of the variance with only two or three motor items achieving significance. Because the variables reflecting maturity at birth are correlated with CNS injury ($r = .44$), some relationship to neurobehavioral performance should exist. This finding not only reinforces the construct validity of the procedure with respect to CNS injury but also provides evidence of its greater discriminant validity when compared to neurobehavioral procedures based mainly on maturity and status at birth.

DEVELOPMENTAL MODEL

Atypical changes can occur in the CNS when any event or series of events causes biochemical, structural, or functional alterations. However, understanding of subsequent developmental disabilities remains one of the most perplexing problems facing developmental study. Although many infants appear to resolve from CNS damage with little or no intervention, others with apparently similar etiologies do not. Using a developmental neurofunctional assessment as a generalized approach to evaluation of brain–behavior relations assumes that behavioral organization represents the interaction of biological and environmental processes within a dynamically changing CNS that is multidetermined and nonlinear. Behavioral information obtained from performance on the neonatal neurobehavioral assessment is used as a converging source of information with nonbehavioral information obtained from US and ABR measures. These three sources of information about neurofunctional organization (US, ABR, and neurobehavior) during the neonatal period are essential for predicting recovery by providing an in-depth, early differentiation of the at-risk population against which current function as well as subsequent development can be judged. Such differentiation is presumed useful by providing contrasts for tracking developmental sequelae of CNS pathology and neurotoxicity, designing specific intervention strategies, and understanding normal brain–behavior relationships (see also Gardner, Karmel, & Dowd, 1984; Karmel et al., 1978; Karmel & Maisel, 1975).

How early behavior forms the basis for later functioning is an important issue with respect to how one behavior transforms over time to higher-level functioning or forms the basis for subsequent complex functioning. An assumption is that developmental projection should have its origins in early information about CNS pathology, if later performance is related to initial neurofunctional organization. Information from multiple domains should be used that can clearly be shown to reflect pathology in order to increase the precision by which early CNS injury could be detailed as long as these domains are not totally redundant (Karmel et al., 1978). Too strong an emphasis on prediction, however, may mask understanding the neonate's current status and be a detriment to immediate behavioral and medical remediation.

Another issue in attempting to predict outcome is determining the effect of the CNS involvement versus the effect of normal maturational processes. Although perturbances to the CNS can result from a variety of causes, normal maturation after early injury can produce improvement independently, even though such normalization is less likely the greater the injury. In addition, there are difficulties in predicting the time course of improvement using only standardized measures of later performance such as the Bayley Scales of Infant Development (BSID; Bayley, 1969, 1993) because differential brain growth and reorganization are not linear over time. Different brain regions mature at different rates and show differing plasticity with respect to environmental experience. Therefore, relations to outcome measures designed to detect more global competence such as the BSID may not be the best test of the validity of the neurobehavioral procedure (however, see predictive findings described later).

THEORETICAL POTENTIAL FOR PREDICTIVE VALIDITY OF NEUROBEHAVIORAL PROCEDURES

Despite being interested in studying the relationship between severity of damage to different brain regions and emerging behavioral organization, a one-to-one relationship is not posited between different levels of organization. Infants with abnormal behavior may have no identifiable CNS pathology and infants with normal behavior may be masking severe pathology. Nonetheless, different brain regions and their interconnecting pathways do form substrates and provide underlying mechanisms for different behaviors. Therefore, it is logical to presume that damage to particular regions may be likely to disrupt some behaviors more than others, even when such factors as immaturity, medical complications, and CNS plasticity are taken into account. On the other hand, if regional specificity has not been completely established, specificity about neurobehavioral abnormality during the neonatal period may not persist with the same regional specificity as identified in older children and adults. Because of greater plasticity, other regions may assume functions for a damaged area, or new pathways and connections may be laid down circumventing the damage.

There also are timing issues in that injury at an early level of organization would directly affect systems already organized but may not have a direct effect on emergent function depending on the degree of organizational interaction with the modified CNS. With continued development, further reintegration into higher levels of CNS order would be expected but may depend on whether the injury occurred before myelination, neural cell proliferation or pruning (i.e., apoptosis), or the encoding of experience cortically.

REEVALUATING NEUROBEHAVIORAL PERFORMANCE AT 1-MONTH POSTTERM AGE: TEST–RETEST RELIABILITY OR DEVELOPMENTAL CHANGE

Infants were reevaluated at 1-month postterm age (44 weeks postconceptional age). The infant's behavioral repertoire is assumed to remain similar during the neonatal period between 36 and 44 weeks postconceptional age. While the categories of behavior judged retain their validity, there is no reason to believe that the infant's behavior remains static during this period. In fact, even in healthy term infants any abnormality seen at birth, such as head lag, should certainly resolve by 1 month. For risk infants, as a recovery function from an initial injury is assumed, less abnormality in behavioral repertoire would be predicted the further in time from the initial injury. For infants with more severe CNS involvement, not only the initial injury but the nature and timing of resolution, if any, may be of utmost importance for predicting outcome.

Analyses of the neurobehavioral data at 1 month using stepwise linear regression indicated similar areas of abnormalities persisting in the CNS injury groups as at newborn, but with lowered incidence and less significant correlations to criterion groups. Most motor and attention problems appeared to resolve, especially in infants with less severe problems, and the

NICU normal infants were now almost identical to the term nursery normal infants. The exceptions were a tendency toward increased hypertonicity in the arms but not the legs with any CNS injury and increased incidence of visual asymmetry with slight, mild/moderate, and severe CNS involvement. Table 20.4 shows the proportion of infants in the various groups with abnormalities at 1-month postterm age.

The current data also indicate that the findings of jitteriness and hypertonicity peculiar to cocaine exposure persist from the neonatal period at least to 1 month, while visual attention problems appear to bifurcate, either resolving or becoming more apparent as visual asymmetry. In contrast, behaviors associated with no prenatal care are not as robust at 1 month, indicating the possibility that inadequate prenatal care, as a source of intrauterine stress, has a more transient effect in contrast to more long-lasting effects on the developing nervous system due to neurotransmitter system changes, most likely dopaminergic, from prenatal cocaine exposure. This intrauterine stress hypothesis is supported by increased transient abnormalities in other stress *in utero* conditions such as intrauterine growth retardation, postdates, and tobacco exposure, which also show resolution by 1 month of age. Infants who are intrauterine growth retarded, who are postdates, or who have been exposed to chronic maternal hypertension or placental insufficiency all appear to share similar characteristics, such as extremity hypertonicity, as long as they have not been asphyxiated or suffered apparent structural CNS injury. Thus, there are early neurobehavioral abnormalities due to stress factors *in utero* that may not be differentiated by type of stress and may have a common underlying etiology. Stress factors should be differentiated from neurotoxic effects and from CNS injury effects that take longer to resolve.

Determining persistence of abnormality, in what ways for which behaviors in which infants, then becomes a major concern. In comparing infants' behavior across examinations to reflect injury and extent of recovery, one approach is to sum the number of abnormalities at each age for the different groups and to evaluate the degree of recovery between exams. Figure 20.2 plots the average scores across groups for the two ages. Another approach may be to assume that abnormalities displayed later in development should carry more weight than earlier ones because they might reflect poorer or slower recovery. Conceptualizing and depicting this rate of recovery function must consider the interaction between the nature of recovery and variations in typology of injury and age of onset. For example, creating a weighted-sum score that doubles the value of an abnormality detected at the second exam can yield a composite score across behavioral categories that increases exponentially as abnormality persists.

However, the real-time delay between exams is not considered, which can itself reflect differential effects. The ages and times of testing cannot always be controlled in a clinical population. For example, sick term infants

TABLE 20.4. Proportion of Infants with Abnormalities in Neurobehavioral Performance at 1-Month Test Age

| | Term nursery | | | | Neonatal intensive care unit[a] | | | | | |
| | No cocaine exposure | | Cocaine exposure | | | | | | | |
	PC	No PC	PC	No PC	NICU normal	ABR-only	Slight	Mild/ moderate	Strong	Severe
Total ($n = 754$)	$n = 110$	$n = 33$	$n = 31$	$n = 44$	$n = 222$	$n = 119$	$n = 67$	$n = 63$	$n = 31$	$n = 40$
Attention										
Visual	.05	.03	.00	.07	.03	.07	.04	.08	.06	.13
Auditory	.00	.00	.00	.00	.00	.02	.00	.02	.03	.05
Sensory asymmetry	.11	.09	.10	.09	.08	.14	.19	.30	.10	.35
Lateral motor asymmetry	.04	.03	.06	.16	.03	.02	.09	.13	.19	.18
Head/neck control										
Flexion	.20	.12	.10	.20	.14	.18	.22	.16	.32	.40
Extension	.07	.03	.10	.07	.10	.12	.09	.14	.13	.25
Movement/tone										
Hypotonia—arms	.15	.06	.06	.14	.13	.17	.09	.14	.19	.30
Hypotonia—legs	.00	.00	.06	.00	.01	.00	.00	.00	.00	.02
Hypertonia—arms	.16	.30	.26	.39	.15	.24	.25	.29	.26	.35
Hypertonia—legs	.05	.24	.17	.32	.14	.17	.27	.37	.45	.33
Difference	.38	.45	.35	.59	.38	.52	.43	.59	.65	.65
State										
Alertness	.02	.00	.00	.00	.02	.03	.00	.03	.03	.05
Peak excitement	.01	.00	.00	.00	.01	.03	.00	.02	.00	.02
Feeding behavior	.03	.00	.00	.00	.00	.00	.01	.02	.07	.10
Jitteriness	.02	.06	.18	.25	.04	.08	.03	.09	.07	.11

Note. NICU, neonatal intensive care unit; ABR, auditory brainstem evoked response; PC, prenatal care.

[a] No cocaine-exposed infants included in this NICU sample.

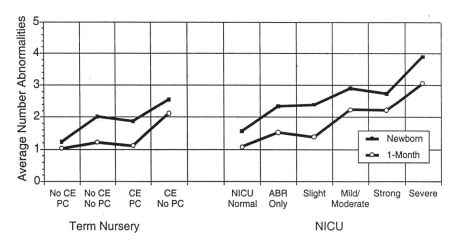

FIGURE 20.2. Average number of abnormalities summed across behavioral categories for risk groups at newborn and 1-month test ages. CE, cocaine-exposed; PC, prenatal care; NICU, neonatal intensive care unit; ABR, auditory brainstem evoked response.

may be tested for the first time a few weeks after birth whereas healthy preterm infants may have longer delays between tests because they typically are ready for discharge, and therefore testing, earlier at about 35–37 weeks postconceptional age. Although the delay as well the postconceptional age at each test can be regressed into the prediction, when dealing with large populations the amount of variance accounted for by these variables tends to be swamped by the data from the majority of infants with average delays and ages at test and therefore they drop out of any analyses. How to handle these types of data, especially over time, poses an interesting statistical problem. Thus, especially difficult to handle both statistically and theoretically is the rate of resolution of the different categories of behavior by the different groups across age. Considering the issue of any transitions of one type of behavioral abnormality to another, the problem of appropriate and accurate analysis of the data becomes even more intriguing.

LONG-TERM PREDICTION OF NEUROBEHAVIORAL PERFORMANCE TO LATER STANDARDIZED ASSESSMENTS

Despite these problems, a generalized linear model was used to determine the degree of association of early neurobehavioral performance to later outcome using a composite score generated from the neurobehavioral exam. As the infant displays more and more neurobehavioral abnormality, a lowered level of performance on standardized scores was shown between this value and development for BSID Mental Development Index (and less so for Psychomotor Development Index) scores when evaluated every 3 months between 4 and 25 months (range of r = .22 to .39) (see also Karmel, Gardner, & Freedland, 1998). These effects were true even when the BSID is recalibrated for our population to eliminate the age trends inherent to both the original (BSID-I) and subsequent (BSID-II) standardization samples. Also, significant relations to the Griffiths Mental Development Scale DQ (Griffiths, 1984) at 34 months were found (range of r = .18 to .20) (see also Gardner, Karmel, Freedland, & Geva, 1998).

Of interest, significant predictions of the neurobehavioral categories with BSID performance were best after 1 year of age, with the most consistent and heavily weighted predictor being visual attention. Attention may be more related to cognitive function after a year than motor skills, which might be more relevant earlier when the infant with CNS involvement is still in a state of recovery. This finding is consistent with that of Wallace et al. (1995) showing relations between cognitive outcome through 6 years and newborn neurobehavioral performance, with visual orienting being the best overall predictor at all ages. The finding that visual functioning is a more robust variable both within the newborn period and as a predictor is consistent with studies showing the importance of visual attention during the newborn period and throughout the early years (Fagan & Singer, 1983; Gardner, Feldman, Karmel, & Freedland, 2000; Gardner & Karmel, 1983; Gardner, Karmel, & Magnano, 1992; Geva, Gardner, & Karmel, 1997, 1999; Karmel & Gardner, 1996; Karmel, Gardner, & Freedland, 1996; Karmel, Gardner, & Magnano, 1991; Lawson & Ruff, Chapter 14, this volume; Rose, 1983; Rose, Feldman, Wallace, & McCarton, 1989; Rose & Orlian, Chapter 13, this volume; Rose & Wallace, 1985; Sigman, Cohen, Beckwith, & Parmelee, 1986; Singer et al., 2000).

STRUCTURAL AND/OR THEORETICAL
CONSTRAINTS/CONTROVERSIES

We have focused our work on the evaluation of neonates at risk for nonoptimal development. In conducting any evaluation of neonates, it is important to tease apart as many of the confounding conditions as possible in any particular population. Only then can similarities and differences among infants and changes over time be determined. This is especially true for cohort effects, for example, resulting from changing societal conditions that may increase intrauterine cocaine exposure or from changing medical practices that may increase survival of infants weighing less than 500 grams.

Only by using appropriate tests and theory that evaluate multiple areas will an understanding of the behavioral functions of the new cohorts of infants emerge. In this regard, as the age and conditions for survivability are lowered to younger and sicker infants, the problems that emerge will reflect the earlier level of CNS organization brought under stress by the abrupt or disruptive changes in environment, as well as by underlying conditions that precipitated the delivery. The issue of when CNS damage is manifest as well as which tissue or systems are involved or subsequently become involved because of interactions with development will remain a major defining problem for neurobehavioral assessment as cohorts and practices change.

A potential weakness in our neurobehavioral exam is the restricted range of scoring within a behavioral category.[3] Although there is strength in using a yes–no dichotomy for classifying infants, some of the breadth of behavior may not be evidenced. Thus, despite the criterion cutoffs for abnormality coming from previous research, the consequence of such a system for statistical analyses may be to group the infant with, for example, more mild degrees of head lag with the infant with more severe head lag. Another potential weakness is the underrepresentation of behavioral categories that could be deviant because the behavioral repertoire evaluated may not be exhaustive. Finally, some subtleties within normal functioning may be missed by concentrating on those behavioral categories that are differentially predictive of CNS injury.

TRAINING REQUIREMENTS

Most professionals in health-related disciplines can learn the neurobehavioral procedures rapidly, especially if familiar with neonates. Currently, training is accomplished through individual instruction and workshops. The procedure checklist and basic decision-making table are in the public domain and available free of charge. The tasks employed to reach clinical categorical decisions have been used to study infants by numerous other investigators in various health-related disciplines, including psychologists, physicians, nurses, speech pathologists, and physical and occupational therapists. Learning to perform each task and the basic interpretation for decision making requires specific experience and aptitude in handling neonates. It should be emphasized, however, that performance on any task is not as important as performance across tasks that yields information about a particular category of behavior. If an investigator finds some task especially difficult to interpret and can obtain the information from a different task, then the other task should be performed. Moreover, a hierarchical approach should be taken such that if the infant appears normal in one area (e.g., attention) but questionable in another (e.g., lower extremity tone and movement), concentration should be on further items to delineate the nature of the questionable area rather than wasting time and effort and the infant's staying power on an area found normal. Despite this flexibility in approach, reliability is fairly easy to obtain with practice, probably due to the fact that access to neonates and interpretation of the information tends to be restricted to professionals in health-related disciplines who already have training and skill with neonates. Finally, the best training situation for learning and building confidence about both handling the infant and making decisions is a hands-on tutorial rather than an off-site workshop or viewing of videotapes. Although videotapes can provide basic descriptions of the tasks as well as present a variety of types of responses, it is more difficult to judge many items without actually handling the infant.

IMPLICATIONS: WHAT RESEARCH STUDIES NEED TO BE DONE?

Several areas of research remain. Are there additional behaviors that would prove interesting for concurrent or subsequent prediction such as arousal-modulated attention, response to novelty, or reaction to amodal (multimodal) information? Can current decision making regarding the forced-choice (normal/abnormal) criterion benefit by an extended range of scores psychophysically? How does a neurobehavioral procedure avoid cohort effects in establishing prediction? What are the effects of sustained very early intervention on subsequent short- and long-term outcomes? What are the effects of repeated testing? Does repeated testing encourage facilitation of learning? Does the parent after observing testing then perform similar tasks at home, thereby introducing an informal intervention situation?

Additional types of behavioral evaluations can supplement the neurobehavioral exam if the information derived can be demonstrated to reflect finer resolution of abnormality or to reflect some form of abnormality related to revised or new definitions of CNS injury, neurotoxicity, or adverse medical conditions. For example, studies are being conducted to determine the degree to which arousal-modulated attention behavior fits this criterion so that it could be included in a neonatal assessment battery (Gardner & Karmel, 1983, 1995; Gardner et al., 1992; Karmel & Gardner, 1996; Karmel et al., 1996; Karmel et al., 1991). Thus, tasks requiring more time and effort such as arousal-modulated attention, response to novelty (Geva et al., 1999), and auditory habituation (Zelazo, Weiss, & Tarquino, 1991), require greater refinement prior to incorporation into a categorical neurobehavioral procedure.

Finally, additional validating studies could prove useful, as a method to verify the effect on neurobehavioral performance of particular conditions such as bronchopulmonary dysplasia, abnormal ABR studies, or exposure to prenatal stress conditions, specific or hypothesized neurotoxins, or unavoidable medications. What sensory-specific information might provide useful prediction or understanding that is not currently tested? How do these data relate to other neurometrics such as involving slower potentials reflected in visual (Karmel & Maisel, 1975) or auditory (Molfese & Molfese, Chapter 16, this volume) cortical evoked potentials or heart rate variability measures to assess vagal stability (Porter, Chapter 6, this volume)? Indeed, these questions could be addressed more efficiently and meaningfully if reliable and valid neurobehavioral procedures are used to assess the neurofunctional integrity of all infants during the neonatal period, regardless of their risk status.

ACKNOWLEDGMENTS

This research was supported in part by funds from the New York State Office of Mental Retardation and Developmental Disabilities, by National Institute of Child Health and Human Development Grant No. R01-HD-21784 awarded to Judith M. Gardner, and by National Institute on Drug Abuse Grant No. R01-DA-06644 awarded to Bernard Z. Karmel and No. K21-DA-00236 awarded to Robert L. Freedland. We wish to express our sincere gratitude and appreciation to the medical and nursery staffs of the Neonatal Intensive Care Unit and Newborn Nursery of St. Vincents Catholic Medical Centers of New York, St. Vincent's, Staten Island, New York, under Dr. A. Harin for their cooperation.

NOTES

1. ABRs depict the temporal flow of auditory information from the initial response of the sensory periphery through the first four to seven synaptic junctions of that sensory source in the brainstem in terms of transmission speeds. The functional integrity of afferent neuronal transmission can be evaluated either by determining deviation from the expected normal developmental trajectory or by estimating the likely group membership based on the multivariate discriminant score reflecting the fit of the pattern of observed component latencies to normal or abnormal criterion groups, thereby providing information about early abnormal functioning.
2. We (Lennon, Gardner, Karmel, Freedland, & Phan, 2000) recently expanded our neurobehavioral evaluation to include spontaneous motor behavior using the methodology of the qualitative assessment of general movements developed by Prechtl and colleagues (Einspieler, Prechtl, Ferrari, Cioni, & Bos, 1997).
3. Despite its strengths, expansion of our two-choice decision-making algorithm to incorporate transitional or uncertain categories in behavior is clearly possible and is being studied at present. For instance, expanded decisions of "definitely abnormal," "questionably abnormal," "questionably normal," or "definitely normal," a four-choice categorical-type ordering are being assessed with the ability to collapse to a 3-point scale inherent. Alternatively, other techniques might be used, such as magnitude estimation on the part of the examiner, so that an estimate of the "quantities" of abnormality could be decided along some examiner-referenced scale. This procedure might enhance decision making and control for specific examiner effects while still relying on detecting manifestations of CNS abnormality as its basic core.

REFERENCES

Allen, M., & Capute, A. (1989). Neonatal neurodevelopmental examination as a predictor of neuromotor outcome in premature infants. *Pediatrics, 83*, 498–506.

Amiel-Tison, C., & Grenier, A. (1986). *Neurological assessment during the first year of life*. New York: Oxford University Press.

Bayley, N. (1969). *The Bayley Scales of Infant Development: Birth to two years*. New York: Psychological Corporation.

Bayley, N. (1993). *The Bayley Scales of Infant Development* (2nd ed.). San Antonio, TX: Psychological Corporation.

Brazelton, T. B. (1984). *Neonatal Behavioral Assessment Scale*. London: Heineman; Philadelphia: Lippincott.

Dubowitz, L. M. S., & Dubowitz, V. (1981). *The neurological assessment of the preterm and fullterm newborn infants*. London: Heineman; Philadelphia: Lippincott.

Einspieler, C., Prechtl, H. F. R., Ferrari, F., Cioni, G., & Bos, A. F. (1997). The qualitative assessment of general movements in preterm, term and young infants: Review of the methodology. *Early Human Development, 50*, 47–60.

Fagan, J. F., & Singer, L. T. (1983). Infant recognition memory as a measure of intelligence. In L. P. Lippsitt (Ed.), *Advances in infancy research* (Vol. 2, pp. 31–78). Norwood, NJ: Ablex.

Fawer, C., Dubowitz, L. M. S., Levene, M. I., & Dubowitz, V. (1983). Auditory brainstem responses in neurologically abnormal infants. *Neuropediatrics, 14*, 88–92.

Gardner, J. M., Feldman, I. J., Karmel, B. Z., & Freedland, R. L. (2000, September). *Development of focused attention from 10 to 16 months: Effects of CNS pathology due to brain injury and intrauterine cocaine exposure*. Brain Development and Cognition in Human Infants: Euroconference on Normal and Abnormal Cortical Functional Specialization. La Londe les Maures, France.

Gardner, J. M., & Karmel, B. Z. (1983). Attention and arousal in preterm and full-term neonates. In T. Field & A. Sostek (Eds.), *Infants born at risk: Behavior and development* (pp. 69–98). New York: Grune & Stratton.

Gardner, J. M., & Karmel, B. Z. (1995). Development of arousal/attention preference interactions in early infancy. *Developmental Psychology, 31*, 473–482.

Gardner, J. M., Karmel, B. Z., & Dowd, J. M. (1984). Relationship of infant psychobiological development to infant intervention programs. *Journal of Children in Contemporary Society, 17*, 93–108.

Gardner, J. M., Karmel, B. Z., & Magnano, C. L. (1992). Arousal/visual preference interactions in high-risk neonates. *Developmental Psychology, 28*, 821–830.

Gardner, J. M., Karmel, B. Z., Magnano, C. L., Norton, K. I., & Brown, E. G. (1990). Neurobehavioral indicators of early brain insult. *Developmental Psychology, 26*, 563–575.

Gardner, J. M., Karmel, B. Z., Freedland, R. L., & Geva, R. (1998). Neonatal neurobehavioral assessment and its relation to developmental outcome in infants with CNS injury. In M. V. Perat (Ed.), *Eighth International Child Neurology Congress: New developments in child neurology* (pp. 83–87). Bologna, Italy: Monduzzi Editore.

Geva, R., Gardner, J. M., & Karmel, B. Z. (1997, September). Neuropsychological sequelae of neonatal compromise. In M. Kalmar & J. M. Gardner (Chairs), *Differential outcome in developmentally at-risk infants*. Symposium conducted at the meeting of the VIIIth European Conference on Developmental Psychology, Rennes, France.

Geva, R., Gardner, J. M., & Karmel, B. Z. (1999). Feeding-based arousal effects on visual recognition memory in early infancy. *Developmental Psychology, 35,* 640–650.

Graziani, L., Pasto, M., Stanley, C., Steben, J., Desai, H., Desai, S., Foy, P., Branca, P., & Goldberg, B. (1985). Cranial ultrasound and clinical studies in preterm infants. *Journal of Pediatrics, 106,* 269–276.

Griffiths, R. (1984). *The Abilities of Young Children. A comprehensive system of mental measurement for the first eight years of life.* Oxon, UK: Test Agency.

John, E. R., Karmel, B. Z., Corning W. C., Easton, P., Brown, D., Ahn, H., John, M., Harmony, T., Prichep, L., Toro, A., Gerson, I., Bartlett, F., Thatcher, R., Kaye, H., Valdes, P., & Schwartz, E. (1977). Neurometrics: Numerical taxonomy identifies different profiles of brain functions within groups of behaviorally similar people. *Science, 196,* 1393–1410.

Karmel, B. Z. & Gardner, J. M. (1996). Prenatal cocaine exposure effects on arousal modulated attention during the neonatal period. *Developmental Psychobiology, 29,* 463–480.

Karmel, B. Z., Gardner, J. M., & Freedland, R. L. (1996). Arousal-modulated attention at 4–months as a function of intrauterine cocaine exposure and CNS injury. *Journal of Pediatric Psychology, 21,* 821–832.

Karmel, B. Z., Gardner, J. M., & Freedland, R. L. (1998). Neonatal neurobehavioral assessment and Bayley I & II scores of CNS-injured and cocaine-exposed infants. In J. A. Harvey & B. E. Kosofsky (Eds.), Cocaine: Effects on the developing brain. *Annals of the New York Academy of Sciences, 846,* 391–395.

Karmel, B. Z., Gardner, J. M., & Magnano, C. L. (1991). Attention and arousal in early infancy. In M. J. Weiss & P. R. Zelazo (Eds.), *Newborn attention: Biological constraints and the influence of experience* (pp. 339–376). Norwood, NJ: Ablex.

Karmel, B. Z., Gardner, J. M., Zappulla, R. A., Magnano, C. L., & Brown, E. G. (1988). Brainstem auditory evoked responses as indicators of early brain insult. *Electroencephalography and Clinical Neurophysiology, 71,* 429–442.

Karmel, B. Z., Kaye, H., & John, E. R. (1978). Developmental neurometrics. In W. A. Collins (Ed.), *Minnesota Symposium in Child Development* (Vol. 11, pp. 141–198). Hillsdale, NJ: Erlbaum.

Karmel, B. Z., & Maisel, E. B. (1975). A neuronal activity model for infant visual attention. In L. Cohen & P. Salapatek (Eds.), *Infant perception: From sensation to cognition* (Vol. 1, pp. 77–131). New York: Academic Press.

Katona, F. (1983). An orienting diagnostic system in neonatal and infantile neurology. *Acta Paediatrica Hungarica, 24,* 299–314.

Katona, F. (1988). Developmental clinical neurology and neurorehabilitation in the secondary prevention of pre- and perinatal injuries of the brain. In P. M. Vietze & H. G. Vaughan, Jr. (Eds.), *Early identification of infants with developmental disabilities* (pp. 121–144) Philadelphia: Saunders.

Kurtzberg, D., Vaughan, H., Daum, C., Grellong, B., Albin, S., & Rotkin, L. (1979). Neurobehavioral performance of low birthweight infants at 40 weeks conceptional age: Comparison with normal full term infants. *Developmental Medicine and Child Neurology, 21,* 590–607.

Leech, R. W., & Alvord, E. C. (1977). Anoxic–ischemic encephalopathy in the human neonatal period. *Archives of Neurology, 34,* 109–113.

Lennon, E. M., Gardner, J. M., Karmel, B. Z., Freedland, R. L., & Phan, H. T. T. (2000, July). *Evaluation of spontaneous and elicited motor performance in high-risk infants from birth to 4 months.* Twelfth Biennial International Conference on Infant Studies, Brighton, UK.

Levene, M. I., Wigglesworth, J. S., & Dubowitz, V. (1981). Cerebral structure and intraventricular hemorrhage in the neonate: A real-time ultrasound study. *Archives of Disabilities in Childhood, 56,* 416–424.

Majnemer, A., Rosenblatt, B., & Riley, P. (1988). Prognostic significance of the auditory brainstem evoked response in high-risk neonates. *Developmental Medicine and Child Neurology, 30,* 43–52.

Papile, L. A., Burstein, J., Burstein, R., & Koffler, H. (1978). Incidence and evaluation of subependymal and intraventricular hemorrhage. A study of infants with birth weights less than 1500 g. *Journal of Pediatrics, 92,* 529–534.

Rose, S. A. (1983). Differential rates of visual information processing in fullterm and preterm infants. *Child Development, 54,* 1189–1198.

Rose, S. A., Feldman, J. F., Wallace, I. F., & McCarton, C. (1989). Infant visual attention: Relation to birth status and developmental outcome during the first 5 years. *Developmental Psychology, 25,* 560–576.

Rose, S. A., & Wallace, I. F. (1985). Visual recognition memory: A predictor of later cognitive functioning in preterms. *Child Development, 56,* 843–852.

Rumack, C. M., & Johnson M. L. (1984). *Perinatal and infant brain imaging.* Chicago: Year Book Medical Publishers.

Sigman, M., Cohen, S. E., Beckwith, L., & Parmelee, A. H. (1986). Infant attention in relation to intellectual abilities in childhood. *Developmental Psychology, 22,* 788–792.

Singer, L. T., Arendt, R., Minnes, S., Farkas, K., & Salvator, A. (2000). Neurobehavioral outcomes of cocaine-exposed infants. *Neurotoxicology and Teratology, 22* 653–666.

Starr, A., Amlie, R. N., Martin, W. H., & Sanders, S. (1977). Development of auditory function in newborn infants revealed by auditory brainstem potentials. *Pediatrics, 60,* 831–839.

Stewart, A., Hope, P. L., Hamilton, P., Costello, A. M., Baudin, J., Bradford, B., Amiel-Tison, C., & Reynolds, E. O. (1988). Prediction in very preterm infants of satisfactory neurodevelopmental progress at 12 months. *Developmental Medicine and Child Neurology, 30,* 53–63.

Volpe, J. J. (2001). *Neurology of the newborn* (4th ed.). Philadelphia: Saunders.

Wallace, I. F., Rose, S. A., McCarton, C. M., Kurtzberg, D., & Vaughan, H. G. (1995). Relations between infant neurobehavioral preformance and cognitive outcome in very low birth weight preterm infants. *Journal of Developmental and Behavioral Pediatrics, 16,* 309–317.

Zelazo, P. R., Weiss, M. J. S., & Tarquino, N. (1991). Habituation and recovery of neonatal orienting to auditory stimuli. In M. J. Weiss & P. R. Zelazo (Eds.), *Newborn attention: Biological constraints and the influence of experience* (pp. 120–141). Norwood, NJ: Ablex.

21

Motor Assessment

JANE CASE-SMITH
ROSEMARIE BIGSBY

HISTORY

Motor assessment of infants has been based on the neuromaturation theory that motor development directly follows the hierarchical progression of central nervous system development. Normal infant development is not as predictable as was previously believed and can be influenced by interrelated biological, biomechanical, environmental, and motivational factors (Kelso, Holt, Rubin, & Kugler, 1981; Kugler & Turvey, 1988; Thelen, 1995; Thelen & Ulrich, 1991). There has been a resurgence of interest in studying motor development and assessment using a dynamical systems approach. Three of these recently published infant motor assessments described in this chapter identify specific variables that influence movement patterns, describe the phases of motor acquisition, and relate motor skills to function in the infant's natural environment.

In neuromaturation theory, movement patterns, particularly those that enable the infant to gain upright posture and locomotion, develop in a well-defined sequence relatively unaffected by the infant's experiences (McGraw, 1945). The first neuromaturation theorists (Gesell, 1945; Gesell et al., 1940; McGraw, 1945) documented the sequence of motor development, and their work has been the basis for the selected items on most motor tests published in the last 60 years. Gesell believed that variations in the normal sequence of development indicated central nervous system dysfunction (e.g., "mental retardation") and a specific purpose of the Gesell Developmental Schedules (Knobloch, Stevens, & Malone, 1980) was to identify children whose neuromaturation was deficient.

Based on neuromaturational theory, brainstem structures develop first, as evidenced by reflexive responses of the neonate (e.g., automatic grasp and asymmetrical tonic neck reflex), and cortical structures develop later, as evidenced by the coordinated patterns of the toddler. Increasing motor control indicates development and myelination of the midbrain and cortical structures and of simultaneous inhibition of brainstem control of movement. Three principles, largely based on the work of Gesell (1945) and McGraw (1945), have dominated neuromotor assessment and intervention; that is, movement progresses from primitive reflex patterns to voluntary, controlled movement and the sequence and rate of motor development develop in a cephalocaudal direction and are consistent.

In the typically developing infant, reflex patterns subside as balance, postural reactions, and voluntary motor control emerge, supporting the infant's learning to roll, sit, creep, stand and walk. The infant with central nervous system (CNS) impairment exhibits reflexive responses well beyond the time that integration is expected. Evaluation of reflexes, their persistence or integration, is used to assess the neurological integrity of the young infant (e.g., Ellison, 1994; Milani-Comparetti & Gidoni, 1967).

The developmental scales of Gesell (1945), Illingworth (1966, 1984), Bayley (1993), and others are based on a typical rate and sequence of development. By assuming a constant, predictable sequence of motor milestones, standard scores derived from normative data can identify infants with dysfunction.

The infant first develops control of neck, shoulder girdle, and upper extremity movements then control of pelvic and lower extremity movement. The first movements of the 1-month-old infant involve head lifting to visualize the environment. By 6 to 7 months of age, trunk and pelvis control are sufficient for upright sitting and later (12–13 months) for independent stance and locomotion.

GENERAL DESCRIPTION

Neuromotor Assessment

The purpose of infant neuromotor assessment is to identify CNS impairment by demonstrating an infant's deviance from the normal sequence of motor milestones and to predict, as early as possible, which infants would later be diagnosed with cerebral palsy or mental retardation. Neuromotor assessments identify specific neurological signs hypothesized or demonstrated to be predictors of cerebral palsy (Ellenberg & Nelson, 1981; Harris, 1987). The assessments described in Table 21.1 are based on neuromaturational theory; their common characteristics include the following:

TABLE 21.1. Neuromaturational-Based Assessments for Infants and Preschool Children

Assessment tool	Age range	Purpose	Design and properties
Infant Neurological International Battery (INFANIB; Ellison, 1994)	Birth to 18 mo	Items include muscle range and resistance, reflexive responses and the quality of milestones (e.g., sitting position).	The examiner elicits responses to a criterion-referenced battery of 20 items. The scoring sheet includes the infant's performance, item, factor and total scores. Interrater reliability is estimated to be $r = .97$ and test–retest reliability is estimated at $r = .95$. INFANIB demonstrated the ability to discriminate between typical and disabled populations with over 80% correctly classified scores.
Movement Assessment of Infants (MAI; Chandler, Swanson, & Andrews, 1980)	Birth to 12 mo	Screening tools for follow-up of high-risk infants. Items use a six-level rating scale to evaluate muscle tone, primitive reflexes, automatic reactions, and volitional movement.	Standardized measure, in which child is observed and handled in prone, supine, sitting, and standing. The MAI at 4 mo correctly predicted group category at 3 years into cerebral palsy (73% of the time) and typically developing children (63%). Predictive validity was low when compared to the PDMS at 4.5 years of age. In another study, 4- and 8-mo scores on the MAI were moderately correlated ($r = .52$ to $.68$) with scores in the BSID at 18 mo of age.
Milani-Comparetti Development Screening Test—Revised (Milani-Comparetti & Gidoni, 1967)	1 mo to 16 mo	Intended as a diagnostic tool to identify children who are at risk for developmental delays, especially cerebral palsy. Items assess primitive reflexes, tilting, righting, and protective reactions, spontaneous posture, and movement through attainment of independent ambulation.	This norm-referenced, standardized screening tool consists of 27 items, scored as present or absent. All items are elicited by the examiner. Items can be completed in 10–15 min. Interrater agreement on the revised edition ranged from 90 to 93%. Interrater reliability, examined after a 1-wk interval was between 80 to 100% agreement on individual items. Validity has not been investigated in the revised edition.

1. Each is based on a hierarchy of brain function in which the infant first demonstrates primitive reflexes, which are later integrated into voluntary patterns of movement.
2. Each rates typical and *atypical* movements. The atypical movement patterns characterize infants with neurological dysfunction (e.g., spasticity and tonic reflex patterns).

3. Each quantifies neurologically based indicators that discriminate motor dysfunction (e.g., muscle tone, primitive reflexes, and postural reactions).

Constraints

Although these evaluations are useful in identifying infants with deviant movement patterns, they fail to provide insight into individual differences or in-depth investigation of movement patterns. These assessments specify normal movement without accounting for the great variability observed in typically developing infants.

Although these tests were developed to identify infants with neurological dysfunction, they have not been consistently accurate in discriminating infants with CNS impairment and long-term developmental problems. Because items were selected to detect CNS impairment, they often have minimal relevance to the child's functional abilities and may have limited clinical value for intervention.

The poor predictive validity of these tests may be due to several factors (Chandler, 1990). The infant behaviors tested are inconsistent across time and different raters, demonstrating only fair test–retest and interrater reliability. Because the tests involve extensive handling and examiners tend to use different levels of touch for the same items, the infant's responses tend to vary in response to the level of sensory input. In addition, the intrusive handling required during test administration can produce aversive responses and behaviors (e.g., arching, startle, and crying) that are difficult to interpret.

A second problem is the variation in normal motor development that is not adequately expressed in the scoring criteria. Infants acquire motor skills at different developmental ages, (Stout, 1994), in varying sequences, with high variability in motor skill acquisition (Heriza, 1991).

The utility of these assessments might be questioned by examining the validity of the neuromaturation theory itself. The recent work of Kugler and Turvey (1988), Thelen and Ulrich (1991), Thelen (1995), and Heriza (1988, 1991) has demonstrated that the CNS is only one factor that determines the motor development of the infant. The rate and sequence of motor development are not invariant and are highly related to a multitude of internal and external variables, including the infant's home environment, caregiving experiences, ethnic background, health, body composition and structure, temperament, motivation, and cognition. Among these, sensory function, perception, cognition, temperament, and emotional development (e.g., Als, 1986; Connolly, 1973; Gibson, 1979, 1988; Lord & Hulme, 1987; Umphred, 1991) have direct effects on motor development and should be included in evaluation of motor skills (Case-Smith, 1997; Miller & Roid, 1994). Rather than emphasizing the infant's deviation from average behavior, infant functional abilities are best understood by identifying unique patterns of posture and movement and the individual variations observed across environments and situations.

The assumption that normal motor development proceeds in a cephalo-caudal direction might also be questioned, because all movements are a result of coordinated body actions. The sequence of motor development is best characterized as a spiraling and interweaving of total body movements and actions. Many body parts function to support the development of the first motor skills, with increasing levels of full body coordination throughout the first years of life (Gilfoyle, Grady, & Moore, 1990).

Dynamical Systems Assessment

The Alberta Infant Motor Scale (AIMS; Piper & Darrah, 1994), the Toddler and Infant Motor Evaluation (TIME; Miller & Roid, 1994), and the Test of Infant Motor Performance (TIMP; Campbell, Kolobe, Osten, Girolami, & Lenki, 1994), based on dynamical systems theory, have similar purposes (see Table 21.2). Each measures functional movements in the infant's natural environment, presents a system for quantifying qualitative aspects of movement, and has flexibility in item administration so that sensory input can be adapted to support the infant's best performance. The tests allow the examiner to make modifications in the environment and task to accommodate the infant's best performance and increase validity. The lack of sensitive instruments to measure the types of movement typically emphasized in intervention programs has been well documented (Campbell, 1991; Miller & Roid, 1994). Each also provides measurement of change in motor activity over time.

Alberta Infant Motor Scale

The AIMS (Piper & Darrah, 1994) is an observational assessment of gross motor and posture in infants, 0–18 months. The 58 items, divided into four positions—supine, prone, sitting, and standing—are constructed to discriminate immature or atypical performance and to evaluate change in motor skill development. Because the AIMS appears to be sensitive to small increments of motor development, the authors recommended its use in longitudinal documentation of the infant's development.

Infants are evaluated as they move freely about the environment. The situation is designed to be as naturalistic as possible with the parents encouraged to stay near the infant and the therapist as observer.

The AIMS documents progress within a skill area (e.g., can show changes in postural control in prone). The items rate transitional patterns of movement that are often the focus of intervention (see Table 21.3). Each item identifies qualitative indicators consistent with functional movement, in-

TABLE 21.2. Dynamical Systems-Based Assessments

Assessment tool	Age range	Purpose	Design and properties
Toddler and Infant Motor Evaluation (TIME; Miller & Roid, 1994)	4 mo to 3.5 yr	Designed to provide a comprehensive assessment of motor abilities. Diagnostic motor assessment that measures the quality of movement. Subtests evaluate mobility, stability, motor organization, social/emotional abilities and functional performance.	Evaluative standardized and normative measure, which uses parent-elicited play and naturalistic observations. Normative data were based on 875 children and parents from a wide geographic and ethnic background. Interrater reliability is $r = 90$ to .99 on all subtests, internal consistency is $r = .72$ to .97 on all subtests, test–retest $r = .96$ to .99 on all subtests. Construct validation shows appropriate age trends, and unidimensionality for the motor organization subset. TIME reasonably discriminates between typically developing and disabled peers, and accurately classifies children into motor delay or no motor delay.
Alberta Infant Motor Scale (AIMS; Piper & Darrah, 1994)	Birth to 18 mo	Identification of motor delays in infants, monitor individual development, and evaluate intervention to remediate motor delays. Fifty-eight items are broken down into four positions, prone, supine, sitting, and standing.	Evaluative, standardized, normative measure which uses skilled observations of a child's spontaneous movement repertoire. Normative data are based on a sample of 2,202 typically developing infants. Interrater reliability was .96 or higher between trained therapists. Test–retest reliability was .86 to .99 until 12 m of age. Construct validation showed excellent fit of test items to a unidimensional scale and conformity of the items for the expected sequence. AIMS discriminates children with abnormal motor development from healthy peers.
Test of Infant Motor Performance (TIMP; Campbell, Osten, Kolobe, & Fisher, 1993)	Birth to 4 mo	Designed to assess the postures and movements used by preterm and full-term infants.	The TIMP consists of 28 observational items scored dichotomously and 25 elicited items scored on a 4-, 5-, or 6-point hierarchical scale. Elicited items require handling of the infant. The TIMP requires 30 to 40 min to administer. Good content validity of a measure of posture and motor responses. TIMP scores increase with increasing age and decrease with medical complications. Internal consistency is .98. Intra- and interrater reliability trained in test administration had reliability coefficients of .95 to .99.

cluding weight-bearing position, postural alignment, and antigravity movements. Each describes how the infant's posture is influenced by gravity and how well he or she moves against gravity.

The AIMS manual includes drawings and photographs of infants in each of the postures assessed with a graph showing the percentage of infants at each month who passed that item. The most and least mature pos-

TABLE 21.3. Examples of Items from the Alberta Infant Motor Scale

Posture items	Movement items
Prone	Prone
Forearm support	Reaching with forearm support
Four-point kneeling	Rolling prone to supine with rotation
Sidelying	Prone
Propped lying on side	Reciprocal creeping
Supine	Supine
Sitting with support	Hands to feet
Sitting without arm support	Sitting to four-point kneeling
Standing	Standing
Supported standing	Cruising with rotation
Half kneeling	Pulls to stand

ture and movement patterns demonstrated by the infant are recorded, with the items between representing the infant's possible motor repertoire in that position or a "window" of current skills. When an infant's window crosses a wide range of items representing different skill levels, the infant may be in a transition phase of new skill acquisition.

Toddler and Infant Motor Evaluation

The TIME (Miller & Roid, 1994), a comprehensive assessment of the motor abilities of children 4–42 months old, includes five standardized subscales: mobility, stability, motor organization, social/emotional abilities, and functional performance. Three clinical subtests were designed for more in-depth analysis of atypical movement patterns.

The primary goal of the TIME is to measure qualitative aspects of movement. The Mobility, Stability, and Motor Organization subscales measure infant ability to perform, sequence, and organize components of movement. The Mobility subscale records the ability to move within and from five starting positions appropriate to the infant's developmental age (e.g., prone, sitting, and supported standing). The scale rates (1) the maturity and number of variations within a position, (2) the maturity and number of transitions between positions, and (3) the highest developmental pattern obtained from each position. The infant's sequence of movements in a 20-second time period is recorded, providing a measurement of patterns of transitional movements. The score reflects the infant's developmentally highest position and records the total motor repertoire in each position. Transitional movements are categorized as mature/immature, with scores weighted to level of difficulty.

Stability, the ability to control upright postures, observationally is scored from the Mobility and Motor Organization subscales. Four aspects of postural stability are rated as follows: (1) the highest nonlocomoting position without weight shift, (2) the highest nonlocomoting position with weight shift, (3) the highest locomoting position with weight shift, and (4) the highest reach position. Scores for the most mature postures demonstrated by the infant in seven different positions are summed.

Motor organization includes praxis and sequencing or the ability to perform unique motor skills requiring visual/spatial skills, balance, and complex sequential motor abilities. Items rated from the infant's play behaviors include qualitative aspects of the infant's approach and performance of a task and posture in sitting, grasp, and release of a tiny object. Raw scores are converted into standard and scaled growth scores.

The Functional Performance subscale is completed by parent interview. Four domains are rated on a 3-point scale: self-care, self-management and mastery, relationships and interactions, and functioning in the community. This subscale links information about the infant's rate of motor development with information about his or her functional abilities, to identify the motor components that appear to interfere with adaptive skill development.

Before and after the assessment, the examiner completes the Social/Emotional Abilities subtest. Behaviors observed during the test, including state, activity level, emotionality, reactivity, temperament, interaction, and attention span, are rated to gain an understanding of the influence of behaviors associated with social-emotional development.

The TIME provides sections to analyze abnormal as well as normal components of movement. Three clinical subtests, Atypical Positions, Quality Rating, and Component Analysis, are scored to structure and analyze clinical observations. However, scores cannot be converted into standardized scores.

The TIME manual provides only general instructions on how to elicit behaviors, although scoring criteria are explicit giving the examiner flexibility to elicit the infant's best performance. The examiner encourages parental participation in administering the test items and facilitating infant responses.

In dynamical systems theory, the organization of movement appears to be the critical aspect of motor skill that drives the proficient performance. Based on the demands of the task and the environment, movements are organized and reorganized through adaptation of the established motor schemes. The TIME is the first test to use clinical observation to quantify the infant's patterns and sequence of movement. This assessment of the ability to transition between and within postures can be compared to motor organization in specific developmental tasks and functional performance as reported by the parents. Longitudinal studies using the TIME are needed to validate the assumption that the qualitative aspects of movement that distinguish normal development are essential factors in functional performance and skill acquisition.

Test of Infant Motor Performance

The TIMP (Campbell et al., 1994), appropriate for preterm infants (from 32 weeks gestation age) to infants of 4 months gestational age, was developed for physical and occupational therapists to evaluate postural control and movement. TIMP items evaluate the ability to move against gravity, change positions, orient head and body, and measure the presence of ballistic and reaching movements. The test reflects the systems model of motor development as it relates to postural control (Shumway-Cook & Woollacott, 1993) through items that measure the infant's ability to (1) sustain a posture, (2) regain a posture, and (3) transition between postures. Head control is evaluated by the infant's ability to maintain head stability in a variety of spatial orientations, to right the head when the body is tilted, turn the head in various positions, and stabilize or orient the head in response to interesting visual or auditory events.

The TIMP requires 25 to 40 minutes to administer and score. It consists of two scales. The elicited scale contains 25 items, each rated on 5- or 6-point scales. Performance on these items reflects the infant's ability to make coordinated postural responses when placed in a variety of spatial orientations. The elicited scale items require handling of the infant based on standardized procedures consistent with typical caregiving handling (Murney & Campbell, 1998). The observed scale consists of 28 dichotomously scored behaviors that reflect the infant's spontaneously emitted attempts to change positions, orient head and trunk, selectively activate individual body segments, and antigravity control of arm and leg movement.

BIOBEHAVIORAL BASIS OF ASSESSMENT

The tests described are consistent with dynamic system theory as proposed by Bernstein (1967) and further developed by Thelen, Kelso, Turvey, and others. In dynamic systems theory, the CNS functions as a heterarchy, as the various structures of the brain work together and are interdependent in producing movement. Motor acts involve cortical, central brain, cerebellar, and brainstem activation and are not produced in a top-down manner (as defined in the neuromaturational theory) but seem to be generated in the central brain and modulated and adapted by afferent signals from the visual, auditory, tactile, proprioceptive, and vestibular systems. Sensory signals enter the CNS via the brainstem and cerebellum and are further interpreted in the association areas of the cortex. Afferent input influences motor output directly from lower-level structures (e.g., the brainstem) that modulate and organize the input and indirectly from higher-level structures (the cerebrum) that interpret the sensory input. During movement, neural activity forms a loop through the brainstem, cerebellum, central brain, and cortex areas.

Perceptions of visual, tactile, kinesthetic, and vestibular inputs and movement interact in a dynamic way. Infant-initiated movement results in sensory feedback that is compared to sensory memories. Most current theorists recognize that movement patterns previously thought to mature at predictable rates and sequences are actually highly influenced by sensory experiences (Bradley, 1994; Gilfolye et al., 1990; Heriza, 1991; Piper & Darrah, 1994). Motor activity depends on the perceptual capability to recognize affordances within the environment and reveals the infant's sensory preferences and ability to discriminate and interpret sensory input. Because the AIMS, TIME, and TIMP are scored during naturalistic observation and rate qualitative aspects of motor responses, they provide information about motor patterns that reflect infant sensory processing and perception.

The types of sensory information used by the infant vary by the motor activity and the developmental stage of that activity. Visual, vestibular, and proprioceptive information are important to walking and upright stance. In the young infant, visual information appears to be the most important sensory system in attaining upright postures. Later upright posture and locomotion are primarily modulated by the vestibular and proprioceptive systems (Shumway-Cook & Woollacott, 1995). Through mobility, the infant experiences bodily movement through space, the tactile/kinesthetic input of various surfaces, and proprioceptive input from surface slopes and heights.

Manipulation is guided by visual, tactile, and kinesthetic input (Rochat, 1989; Ruff, 1989). Sensory information helps the infant adjust and modify finger movement and force so that precise grasp and manipulation are possible. Through object manipulation the child develops haptic sense. When manipulating objects, sensory information enters the CNS as a unit and is integrated at all levels, affecting neuronal centers for motor, perceptual, and cognitive behaviors. Impairment in sensory responsiveness or perception limits refinement of movement patterns because the child received less feedback from movement. Naturalistic observation of the child allows therapists to analyze whether or not the basis for the motor dysfunction is an underlying perceptual impairment and how the motor dysfunction is influencing perceptual learning.

The infant's experiences during caregiving in early mobility and through object play appear to have strong influences on the rate and sequence of motor skills development. The testing environment and the tasks presented have immediate effects on the infant's motor performance. Items may involve sensory input that constrains performance, such as requiring rapid movement or brisk and strong tactile input. An infant may demonstrate active trunk extension when lying prone on a comfortable surface but not exhibit the same trunk extension when held suspended in the air. The AIMS, TIME, and TIMP help determine how sensory input from the environment affects performance. Each allows flexibility in selection of test environment and task constraints. Questions to guide analysis of the relative influence of perception on action are as follows: What does the infant perceive as he moves? What perceptual deficits are linked to immature, stereotypical, or impaired movement patterns? How might the infant adapt motor patterns when sensory input is altered?

FUNCTIONAL MOVEMENT SYNERGIES

The infant begins life with few constraints on movement, permitting the greatest variability for generation of spontaneous movements and flexibility for motor exploration of the environment. Functional synergistic movement patterns are quickly selected by the infant. From birth, the infant demonstrates a pattern of hand to mouth that involves degrees of flexion at the elbow, wrist, and fingers, which is later adapted to bring a bottle, then cup, spoon, and fork to the mouth. The synergistic hand-to-mouth pattern of shoulder internal rotation and adduction, elbow flexion, forearm pronation followed by supination, and neutral wrist position makes only minimal adaptive changes during the course of development. These synergies are softly assembled, as stable but flexible units with consistent characteristics (e.g., sequences of muscle activation and ratios of joint movement) that can be adjusted to accommodate novel situations. Such adaptable stability appears to be a hallmark of normal movement (Cioni et al., 1997).

The basic units of motor behavior are functional synergies or coordinated structures rather than the actions of specific muscles or muscle groups. Functional synergies are highly adaptable and reliable and are organized around a goal. Therefore, motor assessment should focus on functional synergies in the context of the infant's meaningful play. Documentation of the infant's ability to transition from one posture to another has greater relevance to the infant's function and achievement of play goals than the ability to maintain a posture or demonstrate a specific skill. Each of the assessments described analyzes sequences of movement. The TIME's scoring is based on the infant's ability to move through postures (the Mobility scale) and to organize a sequence of movements (the Motor Organization scale). The AIMS allows for evaluation of underlying motor components. Qualitative indicators measured by the AIMS include the body surfaces used in weight bearing, postural alignment, and degree of antigravity movement. Therefore, the items consider some of the biomechanical and sensory (vestibular and proprioceptive) system inputs, as well as environment constraints, that affect how posture and movement are accomplished.

Each assessment uses spontaneous play to elicit functional synergies to evaluate if the infant's movement patterns allow the achievement of play goals. The tests measure the infant's ability to transition between postures and positions as an essential element of motor development.

RELIABILITY AND VALIDITY

Psychometric Properties of the AIMS

The AIMS was normed using 2,202 infants born in Alberta, Canada, between 1990 and 1992 (Piper & Darrah, 1994). The normative data revealed no differences between genders. Age-equivalent scores and percentile ranks can be obtained.

To estimate reliability, 253 infants were assessed by two therapists simultaneously and evaluated 3 to 7 days later. Interrater reliability ranged from .96 to .99. Intrarater reliability ranged from .85 (for infants over 12 month) to .99 for the total sample.

Concurrent validity was evaluated using the Gross Motor Scale of the Peabody Developmental Motor Scales (PDMS; Folio & Fewell, 1983) and the Psychomotor Scales of Bayley Scales of Infant Development (BSID; Bayley, 1993). Using 52 typical infants, the correlation coefficient between AIMS and PDMS scores was .99 and between AIMS and BSID was .97. Using 68 infants categorized as at risk or abnormal, the correlation coefficients ranged from .93 between the BSID and AIMS and .95 between the PDMS and AIMS.

Thus, the AIMS appears to be a reliable and valid measure of the normal sequence of gross motor and posture in infants 0 to 18 months. Flexible testing methods allow the examiner to elicit best performance, although the lack of instructions for eliciting the items may create difficulty for the inexperienced examiner.

Psychometric Properties of the TIME

Two major studies of the TIME ($n = 100$, $n = 390$) were completed prior to standardization in 1992–1994. The early edition discriminated children with and without motor delays. The standardization study included one of children with motor delays ($n = 144$) and typically developing infants ($n = 731$) seen by 75 therapists trained in 2-day seminars. The sample was stratified by age, ethnicity, gender, and socioeconomic status. Internal consistency for each test section was higher for older children (e.g., .95 for the Mobility subscale).

Four sets of items from the Motor Organization scale were calibrated based on Rasch analysis. Data were aggregated across the age samples and total Rasch ability growth scores were calculated based on the sum of all items passed.

Cronbach alpha coefficients for the five standardized subscales fall between .72 and .97. The Mobility and Stability subscales have the lowest internal consistency. Test–retest reliability ranged from .97 to .99. Interrater reliability for two independent examiners observing a child's performance ranged from .89 to .99 on the different scales. The specificity of the Mobility subscale was 86% using -1.0 SD cutoff and 93% using a -1.5 SD cutoff. Specificity of the Stability subscale was 90% and 87%. Sensitivity of the Mobility subscale was 94% using a –1.0 *SD* cutoff and 88% using –1.5 *SD* as the cutoff; sensitivity of the Stability subscale was 91% and 81%.

Psychometric Properties of the TIMP

Based on Rasch logit values, the TIMP can be separated into more than seven different levels of difficulty across the test age span. Mean scores increase with age, and the correlation coefficient between postconceptual age in days and TIMP-derived scores was .83. Using a sample of 137 infants with high, medium, and low risk; age; medical risk; and ethnicity contributed to 72% of the variance in scores (Campbell, Osten, Kolobe, & Fisher, 1993). Postconceptual age was the most significant variable (beta =.80, p = .00001). The correlation between the TIMP and medical risk as measured by the Problem-Oriented Perinatal Risk Assessment System (POPRAS) scores was –.29. Construct validity of the scale was examined through analysis of typical handling during dressing, bathing, and playing and comparison of the demands placed on infants during these activities as compared to the handling involved in the elicited items. Almost all items (23 of 25) were observed during naturalistic handling. Approximately 50% of caregiving demands were approximations to the actual TIMP-elicited items (Campbell, Kolobe, Osten, Lenki, & Girolami, 1995; Murney & Campbell, 1998). The high relationship of scores to factors known to create high risk for development indicates that the TIMP would be useful in identifying infants at risk for developmental delay. The test authors plan additional studies of reliability and a national normative study.

DEVELOPMENTAL MODEL

Historically, when infants have demonstrated variance and delay in attainment of motor milestones, they were labeled as abnormal and given a diagnosis of motor dysfunction (e.g., cerebral palsy or developmental dyspraxia). However, research has demonstrated that variance in motor skills during infancy did not always predict abnormality in later childhood (Horak, 1991; Paben & Piper, 1987). Traditional assessments of motor skills have shown poor predictive validity (Chandler, 1990; Deitz, Crowe, & Harris, 1987). Assessments that use the dynamical systems model place a different emphasis on variability in motor performance. Variability becomes the focus of investigation rather than an indicator of abnormality.

Thelen et al. (1993) referred to periods of high variability and transition to new patterns of movement as a "phase shift." Through naturalistic observation of the infant's play using measures sensitive to the quality of movement, clinicians gain an appreciation of the unique methods children use to learn new skills. Three phases of motor skill acquisition have been identified (Sporns & Edelman, 1993). The infant's first movements are highly variable and appear as random kicking or swiping. Through these movements, the infant receives sensory input and weights the saliency and success of the movements. Certain motor patterns meet the demands of the environment and help her reach desired goals (e.g., make the bell ring). Following this tuning phase is a practice phase in which the infant has selected a movement that has adaptive value.

In the process of exploration and selection Goldfield, Kay, and Warren (1993) demonstrated these phases in a study of infants when first placed in a Johnny Jump-up bouncer. The infants first demonstrated erratic kicking without sustained bouncing. They rapidly developed some consistency in bouncing but leg movement varied. Once an infant demonstrated a stable pattern of leg movement, sustained bouncing occurred with regular frequency and minimal variability was observed. When motor assessment captures emerging skills (marked by instability in performance) as well as established skills (stable performance), clinicians can analyze factors that constrain and promote development. "Knowing when systems are in transition is important because theory predicts that interventions can only be effective when the system has sufficient flexibility to explore and select new solutions" (Thelen, 1995, p. 94).

The concept of phase shifts places the emphasis of evaluation on how the infant learns new skills rather than on what skills the infant consistently performs. Variability in movement patterns presents a window of opportunity in skill development. When motor behaviors are less stable and more flexibly organized, the clinician can observe how the infant approaches motor learning and what variables constrain and facilitate motor development. The AIMS identifies the inconsistently performed items between basal and ceiling levels as a window of emerging skill, and its authors indicate that this window should become the focus of intervention efforts.

The infant's unique motor patterns are the result of input from multiple systems that interact in dynamic ways to both facilitate and constrain movement. The interacting systems with ongoing influence on motor behavior are internal (bone structure, postural alignment, muscle bulk, weight, motivation, cognition) and external (characteristics of the task and the environment). Through the interaction of all these variables, new movement patterns develop and are refined. The affordances of the environment must fit the intrinsic skills of the infant for new skills to emerge. Developmental progress is contingent upon the presence of stimulating and challenging environmental factors when the infant is neurologically ready to learn new skills.

Motor development is characterized by discontinuity, which can be explained through an understanding that the systems controlling development change over time and vary within individual infants. Although each system appears to follow a linear course of maturation, the motor patterns demonstrated may have irregular and discontinuous development due to the constraining or driving forces of the supporting systems.

An example of a constraining or facilitating force in learning to roll is the infant's weight. A large overweight infant may not roll until 8 months, after he has demonstrated sitting and supported standing. His first roll may be a mature one, characterized by trunk rotation and sequenced movement of body segments (shoulders then pelvis). A small infant may roll at 2 months but use a primitive pattern of simple neck and arm extension. Rolling at 2 months would likely be poorly controlled and inconsistent. Documenting when rolling was achieved therefore cannot be reliably used to determine motor dysfunction without considering other variables such as weight and without analysis from observation of how the roll is performed. Physical size might also influence grasping patterns. An infant with small hands may exhibit a palmar grasp (4-month skill) for a longer time than the infant with large hands who can easily move the toy to the radial fingers for a radial digital grasp (8–9-month skill).

The multiple systems driving or constraining motor development have one common denominator—individual resilience, or, as Gleick (1989) describes it, how well a system can withstand small jolts and continue to function over a range of frequencies. Infants who continually explore movement, even in the face of disorganizing external and internal influences, are more likely to continue this trend in the future and thus to become more highly proficient at movement. Use of the infant's natural environments and typical interactions with the parent allow assessment of the effects of the environment on the infant's movement patterns.

STRUCTURAL AND/OR THEORETICAL
CONSTRAINTS/CONTROVERSIES

Because the instruments reviewed have attempted to move beyond the traditional models of motor assessment, their development should include comprehensive study of validity. Each has initial evidence of reliability and validity. The AIMS meets the purposes for which it was designed and is most appropriate for infants who are at risk for delayed motor development. It is not appropriate for infants with abnormal movement patterns (e.g., spasticity or significant hypotonia) because full credit for each item is based on demonstration of normal movement patterns. For example, children with cerebral palsy can make gains and functional progress without demonstrating the "typical" postures and antigravity movements. The authors note the test's limitations for evaluation of this population. In addition, the AIMS falls short of being a comprehensive test of infant motor development because items focus on gross motor to the exclusion of fine motor skill. Another limitation is its narrow age range, which ends at 18 months. Expansion of the test to older ages and development of items that evaluate arm and hand function would increase its application.

The TIME is a more comprehensive test for an expanded age range and includes several motor domains (stability, mobility, motor planning, and sequencing). The five domains of the test require high-level skill and considerable time to implement. Therapists have reported that they most successfully score the test from a videotape because the detailed scoring is difficult while observing the infant. The TIME has not been widely adopted but appears to be useful as a research tool.

The TIMP appears to be a sensitive measure of motor development in the first 4 months of life. The age range limits its use for measuring longitudinal changes beyond 4 months, but it can establish a baseline of motor function. The number of items suggests high sensitivity and pilot studies have demonstrated that the items discriminate infants at high risk for developmental delays. The TIMP involves frequent handling of the infant in a variety of positions. The authors suggest that the handling required for item administration is consistent with the nurturing and caregiving experiences of very young infants. However, handling by the examiner may produce aversive responses and behaviors.

TRAINING REQUIREMENTS

The manuals for the AIMS, TIME, and TIMP do not specify training requirements. The examiner's clinical expertise is needed to interpret the scores. The AIMS "may be performed by any health professional who has a background in infant motor development." Piper and Darrah (1994) recommend that the evaluator have acquired skill in performing observational assessment of movement. The TIME appears more subjective than the AIMS and TIMP in interpreting the child's posture and movement patterns (Miller & Roid, 1994) and therefore a therapist with expertise in motor development should interpret the scores. The TIMP should be administered by an occupational therapist or physical therapist who has experience in the evaluation of young infants.

In the TIME and the AIMS, parents are encouraged to participate in administering the test and should be asked to verify and explain the infant's behaviors. In contrast, therapists should administer the TIMP's elicited scale to ensure that the standardized procedures are followed.

However, the validity of the AIMS, TIME, and TIMP increases when an occupational or physical therapist participates in the testing procedures and interpretation. A background in normal motor development and atypical development patterns is needed to analyze the infant's behaviors and to identify emerging skills and accessible sensory systems to facilitate new skill development.

FUTURE RESEARCH DIRECTIONS

The validity of the motor assessments presented seems promising, although more research is needed. Concepts and principles that undergird continued development of infant motor assessments include a naturalistic environment (Haley, Baryza, & Blanchard, 1993; Linder, 1993; Miller & Roid, 1994; Piper & Darrah, 1994); analysis of motor components and qualitative analysis; using the infant's play ability to characterize functional movement (Goldfield, 1995; Kugler & Turvey, 1987; Thelen, 1995); attending to phases of apparent disorganization and variation which might represent periods of transition and flexibility; and participation of primary caregivers to evaluate sensory issues, functional performance, and concerns.

Understanding the infant's sensory system functions related to movement and manipulation should be a priority goal of assessment because sensory input is the primary means of intervention designed to enhance motor skills. Therapists provide proprioceptive, vestibular, tactile, and visual stimuli to challenge the infant and encourage higher-level motor responses. Without a clear understanding of what the infant perceives during movement, what sensory input motivates the infant to move, and what types of sensory experiences provide the right challenge to facilitate higher-quality skill, motor assessments remain inadequate for the purposes of promoting motor competence and functional performance.

REFERENCES

Als, H. (1986). A synactive model of neonatal behavioral organization: Framework for the assessment of neurobehavioral development in the premature infant and for support of infants and parents in the neonatal intensive care environment. *Occupational and Physical Therapy in Pediatrics, 6,* 3–53.

Bayley, N. (1993). *Bayley Scales of Infant Development—Revised Edition.* San Antonio, TX: Psychological Corporation.

Bernstein, N. (1967). *Coordination and regulation of movements.* New York: Pergamon Press.

Bradley, N. S. (1994). Motor control: Developmental aspects of motor control in skill acquisition. In S. Campbell (Ed.), *Physical therapy for children* (pp. 39–78). Philadelphia: Saunders.

Campbell, S. K. (1991). Framework for the measurement of neurologic impairment and disability. In M. J. Lister (Ed.), *Contemporary management of motor control problems: Proceedings of the II Step Conference* (pp. 143–154). Alexandria, VA: Foundation for Physical Therapy.

Campbell, S. K., Kolobe, T. H. A., Osten, E., Girolami, G. L., & Lenki, M. (1994). *Test of Infant Motor Performance.* Chicago, IL: University of Illinois, Department of Physical Therapy.

Campbell, S. K., Kolobe, T. H. A., Osten, E., Lenki, M., & Girolami, G. L. (1995). Construct validity of the Test of Infant Motor Performance. *Physical Therapy, 75*(7), 21–28.

Campbell, S. K., Osten, E. T., Kolobe, T. H., & Fisher, A. G. (1993). Development of the Test of Infant Motor Performance. *Physical Medicine and Rehabilitation Clinics of North America: New Developments in Functional Assessment, 4*(3), 541–550.

Case-Smith, J. (1997). Assessment. In J. Case-Smith (Ed.), *Pediatric occupational therapy and early intervention* (pp. 49–82). Andover, MA: Andover Medical Publishers.

Chandler, L. S. (1990). Neuromotor assessment. In E. D. Gibbs & D. M. Teti (Eds.), *Interdisciplinary assessment in infants: A guide for early intervention professionals* (pp. 45–61). Baltimore: Brookes.

Chandler, L. S., Andrews, M. S., & Swanson, M. W. (1980). *Movement assessment of infants.* Rolling Bay, WA: Authors.

Cioni, G., Ferrari, F., Einspieler, C., Paolicelli, P., Barbiani, T., & Prechtl, H. F. (1997). Comparison between the observation of spontaneous movements and neurologic examination in preterm infants. *Journal of Pediatrics, 130,* 740–711.

Connolly, K. (1973). Factors influencing the learning of manual skills by young children. In R. A. Hinde & J. Stevenson-Hinde (Eds.) *Constraints on learning.* London: Academic Press.

Deitz, J. C., Crowe, T. K., & Harris, S. R. (1987). Relationship between infant neuromotor assessment and preschool motor measures. *Physical Therapy, 67*(1), 14–17.

Ellenberg, J. H., & Nelson, K. B. (1981). Early recognition of infants at high risk for cerebral palsy: Examination at age four months. *Developmental medicine and Child Neurology. 23,* 705–716.

Ellison, P. (1994). *The INFANIB: A reliable method for the neuromotor assessment of infants.* Tuscan, AZ: Therapy Skill Builders.

Folio, M. R., & Fewell, R. R. (1983). *Peabody Developmental Motor Scales.* Austin, TX: Pro-Ed.

Gesell, A. (1945). *The embryology of behavior: The beginnings of the human mind.* New York: Harper & Bros.

Gesell, A., Halverson, H. M., Thompson, H., Ilg, F. L., Castner, B. M., Ames, L. B., & Amatruda, C. S. (1940) *The first five years of life.* New York: Harper & Row.

Gibson, J. J. (1979). *The ecological approach to visual perception.* Boston: Houghton-Mifflin.

Gibson, J. J. (1988). Exploratory behavior in the development of perceiving, acting, and the acquiring of knowledge. *Annual Review of Psychology, 39,* 1–41.

Gilfolye, E., Grady, A., & Moore, J. (1990). *Children adapt.* Thorofare, NJ: Slack.

Gleick, J. (1989). *Chaos: Making a new science.* New York: Penguin.

Goldfield, E. C. (1995). *Emergent forms: Origins and early development of human action and perception.* New York: Oxford University Press.

Goldfield, E. C., Kay, B. A., & Warren, W. H., (1993). Infant bouncing: The assembly and tuning of action systems. *Child Development, 64,* 1128–1142.

Haley, S. M., Baryza, M. J., & Blanchard, Y. (1993). Functional and naturalistic frameworks in assessing physical and motor disablement. In I. J. Wilhelm (Ed.), *Physical therapy assessment in early infancy* (pp. 225–256). New York: Churchill Livingstone.

Harris, S. R. (1987). Early neuromotor predictors of cerebral palsy in low-birthweight infants. *Developmental Medicine and Child Neurology, 29,* 508–519.

Heriza, C. (1988). Organization of leg movements in preterm infant. *Physical Therapy, 68,* 1340–1346.

Heriza, C. (1991). Motor development: Traditional and contemporary theories. In M. J. Lister (Ed.), *Contemporary management of motor control problems: Proceedings of the II STEP Conference* (p. 99). Alexandria, VA: Foundation for Physical Therapy.

Horak, F. B. (1991). Assumptions underlying motor control for neurologic rehabilitation.

In M. J. Lister (Ed.), *Contemporary management of motor control problems: Proceedings of the II STEP Conference* (pp. 11–27). Alexandria, VA: Foundation for Physical Therapy.

Illingworth, R. S. (1966). The diagnosis of cerebral palsy in the first year of life. *Developmental Medicine and Child Neurology, 8,* 178–194.

Illingworth, R. S. (1984). *The development of the infant and young child.* Edinburgh: Churchill Livingstone.

Kelso, J. A. S., Holt, K. G., Rubin, P., & Kugler, P. N. (1981). Patterns of human interlimb coordination emerge from the properties of non0linear limit cycle oscillatory processes: Theory and data. *Journal of Motor Behavior, 13,* 226–261.

Knobloch, H., Stevens, F., & Malone, A. F. (1980). *Manual of development diagnosis* (rev. ed.). New York: Harper & Row.

Kugler, P. N., & Turvey, M. T. (1987). *Information, natural law, and the self-assembly of rhythmic movement.* Hillsdale, NJ: Erlbaum.

Kugler, P. N., & Turvey, M. T. (1988). Self-organization, flow fields, and information. *Human Movement Science, 7,* 97–129.

Linder, T. (1993). *Transdisciplinary play-based assessment.* Baltimore: Brookes

Lord, R., & Hulme, C. (1987). Kinaesthetic sensitivity of normal and clumsy children. *Developmental Medicine and Child Neurology, 29,* 720–725.

McGraw, M. B. (1945). *The neuromuscular maturation of the human infant.* New York: Macmillan.

Milani-Comparetti, A. M., & Gidoni, E. A. (1967). Routine developmental examination in normal and retarded infants. *Developmental Medicine and Child Neurology, 9,* 631–638.

Miller, L. J., & Roid, R. G. (1994). *The T. I. M. E.: Toddler and Infant Motor Evaluation—A standardized assessment.* Tuscan, AZ: Therapy Skill Builders.

Murney, M., & Campbell, S. (1998). The ecological relevance of the Test of Infant Motor Performance Elicited Scale Items. *Physical Therapy, 78*(5), 479–489.

Paban, M., & Piper, M. C. (1987). Early predictors of one year neurodevelopmental outcome for "at risk" infants. *Physical and Occupational Therapy in Pediatrics, 7,* 17–34.

Piper, M. C., & Darrah, J. (1994). *Motor assessment of the developing infant.* Philadelphia: Saunders.

Rochat, P. (1989). Object manipulation and exploration in 2 to 5 month old infants. *Developmental Psychology, 25,* 871–884.

Ruff, H. A. (1989). The infant's use of visual and haptic information in the perception and recognition of objects. *Canadian Journal of Psychology, 43,* 302–319.

Shumway-Cook, A., & Woollacott, M. (1993). Theoretical issues in assessing postural control. In I. J. Wilhelm (Ed.), *Physical therapy assessment in early infancy* (pp. 161–172). New York: Churchill Livingstone.

Shumway-Cook, A., & Woollacott, M. (1995). *Motor control: Theory and practical applications.* Baltimore: Williams & Wilkins.

Sporns, O., & Edelman, G. M. (1993). Solving Bernstein's problem: A proposal for the development of coordinated movement by selection. *Child Development, 64,* 960–981.

Stout, J. L. (1994). Gait: Development and analysis. In S. Campbell (Ed.), *Physical therapy for children* (pp. 79–103). Philadelphia: Saunders.

Thelen, E. (1995). Motor development: A new synthesis. *American Psychologist, 50,* 79–95.

Thelen, E., Corbotta, D., Kamm, K., Spencer, J., Schneider, K., & Zernicke, R. (1993). The transition to reaching: Mapping intention and intrinsic dynamics. *Child Development, 64,* 1058–1098.

Thelen, E., & Ulrich, B. D. (1991). Hidden skills: A dynamic systems analysis of treadmill stepping during the first year. *Society for Research in Child Development, 56*, 1–98.

Umphred, D. (1991). Merging neurophysiologic approaches with contemporary theories. In M. J. Lister (Ed.), *Contemporary management of motor control problems: Proceedings of the II Step Conference* (pp. 127–131). Alexandria, VA: Foundation for Physical Therapy.

22

The Bayley Scales of Infant Development

Is There a Role in Biobehavioral Assessment?

MARGARET BENDERSKY
MICHAEL LEWIS

Standardized scales of infant development are the most commonly used infant assessment instruments in both clinical and research settings. The most widely used in the United States are the Bayley Scales of Infant Development (BSID; Bayley, 1969, 1993). The BSID, unlike many other methods of biobehavioral assessment discussed in this volume, are not a measure of a specific cognitive process but a standardized, developmentally ordered checklist of complex criterion behaviors. These often require multiple underlying process capacities, not least of which are levels of behavioral organization, comprehension, and sociability necessary to perform the tasks.

HISTORY

The scientific climate of the late 19th century in Western Europe was ripe for the development of tests of mental capacity, with major advances in medicine, a more humane attitude toward the mentally deficient and insane, and an interest in evolution (Brooks-Gunn & Weinraub, 1983). Six factors that converged in this period as enumerated by Lewis and Sullivan (1985), are as follows:

1. Scientific study of psychological processes of perception, sensation, reaction time, and memory originating in German laboratories.
2. British scientific interest in the hereditary aspects of intelligence.
3. U.S. interest in individual differences and the prediction of scholastic achievement.
4. Interest in early human behavioral development.
5. Medical and educational progress in the diagnosis and training of the mentally deficient in France and in the United States.
6. The need for standardized testing and placement criteria demanded by the establishment of compulsory public school in France and in the United States. (p. 506)

In the late 19th century, practitioners used anthropometric measures and sensory functioning to assess "intelligence" (Lewis & Sullivan, 1985). Alfred Binet is credited as the first to declare higher mental functions (e.g., judgment, reasoning, and comprehension) to be the essentials of intellectual ability that are likely to differentiate individuals (Binet & Henri, 1895, 1896). Binet found that simple sensory and motor tasks did not change over age and were unrelated to one another and to school performance. He therefore did not include them in the first test he devised to identify mentally deficient individuals who could benefit from special education. His instrument became the prototype for intelligence tests, generating types of measurable skills and the notion of a single summary score. Infant items, originally for assessment of severely retarded individuals, were omitted from the final 1911 version, because they were not considered relevant for school-age children (Lewis & Sullivan, 1985). The Binet test and its English versions were widely adopted by special educators as compulsory education laws, beginning at the turn of the century, led to the development of special education classes for slower students. The Stanford–Binet (Terman, 1916) became the standard in this country (Brooks-Gunn & Weinraub, 1983).

The realization that different infants of the same age had distinguishable functional capacities came from observational studies first documented in infant diaries kept by eminent scientists such as Charles Darwin (1877). About 30 baby biographies, published between 1877 and 1907 (Papalia & Olds, 1975), influenced the development of infant assessment tools in several ways. They legitimized infants as appropriate subjects of study, described a sequence of maturational development and individual differences in the rate of maturation, and described situations later translated into test items (Lewis & Sullivan, 1985).

The confluence of these interests and events led to the development of assessments to evaluate infants and young children in the 1920s and 1930s (see Brooks-Gunn & Weinraub, 1983). Arnold Gesell's intensive observational studies of development provided an important basis for many infant assessments (Gesell, 1925; Gesell & Amatruda, 1947; Gesell & Thompson, 1938). *Developmental Diagnosis* (Gesell & Amatruda, 1941), the first manual for administering, scoring, and interpreting infant test performance, included comprehensive normative data from 1 to 42 months of age. A major portion of the book detailed the identification of possible developmental delays in children with sensory handicaps, convulsive disorders, and cerebral injury (Kopp, 1994). Gesell used naturally occurring test situations, stimuli that appealed to infants, and parents as informants. He emphasized a sequence of biologically determined behavioral milestones in several distinct functional domains: motor, adaptive (mental), language and personal–social. Although psychometric properties of these developmental schedules were never adequately studied, it served as the main source of test items for subsequent infant assessments (Stott & Ball, 1965). Gesell regarded this instrument as useful for describing developmental progress and as an adjunct to clinical assessments for diagnosing problems in specific functional domains, but he was not concerned with evaluating intelligence or predicting future mental capacity (Brooks-Gunn & Weinraub, 1983; Lewis & Sullivan, 1985).

Other instruments emerging in this period were devised by Nancy Bayley for the Berkeley Growth Study. They were, and continue to be, the most thoroughly studied infant assessment tools (Brooks-Gunn & Weinraub, 1983; Lewis & Sullivan, 1985). Three earlier scales became the basis of the 1969 BSID, which were revised in 1993 (the Bayley Scales of Infant Development—II [BSID-II]). The BSID have been widely adopted as diagnostic and research tools.

GENERAL DESCRIPTION

The 1969 BSID consisted of the Mental and the Motor Scale and the Infant Behavior Record (IBR), a checklist of responses to people, toys, and test situations completed by the examiner following assessment. Items that comprised the scales were not theory driven but derived from other scales to provide observable behavioral responses that placed the child in a developmental sequence (Bayley, 1993). The Mental and Motor Scales were standardized for ages 2 through 30 months. The 163 items on the Mental Scale assessed sensory perception, discrimination, sensory–motor integration, social cognition, object constancy, imitation, and early language skills. Motor Scale items examined gross and fine motor abilities, muscle control, and coordination. Correlations between Mental and Motor Scales at various ages over the first year ranged from .50 to .80 (Bayley, 1969), as many early items on the Mental Scale required controlled movement and manipulation of materials. Some items were observational, but most had specified administration procedures which sometimes required materials provided in the kit. The subject was assigned pass/fail for each item according to the scoring criterion.

Scale items were administered until the basal and ceiling levels were reached. Although Bayley left the determination of those levels to examiner judgment, she offered 10 consecutive items passed or failed on the Mental Scale and 6 on the Motor Scale as a guide. Although items were arranged in order of difficulty, the number of items falling into each age varied considerably from month to month (from 0–15 on the Mental Scale; 0–8 on the Motor Scale). The largest numbers of items per month were clustered at the earliest age levels. Many items had different criteria for passing at various age levels and could be scored based on a single administration (Bayley, 1969).

Raw scores were converted to normalized standard scores, the Mental Development Index (MDI) and the Psychomotor Development Index (PDI), comparable to a deviation IQ with a mean of 100, a standard deviation of 16, and range of 50–150.

The IBR documented examiner impressions of the child's social orientation, emotional tone, attention, and activity level. Infants were scored on 24 items, with ratings and yes/no and open-ended questions. The IBR was not standardized, but its intended use was as an aid in interpreting other Bayley test scores in clinical settings.

The Bayley Scales of Infant Development-II (1993) updated the normative data to achieve representation of the U.S. population in race/ethnicity, gender, parent's education, and geographic location; to extend the age range from 1 month to 42 months; to improve content coverage and identify subscales ("facets"); to update stimulus materials to make them more attractive to children; to improve psychometric quality; and to improve clinical utility by providing data for children with high-incidence clinical diagnoses (e.g., Down syndrome, prematurity, and drug exposure).

Seventy-six percent of the Mental Scale items and 84% of the Motor Scale items remained unchanged from the 1969 version. A number of items were added (e.g., object retrieval from a plexiglass box with an open side, habituation, and novelty preference) which are of theoretical interest, in addition to having predictive validity and clinical implications. Items were deleted to eliminate racial or gender bias, if they showed no strong age trends or were redundant, were unrelated to other items in the scale, or had administration or scoring problems. Four "facets" were developed to increase the utility of the BSID in clinical settings and for developing treatment plans (Bayley, 1993). Nine expert reviewers categorized each item as measuring cognitive, language, personal/social, or motor ability. Final placement into facets was based on reviewer agreement and the correlation of the item to the total facet scores. The appropriate developmental age placement was then determined.

The IBR underwent considerable revamping and was renamed the

Behavior Rating Scale (BRS). The BRS has a standard 5-point scoring system. Items are grouped into three age levels: 1–5 months, 6–12 months, and 13–42 months, on four empirically derived factors (i.e., attention/arousal, orientation/engagement, emotional regulation, and motor quality). Cutoff scores for normal, questionable, and nonoptimal ratings for each factor and the total score were based on the standardization sample. Scores above the 25th percentile are considered normal, between the 11th and 25th questionable, and at or below the 10th percentile nonoptimal.

The major change in administration of the BSID-II is the introduction of item sets. To facilitate comparisons of children of the same age, an effort was made to ensure that a uniform subset of items is administered. Item sets are defined for monthly increments in age through 13 months, 3-month increments from 14–37 months, and a group spanning 5 months from 38–42 months for both the Mental and Motor Scales. In each set, items range in difficulty from those which 90% to 15% of the standardization sample at that age passed. Within each set, the basal rule is five or more items passed in the Mental Scale and at least four items in the Motor Scale, and the ceiling rule is at least three failed items on the Mental and at least two failed on the Motor Scale. If the basal is not met, the examiner must drop down through successive item sets until a basal is achieved and, similarly, must administer higher sets until a ceiling level is established. The concept of basal and ceiling used here differs from that usually applied to tests in which items are sequenced according to difficulty. On the BSID-II, a child can fail lower items within the set but still achieve a basal level if he or she passes at least five (mental) or four (motor) higher level items within the set. This may be disquieting to users because they must assume that the child has met the criterion for every item below the first item in a set, which may be questionable. Similarly, it may make deriving facet scores difficult because items placed at the same or similar developmental levels on the facet may actually cross item sets. There are also large gaps on specific facets at certain age levels. Thus, the examiner interested in facet scores must administer specific items below or above an item set to complete a facet (but not figure those items into the raw score for MDI and PDI).

In addition to the normative sample, the BSID-II provide data on 365 children from seven high-risk groups as evidence for clinical validity to increase the utility of the instrument in clinical settings. One study that compared performance on the BSID and BSID-II in a relatively small sample of high-risk preterm infants in the second year found an average MDI difference of 7.29 and a PDI difference of 9.31 between the first and second editions (Goldstein, Fogle, Wieber, & O'Shea, 1995). Correlations between scores derived from the old and new versions were .95 for both MDI and PDI. Similarly, there was agreement between the versions for 46 of 49 subjects on the MDI clinical classifications (kappa = .85). Agreement was only fair for PDI scores, however (34 of 49, kappa = .46). For both index scores a higher number of subjects were classified as suspect or abnormal by the BSID-II. The clinical implication of these findings is that a greater number of high-risk children may meet criteria for state and federally funded intervention services when the second edition is used.

Mean MDI scores were about 12 points lower, whereas the mean PDI was about 7 points lower on the 1993 compared to the 1969 edition in a representative sample of normal children. Given its widespread use, the updated and improved norms and the extended age range of the new version of the BSID are positive developments. The manual is excellent and provides several new interpretive guides. However, the facets are sadly inadequate. In addition to the difficulty of arriving at a developmental level within the item set format of the test, there are too few or no items in many age ranges, and the directions for deriving the facet scores are ambiguous. For example, the examiner is to identify the highest developmental age at which the child achieves mastery by determining at which level the child passes "a predominant number of items at that level" (Bayley, 1993, p. 49). However, the examiner is not told what level should be assigned if the child passes exactly half of the items at an age level or fails items below the "mastery" level. In addition, the Social facet is apparently only useful at a developmental level of 6 months or less. It is still too soon to be able to evaluate how much of an improvement in content the BSID-II offers over the BSID, and in particular, the predictive validity of the new MDI and PDI scores.

BIOBEHAVIORAL BASIS OF ASSESSMENT

Bayley was interested in determining the set of behaviors which were predictive of future capacities, as well as in determining the stability of mental ability during infancy (Bayley, 1933a). The California First-Year Mental Scale (Bayley, 1933b), the California Preschool Mental Scale (Jaffa, 1934), and the California Infant Scale of Motor Development (Bayley, 1936) included many items found on the Gesell schedules. Extensive psychometric studies of the scales indicated adequate reliability but poor predictive validity. Bayley concluded that the behaviors indicative of early infant development, until the age of 2, are unrelated to "aggregations of traits constituting intelligence" (1933a, p. 82). In addition, she came to believe that early development proceeded in discontinuous shifts in function (Bayley, 1933a, 1970). These findings prompted the debate about the continuous nature of developmental progress. Support for such a "stage theory" of development came from animal research and brain-imaging studies that indicated discontinuities in brain development that correspond to periods of cognitive transition (Fisher, 1987; Goldman-Rakic, 1987). For example, new peak frequencies emerge in electroencephalograms at 4 and 8 months of age, especially in the occipital–parietal region (Fox, & Bell, 1990; Hagne, Persson, Magnusson, &

Petersen, 1973). These ages have been widely recognized as coinciding with the onset of the control of a single action to accomplish a simple goal at 2 to 4 months and the qualitatively different ability to coordinate several actions to accomplish a goal at 7 to 8 months (Piaget, 1952).

Bayley believed that a lack of correspondence over time in mental test scores was due to these changes in the nature of mental processes as they progress from simple sensorimotor skills to increasingly complex reasoning processes. She saw no logical necessity that the simpler would predict the more complex (Bayley, 1970). She argued that a child's performance is the result of complex interactions among multiple determinants of development (Bayley, 1970), including genetic endowment of the child which results not only in neurons, perceptors, reactors, hormones, enzymes, and the like but also tendencies to react to the environment and inherent differences in rates of maturation; the prenatal/perinatal environment which might interfere with the potential for optimal development; and the great variety of postnatal environmental factors, including physical, such as adequate nutrition, as well as the social and emotional climate in which the child is raised. This perspective suggests that it would be necessary to understand environmental factors that continually affect the child's developmental trajectory to improve the prediction of functional capacity over time.

RELIABILITY AND VALIDITY

The BSID (and BSID-II) are the acknowledged gold standard of standardized infant assessment instruments. The Bayley scales, particularly the 1993 edition, amassed a large number of children (100 at each of 17 ages) from a scientifically determined cross-section of the recent U.S. population for standardization. The norms are therefore valid and useful for most samples of U.S. children.

The BSID and BSID-II have adequate reliability. The average reliability coefficient (alpha) for the BSID-II Mental Scale is .88, and .84 for the Motor Scale. The reliability of the BRS also was found to have an average of .88. Test–retest stability, measured from 1 to 16 days apart (median of 4 days), was .83 at 1 and 12 months for the Mental Scale, .77 at 1 and 12 months for the Motor Scale, and .55 at 1 month, .90 at 12 months for the BRS. Interscorer agreement is provided for the BSID-II, although it is based on the duplicate scoring of only 51 children across a 2–30 month age span. The correlation between two scorers, one who administered the items and one who observed, is .96 for the Mental and .75 for the Motor Scales. Because the second scorer did not actually administer the items, it may have been a disadvantage because motor items require physical manipulation of the child. An interscorer correlation of .80 is desirable (Sattler, 1988). The BRS has a lower interscorer reliability of .70 for the total score for infants in the 1–5 month age range, and .88 for children above. Test–retest and interscorer reliability are difficult to establish when assessing young infants. Performance on a given occasion may be influenced enormously by such factors as the time of day, the infant's state of hunger, alertness, general temperament, and sociability. Assessment of motor abilities that are often qualitative and difficult to describe in behavioral terms requires an examiner with wide experience in handling, interacting with, and observing infants. Except for the BRS, the Mental and Motor Scales have moderate to excellent reliability. Multiple assessments using several measures on any single occasion, repeated over time, will increase the confidence that an infant's abilities have been accurately determined (Bayley, 1993; Lewis & Fox, 1986).

The manual (Bayley, 1993) provides evidence of adequate internal validity of the content and construction of the BSID-II scales. In the younger age range, the only comparison of concurrent performance presented in the new edition is to the earlier BSID. Moderate correlations (.62 between MDIs; .63 between PDIs), reflect the significance of the changes made in the new edition but do not necessarily imply improved content validity.

Older research studies that compared BSID performance to other measures of infant mental capacity found relatively low correlations (King & Seegmiller, 1973; Lewis & Brooks-Gunn, 1981; Lewis & McGurk, 1972; Rose & Wallace, 1985; Singer & Fagan, 1984; Uzgiris, 1983). Lewis and Brooks-Gunn (1981) in a study comparing Bayley performance with measures of information processing at 3 months of age reported correlations for two separate samples of –.27 and .22 between MDI and visual habituation scores, and –.01 and –.15 between MDI and recovery of attention to a novel stimulus. They also compared 3-month MDI to a test of sensorimotor functioning based on Piaget's stages (Corman & Escalona, 1969) and found a correlation of just .24.

The lack of a strong relation between Bayley Mental Scale items and more specific measures of cognitive function is not surprising. Successful performance of a Bayley item generally depends on the integration of a number of cognitive and fine motor skills, as well as attention and motivation. Performance can be affected by deficits in a number of different domains, whereas more specific measures require more circumscribed sets of abilities and are often relatively motor free and less dependent on general performance variables.

Extensive evidence of the poor predictive validity of the Bayley and other similar infant test measures to later measures of intelligence, and even later MDI scores, has been presented (for reviews, see Brooks-Gunn & Weinraub, 1983; Fagan & Singer, 1983; Honzik, 1983; Lewis & Sullivan, 1985; McCall, 1979). Only after 2 years of age do test scores moderately relate to IQ scores at 4 years or older. Fagan and Singer (1983) in a review of studies of normal infants reported the median correlation of developmental test scores at 0–4 months with intelligence test scores at 3–6+ years to be about .06. The median correlation between 5–7-month developmental test scores and IQ scores at 3 years was .25, and only .06 with IQ at 6+ years. McCall (1979) found similar cross-age correlations for infant performance to IQ at older ages in a review of 19 studies. Prior to 19 months the median correlation between infant scores and 3–4-year IQ was at most .26. It was only at 19–30 months did studies find a median correlation of .49 to later IQ.

There is evidence that concurrent and predictive validity are greater for infants known to be at high risk of developmental delay or dysfunction due to early medical or environmental conditions (e.g., Brooks-Gunn & Lewis, 1988; Knobloch & Pasamanick, 1967; Lewis & Brooks-Gunn, 1984; McCall, Hogarty, & Hurlburt, 1972; Werner, Honzik, & Smith, 1968). Lewis and Brooks-Gunn (1984) reported that handicapped infants from four different diagnostic groups with low mental ages determined by the BSID also did not show habituation to a redundant stimulus. The correlation between mental age and response decrement was .52 (Brooks-Gunn & Lewis, 1988). Similarly, in a recent study of preterm infants in our laboratory, there was a correlation of .58 between the MDI and response decrement to a visual stimulus at 3 months of age. Moreover, the greater the number of medical complications of prematurity suffered by the infant, the more likely that MDI and habituation were depressed ($r = -.25$ for MDI, and $r = -.49$ for habituation).

More accurate prediction from infant test scores for low-scoring compared to normal subjects has been confirmed by many investigators (e.g., Crowe, Dietz, & Bennett, 1987; Drillien, 1961; Erickson, 1968; Farran & Harber, 1989; Holden, 1972; Honzik, 1983; Honzik, Hutchings, & Burnip, 1965; Illingworth, 1961, 1972; Ireton, Thwing, & Gravem, 1970; Knobloch & Pasamanick, 1967; McCall et al., 1972; Rubin & Balow, 1979; Vanderveer & Schweid, 1974; Werner et al., 1968). In our study of preterm infants, the correlation between 3- and 12-month MDI was .44, compared to a median of .29 that McCall (1979) reported in his meta-analysis of normal samples. Stability in performance across age, as well as greater consistency across assessments at a given age, tend to be stronger for infants who are more severely organically compromised, such as those with Down syndrome or multiple congenital anomalies (Fischler, Graleker, & Koch, 1964).

In other at-risk samples, correlations often vary widely depending on initial diagnosis (Fagan & Singer, 1983). A lack of correspondence across different measures of the young infant's capacities and poor prediction have been found in samples of infants at risk due to preterm birth, other early medical complications, or prenatal exposure to toxicants. Rose and Wallace (1985) reported a correlation of −.24 between visual recognition memory and MDI at 6 months in preterm infants. In our preterm sample, although the short-term prediction was better than that reported for normal samples, the correlation between 3-month MDI and 36-month Stanford–Binet IQ was just −.12, and .20 between 12-month MDI and 3-year IQ.

Another limitation to prediction is that the correlations between single early and later test scores, for normal or handicapped children, are not so high that they yield accurate prediction for any individual. A severely handicapped infant who is very low functioning at 6 months is highly likely to remain so at 2 or 4 years of age. However, a standardized assessment is neither appropriate nor necessary for such a determination, nor would it be sensitive to variation in functional status among the severely handicapped. For the majority of infants, functioning at normal or mild to moderate delay, individual prediction is likely to be quite inaccurate.

Other cogent arguments have been raised against the expectation that prediction of mental ability from infancy would be high. One of the most pervasive has been the apparent discontinuity between early milestone behaviors and later intellectual skills despite individual differences in skills in infancy and later in life (e.g., Bayley, 1970; Fagan & Singer, 1983; McCall, Eichorn, & Hogarty, 1977; Piaget, 1952; Stott & Bell, 1965). Others have argued that there is continuity in mental development from infancy, but more enduring underlying process variables, cognitive as well as attentional and affective, must be measured rather than the complex, age-related criterion skills typically found on infancy tests. A large body of research supports this proposition (for reviews, see Bornstein & Sigman, 1986; Fagan & Singer, 1983).An additional explanation is that there are changes over time that are functions of environmental conditions and social relationships (e.g., Bayley, 1993; Lewis, 1983; Lewis & Fox, 1980; McCall et al., 1977). Therefore, knowing a child's earlier test score is only part of the developmental equation.

Poor predictive validity does not necessarily imply low sensitivity to high-risk conditions. As an outcome measure, the Bayley scales are relatively sensitive. Bayley performance may be affected by deficits in a variety of different domains and therefore by a broad range of impairments (Jacobson & Jacobson, 1995). MDI scores have been found to be sensitive to differences in exposure to alcohol, cocaine, lead, methadone, and polychlorinated biphenyls (Alessandri, Bendersky, & Lewis, 1998; Arendt, Angelopoulos, Salvator, & Singer, 1999; Jacobson & Jacobson, 1985; Jacobson et al., 1993; Singer et al., 1997a; Streissguth, Barr, Martin, & Herman, 1980), prematurity and low birthweight (e.g., Ross, 1985; Singer, Yamashita, Lilien, Collin, & Baley, 1997b; Wilson, 1985), and low neonatal heart rate variability (Fox & Porges, 1985).

The BSID-II manual presents evidence of sensitivity through studies of 365 children from seven high-risk groups. Mean index scores were significantly lower for high-risk infants compared to normals. There was some specificity of deficit across different diagnostic categories. Infants who were preterm, were HIV positive, were asphyxiated at birth, had Down syndrome, or had developmental delay or autism had mean MDIs and PDIs 1 to 3 standard deviations below the mean.

DEVELOPMENTAL MODEL

Maturational unfolding is the dominant underlying developmental model on which the BSID is based. The scales describe a progression of functional abilities expected to appear as the infant matures. These capacities become apparent at a relatively uniform age in normal children. Deviation from this timetable implies a delay or acceleration in maturation at that time point but does not have implications about the timing or ability to attain later developmental milestones.

Bayley (1970) wrote that development has multiple determinants. However, the nature of a checklist of criterion behaviors suggests that though there may be different paths of arriving at a given developmental level, or factors extrinsic to the child that facilitate or suppress development, there is still a biologically programmed set progression of capacities. This is similar to the canalization model described by McCall (1981). There is a species-typical developmental path followed by most humans over the first 2 years of life. Only major organismic or environmental disruptions can push the infant out of this path.

STRUCTURAL AND THEORETICAL CONSTRAINTS

One of the major features of the BSID is the provision of the index scores. This has been seen as a blessing to those who need a single number which indicates that child X is showing a significant delay and is thus eligible for special services, or group A is significantly delayed compared to group B in a research study, or that intervention Q improved developmental status. These uses of the BSID are noted to be legitimate in the manual (Bayley, 1993). However, use of such scores presumes they are valid descriptions of a child's development comparable across children at a given age, or across ages. Bayley (1993) claims that the BSID assesses "the child's current level of cognitive, language, personal-social, and fine and gross motor development" (p. 1). However, an MDI only indicates the sum of items passed on the scale. One child could achieve an MDI of 100 by passing every item up to her age and failing every item above it, whereas another child could achieve the same score by passing items scattered below and above his or her age level. Because items measuring different abilities are integrated into one sequence, a child may perform poorly on language items but well on visual–motor items and achieve a normal MDI because the examiner continues to test until a ceiling is achieved. Similarly, children can obtain identical MDI scores but have entirely different skills profiles. The item set format will help attenuate the inflation of the index scores due to widely scattered performance, but there are still a sufficient number of items of different types within each set to allow achievement of the same index scores by different combinations of competencies. This situation is more true for the MDI than for the PDI. Items on the Motor Scale are much more coherent than those on the Mental, and motor skills are more constrained by biological maturation.

This property of the MDI score calls into question its value for even those uses mentioned previously. For example, what if there were a criterion of a certain extent of developmental delay before a child becomes eligible for special services. A young infant who is sociable and responsive to sensory stimulation may score reasonably well despite a severe delay in early visual–motor coordination manifested by an inability to reach for and grasp objects. That problem, for which an intervention might be appropriate, might not be sufficient for the infant to qualify for publicly funded special services because the total MDI was not low enough. The BSID-II manual cautions that the instrument should only be a component of a complete developmental assessment battery to diagnose a child.

The manual (Bayley, 1993) also points out that the BSID commonly is used to plan and chart a child's progress in intervention programs. It states that "while not providing information about specific gains made by the child [it] is often the instrument of choice due to its superior psychometric properties and quantitative scoring system" (p. 3). Should an intervention program not be interested in specific gains? What if an infant's MDI improves because he is developing an interest in and ability to manipulate toys but interpersonal and communicative behaviors remain unchanged. Is this the kind of progress an intervention program should report? How much improvement in an MDI score is a guarantee that a particular intervention is helping? Furthermore, children with developmental problems often show scattered performance in normal milestone development, making the MDI a particularly meaningless statistic.

A general, global index score cannot adequately describe an infant's abilities. Several attempts have been made to define subscales by assigning items to categories which are different on face value. Kohen-Raz (1967) assigned items to five subscales: eye–hand, manipulation, object relations, imitation–comprehension, and vocalization–social contact–active vocabulary. These may have some value in directing therapeutic interventions to specific areas of deficit or in research studies. Ross (1985) found that preterm infants scored significantly lower than full-term on the MDI at 12 months. Examination of performance on the Kohen-Raz subscales, however, indicated that the difference between groups was not in all areas of functioning but only on eye–hand, imitation–comprehension, and vocalization–social contact–active vocabulary subscales.

A number of studies have tried to define empirically a subscale structure of the Mental Scale using factor analysis. Lewis, Jaskir, and Enright (1986) subjected Bayley Mental Scale data collected at 3, 12, and 24 months of age to factor analyses using oblique rotations so that multiple factors, rather than just a principal component or "g" factor, might emerge. A four-factor solution at 3 months found factors labeled manipulation, social attention, auditory production, and search. At 12 months, three factors, means–end, imitation, and verbal skill, contributed significant variance. At 24 months, four factors were identified: lexical, spatial, verbal/symbolic, and imitation. Correlations of factors at each age with those at the other ages, and with 36-month Stanford–Binet IQ scores, suggest a relatively continuous developmental path for verbal skill. Auditory production at 3 months was significantly related to the 12-month verbal skill factor, which in turn was significantly correlated with the verbal/symbolic and lexical factors at 24 months and 36-month IQ. Both the verbal/symbolic and lexical factors at 24 months were significantly associated with IQ as well.

A second path was identified which began with the social–attention factor at 3 months and was significantly related to the 24-month lexical factor as well as 36-month IQ. This social–attention factor may indicate an affective or temperamental dimension of the infant's behavior that may facilitate mental development in the social context in which it is embedded.

A third strand was found for nonverbal factors beginning at 12 months. Imitation and means–end factors correlated with the 24-month imitation and spatial factors, respectively, and were associated with IQ. The 12-month means–end factor also correlated directly with IQ.

Thus, identifiable subscale-like factors of the Bayley Mental Scale may exist and verbal, social, and nonverbal components of the BSID may have better predictability over time than the global MDI.

The utility of these factor structures can be seen in a study of preterm infants, some of whom had intraventricular hemorrhage (IVH), and full-term infants, who were given the BSID at 3 months (Fantauzzo, Bendersky, & Lewis, 1988). The two preterm groups, those with and without IVH, had significantly lower MDIs (see Table 22.1), as well as lower scores on all four factors, than did full-term infants. Preterms without IVH had scores intermediate in value between term and preterms with IVH and were higher in manipulation and auditory production scores than those with IVH. This is particularly important, in light of the finding that auditory production is associated with later language skills and IQ. In addition, the manipulation factor may be an indicator of early fine motor difficulties.

Another approach is to identify the set of items reflecting the predominant developmental tasks at a given age. McCall et al. (1977) identified item sets by using principal-components analysis and found that the components at 1–2 months of age are simple sensory/perceptual responses, at 4–7 months, exploration of perceptual contingencies; and at 10–13 months, imitative and vocal behaviors.

Such approaches may make the information generated by the BSID more useful for both clinical and research applications. The manual (Bayley,

TABLE 22.1. MDI and Factor Scores by Group

	Full term	Preterm	IVH
	(N = 189)	(N = 75)	(N = 48)
MDI*	124[a]	98[b]	93[b]
	(15)	(12)	(12)
Manipulation*	0.26[a]	0.11[b]	0.04[c]
	(0.24)	(0.15)	(0.07)
Social Attention*	0.56[a]	0.31[b]	0.26[b]
	(0.21)	(0.20)	(0.14)
Search*	0.75	0.54	0.47
	(0.23)	(0.21)	(0.19)
Sound Production*	0.30[a]	0.12[b]	0.08[c]
	(0.20)	(0.12)	(0.05)

Note. Mean values with different superscripts are significantly different, $p \leq$ .05. Standard deviations are given in parentheses.

*$p < .001$.

1993) cautions that a diagnosis of a deficit in a specific area should not be based on a relatively low facet score.

TRAINING REQUIREMENTS

The BSID-II are standardized, comprehensive individual assessment instruments; therefore, examiners must be trained prior to administering them. There is no specific formal training procedure. Examiners should have completed some graduate or professional training in individual assessment. A trained technician could administer these instruments under supervision, providing the guidelines enumerated in *Standards for Educational and Psychological Testing* (American Psychological Association, 1985) are followed.

Administering the BSID-II is more difficult than a standardized IQ test targeting older children. It is not always easy or possible to ensure an alert, happy, cooperative subject. A tired, hungry, or irritable infant will not perform at a level indicative of true capacity. Scheduling the evaluation at an optimal time of day can help. Most infants and toddlers have daily eating and sleeping routines. Having a well-fed, well-rested subject is critical when assessing young children.

Although administration procedures for each item must be followed strictly, the order of item administration is flexible. It might be best to "warm up" an infant by administering preferred items early in the session. It might be necessary to readminister items once rapport has been established, or after a hungry infant has been fed. Similarly, the parent may be asked to help elicit responses.

Experience in handling infants is a prerequisite for valid administration, particularly for the early motor items. The head control and sitting sequences require manipulations of infant position and judgments about muscle tension. The examiner must have adequate guidance and many opportunities to handle infants of different ages to establish interrater reliability.

The BSID-II cover a tremendous range of developmental capacities. In testing children over a wide age range, the examiner must become familiar with many, qualitatively different items, unlike a typical IQ test with qualitatively similar items of increasing difficulty. The examiner needs to be adaptable, have an appropriate manner, and be knowledgeable about a wide range of normal infant behavior.

IMPLICATIONS

Factor-analytic studies, and the principal-component analyses that preceded them (e.g., McCall et al., 1977), confirm that infant intelligence is not a unitary construct but multidimensional and changing rapidly. The BSID at any age is sampling a limited number of competencies, which may in part explain the poor correspondence of scores over time. The BSID should be supplemented by other measures of cognitive functioning, ideally process-oriented measures, such as those described in this volume, that reflect underlying cognitive and affective capacities.

Developmental paths are shaped by the interaction of a child's innate capacities and environmental factors. Socioeconomic status (SES) is the single most informative variable for any individual child's prognosis (e.g., Broman, Nichols, & Kennedy, 1975; Caputo, Goldstein, & Taub, 1981; Cohen, Parmelee, Beckwith, & Sigman, 1986). Although better than no consideration of environmental factors, SES is a conglomerate environmental measure within which there is much variation in more specific variables describing particular aspects of the physical and social environment which directly affect the child (Bendersky & Lewis, 1994; Sameroff, Seifer, Baldwin, & Baldwin, 1993). SES has been shown to become more related to developmental status beginning at about 2 years of age (Gottfried & Gottfried, 1984; Wilson, 1985). A family-risk variable, developed in our longitudinal study of preterm infants, and consisting of measures of parent–child interaction, the physical and social composition and organization of the environment, maternal social support, and life stresses was highly related to developmental outcomes at age 2. It was more predictive of MDI, receptive and expressive language than early medical complications including IVH (Bendersky & Lewis, 1994). Even in the first year, the family-risk measure contributed to the prediction of 12-month MDI, when 3-month MDI, IVH, medical complications, and SES were controlled. SES had no independent relation to 12-month MDI in these analyses.

Thus, a comprehensive evaluation to determine a child's current status, as well as a prognosis of what abilities or disabilities might be anticipated in the future, requires multiple assessments generating a profile of abilities in different areas and detailed consideration of the environment. In addition, as the child develops and social interaction and other environmental conditions change, it will be necessary to reevaluate repeatedly to have any confidence in a child's developmental trajectory.

REFERENCES

Alessandri, S., Bendersky, M., & Lewis, M. (1998). Cognitive functioning in 8- to 18-month-old drug-exposed infnats. *Developmental Psychology, 34*, 565–573.

American Psychological Association. (1985). *Standards for educational and psychological testing*. Washington, DC: American Psychological Association.

Arendt, R., Angelopoulos, J., Salvator, A., & Singer, L. T. (1999). Cocaine-exposed infants: Motor development at age two. *Pediatrics, 103*, 86–92.

Bayley, N. (1933a). Mental growth during the first three years: A developmental study of 61 children by repeated tests. *Genetic Psychology Monographs, 14*, 1–92.

Bayley, N. (1933b). *The California First-Year Mental Scale*. Berkeley: University of California Press.

Bayley, N. (1936). *The California Infant Scale of Motor Development*. Berkeley: University of California Press.

Bayley, N. (1969). *Manual for the Bayley Scales of infant development*. San Antonio, TX: Psychological Corporation.

Bayley, N. (1970). Development of mental abilities. In P. Mussen (Ed.), *Carmichael's manual of child psychology* (Vol. 1, pp. 1163–1209). New York: Wiley.

Bayley, N. (1993). *Manual for the Bayley Scales of Infant Development* (2nd ed.). San Antonio, TX: Psychological Corporation.

Bendersky, M., & Lewis, M. (1994). Environmental risk, medical risk and cognition. *Developmental Psychology, 30*, 484–494.

Binet, A., & Henri, V. (1895). La mémoire des phrases. *L'Année Psychologique, 1*, 24–59.

Binet, A., & Henri, V. (1896). La psychologie individuelle. *L'Année Psychologique, 2*, 411–465.

Bornstein, M., & Sigman, M. (1986). Continuity in mental development from infancy. *Child Development, 57*, 251–274.

Broman, S. H., Nichols, P. L., & Kennedy, W. A. (1975). *Preschool IQ: Prenatal and early developmental correlates*. New York: Wiley.

Brooks-Gunn, J., & Lewis, M. (1988). The prediction of mental functioning in young handicapped children. In P. M. Vietze & H. G. Vaughan, Jr. (Eds.), *Early identification of infants with developmental disabilities* (pp. 331–355). Philadelphia: Grune & Stratton.

Brooks-Gunn, J., & Weinraub, M. (1983). Origins of infant intelligence testing. In M. Lewis (Ed.), *Origins of intelligence: Infancy and early childhood* (2nd ed., pp. 25–66). New York: Plenum Press.

Caputo, D., Goldstein, K., & Taub, H. (1981). Neonatal compromise and later psychological development: A ten-year longitudinal study. In S. Friedman & M. Sigman (Eds.), *Preterm birth and psychological development* (pp. 353–386). New York: Academic Press.

Cohen, S., Parmelee, A., Beckwith, L., & Sigman, M. (1986). Cognitive development in preterm infants: Birth to 8 years. *Journal of Developmental and Behavioral Pediatrics, 7,* 102–110.

Corman, H. H., & Escalona, S. K. (1969). Stages of sensorimotor development: A replication study. *Merrill–Palmer Quarterly, 15,* 351–361.

Crowe, T. K., Dietz, J. C., & Bennett, F. C. (1987). The relationship between the Bayley Scales of Infant Development and preschool gross motor and cognitive performance. *American Journal of Occupational Therapy, 41,* 374–378.

Darwin, C. (1877). A biographical sketch of an infant. *Mind, 2,* 285–294.

Drillien, C. M. (1961). Longitudinal study of growth and development of prematurely and maturely born children: VII. Mental development, 2–5 years. *Archives of Diseases of Childhood, 36,* 233–240.

Erickson, M. T. (1968). The predictive validity of the Cattell Infant Intelligence Scale for very young mentally retarded children. *American Journal of Mental Deficiency, 72,* 728–733.

Fagan. J. F., & Singer, L. T. (1983). Infant recognition memory as a measure of intelligence. In L. P. Lipsitt (Ed.), *Advances in infancy research* (Vol. 2, pp. 31–78). Norwood, NJ: Ablex.

Fantauzzo, C., Bendersky, M., & Lewis, M. (1988). *Three-month developmental status as a function of maturity at birth and intraventricular hemorrhage.* Poster presented at the International Conference on Infant Studies, Washington, DC.

Farran, D. C., & Harber, L. A. (1989). Responses to a learning task at 6 months and IQ test performance during the preschool years. *International Journal of Behavioral Development, 12,* 101–114.

Fischler, K., Graleker, B., & Koch, R. (1964). The predictability of intelligence with Gesell Developmental Scales in mentally retarded infants and young children. *American Journal of Mental Deficiency, 69,* 515–525.

Fisher, K. (1987). Relations between brain and cognitive development. *Child Development, 58,* 623–632.

Fox, N., & Bell, M. (1990). Electrophysiological indices of frontal lobe development and neural bases of higher cognitive functions. *Annals of New York Academy of Sciences, 608,* 677–704.

Fox, N., & Porges, S. (1985). The relation between neonatal heart period patterns and developmental outcome. *Child Development, 56,* 28–37.

Gesell, A. (1925). *The mental growth of the preschool child: Infancy through adolescence.* New York: Macmillan.

Gesell, A., & Amatruda, C. S. (1941). *Developmental diagnosis.* New York: Hoeber.

Gesell, A., & Amatruda, C. S. (1947). *Developmental diagnosis: Normal and abnormal child development: Clinical methods and pediatric applications* (2nd ed.). New York: Hoeber.

Gesell, A., & Thompson, H. (1938). *The psychology of early growth.* New York: Macmillan.

Goldman-Rakic, P. (1987). Development of cortical circuitry and cognitive function. *Child Development, 58,* 601–622.

Goldstein, D., Fogle, E., Wieber, J., & O'Shea, T. M. (1995). Comparison of the Bayley Scales of Infant Development—Second Edition and the Bayley Scales of Infant Development with premature infants. *Journal of Psychoeducational Assessment, 13,* 391–396.

Gottfried, A. W., & Gottfried, A. E. (1984). Home environment and cognitive development in young children of middle socioeconomic status families. In A. W. Gottfried (Ed.),

Home environment and early cognitive development: Longitudinal research (pp. 57–112). New York: Academic Press.

Hagne, I., Persson, J., Magnusson, R., & Petersen, I. (1973). Spectral analysis via fast Fourier transform of waking EEG in normal infants. In P. Kellaway & I. Petersen (Eds.), *Automation of clinical electroencephalography* (pp. 103–143). New York: Raven.

Holden, R. (1972). Prediction of mental retardation in infancy. *Mental Retardation, 10,* 28–30.

Honzik, M. P. (1983). Measuring mental abilities in infancy: The value and limitations. In M. Lewis (Ed.), *Origins of intelligence: Infancy and early childhood* (2nd ed., pp. 67–106). New York: Plenum Press.

Honzik, M. P., Hutchings, J. J., & Burnip, S. R. (1965). Birth record assessments and test performance at eight months. *American Journal of Diseases of Childhood, 109,* 416–426.

Illingworth, R. S. (1961). The predictive value of developmental tests in the first year, with special reference to the diagnosis of mental subnormality. *Journal of Child Psychology and Psychiatry, 2,* 210–215.

Illingworth, R. S. (1972). *The development of the infant and young child, normal and abnormal.* Baltimore: Williams & Wilkins.

Ireton, H., Thwing, E., & Gravem, H. (1970). Infant mental development and neurological status, family socioeconomic status, and intelligence at age four. *Child Development, 41,* 937–946.

Jacobson, J., & Jacobson, S. (1995). Strategies for detecting the effects of prenatal drug exposure: Lessons from research on alcohol. In M. Lewis & M. Bendersky (Eds.), *Mothers, babies and cocaine: The role of toxins in development* (pp. 111–127). Hillsdale, NJ: Erlbaum.

Jacobson, J., Jacobson, S., Sokol, R., Martier, S., Ager, J., & Kaplan-Estrin, M. (1993). Teratogenic effects of alcohol on infant development. *Alcoholism: Clinical and Experimental Research, 17,* 174–183.

Jaffa, A. S. (1934). *The California Preschool Mental Scale.* Berkeley: University of California Press.

King, W., & Seegmiller, B. (1973). Performance of 14- to 22-month-old black, first-born infants on two tests of cognitive development: The Bayley scales and the Infant Psychological Development Scale. *Developmental Psychology, 8,* 317–326.

Knobloch, H., & Pasamanick, B. (1967) Prediction from the assessment of neuromotor and intellectual status in infancy. In J. Zubin, & G. A. Jervis (Eds.), *Psychopathology of mental development* (pp. 28–241). New York: Grune & Stratton.

Kohen-Raz, R. (1967). Scalogram analysis of some developmental sequences of infant behavior as measured by the Bayley Infant Scales of Mental Development. *Genetic Psychology Monographs, 76,* 3–21.

Kopp, C. (1994). Infant assessment. In C. B. Fisher & R. Lerner (Eds.), *Applied developmental psychology* (pp. 265–293). New York: McGraw-Hill.

Lewis, M. (1983). On the nature of intelligence: Science or bias? In M. Lewis (Ed.), *Origins of intelligence: Infancy and early childhood* (2nd ed., pp. 1–24). New York: Plenum Press.

Lewis, M., & Brooks-Gunn, J. (1981). Visual attention at three months as a predictor of cognitive functioning at two years of age. *Intelligence, 5,* 131–140.

Lewis, M., & Brooks-Gunn, J. (1984). Age and handicapped group differences in infants' visual attention. *Child Development, 55,* 858–868.

Lewis, M., & Fox, N. (1980). Predicting cognitive development from assessments in infancy. *Advances in Behavioral Pediatrics, 1,* 53–67.

Lewis, M., & Fox, N. (1986). Infant assessment: Challenges for the future. In M. Lewis (Ed.), *Learning disabilities and prenatal risk* (pp. 307–331). Urbana: University of Illinois Press.

Lewis, M., Jaskir, J., & Enright, M. K. (1986). The development of mental abilities in infancy. *Intelligence, 10,* 331–354.

Lewis, M., & McGurk, H. (1972). Evaluation of infant intelligence. *Science, 178,* 1174–1177.

Lewis, M., & Sullivan, M. W. (1985). Infant intelligence and its assessment. In B. Wolman (Ed.), *Handbook of intelligence: Theories, measurements, and applications* (pp. 505–599). New York: Wiley.

McCall, R. B. (1979). The development of intellectual functioning in infancy and the prediction of later IQ. In J. D. Osofsky (Ed.), *Handbook of infant development* (pp. 707–741). Hillsdale, NJ: Erlbaum.

McCall, R. B. (1981). Early predictors of later IQ: The search continues. *Intelligence, 5,* 141–147.

McCall, R. B., Eichorn, D. H., & Hogarty, P. S. (1977). Transitions in early mental development. *Monographs of the Society for Research in Child Development, 42*(3, Serial No. 171).

McCall, R. B., Hogarty, P., & Hurlburt, N. (1972). Transitions in infant sensorimotor development and the prediction of childhood IQ. *American Psychologist, 27,* 728–748.

Papalia, D. E., & Olds, S. W. (1975). *A child's world: Infancy through adolescence.* New York: McGraw-Hill.

Piaget, J. (1952). *Origins of intelligence.* New York:Norton.

Rose, S., & Wallace, I. (1985). Visual recognition memory: A predictor of later cognitive functioning in preterms. *Child Development, 56,* 843–852.

Ross, G. (1985). Use of the Bayley scales to characterize abilities of premature infants. *Child Development, 56,* 835–842.

Rubin, R. A., & Balow, B. (1979). Measures of infant development and socioeconomic status as predictors of later intelligence and school achievement. *Developmental Psychology, 15,* 225–227.

Sameroff, A., Seifer, R., Baldwin, A., & Baldwin, C. (1993). Stability of intelligence from preschool to adolescence: The influence of social and family risk factors. *Child Development, 64,* 80–97.

Sattler, M. M. (1988). *Assessment of children* (3rd ed.). San Diego, CA: Jerome Sattler.

Singer, L. T., & Fagan, J. F. (1984). The cognitive development of the failure-to-thrive infant: A three-year longitudinal study. *Journal of Pediatric Psychology, 9,* 363–384.

Singer, L., Arendt, R., Farkas, K., Minnes, S., Huang, J., & Yamashita, T. (1997a). Relationship of prenatal cocaine exposure and maternal postpartum psychological distress to child developmental outcome. *Development and Psychopathology, 9,* 473–489.

Singer, L., Yamashita, T., Lilien, L., Collin, M., & Baley, J. (1997b). A longitudinal study of developmental outcome of infants with bronchopulmonary dysplasia and very low birth weight. *Pediatrics, 100*(6), 987–993.

Stott, L. H., & Ball, R. S. (1965). Infant preschool and mental tests: Review and evaluation. *Monographs of the Society for Research in Child Development, 30*(3, Serial No. 101).

Streissguth, A., Barr, H., Martin, D., & Herman, C. (1980). Effects of maternal alcohol, nicotine, and caffeine use during pregnancy on infant mental and motor development at 8 months. *Alcoholism: Clinical and Experimental Research, 4,* 152–164.

Terman, L. M. (1916). *The measurement of intelligence*. Boston: Houghton-Mifflin.

Uzgiris, I. (1983). Organization of sensorimotor intelligence. In M. Lewis (Ed.), *Origins of intelligence: Infancy and early childhood* (2nd ed., pp. 135–189). New York: Plenum Press.

Vanderveer, B., & Schweid, E. (1974). Infant assessment: Stability of mental functioning in young retarded children. *American Journal of Mental Deficiency, 79*, 1–14.

Werner, E. E., Honzik, M. P., & Smith, R. S. (1968). Prediction of intelligence and achievement at 10 years from 20–month pediatric and psychological examinations. *Child Development, 39*, 1063–1075.

Wilson, R. (1985). Risk and resilience in early mental development. *Developmental Psychology, 21*, 795–805.

Index

learning assessment, 256, 257t, 444, 451, 455
visual recognition memory, 274
visual recognition memory
  instrument assessment, 274–275, 277, 282, 283, 287
  mental retardation, 287–288
Interaction models, 19–20
Interburst interval (IBI), 257–260

Joint Committee on Infant Hearing, 95

Kaufman Assessment Battery for Children (K-ABC), 256, 257t

Laboratory Assessment of Infant Temperament (LTS), 198, 199t
Laboratory Temperament Assessment Battery (LAB-TAB), 199t
Language processes; *see* Event-related potential (ERP)
Law of initial values (LIV), 182
Law of performance, 253
Learning assessment
  at-risk infants
    expectancy formation, 252
    habituation, 241–244
    instrumental conditioning, 260–264
  attention, 235, 244–245, 246, 266–267
  cerebral palsy infants, 243–244
  Down syndrome infants
    habituation, 242–244
    instrumental conditioning, 263–265
  drug exposure
    expectancy formation, 252
    habituation, 243–244
    instrumental conditioning, 264
  expectancy formation
    anticipation measure, 246–252
    at-risk infants, 252
    biobehavioral basis, 248
    constraints, 251
    defined, 246–247
    description, 247–248
    developmental model, 249–251
    drug exposure, 252
    facilitation measure, 248
    history, 247
    implications, 252
    information acquisition, 246–247
    information processing, 247, 248, 249, 251
    intelligence, 248–249, 251

memory, 248
minimum latency, 250
overview, 233–234, 246–247
reaction time (RT) measure, 248–252
reliability, 248–249
summary, 266–267
training requirements, 251–252
validity, 248–249
videotaping, 247–248, 251–252
visual expectation paradigm (VExP), 247, 248–252, 265–266
Wechsler Preschool and Primary Scales of Intelligence, (Revised), 249
focused attention assessment, 295, 296–297, 305–306, 308
habituation
  at-risk infants, 241–244
  attention, 235, 244–245, 246, 266–267
  Bayley Scales of Infant Development (BSID), 245
  biobehavioral basis, 237
  Bronstein effect, 240–241
  cardiac system, 242
  cerebral palsy infants, 243–244
  constraints, 244–245
  corneal reflection photography, 245
  description, 236–237
  dishabituation, 236, 242
  Down syndrome infants, 242–244
  drug exposure, 243–244
  dual-process theory, 234, 235, 236, 246
  fixation duration, 238, 239–240, 241, 242–243
  fixed-trial procedure, 237–239, 241
  habituation function, 238, 241, 246
  habituation pattern, 238–239, 242, 246
  habituation rate, 238, 239, 241, 242
  history, 234–235
  implications, 245–246
  indirect memory assessment, 253
  information acquisition, 247
  information processing, 234, 237, 243, 244–245, 251, 266–267
  intelligence, 240, 243–244, 245–246, 249, 251, 266–267
  intertrial procedure, 237–239, 241
  irrelevant stimuli, 237
  long vs. short lookers, 238, 244–245
  memory, 235, 251, 253, 266–267
  neonatal infants, 240–241
  neuronal model, 234–235, 246
  overview, 233–234